BONE MARROW TRANSPLANTATION: FOUNDATIONS FOR THE 21ST CENTURY

ANNALS OF THE NEW YORK ACADEMY OF SCIENCES
Volume 770

BONE MARROW TRANSPLANTATION: FOUNDATIONS FOR THE 21ST CENTURY

Edited by Robert Sackstein, William E. Janssen, and Gerald J. Elfenbein

The New York Academy of Sciences
New York, New York
1995

Library of Congress Cataloging-in-Publication Data

Bone marrow transplantation: foundations for the 21st century / edited
   by Robert Sackstein, William E. Janssen, and Gerald J. Elfenbein.
      p.   cm. — (Annals of the New York Academy of Sciences, ISSN
0077-8923 ; v. 770)
   Includes bibliographical references and index.
   ISBN 0-89766-993-2 (cloth : alk. paper). — ISBN 0-89766-994-0
(paper : alk. paper).
   1. Bone marrow—Transplantation—Congresses. I. Sackstein,
Robert. II. Janssen, William Earl. III. Elfenbein, Gerald J.
IV. New York Academy of Sciences. V. Series.
   [DNLM: 1. Bone Marrow Transplantation—congresses. W1 AN626YL
v.770 1995 / WH 380 B711921226 1995]
Q11.N5 vol. 770
[RD123.5]
500 s—dc20
[617.4′4]
DNLM/DLC
for Library of Congress   95-45313
                                                           CIP

PCP
Printed in the United States of America
ISBN 0-89766-993-2 (cloth)
ISBN 0-89766-994-0 (paper)
ISSN 0077-8923

ANNALS OF THE NEW YORK ACADEMY OF SCIENCES
Volume 770
December 29, 1995

BONE MARROW TRANSPLANTATION: FOUNDATIONS FOR THE 21ST CENTURY[a]

Editors and Conference Organizers
ROBERT SACKSTEIN, WILLIAM E. JANSSEN, and GERALD J. ELFENBEIN

CONTENTS

---

[a]This volume is the result of a conference entitled **Bone Marrow Transplantation in the 90s: Into the 21st Century,** which was held by the New York Academy of Sciences on March 15–18, 1995 in Orlando, Florida.

Financial assistance was received from:

Major Funders

- AMGEN, INC.
- H. LEE MOFFITT CANCER CENTER AND RESEARCH INSTITUTE

Supporters

- BRISTOL-MYERS SQUIBB
- SANDOZ PHARMACEUTICAL CORPORATION

Contributors

- ALPHA THERAPEUTICS CORPORATION
- ARMOUR PHARMACEUTICAL COMPANY
- BAYER CORPORATION
- CHIRON THERAPEUTICS
- COULTER CORPORATION
- GENENTECH, INC.
- GLAXO, INC.
- HOFFMANN-LA ROCHE, INC.
- IMMUNEX CORPORATION
- INTEGRATED THERAPEUTICS CORPORATION
- NATIONAL CANCER INSTITUTE/NATIONAL INSTITUTES OF HEALTH
- ONCOLOGY BIOTECH
- ORTHO BIOTECH
- PFIZER, INC.
- THE UPJOHN COMPANY
- XOMA CORPORATION

Preface

ROBERT SACKSTEIN, WILLIAM E. JANSSEN, AND
GERALD J. ELFENBEIN

Division of Bone Marrow Transplantation
H. Lee Moffitt Cancer Center and Research Institute
at the University of South Florida
Tampa, Florida 33612

The rapid growth in our understanding of immunology and the molecular basis of hematopoiesis, compounded by the increasing clinical indication for high dose chemoradiotherapy in the treatment of solid malignancy, has markedly advanced the use of bone marrow transplantation over the last decade. Although bone marrow transplantation has become the paradigm for the symbiotic interplay of basic science research, clinical research, and medical practice, there are limited opportunities for open discussion of relevant research and clinical issues among both investigators and practitioners. In organizing this conference, we attempted to provide a framework for such discussion, specifically to promote a look back, a current assessment, and a future view of the status of bone marrow transplantation. We felt that the success of this goal depended critically on the participation of senior clinician-scientists such as E. Donnall Thomas, Robert A. Good, and George W. Santos, each of whom presented historical perspectives and contributed fully to the discussions of all presentations that followed. Clearly, a conference limited to $2\frac{1}{2}$ days could not cover the total scope of the complex questions in the field, and we apologize for our inability to be all-inclusive. However, our aim was to bridge the basic science and clinical aspects of issues most central to the future of bone marrow transplantation in clinical practice, and the section titles are reflective of this emphasis.

We anticipate that the published proceedings of this conference will serve as a useful resource to help guide both clinicians and scientists in understanding the applications, limitations, and unresolved questions in the use of bone marrow transplantation in the therapy of life-threatening diseases. More importantly, it is our hope that the research efforts reported here will provide the needed insights to yield improved outcomes for our patients in the next few years and the coming millenium.

A Tribute to George W. Santos

GERALD J. ELFENBEIN

Division of Bone Marrow Transplantation
H. Lee Moffitt Cancer Center and Research Institute at the
University of South Florida
Tampa, Florida 33612

This volume of the *Annals of the New York Academy of Sciences* is dedicated to my first medical scientific mentor, George W. Santos, MD. The conference, entitled "Bone Marrow Transplantation in the 90s: Into the 21st Century," provided a rare opportunity to bring together 23 extraordinarily talented investigators from North America and Europe with three of its most influential senior investigators, E. Donnall Thomas, Robert A. Good, and George W. Santos, considered founders of the field of bone marrow transplantation in the United States, to discuss research and share their views about the future of the field.

The conference enabled noted experts at the forefront of the most relevant basic science and clinical aspects of stem cell transplantation to explore the science behind a variety of clinical questions, with emphasis on its most rapidly evolving aspects, including the molecular basis of alloreactivity and graft versus tumor effects, the physiology of the hematopoietic stem cell and stroma, the biology of cytokines, and the selected clinical indications for marrow transplant therapy. The laboratory and clinical research presented at this meeting hopefully will form the basis for future clinical trials and practices in bone marrow transplantation.

In a very real way, the objectives of the conference are in fact a summary of the life and career of George Santos in the field of bone marrow transplantation. George is a graduate of the Massachusetts Institute of Technology and received his medical education at Johns Hopkins. After an internship on the Osler Medical Service, he spent two formative years at the U.S. Radiological Defense Laboratory in San Francisco, where his research career in bone marrow transplantation actually began. He spent the remainder of his professional training and academic career at Johns Hopkins until his retirement in 1994, 43 years after he entered medical school there. George was Professor of Medicine and Oncology for 21 of those years at Johns Hopkins. He has received many honors and much recognition for his seminal ideas and creative work. What he may not be as well known for is the many people he mentored who went on to other venues and made significant contributions of their own.

I first met George in 1967. Because of my interest in clinical pharmacology, I was directed to George who was developing high dose chemotherapy with allogeneic bone marrow transplantation for the treatment of acute leukemia, non-Hodgkin's lymphoma, and severe aplastic anemia. Because of his deep and abiding interests in transplantation immunology and experimental hematology, the fundamental fields underpinning allogeneic bone marrow transplantation, I studied these fields as well. What I remember most about George from the very early days was his enthusiasm, his energy, his vision, his optimism, and his joy in acquiring scientific information.

He was the epitome of the renaissance man in medicine. He truly went from the bench to the bedside, virtually on a daily basis. He believed that it was possible to have a career as both a basic scientist and a clinical investigator. He was a role model worth emulating. He was a builder, a prophet, and a pioneer. He translated basic research into clinical practice. He made a great difference and will not go unremembered. I am deeply indebted to him as are many other transplanters around the country.

A man's legacy is not only the worthy work he has done that will be remembered by those who follow in the field but also how many disciples he has prepared to carry future work to even greater heights, long after he has left the field.

Preparative Regimens: Chemotherapy versus Chemoradiotherapy

A Historical Perspective

GEORGE W. SANTOS[a]

Professor Emeritus, Johns Hopkins University
Baltimore, Maryland

INTRODUCTION AND EARLY HISTORY

In 1922 Fabricious-Moeller, a Danish investigator, reported that shielding the legs of guinea pigs undergoing high doses of total body irradiation (TBI) protected these animals from the radiation-induced hemorrhagic diathesis.[1] The implications of these observations were not appreciated and largely forgotten.

The detonation of a nuclear device on July 16, 1945, near Almagordo, New Mexico, was a major stimulus for further research into the pathophysiology of radiation-induced injury. Working under this stimulus, Jacobson *et al.*[2] rediscovered the principles of the observations made 25 years earlier by Fabricious-Moeller in another setting. They reported that the lethal effects of TBI given to mice could be prevented by shielding the spleen (a hematopoietic organ in the mouse) during the administration of radiation. In insightful experiments these workers showed that protection from the lethal effects of TBI could be provided by intraperitoneal injection of spleen cells following radiation.[3] In the same year Lorenz *et al.*[4] reported that mice and guinea pigs could be protected from lethal doses of TBI when given syngeneic marrow intravenously. The results of the latter experiment were soon confirmed in a variety of mammalian species.[5]

TOTAL BODY IRRADIATION ALONE

Given this background, it is not surprising that TBI was the earliest preparative regimen to be developed for use in the clinic. In 1957 Thomas *et al.*[6] reported the safety of administering large amounts of allogeneic marrow following a single dose of TBI. Transient engraftment was seen in this patient. In 1963 Mathé *et al.*[7] reported the first long-term engraftment in a 26-year-old patient with acute leukemia following

---

[a] Address for correspondence: George W. Santos, MD, 307B Mariners Point, Hilton Head Plantation, Hilton Head, SC 29926.

a single dose of TBI. Unfortunately the patient died of varicella encephalitis free of leukemia 20 months later.

TOTAL BODY IRRADIATION AND CHEMOTHERAPY

Because of the high relapse rate following bone marrow transplantation (BMT) with TBI alone, the Seattle group employed a regimen of 120 mg/kg of cyclophosphamide (CY) given over 2 days prior to 1,000 Gy of TBI. In 1977, in a now classic paper, the Seattle group reported the results of allogeneic BMT in 54 patients with acute myelogenous leukemia and acute lymphocytic leukemia in patients considered to be in a clinical end stage of their disease.[8] All patients received 1,000 Gy. One group of 43 patients received 120 mg/kg of CY over 2 days before TBI. Another group of 31 received additional chemotherapy before CY and TBI. A third group of 19 received BCNU before CY and TBI, and a fourth group of seven patients received other chemotherapy before TBI. All patients except one had sustained engraftment. This study illustrated the potential curative effect of BMT in acute leukemia with 13 very long-term disease-free survivors. The Seattle group continued to employ CY as just noted, but administered TBI as daily fractions rather than as a single dose.[9] With minor modifications this has been the primary regimen used by the Seattle group for BMT in hematologic malignancies. Other groups have used either this "standard" regimen or a modification of it by employing other chemotherapeutic agents preceding fractionated TBI or by employing hyperfractionated TBI.[10]

SINGLE CHEMOTHERAPEUTIC AGENTS

The use of single chemotherapeutic agents as preparative regimens has been explored in malignancy primarily to define dose-limiting toxicities following autologous BMT in phase I studies.[11] Phase II studies have been performed with a few of the agents but only with very small series of patients. Cyclophosphamide is the exception and has been studied extensively in the clinic.

Investigations begun in the mid 1960s indicated that CY was a powerful immunosuppressive agent in animals and man and could prepare them for BMT.[12] The limiting toxicity, rarely seen at currently employed doses, is cardiomyopathy. These very high doses do not produce fatal myeloablation. The CY regimen was initially developed for BMT in acute leukemia. It was soon abandoned for that purpose because of a very high relapse rate.[13]

The Seattle group successfully adopted this regimen with minor modification for BMT in severe aplastic anemia.[14] With this regimen patients are given 50 mg/kg of CY intravenously on each of 4 successive days for a total dose of 200 mg/kg. At this total dose both rodents and man given allogeneic BMT show mixtures of host and donor hematopoietic cells, but eventually with the passage of time most become complete donor type chimeras.[15] This regimen is presently the most commonly used preparative regimen for severe aplastic anemia. The addition of cyclosporine[16] or antithymocyte immunoglobulin[17] has improved the therapeutic results.

BUSULFAN AND CYCLOPHOSPHAMIDE

In animal investigations busulfan was markedly myeloablative and an excellent "space" maker, but it was not immunosuppressive. Without BMT the dose-limiting toxicity in rodents is marrow aplasia. With syngeneic BMT in rodents the dose-limiting toxicities are gastrointestinal and central nervous system damage. Only syngeneic marrow can provide protection from otherwise lethal doses of BU. Allogeneic BMT affords excellent protection from lethal doses of BU when potent immunosuppressive agents such as antithymocyte globulin or CY are added to the preparatory regimen.[18]

Based on preceding animal data, a preparative regimen of BU and CY for BMT in acute myelogenous leukemia was evaluated in a phase I-II clinical study.[19] The final regimen consisted of BU 1 mg/kg orally every 6 hours for a total dose of 16 mg/kg followed on the fifth day by 50 mg/kg of CY intravenously on each of 4 consecutive days for a total dose of 200 mg/kg. Busulfan crossed the blood-brain barrier, and initially grand mal seizures were seen in about 10% of patients. This toxicity was eliminated by the prophylactic administration of phenytoin. Fatal venoocclusive disease may occur in some cases; however, the incidence of this toxicity was markedly reduced when dose adjustments were made on the basis of pharmacokinetic studies of the initial doses.[20] Adequate blood levels of BU may not be obtained in children if doses are not adjusted as dictated by pharmacokinetic studies of initial doses.[21]

To decrease the toxicity of the BUCY regimen, Tutschka and colleagues designed a protocol that differed from the original in that the dose of CY was decreased to 60 mg/kg given on 2 successive days.[22] Thereafter, the original BUCY was designated big BUCY, or BUCY4, versus little BUCY, or BUCY2, for the modified regimen. Despite the original intent, subsequent data suggest little significant difference in toxicity between BUCY2, BUCY4, and CYTBI.[23]

BUSULFAN/CYCLOPHOSPHAMIDE VERSUS CYCLOPHOSPHAMIDE/TOTAL BODY IRRADIATION

Few clinical studies have made direct comparisons between various preparatory regimens; however, reports from nonrandomized studies suggest that BUCY regimens are therapeutically equivalent to CYTBI regimens for hematologic malignancies.[24-27] BUCY2 was compared to CYTBI as a preparative regimen in chronic myelogenous leukemia by the Seattle group. No significant differences were noted in therapeutic outcome as measured by survival, speed of engraftment, relapse, or incidence of venoocclusive disease of the liver.[28]

In the first of three randomized comparisons between BUCY2 and TBI regimens, Ringden et al.[29] reported no difference in overall relapse-free survival in patients with early disease (CRI of leukemia, first chronic phase of chronic myelogenous leukemia). Patients with advanced disease, however, showed better relapse-free survival after CYTBI.[29]

In the second study, a comparison was made between BUCY2 and CYTBI as regimens for BMT in adult patients with acute myelogenous leukemia in first remission. Probabilities for survival and disease-free survival were better after the CYTBI regimen which also resulted in a lower relapse rate.[30] In a nonrandomized study of children with acute myelogenous leukemia in first remission, however, the same group found that the CYTBI and BUCY4 regimens were equivalent but better than the BUCY2 regimen primarily because of the increased relapse rate with BUCY2.[31]

In a third randomized study, BUCY2 was compared to a regimen of fractionated TBI and etoposide as preparation for allogeneic BMT in "good risk" or "poor risk" patients with acute myelogenous, acute lymphocytic, and chronic myelogenous leukemia. The two regimens did not differ significantly with respect to toxicity, incidence of acute graft-versus-host disease, overall survival, or relapse-free survival.[32]

The BUCY regimens have been used successfully in lymphomas, genetic storage diseases, thalassemia major, immunodeficiency diseases, and osteopetrosis.[10] The combination of etoposide with BU or BUCY appears to be particularly useful in autologous BMT for acute myelogenous leukemia[33] or lymphoid malignancies, respectively.[34]

BACT-DERIVED REGIMENS

In 1972 Graw *et al.*[35] described a regimen composed of carmustine (BCNU), cytarabrine, cyclophosphamide, and 6-thioguanine (BACT) for BMT in acute leukemias. Later, others used the BACT regimen, variations of it, or other combination chemotherapy and reported long-term disease-free survival in patients with lymphoma following BMT.[36] The BACT regimen or its derivatives such as BAVC, CBV, LACE, and BEAM developed at other centers were never extensively evaluated as conditioning regimens.[37] Furthermore, in the absence of randomized or even comparative studies it is unclear which regimen(s) produces the best overall survival.

BACT-derived regimens have been used primarily as preparation for autologous BMT in lymphomas. The most extensive experience has been with CBV for which a number of drug dose and schedules have been examined. In nonrandomized studies of CYTBI and BACT-derived regimens for autologous BMT in lymphoid malignancies, similar outcomes were found.[38] It seems that the choice of a particular regimen should be guided by toxicity considerations as well as the previous experience of the treatment center.

REFERENCES

1. FABRICIOUS-MOELLER, J. 1992. Experimental Studies of Hemorrhagic Diathesis from X-ray Sickness. Levin and Munksgaard. Copenhagen.
2. JACOBSON, L. O., E. K. MARKS, E. O. GASTON & R. E. ZIRKLE. 1949. Effects of spleen protection on mortality following X-irradiation. J. Lab. Clin. Med. **34:** 1538–1543.
3. JACOBSON, L. O., E. L. SIMMONS, E. K. MARKS & J. H. ELDREDGE. 1951. Recovery from radiation injury. Science **113:** 510–511.
4. LORENZ, E., D. E. UPHOFF, T. R. REID & E. SHELTON. 1951. Modification of acute irradiation injury in mice and guinea pigs by bone marrow injection. Radiology **58:** 863–877.
5. VAN BEKKUM, D. W. & J. J. DEVRIES. 1967. Radiation Chimaeras. 1–272. Logas. London.

6. THOMAS, E. D., H. L. LOCHTE, Jr., W. C. LU & J. W. FERREBEE. 1957. Intravenous infusion of bone marrow in patients receiving radiation and chemotherapy. N. Engl. J. Med. **257:** 491-496.

7. MATHÉ, G., J. L. AMIEL, L. SCHWARZENBERG, A. CATTAN & M. SCHNEIDER. 1963. Hematopoietic chimera in man after allogeneic (homologous) bone marrow transplantation. Br. Med. J. **ii:** 1633-1635.

8. THOMAS, E. D., C. D. BUCKNER, M. BANAJI, R. A. CLIFT, A. FEFER, N. FLOURNOY, B. W. GOODELL, R. O. HICKMAN, K. G. LERNER, P. E. NEIMAN, G. E. SALE, J. E. SANDERS, J. SINGER, M. STEVENS, R. STORB & P. I. WEIDEN. 1977. One hundred patients with acute leukemia treated by chemotherapy, total body irradiation, and allogeneic marrow transplantation. Blood **49:** 511-533.

9. THOMAS, E. D., C. D. BUCKNER, R. A. CLIFT, A. FEFER, F. L. JOHNSON, P. E. NEIMAN, G. E. SALE, J. E. SANDERS, J. W. SINGER, H. SCHULMAN, R. STORB, & P. L. WEIDEN. 1979. Marrow transplantation for acute nonlymphoblastic leukemia in first remission. N. Engl. J. Med. **301:** 597-599.

10. SANTOS, G. W. 1991. Bone marrow transplantation: Current studies. *In* Year Book of Hematology. J. L. Spivak, W. R. Bell, P. M. Ness, P. J. Quesenberry & P. H. Wiernik, Eds.: 181-201. Year Book Medical Publishers, Inc. Chicago, IL.

11. APPELBAUM, F. R. & C. D. BUCKNER. 1986. Overview of the clinical relevance of autologous bone marrow transplantation. Clin. in Haematol. **15:** 1-18.

12. SANTOS, G. W., P. J. BURK, L. L. SENSENBRENNER & A. H. OWENS, Jr. 1970. Rationale for the use of cyclophosphamide as an immunosuppressant for marrow transplants in man. *In* Proceedings of the International Symposium on Pharmacological Treatment in Organ and Tissue Transplantation. A. Bertelli & A. P. Monaco, Eds.: 24-31. Exerpta Medica Foundation. Amsterdam.

13. SANTOS, G. W. 1983. History of bone marrow transplantation. Clin. Haematol. **12:** 611-639.

14. STORB, R., E. D. THOMAS, C. D. BUCKNER, R. A. CLIFT, F. L. JOHNSON, A. FEFER, H. GLUCKSBERG, E. R. GIBLETT, K. G. LERNER & P. NIEMAN. 1974. Allogeneic marrow grafting for treatment of aplastic anemia. Blood **43:** 157-180.

15. SANTOS, G. W., L. L. SENSENBRENNER, P.J. BURKE, G. M. MULLINS, W. B. BIAS, P. J. TUTSCHKA & R. E. SLAVIN. 1972. The use of cyclophosphamide for clinical transplantation. Transplant. Proc. **4:** 559-564.

16. HOWS, J. W., J. C. MARSH, J. L. YIN, S. DURANT, D. SWIRSKY, A. WORSLEY *et al.* 1989. Bone marrow transplantation for severe aplastic anemia using cyclosporin: Long-term follow-up. Bone Marrow Transplant. **4:** 11-16.

17. STORB, R., G. LONGTON, C. ANASETTI, F. R. APPELBAUM, P. BEATTY, W. BENSINGER *et al.* 1992. Changing trends in marrow transplantation for aplastic anemia. Bone Marrow Transplant. **10:** 45-52.

18. SANTOS, G. W. 1993. The development of busulfan/cyclophosphamide preparative regimens. Semin. Oncol. **20** (suppl. 4): 12-16.

19. SANTOS, G. W., P. J. TUTSCHKA, R. BROOKMEYER, R. SARAL, W. E. BESCHORNER, W. B. BIAS, H. G. BRAINE, W. H. BURNS, G. J. ELFENBEIN, H. KAIZER, D. MELLITS, L. L. SENSENBRENNER, R. K. STUART & A. M. YEAGER. 1983. Marrow transplantation for acute non-lymphocytic leukemia after treatment with busulfan and cyclophosphamide. N. Eng. J. Med. **309:** 1347-1353.

20. GROCHOW, L. B. 1993. Busulfan disposition: The role of therapeutic monitoring in bone marrow transplantation induction regimens. Semin. Oncol. **20** (suppl. 4): 18-25.

21. YEAGER, A. M., J. E. WAGNER, M. L. GRAHAM, G. W. SANTOS & L. B. GROCHOW. 1992. Optimization of busulfan dosage in children undergoing bone marrow transplantation: A pharmacokinetic study of dose escalation. Blood **80:** 2425-2428.

22. TUTSCHKA, P. J., E. A. COPELAN & J. P. KLEIN. 1987. Bone marrow transplantation for leukemia following a new busulfan and cyclophosphamide regimens. Blood **70:** 1382-1388.

23. DEVINE, S. M., R. B. GELLER, H. K. HOLLAND, J. R. WINGARD & R. SARAL. 1993. New preparative regimens with diaziquone or cytarabine in combination with busulfan and cyclophosphamide. Semin. Oncol. **20** (suppl. 4): 56–63.

24. BRODSKY, I., J. C. BIGGS, J. SZER, P. CRILLEY, K. ATKINSON, K. DOWNS, A. DODDS, A. J. CONCANNON, B. R. AVALOS, P. TUTSCHKA, N. KAPOOR, D. TOPOLSKY, S. I. BULOVA & E. A. COPELAN. 1993. Treatment of chronic myelogenous leukemia with allogeneic bone marrow transplantation after preparation with busulfan and cyclophosphamide (BUCY2): An update. Semin. Oncol. **20** (suppl. 4): 27–31.

25. COPELAN, E. A., J. C. BIGGS, J. SZER, J. M. THOMPSON, P. CRILLEY, I. BRODSKY, J. L. KLEIN, N. KAPOOR, G. S. HARMAN & B. R. AVALOS. 1993. Allogeneic bone marrow transplantation for acute myelogenous leukemia, acute lymphocytic leukemia, and multiple myeloma following preparation with busulfan and cyclophosphamide (BUCY2) [Review]. Semin. Oncol. **20** (suppl. 4): 33–38.

26. GELLER, R. B., R. SARAL, S. PIANTADOSI, M. ZAHURAK, G. B. VOGELSANG, J. R. WINGARD, R. AMBINDER, W. B. BESCHORNER, H. G. BRAINE, W. H. BURNS, A. D. HESS, R. J. JONES, W. S. MAY, S. D. ROWLEY, J. D. WAGNER, A. M. YEAGER & G. W. SANTOS. 1989. Allogeneic bone marrow transplantation after high dose busulfan and cyclophosphamide in patients with acute non-lymphocytic leukemia. Blood **73:** 2209–2218.

27. SANTOS, G. W. Marrow transplantation in acute non-lymphocytic leukemia. Blood **74:** 901–908.

28. CLIFT, R. A., C. D. BUCKNER, E. D. THOMAS, W. I. BENSINGER, R. BOWDEN, E. BRYANT, H. J. DEEG, K. C. DONEY, L. D. FISHER, J. A. HANSEN, P. MARTIN, G. B. McDONALD, J. E. SANDERS, G. SCHOCH, J. SINGER, R. STORB, K. M. SULLIVAN, R. P. WITHERSPOON & F. R. APPLEBAUM. 1994. Marrow transplantation for chronic myeloid leukemia: A randomized study comparing cyclophosphamide and total body irradiation with busulfan and cyclophosphamide. Blood **84:** 2036–2043.

29. RINGDEN, O., T. RUUTU, M. REMBERGER, J. M. NIKOSKELAINEN, J. VOLIN, L. VINDELEV, T. PARKKAL, S. LENHOFF, B. SALLERFORS, P. LJUNGMAN, L. MELLANDER & N. JACOBSEN for the Nordic bone marrow transplantation group. 1994. A randomized trial comparing busulfan with total body irradiation as conditioning in allogeneic marrow transplant recipients with leukemia: A report from the Nordic Bone Marrow Transplantation Group. Blood **83:** 2723–2730.

30. BLAISE, D., D. MARANINCHI, E. ARCHINBAUD, J. REIFFERS, A. DEVERGIE, J. P. JOUET, N. MILPIED, M. ATTAI, M. MICHALLET, N. IFRAH, M. KUENTZ, C. DAURIAC, P. BORDIGONI, N. GRATECOS, F. GUILHOT, D. GUYOTAT, J. GOUVERNET & E. GLUCKMAN for the group d'Etude de la Greffe de Moella Osseuse. 1992. Allogeneic bone marrow transplantation for acute myeloid leukemia in first remission: A randomized trial of busulfan-cytoxan versus cytoxan-total body irradiation as preparative regimen: A report from the Groupe d'Etudes de la Greffe de Moelle Osseuse. Blood **79:** 2578–2582.

31. MICHEL, G., E. GLUCKMAN, H. ESPEROU-BOURDEAU, J. REIFFERS, J. L. PICO, P. BORDIGONI, I. THURET, D. BLAISE, F. BERNAUDIN, J. P. JOUET, S. LEMERLE, H. RUBIE, N. MILPIED, J. P. VANNIER, F. DEMEOCQ, X. TROUSSARD, N. GRATECOS, E. PLOUVIER, C. BERGERON, M. GARDEMBOS, J. GOUVERNET & D. MARANINCHI. 1994. J. Clin. Oncol. **12:** 1217–1222.

32. BLUME, K. G., K. J. KOPECKY, J. P. HENSLEE-DOWNEY, S. J. FORMAN, P. J. STIFF, C. F. LeMAISTRE & F. R. APPELBAUM. 1993. A prospective randomized comparison of total body irradiation-etoposide versus busulfan-cyclophosphamide as preparatory regimens for bone marrow transplantation in patients with leukemia who were not in first remission: A Southwest Oncology Group Study. Blood **81:** 2187–2193.

33. LINKER, C. A., L. E. DAMON, C. A. RIES, H. S. RUGO & J. L. WOLF. 1993. Busulfan plus etoposide as a preparative regimen for autologous bone marrow transplantation for acute myelogenous leukemia: An update. Semin. Oncol. **20** (suppl. 4): 40–48.

34. CRILLEY, P., H. LAZARUS, D. TOPOLSKY, N. CIOBANU, R. J. CREGOR, R. M. FOX, S. I. BULOVA, D. C. SHINA, R. GUCALP, B. W. COOPER, W. SOEGIARSO, M. STYLER & I. BRODSKY. 1993. Comparison of preparative transplant regimens using carmustine/

etoposide/cisplatin or busulfan/etoposide/cyclophosphamide in lymphoid malignancies. Semin. Oncol. **20** (suppl. 4): 50-54.

35. GRAW, R. G., R. A. YANKEE, G. N. ROGENTINE, B. G. LEVENTHAL, G. P. HERZIG, R. H. HALTERMAN, C. B. MERRITT, M. H. McGINNISS, G. R. D. KRUEGER, J. WHONG-PENG, P. L. CAROLLA, D. S. GULLIAN, M. E. LIPPMAN, H. R. GRALNICK, G. W. BERARD, P. I. TERASAKI & E. S. HENDERSON. 1972. Bone marrow transplantation from HLA-matched donors to patients with acute leukemia: Toxicity and antileukemic effect. Transplantation 79-90.

36. APPELBAUM, F. R. & C. D. BUCKNER. 1986. Overview of the clinical relevance of autologous bone marrow transplantation. Clin. Haematol. **15:** 1-18.

37. KANFER, E. 1992. Bone marrow transplant conditioning schedules. *In* Bone Marrow Transplantation in Practice. J. Treleaven & J. Barrett, Eds.: 247-255. Churchhill Livingston. Edinburgh, London, Madrid, Melbourne, New York and Tokyo.

38. CHOPRA, R. & A. GOLDSTONE. 1992. The role of bone marrow transplantation in Hodgkin's disease and non-Hodgkin's lymphoma. *In* Bone Marrow Transplantation. J. Treleaven & J. Barrett, Eds.: 87-104. Churchhill Livingston, Edinburgh, London, Madrid, Melbourne, New York, and Tokyo.

Organization and Development of the Immune System

Relation to its Reconstruction

ROBERT A. GOOD

University of South Florida
All Children's Hospital
801 Sixth Street South
St. Petersburg, Florida 33701-4899

Our work to define the immune system in cellular terms began in Minnesota in 1937-1938 when Fred Kolouch first became interested in the plasma cell.[1,2] Bing and Plum[3] in Denmark had observed that patients with primary neutropenia sometimes had a remarkable bone marrow plasmacytosis that was associated with hyperglobulinemia. Kolouch, a hematologic fellow, had followed up a patient with lethal subacute bacterial endocarditis and at postmortem examination was struck by the abundance of plasma cells in the bone marrow and spleen, and he was further surprised by the plasmacytosis seen in the lesions and hematopoietic tissues of patients with tuberculosis or serum sickness. Not being content with the speculations about plasma cell function by his teachers and professors of hematology and pathology, Kolouch made a killed vaccine of the streptococci that had led to his patient's death, and injecting this vaccine into rabbits produced massive plasmacytosis which often was associated with anaphylactic shock. From these experiments he concluded that plasma cells, which were abundant after anaphylactic shock, may be antibody-producing cells. Several years later, Kolouch, then a surgical resident, asked me to help him with his experiments. I was studying neurophysiology at the time and was timing the two neuron-two axon reflex using the cathode ray oscilloscope in rabbits that had been infected with herpes simplex virus via the femoral nerve.

From the little immunology I had learned through experimentation with virus infection I suggested that comparing the secondary antibody responses to the primary response using either passive or active anaphylaxis to see which produced plasmacytosis might help develop Kolouch's linkage of plasma cells to antibody production. The result of my experiment was clear-cut. Dramatic plasmacytosis of bone marrow was generated by secondary antigenic stimulation which led to active anaphylactic shock. By contrast, few plasma cells were generated by primary stimulation, even when accompanied by a passive anaphylactic reaction.[4] From the time of those experiments in late 1944 and 1945, I have always considered myself to be an immunologist. I then showed that plasmacytosis in brain and other tissues was a reliable sign of local immunity and probably reflected local antibody production. I also observed that plasmacytosis in many tissues accompanied immune responses to several different antigens.[5-7] I further found that bone marrow plasmacytosis could be related precisely to the slope of the curve represented by the accumulation of serum IgG immunoglobulin (gammaglobulin) in patients with rheumatic fever.[8] From my investigation,

8

Kolouch's scholarly and experimental analysis, and my research on the thesis for my PhD, we became conversant with a substantial literature that linked plasma cells to antibody production.[9-12] This association represented an important preparation for future events.

While studying at the Rockefeller Institute in New York, I was working with patients who had two diseases in which immunodeficiency was a part, Hodgkin's disease and multiple myeloma. In obtaining blood and blood serum from patients with myeloma with which to compare the immunochemistry of myeloma proteins[13] and normal gammaglobulins and also in research, to obtain pleural and peritoneal effusions from patients with Hodgkin's disease for trying to crystalize C-reactive protein,[14] I was impressed with the different kinds of infection that frequently caused major trouble in these two groups of patients. Patients with myeloma had frequent infections due to high grade encapsulated extracellular bacterial pathogens such as *Streptococcus pneumoniae, S. pyogenes, Haemolphilus influenzae,* and *Pseudomonas aeruginosa* to which they were very susceptible because they could not form antibodies. They did not have much clinically apparent trouble with infections by fungi, atypical acid fast organisms, most viruses, BCG, or the tubercle bacillus. By contrast, patients with Hodgkin's disease frequently had viral infections, such as Herpes viruses and infections with fungi, and they were also susceptible to tuberculosis and atypical acid fast injections. Thus, patients with Hodgkin's disease and those with multiple myeloma appeared to bisect the microbial universe into two components, and their susceptibility to disease (as through a haze at that time) seemed also to bisect the universe of bodily defenses. During the same period of these clinical and laboratory experiments, Astrid Fragraeus, whose interest had also been aroused by multiple myeloma, did experiments to prove that plasma cells produce antibodies.[15]

Thus, when Colonel Ogden Bruton described agammaglobulinemia,[16] we were prepared to act promptly. Within a year we were able to study eight patients with agammaglobulinemia. Three of these patients were already being treated on wards at the University of Minnesota Hospitals and two additional patients in the clinics. All of our initial patients, save one, were males and one had a disease of late onset which had appeared abruptly following an apparently initiating infection in the patient's early twenties.[17,18] Three of these agammaglobulinemic patients also had family histories suggestive of X-linked disease. Several of them had little or no gammaglobulin in their blood, and they could not make any antibodies following numerous, otherwise effective antigenic stimulations. Furthermore, most of these agammaglobulinemic patients exhibited perfectly normal delayed type hypersensitivity reactions. They usually rejected skin grafts and exhibited susceptibilities to the same kinds of bacterial infections that troubled the patients with myeloma. These agammaglobulinemic patients, at least some of whom had apparent X-linked recessive disease, like the myeloma patients, exhibited frequent infections with *Pneumococci, Streptococci, H. influenzae,* and other pyogenic pathogens such as *P. aeruginosa.* They impressively resisted infections with numerous viruses, fungi, lower grade pyogenic bacterial pathogens, BCG. Analysis of bone marrow aspirates, of antigen-stimulated regional lymph nodes, and of chronic inflammatory exudates from patients with apparent "X-linked agammaglobulinemia" (XLA) showed that lymphocytes were deficient and almost completely lacking in the far cortical regions of the nodes, and no secondary follicles or germinal centers were present in the antigen stimulated nodes. No plasma cells were found in either bone marrow, nodes, or inflamed tissues. The zones in the node that were later found preferentially to house B lymphocytes were virtually devoid of all lymphoid cells.[17-23] The spongy deep cortical areas of the lymph nodes contained plenty of lymphocytes. These areas were later called the paracortical regions by Turk[23] and were also later shown to house primarily T lymphocytes.[24] Total lymphocyte counts in the peripheral blood were normal, but these patients lacked plasma cells completely in bone marrow, bowel, and inflammatory sites.[17-22,24,25] Thus, patients with XLA were found to bisect not only the microbial universe into the high grade encapsulated bacterial pathogens, on the one hand, and fungi viruses and lower grade pyogenic pathogens, on the other, but also to bisect the lymphoid system into germinal centers (secondary follicles) and plasma cells, on the one hand, and ordinary small lymphocytes, on the other.[18,20b-22,24,25] These patients also bisected the immune system functionally into the cell-mediated immunities which were intact in the XLA patients and antibody production which was completely or almost completely lacking in these patients. This dissection of microbial, lymphoid, and immunologic universes by the findings in immunodeficient patients was thus first revealed clearly by our agammaglobulinemic patients as Experiments of Nature[17,18,20-22] These findings from our clinical and pathological research proved to be prophetic of our subsequent experimental analyses. The contribution of these patients, especially those with XLA, represented a unique and impressive legacy which prophesied many of the experimental scientific developments in the two-component cellular definition of the basic immunity systems.

The molecular genetic basis of the primary immunodeficiency diseases is developing rapidly. Perhaps incorrectly as it turns out, it has been considered the ultimate goal in the study of the pathogenesis of disease. We are learning with considerable dismay that this new information may not necessarily yield the level of understanding of the pathogenesis of disease that some of us were expecting. For example, Ohta *et al.* working with Gary Litman[26] and associates in the molecular genetics laboratories at All Children's Hospital in St. Petersburg, recently analyzed, defined, and described in detail the organization of the entire gene that Rawlings *et al.*[27] with Witte and Vetrie *et al.*[28] had discovered to be the gene on the X chromosome, the mutations of which are responsible for XLA. We now know for sure that this is a gene called *BTK,* the mutations of which are responsible for XLA. More than 150 different mutations of the gene that underlie XLA have already been described.[26] Although it is known that a product of this gene functions as a nonmembrane tyrosine kinase, just what the *BTK* gene normally provides for or promotes in cellular function and how the many mutations of this gene actually cause XLA are not at all clear. That this gene codes for tyrosine kinase is not in question, but just how this tyrosine kinase functions to promote B cell and plasma cell development and why patients with the mutated *BTK* genes cannot develop mature B cells or plasma cells remain enigmatic. Approximately 150 single nucleotide substitutions that lead to nonsense and missense genetic consequences, premature terminations, framework shifts, stop codons, as well as multiple nucleotide deletions and insertions all involving the *BTK* gene have already been described as the genetic basis of the disease in XLA.[29] Each of these mutations, we know, can give rise to XLA, but we still do not know how the normal gene functions to make possible normal B cell and plasma cell development and how each of the mutations interrupts B-cell maturation at a precise pre-B to

B-cell developmental stage. Furthermore, we have not yet been able to ascertain why between families different gene mutations yield different clinical expressions and how within a family a single mutation can sometimes yield a high degree of variation in clinical pathologic expression.[29] Such variation may be reflected in the time of clinical presentation of the disease and the severity of the disease presented.[26,29,30] Nonetheless, we will soon learn how to link the molecular genetic abnormalities responsible for XLA and how these molecular genetic abnormalities account for the dramatic cellular pathology of XLA, one of the first, if not the first, primary immunodeficiencies of man.[26,29] By contrast, we have learned much not only about XLA, but also about how the immunity systems work and how the different cellular components of the immunity systems work together to subserve the bodily defenses from cellular, immunopathologic, immunologic, and immunogenetic analyses of immunodeficiency diseases. We can be sure that the new molecular genetic information being derived from the molecular genetic analyses of the immunodeficiency diseases will also ultimately open doors to additional understanding, even perhaps to gene therapy for primary immunodeficiencies.

The next crucial contribution of our clinical and pathologic studies was presented to us by a farmer from Western Minnesota. This man, who proved to represent an important Experiment of Nature, had a profound primary immunodeficiency. He was the very first patient to be recognized as having the thymoma-agammaglobulinemia syndrome.[17,20b,21,31,32] Subsequently, more than 100 such cases have been described.[33] The patient (F.H.) came to our surgical clinic in 1952 believing that he was addicted to terramycin, because every time he felt poorly he would medicate himself with terramycin, the first of the tetracylines, and soon he would feel better. When he discontinued terramycin treatment, his disease in the form of pneumonias, sinusitis, skin, and septic infections returned. His clinical course was due to the fact that he was treating himself with a relatively new antibiotic for pneumonia, sinusitis, septicemia, or other bacterial disease to which he was very susceptible. This man had a huge thymic tumor of the mediastinum which proved to be a 500-g stromal epithelioma of the thymus made up largely of ''spindle-shaped'' stromal thymic epithelial cells. He had agammaglobulinemia, a markedly deficient ability to produce antibodies, and significant deficits of the cell-mediated immunities as well.[17,18,20b,21,31,33] Delayed allergy to common antigens was deficient or absent, and he rejected a skin graft much more slowly than normal. Surgical removal of the huge tumor did not correct any of the apparent immunodeficiencies. The epithelioma, which was benign, was found histologically to occupy almost all of the thymic gland. However, the association of this thymic abnormality with the profound and broadly based immunodeficiency provoked us to question the role of thymus in bodily defenses or, even better, the role of the thymus in immunologic development.[31] This patient thus caused us to launch an analysis of the role of the thymus in immunity. These studies revolutionized modern immunology. At first we removed the thymus in young 4-5-week-old rabbits. These initial experiments failed, probably because our studies were performed with rabbits that were just too old to reveal a crucial role of the thymus in early developmental immunology.[32] But by personal communication, we soon found out from Harold Wolfe at Wisconsin that Glick, Chang, and Jaap[34-36] rather accidentally had discovered that removal of the bursa of Fabricius from chickens inhibited the ability to make antibody. The bursa of Fabricius in the chicken proved to be the site of origin for a cell system represented in peripheral tissues by larger lymphocytes, germinal centers, and plasma cells. Wolfe and his students[37–39] confirmed the discovery of Glick *et al.* This research on the bursa of Fabricius especially alerted me, because Hal Downey, my teacher of hematology, had taught me earlier that in 1911[40] and 1914.[41] Jolly had concluded from his research and observations that the bursa of Fabricius may be the "cloacal thymus." The bursa of Fabricius, like the thymus, is a lymphoepithelial organ, but it is derived from the posterior end of the gastrointestinal tract. We now know (see below) that this is the site of differentiation of B lymphocytes, which later develop into antibody-producing plasma cells. Because Glick and colleagues' experiments employing early bursectomy in newly hatched chickens[34–36] had interfered with the development of immune capacity, we immediately began to remove the thymus from newborn rather than the 4-week-old rabbits that had been the subject of our initial experiments.[31,32] Furthermore, in addition to the studies in rabbits, we also had begun extensive experimentation on the influence of neonatal thymectomy in mice and rats and later also in dogs and hamsters. Our experiments focused in this way quickly showed that the thymus plays a crucial role in the development and maintenance of the lymphoid system as well as all immunologic functions. Its influences included a crucial role in the development of cell-mediated immunities and also in the ability to produce many kinds of antibodies.[42,43] Once we knew from Glick's experiment[34–36] that removing the bursa of Fabricius from newly hatched chickens interferes with antibody production, it was possible to do the correct experiments in rabbits and mice.[42–46] This critical function in lymphoid development was also demonstrable in rats and hamsters.[48] When we removed the thymus in the immediate neonatal period in mice, we produced deficiency of both antibody-producing function and ability to develop all cell-mediated immunities.[44–46] By neonatal thymectomy, particularly in mice, we inhibited allograft rejection, for example, rejection of tumors and skin grafts,[44,46,49,50] as well as production of antibodies.[43,46,47]

At exactly this same time, Miller in England apparently independently was approaching analyses of thymic function from a different perspective. Earlier, McEndy *et al.*[51] and Furth[52] had shown that thymectomy in newborn AKR mice, a leukemia-prone mouse strain that Furth had developed, prevented the development of a genetically based leukemia. Miller[53,54] in London was seeking further resolution of this antileukemic effect of neonatal thymectomy. He too examined the immune system and the immune consequence of early thymectomy and showed that neonatal thymectomy prevented the development of cell-mediated immunities and inhibited the development of certain lymphocytes in the mouse.[58,59] There has always been an argument as to whether we or Miller discovered the key role of the thymus in immunologic development.[57–59] However, we contend that our research could not have followed or confirmed Miller's discovery, because my young associate, Olga Archer, a master's degree fellow, and a young surgical resident, J. C. Pierce, submitted to the Federation Proceedings in December 1960 the very first results of the studies in our laboratory which showed that neonatal thymectomy in rabbits inhibits antibody production. The abstract was published in April 1961[42] before any report of experiments from Miller's laboratory. In addition, in the discussion of Archer's presentation, I presented a review of our already abundant evidence that tumor immunities as well as skin allograft rejection within and across MHC barriers and antibody production were inhibited from developing normally by neonatal thymectomy.[44] Miller's first publication was in the Lancet in November 1961.[56] In several different inbred strains of mice both groups showed clearly that neonatal thymectomy inhibited both antibody production and the cell-mediated immunities represented by delayed type hypersensitivity allograft rejection within and across MHC barriers and also prevented normal development of lymphoid tissues.[42,44,46,55,56]

We then organized an international conference in Minneapolis in November 1962 on the role of the thymus in immunology, at which each of the several groups working on the thymus had his or her say.[46,49,50,57] Warner and Szenberg[60,61] argued that the thymus and the thymus-like bursa of Fabricius in chickens played different roles in developmental immunology.

They believed that the thymus was responsible for the development of allograft rejection, the bursa was responsible for the development of both antibodies and also delayed allergy, while the ability to launch a graft-versus-host reaction was not under the influence by either of these central lymphoid organs. We considered their division of functions in the development of immunity responses between the thymus and bursa, as presented at that international conference, to be incorrect.

Because our results from clinical studies of patients with immunodeficiencies and results of our many experiments did not exactly fit the view that had been presented at the Minneapolis Thymus Conference by Warner and Szenberg,[60,61] Ray Peterson and I resolved to reinvestigate the role of the thymus and bursa in the chicken model. Max Cooper, then an allergist-pediatrician, had just come to our laboratory to begin his immunology postdoctorate fellowship training. He decided to revisit in laboratory studies the roles played by the thymus and bursa on lymphoid development in the chicken. It was only a few months before these experiments hit paydirt. Removal of the thymus from x-irradiated, newly hatched chickens, removal of the bursa of Fabricius from similarly sublethally irradiated newly hatched chickens, or removal of both thymus and bursa from such newly hatched chickens each produced very different results. Removal of the thymus so early in life prevented the development of lymphocytes in the blood and in the dense aggregates of lymphocytes in the white pulp of chicken spleen, leaving the germinal center and plasma cell development impressively intact.

Cooper initially presented these experimental analyses of the development of lymphocytes to the American Pediatric Society meeting in 1964.[62] He described our definition of two distinct arms of the immunity system. According to the new view of lymphoid development, cell-mediated immunities and certain small lymphocytes were dependent on the thymus, and antibody production, germinal center formation, other lymphocytes, and plasma cell formation depended on the bursa of Fabricius. Thus, from these studies, we presented the results of our extensive experiments and at the same time formulated more definitively our revolutionary two-component concept of immunity.[63–67] The thymus, we had found, was related to the development of a population of small lymphocytes, which we called thymus-dependent cells and were later named T cells by Ivan Roitt. They were located especially in blood, in splenic white pulp aggregates, and in specific regions of the small lymph nodes and gastrointestinal lymphoid aggregates in the chicken. They appeared responsible for the ability to mount all of the major cell-mediated immunities such as delayed type hypersensitivity, allograft rejection, and capacity to initiate graft-versus-host reactions. By contrast, we showed that the bursa of Fabricius was essential for the development of normal levels of all the immunoglobulins, for the development of capabilities for all antibody production, for germinal center development, and for plasma cell formation in spleen, lymph nodes, and intestinal mucosa. Cooper et al.[62] presented these results and interpretations, the first of our numerous presentations of this material at the American Pediatric Society meetings in 1964.

Immediately following Cooper's presentation, DiGeorge from St. Christopher's Hospital in Philadelphia described his observations on children born without thymus or parathyroid glands who often exhibited these defects together with congenital cardiac defects and especially with abnormalities of the outflow tracts of the heart.[68,69] These children often lacked intact cell-mediated immunity and lacked normal lymphoid cell population development in the deep cortical regions of the lymph nodes.[24] By contrast, these children whose lymph nodes were almost a mirror image of those of patients with XLA described earlier possessed abundant cells in the peripheral cortical regions of the lymph nodes but did not develop morphologically and functionally normal germinal centers. Although they usually had normal immunoglobulin levels, they could not make antibodies well, and even with repeated antigenic stimulation, they never did form decent germinal centers. However, they did have plasma cells in bone marrow and nodes. I promptly named the clinical immunodeficiency disease he described as the DiGeorge syndrome. Ray Peterson, Cooper, and I[70] wrote a paper in which we applied all of these experimental and clinicopathologic findings and insights to define the pathogenesis of the then major forms of primary immunodeficiency diseases of man.[70] Our experiments with irradiated bursectomized chicken combined with our similarly extensive histopathologic studies of patients with primary immunodeficiency diseases provided a clear perspective for understanding several of these immunodeficiency diseases and also the entire lymphoid system in both chickens and humans. We reasoned that XLA patients represented the same lymphoid system deficiency as that produced in chickens that had been irradiated and bursectomized at hatching and that consequently lacked development of both plasma cells and germinal centers. Patients with Swiss type agammaglobulinemia as originally described by Glanzman and Riniker[71] and extensively studied by Hitzig and Willie[72] and Tobler and Cottier[73] lacked thymus, lymphocytes, germinal centers, white pulp aggregates in spleen, and other thymus-dependent aggregates in nodes and other sites such as bowel. These patients were comparable to the irradiated newly hatched chickens that had been subjected to both thymectomy and bursectomy. The newly hatched irradiated thymectomized chickens, we reasoned, were equivalent to the athymic patients that DiGeorge and his coworkers were studying at St. Christopher's Hospital in Philadelphia. Thus, from both bedside and autopsy and necropsy studies, and from experimental analysis, it now seemed clear that immunodeficiency diseases could be critically viewed in a context that included two major arms of the immunity systems, a thymus arm and a bursal arm (or bursal equivalent arm) with central lymphoid and peripheral lymphoid development sites for each.[64,70,74] Since no bursa could ever be found in any mammal or at any stage of development in man, the fetal liver and, later, the bone marrow were shown to be the central sites for spawning cells of B lymphocyte lineage which subserved the differentiation of both B lymphocytes and plasma cells—the major factories for antibody production.

To remove the potentially confounding role of irradiation from the chicken model, Van Alten, an embryologist from Illinois, took a sabbatical leave to work in our laboratory. With great effort he operated directly on the chick embryo in the egg to remove all of the thymus, the entire bursa, or both sufficiently well to show that the sublethal irradiation we had used in the chicken experiments was not essential to our model of lymphoid development.[75]

Recently, Haire and associates in Litman's molecular genetics group[76] found that patients with the complete DiGeorge syndrome do not exhibit the essential somatic mutations of the genes responsible for antibody development during repeated immune responses. Such somatic mutations normally occur abundantly in the germinal centers, where essential development of antibodies occurs. This development includes isotype class switching and the somatic mutations that leads to production of antibodies with the high affinities for antigen. It is such antibodies that characteristically are generated during secondary and tertiary immune responses.

LAUNCHING BONE MARROW TRANSPLANTATION TO CURE HUMAN DISEASE

In the midst of all the excitement generated by these insights into the cellular development of the immunity systems and the putative cellular developmental pathogenesis of many of the primary immunodeficiency diseases, I felt that we had learned enough to begin to making an effort to use this incredibly increasing understanding to develop a form of cellular engineering that might cure some of our patients with primary immunodeficiency diseases.

We followed evidence that in experimental animals bone marrow transplantation from an MHC-matched donor could correct the hematopoietic and immunologic abnormalities produced by lethal doses of total body x-irradiation.[77] Main and Prehn[78] showed that when they achieved successful allogeneic bone marrow transplantation in mice, they also produced lasting immunologic tolerance of the donor in recipient mice.[78] In these experiments, x-irradiation was given in large doses to destroy all hematopoietic and lymphopoietic cells and their precursors in the recipient. Then donor marrow, syngeneic or allogeneic, that contained hematopoietic and lymphopoietic stem cells could be given to fully reconstitute all blood cell and lymphoid tissue and cellular deficits produced by irradiation. In such a model system, the hematopoietic and lymphoid cells that developed were all shown to be derived from the donor stem cells. Thus, such animals were shown to be fully allogeneic chimeras. Furthermore, Donnall Thomas had already succeeded in a few instances in achieving long-term survival of pen-bred Beagle dogs by bone marrow transplantation after lethal total body irradiation.[79-81]

From these experimental studies, from analysis of our diseased patients, and from our postmortem findings in lymphoid tissues, we concluded that it might be possible to correct the immunodeficiency disorder associated with severe combined immunodeficiency (SCID) by bone marrow transplantation. We reasoned that perhaps because of the profound immunodeficiency in patients with SCID even without further preparations, such as x-irradiation or administration of cytotoxic immunosuppressive drugs, we might successfully transplant patients with severe combined immunodeficiency disease (SCID) without additional myeloablation or immunosuppression. Initially we attempted to use fetal liver as the source of stem cells. That effort, which seemed to be succeeding in one instance, failed when the patient with SCID who had accepted a hematopoietic graft was inadvertently given a blood transfusion by the pediatric staff without inactivating the peripheral lymphocytes by treatment with x-irradiation *in vitro*.[82] This adverse experience was devastating to our entire study group. However, in a paper[83] we discussed the theoretic potential of such treatment and proposed again that marrow transplantation might be treatment of choice in patients with SCID. We proposed that giving marrow cells from an MHC-matched sibling donor should permit constitution of the deficient missing or abnormal lymphoid stem cells in SCID.[83]

Our opportunity came in June 1968 when Dr. Le Heureux, a pediatrician in Meridan, Connecticut, referred a 4-month-old child to us. This child came from a large Italian kindred in which the infant represented the last of 12 male children who had had fatal SCID. Eleven of these children over three generations had died of severe immunodeficiency and its consequent infections. All of these males had apparently had the same genetic form of SCID, X-linked SCID, now known to be attributed to genetic abnormality of the IL-2Rγ or IL-RC, a high affinity receptor for IL-2, IL-4, IL-7, IL-9, and IL-15.[84] This disease was clearly transmitted as an X-linked recessive trait. This patient, a baby boy, the only survivor in his family of those with this disease, had four sisters, and so Dr. Le Heureux, after hearing me speak about the potential to cure the disease by cellular engineering using an MHC-matched sibling donor, referred the entire family to us from Connecticut.

Although tissue typing was not yet perfectly developed, we ascertained that a reasonable tissue match existed between the baby and one of his sisters. The two children matched quite well according to the major histocompatibility determinant that we were just becoming able to define and utilize. The patient and his sister were also well matched according to the undirectional mixed leukocyte culture analyses that we had recently learned from Bach. Thus, my colleague, Richard Hong, my new immunology fellow, Richard Gatti, a senior fellow, Hilaire Meuwissen, our intern, Hugh Allen, and I performed a bone marrow transplantation from the healthy 9-year-old female donor into the patient with lethal immunodeficiency. This transplant very promptly, within 45 days, appeared to correct the infant's severe combined immunodeficiency.[85] Although the immunocorrection was dramatic, the recipient child developed a severe graft-versus-host reaction (GVHR). Everyone advised me to get rid of the bone marrow graft which surely was producing the GVHD. I knew that even if I could eliminate the graft, I would at best only return to the starting place of the clinical trial I knew to be the highly lethal disease SCID. However, the GVHR-GVHD progressed and led to the unusual (in humans) development of a profound complicating aplastic anemia.

At that moment I decided not to retreat, but rather to forge ahead. I reasoned that the best thing to do would be to attempt to cure the complicating aplastic anemia with a second bone marrow transplantation from the same matched sibling donor. That second bone marrow transplant also took promptly. The GVHD subsided, and the little boy became the very first child with otherwise fatal primary immunodeficiency disease to be cured by this form of cellular engineering that used bone marrow transplantation.[85] In this case, we were the first to use bone marrow transplantation as a form of cellular engineering to cure a fatal human disease.[85] In 1968, in this same patient, we had cured for the first time as well, with a second successful bone marrow transplantation, another fatal disease, namely, aplastic anemia.[86,87] Thus, with two successive bone marrow transplantations in this child, we had cured both SCID, a lethal genetically determined disease, and aplastic anemia, a frequently fatal acquired disease that had complicated our initial bone marrow transplant.[85–89]

Both Richard Gatti and I have followed this youngster closely from infancy through childhood to manhood. Throughout his entire life he has remained perfectly healthy. When tested, he has been immunologically and hematologically normal in every way.[90] As analyses improved, we determined that a genetic recombinant event had occurred and probably was responsible for the severity of the GVHD in the infant. We recognized that the child and his sister had been perfectly matched at the HLA B and D loci of the MHC, but mismatched at the A locus. This was surely why the complicating GVHD had been so severe. On repeated testing through the years, we found that in this patient all hematopoietic cells that can be made to divide are of female karyotype. The child has always been a full hematopoietic chimera. All his red cells were shown to be derived from his sister's O precursors rather than having his own original genetic A red cell type origins. All cells that could be made to divide in his blood or bone marrow by phytohemagglutinin or antigenic stimulation are of his donor sister's female karyotype, XX instead of his own XY. His blood cells switched completely from his genetic A to his sister's genetic O type.

Our experience with two separate highly lethal diseases as well as the experience of Bach *et al.*[91] who administered massive doses of cyclophosphamide, 200 mg/kg, plus bone marrow transplantation from an MHC matched sibling donor in a patient with Wiskott-Aldrich syndrome launched bone marrow transplantation as an effective cure for many otherwise fatal hematopoietic or immunologic diseases.[88] In the latter instance, Bach, Bortin, and their colleagues[91] achieved partial immunologic correction of the Wiskott-Aldrich syndrome by bone marrow transplantation from a perfectly MHC-matched sibling donor, and a stable mixed hematopoietic chimerism was produced.[91]

During the next 4 years, we treated five additional children with SCID. Taken together, they represented at least three different fatal genetically based immunodeficiency diseases, each of which could be labeled as SCID. Five of these first six children with immunodeficiency were cured by bone marrow transplantation. Among these five were two whose SCID was X-linked, Swiss type (autosomal recessive and now known in some instances to be due to RAG-1, RAG-2, or RAG-1 + RAG-2 deficiency) and one patient who had SCID due to an enzyme deficiency, adenosine deaminase (ADA deficiency), later identified as the cause of the SCID we had treated.[92] The child with ADA deficiency was noteworthy because of the difficulty in achieving a corrective graft perhaps due to toxic metabolites that pile up behind the ADA enzyme deficiency and inhibit acceptance of the graft from the MHC-matched sibling. Several attempts at bone marrow transplantation were made before a satisfactory chimeric state could be achieved. Once we got engraftment, this patient's immunodeficiency was also cured. This patient therefore represents the first enzyme deficiency to be cured by bone marrow transplantation.[92] This patient has been followed closely for 25 years and has remained completely healthy and immunologically normal. However, she represents a fascinating mixed macrochimerism. Her RBC, neutrophils, and macrophages remain ADA negative; they continue to be products of her own ADA-deficient stem cells. By contrast, the lymphocytes contain normal amounts of ADA and are clearly derived from her healthy ADA-positive sister who was the BMT donor. They surely have derived from donor's lymphoid stem cells that occupied the niche of T cells, B cells, and lymphocyte precursors attributable to the enzyme deficiency and toxic metabolites.

Except for one, all of our patients with SCID, including two females with autosomal recessive SCID, two males probably with X-linked SCID, and the patient with ADA deficiency, have all been cured by cellular engineering using bone marrow transplantation. It was with these five patients with SCID that allogeneic bone marrow transplantation was launched as a long-lasting correction and probably a cure for human diseases. DeKonig, Dooren, van Bekkum *et al.*,[93] following our success, also successfully treated a child with SCID by bone marrow transplantation. This achievement was described a little more than 1 year after our initial report. Last year that patient celebrated 25 years achieved by bone marrow transplantation.[90]

Bone marrow transplantation as a treatment for many otherwise lethal diseases did not stop with these initial successes in patients with SCID. Bone marrow transplantation is now being used worldwide under the strong and steady leadership of Donnall Thomas and his group in Seattle. It has use as life-saving treatment for many forms of drug-resistant leukemias, other malignancies, aplastic anemias, and developmental abnormalities of red cells, leukocytes, and platelets. In addition, as many as 30 different forms of primary immunodeficiency diseases have now been cured by BMT. I can count conservatively more than 60 otherwise highly lethal diseases that can be cured by BMT from an MHC-matched sibling. I know my count is conservative because others have counted as many as 75 otherwise lethal diseases that can be considered curable sometimes by allogeneic bone marrow transplantation from an MHC-matched sibling donor. In addition, under the leadership of George Santos at John's Hopkins,[94,95] autologous marrow transplantation based on stored autologous marrow has also been developed as an important adjunct to chemotherapy for treatment of resistant forms of leukemia and malignancy.

Dependence on allogeneic marrow transplantation which employed only MHC-matched sibling donors placed a serious restriction on the development of bone marrow transplantation. Only 25% of those needing a marrow transplant will have a matched sibling who can be used as suitable donor. However, recognizing this limitation we continued to press the concept that cellular engineering by BMT can more generally be applied when we showed for the first time that nonsibling donors from the extended family[92,96–100] and even a donor in the general population might be employed as the basis for successful treatment of immunodeficiency or other disease by BMT.[101]

Following von Boehmer's lead in pursuing our experimental research,[102] we then showed that if we completely purged all T lymphocytes plus the immediate precursors of T cells from bone marrow preparations of mice, we could transplant bone marrow of mice across multimajor plus multiminor histocompatibility barriers without producing graft-versus-host reaction.[103–106]

Such experimental marrow transplants regularly produced tolerance of donor and tolerance of recipient and permitted expression of impressive immunologic capacity that could reject third party allogeneic cells and tissues with cell-mediated responses of normal vigor. Although such mice transplanted with T-cell purged fully allogeneic marrow across MHC barriers[104–109] showed demonstrable immunodeficiencies, especially in primary immune responses, mice of many strains transplanted across multimajor plus multi-minor histocompatibility barriers could survive well and remain in good health in conventional environments.[103–108] When donor and recipient mice were haploidentical at MHC, primary antibody production as well as all cell-mediated immune responses could be marshalled without problem.[109] Fetal or neonatal liver transplants, when free of mature T cells relatively early in fetal development, T-cell purged marrow, or even neonatal spleen in some experiments could be transplanted without producing GVHR or GVHD.[110–112] To extend the latter findings from mice to humans, we[113] and later one of our prior associates, Jean Louis Touraine,[114] performed fetal liver transplants from very immature donors which were regularly free of fully mature lymphocytes and could in a few instances restore immunologic function to children who had been born with SCID and who had no MHC-matched donor.[113,114] Occasionally these fetal liver transplants, as in inbred mice, restored impressive immunologic function and corrected most if not all of the immunodeficiency with which the children had been born.

At the same time, Reisner from Sharon's laboratory[115,116] had been using a nonimmunologic method of purging mouse marrow cells using plant lectins to aggregate cell populations, plus differential centrifugation of mouse marrow and spleen cells to remove all T cells. These preparations of MHC-mismatched marrow permitted bone marrow or bone marrow plus spleen cell transplantation in mice without inducing GVHD. Because the monoclonal antibodies available at the time did not permit in humans sufficient purging of T cells and T-cell precursors that could develop into T cells that initiated GVH reactions, I invited Reisner to the Sloan Kettering Institute and Memorial Hospital to join in our efforts to advance beyond the limitations of MHC-matched sibling donors in humans. Reisner promptly discovered that the peanut and soybean agglutination method that had worked well to purge bone marrow and spleen cells of most T cells in mice, could not be used to eliminate T cells from human marrow. However, after Reisner changed the lectin-purging technique to one that employed initial aggregation with soybean agglutinin followed by centrifugation and rosetting the T cells with sheep red blood cells (as a second lectin) followed by differential centrifugation, Reisner was able to remove the T cells from human marrow perhaps by a factor of 3 logs.[117]

With this new technique, we could employ parental marrow for successful treatment of SCID.[118] We also used this approach to prepare parental marrow for bone marrow transplantation in patients with leukemia if a matched sibling or perfectly matched relative was not available.[119–124]

Indeed, both O'Reilly *et al.*[125,126] at Memorial Sloan Kettering Cancer Center and Buckley *et al.*[127] at Duke have used these relatively crude preparations of haploidentical marrow stem cells, purged of T cells and T-cell precursors, to treat many patients who have SCID with frequent curative success. The success rate for marrow transplants to correct various forms of SCID with haploidentical donor marrow purged of T cells by the lectin technique under the very best conditions has been comparable or only slightly lower than the rates achieved with MHC-matched sibling donor marrow transplants.[125–127]

As mentioned earlier, haploidentical T-cell purged marrow transplants have also been applied in patients with chemotherapy-resistant high risk leukemias and lymphomas. There is no question that T-cell purging prevents the development of graft-versus-host reactions by these haploidentical marrow transplants. However, recurrence of the leukemic or lymphomatous process has been too frequent and has limited the use of haploidentical T-cell purged bone marrow transplantation for the treatment of leukemia.[128]

More recently, Reisner and Italian coworkers[129] showed that when such T-cell purging of stem cell-enriched bone marrow preparations is employed together with additional stem cell populations prepared from peripheral blood after growth factor stimulation for treatment of patients with high risk leukemias, long-term remissions of the malignant processes as well as durable bone marrow engraftment can be produced.[129]

In our laboratory, Ishii and Gengozian[109] analyzed experimental haploidentical marrow transplants that had been purged of T cells and probably also T-cell precursors following treatment of mice with high dose total body irradiation plus dimethylmyleran. We showed that all cell-mediated immunities and all humoral immune responses, even those known to require exquisite T cell/B cell plus antigen-presenting cell interactions, can be completely normal, and marrow grafts attempted under these conditions are regularly not only successful, but also very durable.[109]

In experiments with mice, fully MHC-mismatched T-cell purged bone marrow transplantation,[130–134] T-cell purged or unpurged MHC-matched marrow transplantation, haploidentical bone marrow transplantation,[135–137] or MHC-matched stem cell-enriched marrow transplantation[138,137] has been used successfully to treat, prevent, and regularly produce apparent long-term cures of most genetically determined autoimmunities. The autoimmune diseases, treated or prevented successfully, include the systemic autoimmunities in B/W, BXSB, and NZB mice, organ-specific autoimmune diseases, such as diabetes in NOD mice, autoimmune thyroid disease in mice, and autoimmune thrombocytopenia and coronary vascular disease in the NZW × BXSB hybrid mice.

Bone marrow transplantation produced significantly prolonged remissions but not permanent cures of the complex developmental Fas defect that controls peripheral tolerance in MRL/*lpr/lpr* mice.[139,140] When allogeneic bone marrow transplants were coupled with bone transplants or with bone transplants that contain stromal cells, the Fas gene-associated autoimmunities (related to failure of peripheral apoptosis,[140,141]) were corrected.[142] Recently, Hisha *et al.*[143] achieved long-term correction of Fas ligand-deficient mice by bone grafting which included bone marrow transplantation within the bone graft.

These data, taken together, to indicate that all forms of experimental autoimmune diseases, be they systemic, organ-specific, or dominantly vasculitic, involved disturbances that reside in the radiosensitive stem cells that can be corrected by complete and very long-lasting or permanent engraftment of the radiosensitive stem cells.[131,133,144–148] On the other hand, transplantation of marrow from autoimmune-prone mice to autoimmune-resistant mice frequently cause autoimmune diseases in these otherwise resistant mice.

Recently, we and many others have made major efforts to test the hypothesis that the stem cells express critical abnormalities in these autoimmune diseases. With Ogata *et al.,*[149] we defined the mouse hematopoietic and lymphoid stem cell as precisely as possible. Our analyses have already permitted us to be certain that we can identify mouse stem cells very well. We found that (1) these true stem cells are nonproliferating cells and thus are not destroyed by high dose 5-fluorouracil, (2) they are negative for markers of all definable hematopoietic and lymphoid lineages, and (3) because they are nondividing, they are transferrin receptor negative (CD71 negative). Further, they express class I MHC in high concentration at their surface, they have low concentration of Thy-1 antigen and are *c-kit* negative. These stem cells also have low density and are wheat germ agglutinin positive. With as few as four or five such stem cells from donor mice, it has been possible to achieve reconstruction of cells in every major hematopoietic and lymphopoietic lineage in the mouse. This production of lineage-specific cells is long-lasting and is demonstrable over a minimum period of 8 months in mice. To demonstrate production of hematopoietic and lymphoid cells from isolated stem cells, it was necessary to assure long-term survival of mice following very high dose total body irradiation. To assure initial survival of the animals, compromised hematopoietic cells that permit long-term hematopoietic reconstruction were employed. Suitable compromising hematopoietic cells can be achieved using cells that have been collected after two cycles of bone marrow transplantation in lethally irradiated mice.

BONE MARROW TRANSPLANTATION AS AN APPROACH TO PRODUCTION OF SPECIFIC IMMUNOLOGIC TOLERANCE

One of the most dramatic influences of successful bone marrow transplantation within and across MHC barriers is that it regularly provides specific immunologic tolerance that is either life-long or lasts as long as the transplanted marrow. Main and Prehn[78] were the first to recognize this striking tolerance-inducing phenomenon attributable to bone marrow transplantation. In their early experience such tolerance was even produced across MHC barriers. This tolerance in successful bone marrow transplantation is bidirectional and is towards donor as well as host MHC determinants.[103–105] This form of immunologic tolerance is remindful of the life-long tolerance that is a consequence of the hematopoietic exchange that accompanies the mutually tolerant state that develops in synchorious fraternal twin cattle during embryonic life.[150,151] Another model of this tolerance may be the neonatal tolerance produced by injections of hematopoietic cells (viable spleen cells) in late embryonic or neonatal mice.[152] Similarly, life-long tolerance was produced regularly by parabiosis in mice; especially those that were matched at the MHC proved a similar model of tolerance.[153,154]

Thus, recipients of successful bone marrow transplantation, whether prepared when donor and recipient are matched or whether they are mismatched at MHC, if prepared correctly, are almost always fully chimeric. They are tolerant of donor MHC determinants, tolerant of recipient MHC determinants, and fully responsive to third party MHC determinants as repeatedly shown by allograft rejection experiments or quantitation of proliferative responses of their lymphocytes to stimulation with allogeneic cells bearing MHC components at their surface. Such fully tolerant bone marrow chimeric mice are often impressively immunocompetent, but immunodeficiencies in both humoral and cell-mediated immune responses can readily be demonstrated if the marrow transplantation bridges MHC barriers.[104,105,155,156] The immunodeficiencies are especially apparent when primary immunologic responses[104,105,155,156] and resistance to certain pathogens are considered.[106,107,157] Partial histocompatibility matching eliminates this immunologic deficiency, that is, haploidentical bone marrow transplants of mice and humans do not exhibit recognizable immunodeficiencies.[109]

To eliminate the immunodeficiencies that do exist in fully allogeneic chimeric mice and rats, Ildstad and Sachs[158] produced stable mixed chimeric animals by simultaneous transplantation of T-cell purged donor plus T-cell purged recipient marrow preparations given to lethally irradiated recipients which differed from one another at minor or major histocompatibility barriers. Such mixed chimeric transplants produce long-lasting tolerance of donor and tolerance of recipient, with full reactivity towards third party cells and tissue grafts. In addition, such mice did not exhibit any evidence of graft-versus-host reaction or of humoral or cellular immunodeficiency.[158]

El-Badri Dajani in my laboratory[159,160] has pursued this line of investigation as well and has established stable mixed chimeras that are tolerant of donor, tolerant of recipient, and fully immunocompetent by transplants of T-cell purged donor plus T-cell purged recipient marrow across entire MHC plus multiminor histocompatibility barriers. These mice retain a most impressive mixed chimeric state. They develop normal structure of thymus and of all peripheral lymphoid tissues and thrive in conventional microbial environments. These chimeric mice exhibit vigorous cell-mediated immunities and have as their only recognizable immunodeficiency a fully tolerant state towards their own genetically defined tissues and also tolerance of the genetically defined tissues of the mice of the donor strain. These mice are perfectly normal in antibody and primary and secondary immune responses and responses to all third party MHC antigens.

When an enriched stem cell population is separated from the rest of the bone marrow cells, the donor stem cells plus recipient stem cells can also be used to establish a mixed chimerism. However, relatively isolated stem cells from donor and recipient whole marrow transplantation are usually unable to bridge the full major histocompatibility barrier.[161] By contrast, such mixed donor and recipient stem cell transplants can readily produce stable mixed chimerism when only minor histocompatibility barriers are to be bridged.

Recently, Ildstad and coworkers[162] succeeded in some instances in achieving stable mixed chimerism even when certain xenogeneic barriers had to be bridged.[162] The Ildstad-Sachs model of stable mixed chimerism has been improved by Sharabi *et al.*[163] and uses bone marrow transplantation after much lower doses of total body irradiation. In this model, an incompletely myeloablating regimen is used, that is, 300 r of total body irradiation plus high dose 800–1,000 R x-irradiation to the thymus followed by preparation of a stable state of chimerism by transplantation of both T-cell purged donor plus T-cell purged recipient marrow.

In another step forward, Kaufman *et al.*[164] in Ildstad's laboratory were able to identify and work with a rather unique cell, which they call a "facilitating" cell. This cell has some characteristics of the large granular lymphocyte population. Using cells of this type together with a relatively crude stem cell preparation from both donor and recipient, it has been possible to achieve stable mixed chimerism in which donor and recipient differ across the entire MHC plus a multiminor histocompatibility barrier. Recently, El-Badri Dajani and I discovered that osteoblasts also act as facilitating cells.[165]

Starzl *et al.*[166,167] have added further considerations to current thinking about organ transplantation. They have been concerned with the role of specific immunologic tolerance in organ transplantation. They ascertained that organ transplantations, especially of liver, kidney, or heart, both contribute and accept cells, perhaps dendritic cells, which establish a long-lasting micro donor-host, host-donor mixed chimerism in the transplanted organ and throughout the host tissues. This micro-mixed chimerism has been demonstrated at many sites throughout the recipient's body, and host-donor chimerism exists within the graft. He and his colleagues believe that such chimerism may add to the development of a tolerant or partially tolerant state that contributes to successful organ transplantation and that may account for some of the long-term successes of organ transplants. Indeed, Starzl proposes that such recipient mixed chimerism may contribute to a tolerant state for organ transplants and may permit allotransplanted organs to persist even without ongoing immunosuppressive therapy. He has presented evidence of a hierarchy of different organ transplants in contributing the tolerance-inducing cells that establish the microchimerism.[108] Recently, extension of this concept has led Starzl and his colleagues to attempt to promote major organ transplants by giving bone marrow transplants at the same time as the organ transplant is performed.[169] Ricordi *et al.* are even trying multiple bone marrow transplants from the donor subsequent to organ transplants in an effort to foster tolerance towards the transplanted organ. Further analyses and experimentation will be needed to establish whether marrow transplantation or multiple marrow transplants can contribute to the success of solid organ transplants.

More time is needed to evaluate how much Starzl's new paradigm will contribute to the further successes of organ transplantation and what role bone marrow transplantation will play in the transplantation of organs other than bone marrow itself. There is experimental evidence that such may be the case, but as yet the jury may still be out. His chapter in this book will describe further the future of this approach to organ transplantation.

ACKNOWLEDGMENT

I thank my editorial assistant, Tazim Verjee, for manuscript preparation.

REFERENCES

1. KOLOUCH, F. 1938. Origin of bone marrow plasma cell associated with allergic and immune states in rabbits. Proc. Soc. Exp. Biol. Med. **39:** 147-148.
2. KOLOUCH, F. 1938. A study of the bone marrow plasma cell of mammals with special reference to its origin in the rabbit under normal and experimental conditions. Thesis, University of Minnesota, pp. 1-84.
3. BING, J. & P. PLUM. 1937. Serum proteins in leucopenia. (Contribution on question about place of formation of serum proteins). Acta Med. Scandinav. **92:** 415-428; also, Ugesk. f. laeger **99:** 738-743.
4. GOOD, R. A. 1948. Effect of passive sensitization and anaphylactic shock on rabbit bone marrow. Proc. Soc. Exp. Biol. Med. **67:** 203-205.
5. GOOD, R. A. 1947. The morphologic mechanisms of hyperergic inflammation in the brain; with special reference to the significance of local plasma cell formation. Ph.D. dissertation, the Graduate School of the University of Minnesota, Minneapolis, MN.

6. GOOD, R. A. 1950. Experimental allergic brain inflammation, a morphological study. J. Neuropathol. Exp. Neurol. **9:** 78–92.

7. KOLOUCH, F., R. A. GOOD & B. CAMPBELL. 1947. The reticulo-endothelial origin of the bone marrow plasma cells in hypersensitive states. J. Lab. Clin. Med. **32:** 749–755.

8. GOOD, R. A. & B. CAMPBELL. 1950. Relationship of bone marrow plasmacytosis to the changes in serum gamma globulin in rheumatic fever. Am. J. Med. **9:** 330–342.

9. MICHAELS, N. A. 1931. The plasma cell: A critical review of its morphogenesis, function, and developmental capacity under normal and abnormal conditions. Arch. Path. Lab. Med. **11:** 775–793.

10. MAS, Y. & F. MAGRO. 1929. Morphologie, Genese, und Physiologie der Zyanophilenzellen (Plasmazellen) der hämatopoetischen Organe. Arch. exp. Zellforsch. **8:** 415–431.

11. GSELL, O. 1939. The significance of serum protein and bone marrow changes in lymphogranuloma inguinale. Klin. Wchnschr. **18:** 778–781.

12. BJOERNEBOE, M. & H. GORMSEN. 1943. Experimental studies on the role of plasma cells as antibody producers. Acta path. microbiol. Scandinav. **20:** 649–692.

13. KUNKEL, H. G., R. J. SLATER & R. A. GOOD. 1951. Relation between certain myeloma proteins and normal gamma globulin. Proc. Soc. Exp. Biol. Med. **76:** 190–193.

14. McCARTY, M. 1947. The occurrence during acute infections of a protein not normally present in the blood. IV. Crystallization of the C-reactive protein. J. Exp. Med. **85:** 491.

15. FAGRAEUS, A. 1948. Antibody production in relation to the development of plasma cells: In vivo and in vitro experiments. Esselte Aktiebolag. Stockholm.

16. BRUTON, O. C. 1952. Agammaglobulinemia. Pediatrics **9:** 722.

17. GOOD, R. A. 1954. Agammaglobulinemia—a provocative experiment of nature. Bull. Univ. Minn. Hosp. Minn. Med. Found. **26:** 1–19.

18. MAZZITELLO, W. F. & R. A. GOOD. 1956. Agammaglobulinemia. Minn. Med. **39:** 308.

19. GOOD, R. A. 1954. Absence of plasma cells from bone marrow and lymph nodes following antigenic stimulation in patients with agammaglobulinemia. Revue d'Hematol. **9:** 502–503.

20. GOOD, R. A. 1955. Studies of agammaglobulinemia. II. Failure of plasma cell formation in the bone marrow and lymph nodes of patients with agammaglobulinemia. J. Lab. Clin. Med. **56:** 167–181.

20a. GOOD, R. A. & R. L. VARCO. 1955. A clinical and experimental study of agammaglobulinemia. *In* Essays on Pediatrics, in Honor of Irvine McQuarrie. R. A. Good & E. S. Platou, Eds.: 103–129. Lancet Publications. Minneapolis.

21. GOOD, R. A. & R. L. VARCO. 1955. A clinical and experimental study of agammaglobulinemia. J. Lancet **75:** 245–271.

22. GOOD, R. A. & S. J. ZAK. 1956. Disturbances in gamma globulin synthesis as "experiments of nature." Pediatrics **18:** 109–149.

23. TURK, J. L. & S. H. STONE. 1963. Implication of the cellular changes in lymph nodes during the development and inhibition of delayed hypersensitivity. *In* Cell-Bound Antibodies. B. Amos & H. Koprowski, Eds.: 51. Wistar Institute Press. Philadelphia.

24. PARROTT, D. V. M., M. DE SOUSA & J. EAST. 1966. Thymus-dependent areas in the lymphoid organs of neonatally thymectomized mice. J. Exp. Med. **123:** 191.

25. GOOD, R. A. 1955. Studies on agammaglobulinemia. II. Failure of plasma cell formation in the bone marrow and lymph nodes of patients with agammaglobulinemia. J. Lab. Clin. Med. **46:** 167–181.

26. OHTA, Y., R. N. HAIRE, R. T. LITMAN, S. M. FU, R. P. NELSON, J. KRATZ, S. J. KORNFELD, R. A. GOOD & G. W. LITMAN. 1994. Genomic organization and structure of the Bruton's tyrosine kinase: Localization of different mutations which are associated with variation in clinical presentation and course in X-linked agammaglobulinemia. Proc. Natl. Acad. Sci. USA **91:** 9062–9066.

27. RAWLINGS, D. J., D. C. SAFFRAN, S. TSUKADA, D. A. LARGAESPADA, J. C. GRIMALDI, L. COHEN, R. N. MOHR, J. F. BAZAN, M. HOWARD, N. G. COPELAND, N. A. JENKINS &

O. N. WITTE. 1993. Mutation of unique region of Bruton's tyrosine kinase in immuno-deficient XID mice. Science **261:** 358-361.

28. VETRIE, D., I. VORECHOVSKY, P. SIDERAS, J. HOLLAND, A. DAVIES, F. FLINTER, L. HAMMARSTROM, C. KINNON, R. LEVINSKY, M. BOBROW, C. I. E. SMITH & D. R. BENTLEY. 1993. The gene involved in X-linked agammaglobulinaemia is a member of the *src* family of protein-tyrosine kinases. Nature **361:** 226-233.

29. VIHINEN, M., M. D. COOPER, G. DE SAINT BASILE, A. FISCHER, R. A. GOOD, R. W. HENDRICKS, C. KINNON, S.-P. KWAN, G. W. LITMAN, L. D. NOTARANGELO, H. D. OCHS, F. S. ROSEN, D. VETRIE, A. D. B. WEBSTER, B. J. M. ZEGERS & C. I. E. SMITH. 1995. BTKbase-Database of XLA causing mutations. Immunology Today. In press.

30. KORNFELD, S. J., R. A. GOOD & G. W. LITMAN. 1994. Atypical X-linked agammaglobuli-nemia (Letter). New Engl. J. Med. **331:** 949-950.

31. MacLEAN, L. D., S. J. ZAK, R. L. VARCO & R. A. GOOD. 1956. Thymic tumor and acquired agammaglobulinemia: A clinical and experimental study of the immune response. Surgery **40:** 1010-1017.

32. MacLEAN, L. D., S. J. ZAK, R. L. VARCO & R. A. GOOD. 1957. The role of the thymus in antibody production: An experimental study of the immune response in thymectomized rabbits. Transplant. Bull. **4:** 21.

33. JEUNET, F. S., H. J. MEUWISSEN & R. A. GOOD. 1970. Fate of *Candida albicans* in neonatally thymectomized rats. Proc. Soc. Exp. Biol. Med. **133:** 53-56.

34. GLICK, B., T. S. CHANG & R. G. JAAP. 1956. The bursa of Fabricius and antibody production. Poultry Sci. **35:** 224.

35. GLICK, B. 1958. Further evidence for the role of the bursa of Fabricius in antibody production. Poultry Sci. **37:** 240.

36. GLICK, B. 1964. The bursa of fabricius and the development of immunologic competence. *In* The Thymus in Immunobiology R. A. Good & A. E. Gabrielsen, Eds.: 343-358. Harper & Row Publishers. New York.

37. ROYAL, F. RUTH, P. C. ALLEN & H. R. WOLFE. 1964. The effect of thymus on lymphoid tissue. *In* The Thymus in Immunobiology. R. A. Good & A. E. Gabrielsen, Eds.: 183-206. Harper & Row Publishers, New York.

38. MUELLER, A. P., H. R. WOLFE & W. P. COTE. 1964. Antibody studies in hormonally and surgically bursectomized chickens. *In* The Thymus in Immunobiology. R. A. Good & A. E. Gabrielsen, Eds.: 359-375. Harper & Row Publishers. New York.

39. ACKERMAN, G. A. & R. A. KNOUFF. 1964. Lymphocytopoietic activity in the bursa of fabricius. *In* The Thymus in Immunobiology. R. A. Good & A. E. Gabrielsen, Eds.: 123-149. Harper & Row Publishers. New York.

40. JOLLY, J. 1911. Sur la function hematopoietique de la burse de fabricius. Comp. Rend. Soc. Biol. **70:** 498.

41. JOLLY, J. 1914. Sur les mouvements amiboides des petites cellules de la bourse de Fabricius et du thymus. C. R. Soc. Biol. **77:** 148.

42. ARCHER, O. K. & J. C. PIERCE. 1961. Role of the thymus in development of the immune response. Fed. Proc. **20:** 26.

43. ARCHER, O. K., J. C. PIERCE, B. W. PAPERMASTER & R. A. GOOD. 1962. Reduced antibody response in thymectomized rabbits. Nature **191:** 191-192.

44. GOOD, R. A. 1961. Discussion of Archer-Pierce presentation at The Federation of American Society of Experimental Biology. Atlantic City, NJ.

45. MARTINEZ, C., J. KERSEY, B. W. PAPERMASTER & R. A. GOOD. 1962. Skin homograft survival in thymectomized mice. Proc. Soc. Exp. Biol. Med. **109:** 193-196.

46. GOOD, R. A., A. P. DALMASSO, C. MARTINEZ, O. K. ARCHER, J. C. PIERCE & B. W. PAPERMASTER. 1962. The role of the thymus in development of immunologic capacity in rabbits and mice. J. Exp. Med. **116:** 773-796.

47. ARCHER, O. K., B. W. PAPERMASTER & R. A. GOOD. 1964. Thymectomy in rabbit and mouse: Consideration of time and lymphoid peripheralization. *In* The Thymus in

Immunobiology: Structure, Function, and Role in Disease. R. A. Good & A. E. Gabrielsen, Eds.: 414-435. Hoeber-Harper, New York.

48. HARD, R. C., C. MARTINEZ & R. A. GOOD. 1962. Intestinal crypt lesions in neonatally thymectomized hamsters. Nature **196:** 836.

49. DALMASSO, A. P., C. MARTINEZ & R. A. GOOD. 1964. Studies of immunologic characteristics of lymphoid cells from thymectomized mice. *In* The Thymus in Immunobiology: Structure, Function, and Role in Disease. R. A. Good & A. E. Gabrielsen, Eds.: 478-491. New York. Hoeber-Harper.

50. MARTINEZ, C., A. DALMASSO & R. A. GOOD. 1964. Homotransplantation of normal and neoplastic tissues in thymectomized mice. *In* The Thymus in Immunobiology: Structure, Function, and Role in Disease. R. A. Good & A. E. Gabrielsen, Eds.: 465-477. New York. Hoeber-Harper.

51. McENDY, D. P., M. C. BOON & J. FURTH. 1944. On the role of thymus, spleen, and gonads in the development of leukemia in a high-leukemia stock of mice. Cancer Res. **4:** 377.

52. FURTH, J. 1946. Prolongation of life with prevention of leukemia by thymectomy in mice. J. Gerontol. **1:** 46.

53. MILLER, J. F. A. P. 1960. Studies on mouse leukaemia. The role of thymus in leukemogenesis by cell-free leukaemic filtrates. Br. J. Cancer **14:** 93.

54. MILLER, J. F. A. P. 1961. Etiology and pathogenesis of mouse leukemia. Adv. Cancer Res. **6:** 291.

55. MILLER, J. F. A. P. 1961. Immunological function of the thymus. Lancet **2:** 748.

56. MILLER, J. F. A. P. 1962. Effect of neonatal thymectomy on the immunological responsiveness of the mouse. Proc. Roy. Soc. B **156:** 415.

57. MILLER, J. F. A. P. 1962. The role of the thymus in transplantation immunity. Ann. N. Y. Acad. Sci. **99:** 340.

57a. MILLER, J. F. A. P. 1964. Effect of thymic ablation and replacement. *In* The Thymus in Immunobiology: Structure, Function, and Role in Disease. R. A. Good & A. E. Gabrielsen, Eds.: 436-464. Hoeber-Harper. New York.

58. GOOD, R. A. 1991. Immunology yesterday—Experiments of nature in the development of modern immunology. Immunol. Today **12:** 283-286.

59. MILLER, J. F. A. P. 1991. Immunology yesterday—The discovery of the immunological function of the thymus. Immunol. Today **12:** 42-45.

60. WARNER, N. L. & A. SZENBERG. 1964. Immunologic studies in hormonally bursectomized and surgically thymectomized chickens: Dissociation of immunologic responsiveness. *In* The Thymus in Immunobiology: Structure, Function, and Role in Disease. R. A. Good & A. E. Gabrielsen, Eds.: 395-414. Hoeber-Harper. New York.

61. WARNER, N. L., A. SZENBERG & F. M. BURNET. 1962. The immunological role of different lymphoid organs in the chicken. I. Dissociation of immunological responsiveness. Australian J. Exp. Biol. Med. Sci. **40:** 373.

62. COOPER, M. D., R. D. A. PETERSON & R. A. GOOD. 1965. A new concept of the cellular basis of immunity. J. Pediat. **67:** 907.

63. COOPER, M. D., R. D. A. PETERSON & R. A. GOOD. 1965. Delineation of the thymic and bursal lymphoid systems in the chicken. Nature **205:** 143-146.

64. COOPER, M. D., D. Y. PEREY, R. D. A. PETERSON, A. E. GABRIELSEN & R. A. GOOD. 1968. The two-component concept of the lymphoid system. *In* Immunologic Deficiency Diseases in Man. D. Bergsma & R. A. Good, Eds.: 7-16. The National Foundation. New York.

65. COOPER, M. D., R. D. A. PETERSON, M. A. SOUTH & R. A. GOOD. 1966. The functions of the thymus system and the bursa system in the chicken. J. Exp. Med. **123:** 75-102.

66. GOOD, R. A., A. E. GABRIELSEN, M. D. COOPER & R. D. A. PETERSON. 1966. The role of the thymus and bursa of Fabricius in the development of effector mechanisms. Ann. N.Y. Acad. Sci. **129:** 130.

67. GOOD, R. A., R. D. A. PETERSON, D. Y. PEREY, J. FINSTAD & M. D. COOPER. 1968. The immunological deficiency diseases of man: Consideration of some questions asked by these patients with an attempt at classification. *In* Immunologic Deficiency Diseases in Man. D. Bergsma & R. A. Good, Eds.: 17–39. The National Foundation (Birth Defects: Original Article Series, Vol. IV, No. 1). New York.

68. DIGEORGE, A. M. 1965. Discussion (following presentation by M. D. Cooper). Perlman and Good. J. Pediat. **67:** 908.

69. DIGEORGE, A. M. 1968. Congenital absence of the thymus and its immunologic consequences: Concurrence with congenital hypoparathyroidism. *In* Immunologic Deficiency Diseases in Man. D. Bergsma & R. A. Good, Eds.: 116. National Foundation Press (Birth Defects: Original Article Series, Vol. IV, No. 1). New York.

70. PETERSON, R. D. A., M. D. COOPER & R. A. GOOD. 1965. The pathogenesis of immunologic deficiency diseases. Am. J. Med. **38:** 579–604.

71. GLANZMANN, E. & P. RINIKER. 1950. Essentielle lymphocytophthise. Ein neues Krankheitsbild aus der Sauglingspatholgie. Ann. Paediat. (Basel) **17:** 1.

72. HITZIG, W. H. & H. WILLIE. 1961. Hereditare lymphoplasmocytare Dysgenesie ("Alymphocytose mit Agammaglobulinamie"). Schweiz. Med. Wchnschr. **91:** 1625.

73. TOBLER, R. & H. COTTIER. 1958. Familiare Lymphopenie mit Agammaglobulinamie und schwerer Moniliasis. Helvet. Pediatr. Acta **13:** 313.

74. GOOD, R. A., J. FINSTAD & R. A. GATTI. 1970. Bulwarks of the bodily defense. *In* Infectious Agents and Host Reactions. S. Mudd, Eds.: 76–114. W. B. Saunders. Philadelphia.

75. VAN ALTEN, P. J., W. A. CAIN, R. A. GOOD & M. D. COOPER. 1968. Gamma globulin production and antibody synthesis in chickens bursecotmized as embryos. Nature **217:** 358.

76. HAIRE, R. N., R. BUELL, R. T. LITMAN, Y. OHTA, T. HONJO, F. MATSUDA, M. DE LA MORENA, J. CARRO, R. A. GOOD & G. W. LITMAN. 1993. Diversification, not utilization of the immunoglobulin Vh gene repertoire is restricted in DiGeorge syndrome. J. Exp. Med. **178:** 825–834.

77. LORENZ, E., D. UPHOFF, T. R. REID & E. SHELTON. 1951. Modification of irradiation injury in mice and guinea pigs by bone marrow injections. J. Natl. Cancer Inst. **12:** 197–201.

78. MAIN, J. M. & R. T. PREHN. 1955. Successful skin homografts after the administration of high dosage X radiation and homologous bone marrow. J. Natl. Cancer Inst. **15:** 1023.

79. STORB, R. & E. D. THOMAS. 1972. Bone marrow transplantation in randomly bred animal species and in man. *In* Proceedings of the Sixth Leucocyte Culture Conference. M. R. Schwarz, Ed.: 805–840. Academic Press. New York.

80. THOMAS, E. D., R. LEBLOND, T. C. GRAHAM & R. STORB. 1970. Marrow infusions in dogs given midlethal or lethal irradiation. Radiat. Res. **41:** 113–124.

81. STORB, R., R. B. EPSTEIN, T. C. GRAHAM & E. D. THOMAS. 1970. Methotrexate regimens for control of graft-versus-host disease in dogs with allogeneic marrow grafts. Transplantation **9:** 240–246.

82. HONG, R., H. E. M. KAY, M. D. COOPER, H. MEUWISSEN, M. J. G. ALLAN & R. A. GOOD. 1968. Immunological restitution in lymphopenic immunologic deficiency syndrome. Lancet **1:** 503–506.

83. HONG, R., R. A. GATTI & R. A. GOOD. 1968. Hazards and potential benefits of blood-transfusion in immunological deficiency. Lancet **2:** 388–389.

84. NOGUCHI, M., H. YI, H. M. ROSENBLATT, A. H. FILIPOVICH, S. ADELSTEIN, W. S. MODI, O. W. MCBRIDE & W. J. LEONARD. 1993. Interleukin-2 receptor γ chain mutation results in X-linked severe combined immunodeficiency in humans. Cell **73:** 147–157.

85. GATTI, R. A., H. F. MEUWISSEN, H. D. ALLEN, R. HONG & R. A. GOOD. 1968. Immunological reconstitution of sex-linked lymphopenic immunological deficiency. Lancet **2:** 1366–1369.

86. GOOD, R. A., R. A. GATTI, R. HONG & H. J. MEUWISSEN. 1969. Graft treatment of immunological deficiency (Letters to the Editor). Lancet 1: 1162.

87. GOOD, R. A., R. A. GATTI, R. HONG & H. J. MEUWISSEN. 1969. Successful marrow transplantation for correction of immunological deficit in lymphopenic agammaglobulinemia and treatment of immunologically induced pancytopenia. Exp. Hematol. 19: 4-10.

88. GOOD, R. A. 1969. Immunologic reconstitution: The achievement and its meaning. Hosp. Pract. 4: 41-47.

89. GOOD, R. A. 1983. Immunologic reconstitution: Achievements and potentials. In The Biology of Immunologic Disease. F. Dixon & D. Fisher, Eds. Sinauer Assoc., Inc.: 359-368.

90. BORTIN, M. M., F. H. BACH, D. W. VAN BEKKUM, R. A. GOOD & J. J. VAN ROOD. 1994. 25th anniversary of the first successful allogeneic bone marrow transplants. Bone Marrow Transplant. 14: 211-212.

91. BACH, F. H., R. J. ALBERTINI, P. JOO, J. L. Y. ANDERSON & M. M. BORTIN. 1968. Bone marrow transplantation in a patient with the Wiskott-Aldrich syndrome. Lancet 1: 1364.

92. KAPOOR, N. & R. A. GOOD. 1986. Bone marrow transplantation in 1985. In Recent Advances in Primary and Acquired Immunodeficiencies. F. Aiuti, F. Rosen & M. D. Cooper, Eds.: 327. Raven Press. New York.

93. DEKONIG, J., L. J. DOOREN, D. W. VAN BEKKUM, J. J. VAN ROOD, K. A. DICKE & J. RADL. 1969. Transplantation of bone marrow cells and fetal thymus in an infant with lymphopenic immunological deficiency. Lancet 1: 1223.

94. SANTOS, G. W. & H. KAIZER. 1981. Current status of autologous marrow transplantation. In Cancer Achievements, Challenges and Prospects for the 1980s. J. H. Buchenal & H. F. Oettgen, Eds.: 673. Grune and Stratton. New York.

95. SANTOS, G. W., L. L. SENSENBRENNER, P. N. ANDERSON, P. J. BURKE, D. L. KLEIN, R. E. SLAVIN, B. SCHACTER & D. S. BORGAONKAR. 1976. HL-A-Identical marrow transplantation in aplastic anemia, acute leukemia, and lymphosarcoma employing cyclophosphamide. In Immunobiology of Bone Marrow Transplantation. B. Dupont & R. A. Good, Eds.: 259-262. Grune and Stratton. New York.

96. KOCH, C., K. HERRIKSEN, F. JUHL, A. WIIK, V. FABER, V. ANDERSEN, B. DUPONT, G. S. HANSEN, A. SVEJGAARD, M. THOMSEN, P. ERNST, S. A. KILLMANN, R. A. GOOD, K. JENSEN & N. MÜLLER-BERAT. 1973. Copenhagen Study Group of Immunodeficiencies: Bone-marrow transplantation from an HL-A non-identical but mixed-lymphocyte-culture identical donor. Lancet 1: 1146-1150.

97. HANSEN, J. A., R. J. O'REILLY, R. A. GOOD & B. DUPONT: 1976. Relevance of major human histocompatibility determinants in clinical bone marrow transplantation. Transplant. Proc. 8: 581-589.

98. O'REILLY, R. J., R. PAHWA, B. DUPONT & R. A. GOOD. 1978. Severe combined immunodeficiency: Transplantation approaches for patients lacking an HLA genotypically identical sibling. Transplant. Proc. 10: 187-199.

99. O'REILLY, R. J., R. PAHWA, D. KIRKPATRICK, M. SORELL, A. KAPADIA, N. KAPOOR, J. A. HANSEN, M. POLLACK, S. E. SCHUTZER, R. A. GOOD & B. DUPONT. 1978. Successful transplantation of marrow from an HLA-A, -B, -D-mismatched heterozygous sibling donor into an HLA-D-homozygous patient with aplastic anemia. Transplant. Proc. 10: 957-962.

100. O'REILLY, R. J., N. KAPOOR, M. POLLACK, M. SORELL, R. S. K. CHAGANTI, R. M. BLAESE, R. WANK, R. A. GOOD & B. DUPONT. 1979. Reconstitution of immunologic function in a patient with severe combined immunodeficiency following transplantation of marrow from an HLA-A, B, C non-identical but MLC-compatible paternal donor. Transplant. Proc. 11: 1934-1937.

101. O'REILLY, R. J., B. DUPONT, S. PAHWA, E. GRIMES, E. M. SMITHWICK, R. PAHWA, S. SCHWARTZ, J. A. HANSEN, F. P. SIEGAL, M. SORELL, A. SVEJGAARD, C. JERSILD. M. THOMSEN, P. PLATZ, P. L'ESPERANCE & R. A. GOOD. 1977. Reconstitution in

severe combined immunodeficiency by transplantation of marrow from an unrelated donor. N. Engl. J. Med. **297:** 1311–1318.

102. VON BOEHMER, H., J. SPRENT & M. NABHOLZ. 1975. Tolerance to histo-compatibility determinants in tetraparental bone marrow chimeras. J. Exp. Med. **141:** 322.

103. ONOÉ, K., G. FERNANDES & R. A. GOOD. 1980. Humoral and cell-mediated immune responses in fully allogeneic bone marrow chimera in mice. J. Exp. Med. **151:** 115–132.

104. KROWN, S. E., R. COICO, M. P. SCHEID, G. FERNANDES & R. A. GOOD. 1981. Immune function in fully allogeneic mouse bone marrow chimeras. Clin. Immunol. Immunopathol. **19:** 268–283.

105. COICO, R., S. E. KROWN, R. A. GOOD & M. K. HOFFMAN. 1982. Helper cell factors restore antibody responses of allogeneic bone marrow chimeras: Evidence for ineffective cellular interactions. J. Immunol. **128:** 1590–1593.

106. ONOÉ, K. & R. A. GOOD. 1979. Immune responses in fully allogeneic chimera. Proc. Japan Soc. Immunol. 9–45.

107. ONOÉ, K., R. YASUMIZU, T. OH-ISHI, M. KAKINUMA, R. A. GOOD & K. MORIKAWA. 1981. Restricted antibody formation to sheep erythrocytes of allogeneic bone marrow chimeras histoincompatible at the K end of the H-2 complex. J. Exp. Med. **153:** 1009–1014.

108. ONOÉ, K., R. YASUMIZU, M. NOGUCHI, K. IWABUCHI, M. OGASAWARA, M. KAKINUMA, H. OKUYAMA, R. A. GOOD & K. MORIKAWA. 1985. Analyses of H-2 restriction specificity of helper T cells in fully allogeneic bone marrow chimera in mice. Immunobiology **169:** 60–70.

109. ISHII, E., N. GENGOZIAN & R. A. GOOD. 1991. Influence of dimethyl myleran on tolerance induction and immune function in major histocompatibility complex-haploidentical murine bone-marrow transplantation. Proc. Natl. Acad. Sci. USA **88:** 8435–8439.

110. YUNIS, E. J., G. FERNANDES, J. SMITH & R. A. GOOD. 1976. Long survival and immunologic reconstitution following transplantation with syngeneic or allogeneic fetal liver and neonatal spleen cells. Transplant. Proc. **8:** 521–525.

111. YUNIS, E. J., R. A. GOOD, J. SMITH & O. STUTMAN. 1974. Protection of lethally irradiated mice by spleen cells from neonatally thymectomized mice. Proc. Natl. Acad. Sci. USA **71:** 2544–2548.

112. TULUNAY, O., R. A. GOOD, & E. J. YUNIS. 1975. Protection of lethally irradiated mice with allogeneic fetal liver cells: Influence of irradiation dose on immunologic reconstitution. Proc. Natl. Acad. Sci. USA **72:** 4100–4104.

113. O'REILLY, R. J., R. PAHWA, M. SORRELL, N. KAPOOR, A. KAPADIA, D. KIRKPATRICK, M. POLLACK, B. DUPONT, G. INCEFY, T. IWATA & R. A. GOOD. 1980. Transplantation of fetal liver and thymus in patients with severe combined immunodeficiencies. *In* The Immune System: Functions and Therapy of Dysfunction: Proceedings of the Seronon Symposia, Vol. 27. G. Doria & A. Eshkol, Eds.: 241–253. New York. Academic Press.

114. TOURAINE, J. L. 1979. T lymphocyte maturation after bone marrow, fetal liver, or thymus transplantation in immunodeficiencies. Transplant Proc. **11:** 494–497.

115. REISNER, Y. & N. SHARON. 1980. Cell fractionation by lectins. Trends Biochem. Sci. **5:** 29.

116. REISNER, Y., L. ITZICOVITCH, A. MESHORER & N. SHARON. 1978. Hemopoietic stem cell transplantation using mouse bone marrow and spleen cells fractionated by lectins. Proc. Natl. Acad. Sci. USA **75:** 2933.

117. REISNER, Y., N. KAPOOR, M. Z. HODES, *et al.* 1982. Enrichment for CFU-C from murine and human bone marrow using soybean agglutinin. Blood **59:** 360.

118. O'REILLY, R. J., N. KAPOOR, D. KIRKPATRICK, S. CUNNINGHAM-RUNDLES, M. POLLACK, B. DUPONT, M. Z. HODES, R. A. GOOD & Y. REISNER. 1983. Transplantation for severe combined immunodeficiency using histoincompatible parental marrow fractionated by soybean agglutinin and sheep red blood cells: Experience in six consecutive cases. Transplant. Proc. **15:** 1431–1435.

119. REISNER, Y., N. KAPOOR, R. J. O'REILLY & R. A. GOOD. 1980. Allogeneic bone marrow transplantation using stem cells fractionated by lectins. VI. *In vitro* analysis of human and monkey bone marrow cells fractionated by sheep red blood cells and soybean agglutinin. Lancet **2:** 1320-1324.

120. REISNER, Y., N. KAPOOR, M. Z. HODES, R. J. O'REILLY & R. A. GOOD. 1982. Enrichment for CFU-C from murine and human bone marrow using soybean agglutinin. Blood **59:** 360-363.

121. REISNER, Y., N. KAPOOR, D. KIRKPATRICK, M. POLLACK, S. CUNNINGHAM-RUNDLES, B. DUPONT, M. Z. HODES, R. A. GOOD & R. J. O'REILLY. 1983. Transplantation for severe combined immunodeficiency with HLA A, B, D, Dr incompatible parental marrow cells fractionated by soybean agglutinin and sheep red blood cells. Blood **61:** 341.

122. O'REILLY, R. J., N. KAPOOR, D. KIRKPATRICK, N. FLOMENBERG, M. S. POLLACK, B. DUPONT, R. A. GOOD & Y. REISNER. 1983. Transplantation of hematopoietic cells for lethal congenital immunodeficiencies. *In* Primary Immunodeficiency Diseases. R. J. Wedgwood *et al.,* Eds.: 129-137. Birth Defects: Original Article Series, Vol. 19, No. 3. Alan R. Liss, Inc. New York.

123. O'REILLY, R. J., N. KAPOOR, D. KIRKPATRICK, S. CUNNINGHAM-RUNDLES, M. POLLACK, B. DUPONT, M. Z. HODES, R. A. GOOD & Y. REISNER. 1983. Transplantation for severe combined immunodeficiency using histoincompatible parental marrow fractionated by soybean agglutinin and sheep red blood cells: Experience in six consecutive cases. Transplant Proc. **15:** 1431-1435.

124. REISNER, Y., N. KAPOOR, S. POLLACK, W. FRIEDRICH, D. KIRKPATRICK, B. SHANK, R. CSURNY, M. S. POLLACK, B. DUPONT, R. A. GOOD & R. J. O'REILLY. 1983. Use of lectins in bone marrow transplantation. *In* Advances in Marrow Transplantation. UCLA Symposia, Vol. 7: 355-398.

125. O'REILLY, R. J., N. H. COLLINS, N. KERNAN, J. BROCHSTEIN, R. DINSMORE, D. KIRKPATRICK, S. SIENA, C. KEEVER, B. SHANK, L. WOLF, B. DUPONT & Y. REISNER. 1985. Transplantation of marrow depleted of T cells by soybean lectin agglutination and E-rosette depletion: Major histocompatibility complex-related graft resistance in leukemic transplant recipients. Transplant. Proc. **17:** 455.

126. O'REILLY, R. J., N. A. KERNAN, I. CUNNINGHAM, J. BROCHSTEIN, H. CASTRO-MALASPINA, J. LAVER, N. FLOMENBERG, D. EMANUEL, S. GULATI, C. KEEVER, T. SMALL, N. H. COLLINS & C. BORDIGNON. 1988. Allogeneic transplants depleted of T cells by soybean lectin agglutination and E-rosette depletion. Bone Marrow Transplant **3:** 3.

127. BUCKLEY, R. H., S. E. SCHIFF, H. A. SAMPSON, R. I. SCHIFF, M. L. MARKERT, A. P. KNUTSEN, M. S. HERSHFIELD, A. T. HUANG, G. H. MICKEY & F. E. WARD. 1986. Development of immunity in human severe primary T cell deficiency following haploidentical bone marrow stem cell transplantation. J. Immunol. **136:** 2398-2407.

128. HANSEN, J. A., C. ANASETTI, P. G. BEATTY, P. J. MARTIN, D. AMOS & E. D. THOMAS. 1988. Marrow transplants from HLA haploidentical donors: Failure to engraft and late graft failure. *In* T Cell Depletion in Allogeneic Bone-Marrow Transplantation. M. F. Martelli, F. Grignani & Y. Reisner, Eds.: 111. Serono Symposia Review No. 13. Rome. Italy.

129. AVERSA, F., A. TABILIO, A. TERENZI, A. VERLARDI, F. FALZETTI, C. GIANNONI, R. IACUCCI, T. ZEI, M. P. MARTELLI, C. GAMBELUNGHE, M. ROSETTI, P. CAPUTO, P. LATINI, C. ARISTEI, C. RAYMONDI, Y. REISNER & M. F. MARTELLI. 1994. Successful engraftment of T-cell depleted haploidentical "three loci" incompatible transplants in leukemia patients by addition of recombinant human granulocyte colony-stimulating factor-mobilized peripheral blood progenitor cells to bone marrow inoculum. Blood **84:** 3948-3955.

130. ISHII, E., N. GENGOZIAN & R. A. GOOD. 1991. Influence of dimethyl myleran on tolerance induction in haploidentical murine bone marrow transplantation. (Abstract 7760).

1991 Meeting of the American Association of Pathologists, Atlanta, GA, April 21–25, 1991. FASEB J. **5:** A1707.

131. IKEHARA, S., R. YASUMIZU, M. INABA, S. IZUI, K. HAYAKAWA, K. SEKITA, J. TOKI, K. SUGIURA, H. IWAI, T. NAKAMURA, E. MUSO, Y. HAMASHIMA & R. A. GOOD. 1989. Long-term observations of autoimmune-prone mice treated for autoimmune disease by allogeneic bone marrow transplantation. Proc. Natl. Acad. Sci. USA **86:** 3306–3310.

132. IWAI, H., S. KUMA, M. M. INABA, R. A. GOOD, T. YAMASHITA, T. KUMAZAWA & S. IKEHARA. 1989. Acceptance of murine thyroid allografts by pretreatment of anti-Ia antibody or anti-dendritic cell antibody *in vitro*. Transplantation **47:** 45–49.

133. IKEHARA, S., M. KAWAMURA, F. TAKAO, M. INABA, R. YASUMIZU, S. THAN, H. HISHA, K. SUGIURA, Y. KOIDE, T. O. YOSHIDA, T. IDA, H. IMURA & R. A. GOOD. 1990. Organ-specific and systemic autoimmune diseases originate from defects in hematopoietic stem cells. Proc. Natl. Acad. Sci. USA **87:** 8341–8344.

134. SUGIURA, K., R. YASUMIZU, H. IWAI, M. N. INABA, J. TOKI, M. OGURA, I. HARA, R. A. GOOD & S. IKEHARA. 1991. Long-term immunologic tolerance induction in chimeric mice after bone marrow transplantation across major histocompatibility barriers: Persistent or redeveloping immunologic responsiveness after prolonged survival. Thymus **18:** 137–153.

135. MIZUTANI, H., R. W. ENGELMAN, Y. KURATA, S. IKEHARA & R. A. GOOD. 1993. Development and characterization of monoclonal antiplatelet autoantibodies from autoimmune thrombocytopenic purpura-prone (NZW x BXSB)F_1 mice. Blood **82:** 837–844.

136. MIZUTANI, H., R. W. ENGELMAN, K. KINJOH, Y. KURATA, S. IKEHARA & R. A. GOOD. 1993. Prevention and induction of occlusive coronary vascular disease in autoimmune (W/B)F_1 mice by haploidentical bone marrow transplantation: Possible role for anticardiolipin autoantibodies. Blood **82:** 3091–3097.

137. KIRZNER, R. P.: Prevention of coronary vascular disease in W/BF_1 autoimmune-prone mice by bone marrow transplantation. Ph.D. Dissertation. University of South Florida, Tampa, Florida, 1995.

138. SARDIÑA, E. E., K. SUGIURA, S. IKEHARA & R. A. GOOD. 1991. Transplantation of WGA$^+$ hematopoietic cells to prevent or induce systemic autoimmune disease. Proc. Natl. Acad. Sci. USA **88:** 3218–3222.

139. HIMENO, K. & R. A. GOOD. 1988. Marrow transplantation from tolerant donors to treat and prevent autoimmune diseases in BXSB mice. Proc. Natl. Acad. Sci. USA **85:** 2235–2239.

140. AHMED, H. 1992. Bone marrow transplantation and dietary manipulation as approaches to the prevention and treatment of autoimmune disease in MRL mice. Ph.D. Dissertation, University of South Florida, Tampa, Florida.

141. NAGATA, S. 1994. Mutations in the Fas antigen gene in *lpr* mice. Semin. Immunol. **6:** 3–15.

142. IKEHARA, S., M. INABA, S. ISHIDA, H. OGATA, H. HISHA, R. YASUMIZU, N. OYAIZU, K. SUGIURA, J. TOKI, F. TAKAO, S. THAN, M. KAWAMURA, N. NISHIOKA, N. NAGATA & R. A. GOOD. 1991. Rationale for transplantation of both allogeneic bone marrow and stromal cells in the treatment of autoimmune diseases. *In* New Strategies in Bone Marrow Transplantation. R. E. Champlin & R. P. Gale, Eds.: 251–257. New York. Wiley-Liss, Inc.

143. HISHA, H., T. NISHINO, M. KAWAMURA, S. ADACHI & S. IKEHARA. 1995. Successful bone marrow transplantation by bone grafts in chimeric-resistant combination. Exp. Hematol. **23:** 347–352.

144. IKEHARA, S., T. NAKAMURA, K. SEKITA, E. MUSO, R. YASUMIZU, H. OHTSUKI, Y. HAMASHIMA & R. A. GOOD. 1987. Treatment of systemic and organ-specific autoimmune disease in mice by allogeneic bone marrow transplantation. Prog. Clin & Biol. Res. **229:** 131–146.

145. IKEHARA, S., H. OHTSUKI, R. A. GOOD, H. ASAMOTO, T. NAKAMURA, K. SEKITA, E. MUSO, Y. TOCHINO, T. IDA & H. KUZUYA. 1985. Prevention of type I diabetes in

non-obese diabetic mice by allogenic bone marrow transplantation. Proc. Natl. Acad. Sci. USA **82:** 7743-7747.

146. IKEHARA, S., H. TANAKA, T. NAKAMURA, F. FURUKAWA, S. INOUE, K. SEKITA, J. SHIMIZU, Y. HAMASHIMA & R. A. GOOD. 1985. The influence of thymic abnormalities on the development of autoimmune diseases. Thymus **7:** 25-36.

147. IWAI, H., R. YASUMIZU, K. SUGIURA, M. INABA, T. KUMAZAWA, R. A. GOOD & S. IKEHARA. 1987. Successful pancreatic allografts in combination with bone marrow transplantation in mice. Immunology **62:** 457-462.

148. YASUMIZU, R., K. SUGIURA, H. IWAI, M. INABA, S. MAKINO, T. IDA, H. IMURA, Y. HAMASHIMA, R. A. GOOD & S. IKEHARA. 1987. Treatment of type 1 diabetes mellitus in non-obese diabetic mice by transplantation of allogeneic bone marrow and pancreatic tissue. Proc. Natl. Acad. Sci. USA **84:** 6555-6557.

149. OGATA, H., W. G. BRADLEY, M. INABA, N. OGATA, S. IKEHARA & R. A. GOOD. 1995. Long term repopulation of hematolymphoid cells with only a few hemopoietic stem cells in mice. Proc. Natl. Acad. Sci. USA **92:** 5945-5949.

150. OWEN, R. D. 1945. Immunogenetic consequences of vascular anastomoses between bovine twins. Science **102:** 400.

151. ANDERSON, D., R. E. BILLINGHAM, G. H. LAMPKIN & P. B. MEDAWAR. 1952. Heredity **5:** 379-397.

152. BILLINGHAM, R. E., L. BRENT & P. B. MEDAWAR. 1953. Actively acquired tolerance of foreign cells. Nature **172:** 603-606.

153. MARTINEZ, C., F. SHAPIRO, H. KELMAN, T. ONSTAD & R. A. GOOD. 1960. Tolerance of F1 hybrid skin homografts in the parent strain induced by parabiosis. Proc. Soc. Exp. Biol. Med. **103:** 266-269.

154. MARTINEZ, C., F. SHAPIRO & R. A. GOOD. 1960. Essential duration of parabiosis and development of tolerance to skin homografts in mice. Proc. Soc. Exp. Biol. Med. **104:** 256-259.

155. ONOÉ, K., G. FERNANDES, F. W. SHEN & R. A. GOOD. 1982. Sequential changes of thymocyte surface antigens with presence or absence of graft-vs-host reaction following allogeneic bone marrow transplantation. Cell. Immunol. **68:** 207-219.

156. ONOÉ, K., R. YASUMIZU, L. GENG, K. IWABUCHI, M. OGASAWARA, M. KAKINUMA, H. OKUYAMA, R. A. GOOD & K. MORIKAWA. 1985. Analyses of Ia restriction specificity of helper T cells in H-2 subregion compatible bone marrow chimera in mice. Immunobiology **169:** 71-82.

157. ONOÉ, K., R. A. GOOD & K. YAMAMOTO. 1986. Anti-bacterial immunity to *Listeria monocytogenes* in allogeneic bone marrow chimera in mice. J. Immunol. **136:** 4264-4269.

158. ILDSTAD, S. T. & D. H. SACHS. 1984. Reconstitution with syngeneic plus allogeneic or xenogeneic bone marrow leads to specific acceptance of allografts or xenografts. Nature **307:** 170.

159. EL-BADRI, N. 1992. Lymphohemopoietic reconstitution and induction of immunological tolerance using WGA hemopoietic stem cell transplantation in a mixed chimerism model. Ph.D. Dissertation. University of South Florida, Tampa, Florida.

160. EL BADRI, N. S. & R. A. GOOD. 1993. Lymphohemopoietic reconstitution using wheat germ agglutinin-positive hemopoietic stem cell transplantation within but not across the major histocompatibility antigen barriers. Proc. Natl. Acad. Sci. USA **90:** 6681-6685.

161. EL-BADRI, N. & R. A. GOOD. 1994. Induction of Immunological tolerance in full major and multiminor histocompatibility-disparate mice using a mixed bone marrow transplantation model. Proc. Soc. Exp. Biol. **205:** 67-74.

162. ILDSTAD, StT., S. S. BOGGS, F. VECCHINI *et al.* 1992. Mixed xenogeneic chimeras (rat + mouse → rat): Evidence of rat stem cell engraftment, strain-specific transplantation tolerance, and skin-specific antigen. Transplantation **53:** 815.

163. SHARABI, Y., V. S. ABRAHAM, M. SYKES & D. H. SACHS. 1993. Mixed allogeneic chimeras prepared by a non-myeloablative regimen: Requirement for chimerism to maintain tolerance. Bone Marrow Transplant. **9:** 191-197.

164. KAUFMANN, C. L., Y. L. COLSON, S. M. WREN, S. WATKINS, R. SIMMONS & S. T. ILDSTAD. 1994. Phenotypic characterization of a novel bone marrow-derived cell that facilitates engraftment of allogeneic bone marrow stem cells. Blood **84:** 2436-2446.

165. EL-BADRI DAJANI, N., B. Y. WANG, D. UCKAN & R. A. GOOD. Osteoblasts promote engraftment of allogeneic marrow stem cells. Unpublished observations, 1995.

166. STARZL, T. E. & A. J. DEMETRIS. 1995. Transplantation milestones: Viewed with one- and two-way paradigms of tolerance. JAMA **273:** 876-879.

167. STARZL, T. E., A. J. DEMETRIS, M. TRUCCO, A. ZEEVI, H. RAMOS, P. TERASAKI, W. A. RUDERT, M. KOCOVA, C. RICORDI, S. ILDSTAD et al. 1993. Chimerism and donor-specific nonreactivity 27 to 29 years after kidney allotransplantation. Transplantation **55:** 1272-1277.

168. FONTES, P., A. S. RAO, A. J. DEMETRIS, A. ZEEVI, M. TRUCCO, P. CARROLL, W. RYBKA, W. A. RUDERT, C. RICORDI, F. DODSON et al. 1994. Bone marrow augmentation of donor-cell chimerism in kidney, liver, heart, and pancreas islet transplantation. Lancet **344:** 151-155.

169. MURASE, N., T. E. STARZL, M. TANABE, S. FUJISAKI, H. MIYAZAWA, Q. YE, C. P. DELANEY, J. J. FUNG & A. J. DEMETRIS. 1995. Variable chimerism, graft-versus-host disease, and tolerance after different kinds of cell and whole organ transplantation from Lewis to brown Norway rats. Transplantation **60:** 158-171.

Bone Marrow Transplantation from Bench to Bedside

E. DONNALL THOMAS [a]

Fred Hutchinson Cancer Research Center
and
Professor of Medicine, Emeritus
University of Washington
Seattle, Washington 98104

THE BEGINNINGS OF MARROW TRANSPLANTATION

In medical school in the 1940s, I learned that it was not possible to transplant tissue or cells from one individual to another of different genetic origin without subsequent rejection of the graft, knowledge that dated back to the studies of Alexis Carrel who received the Nobel prize in 1912. A few years after my graduation in 1946, two different areas of study were reported that were to have a profound effect on my interest in transplantation and hematopoietic diseases. First were the studies of Medawar, Burnett, Hasek, and others showing that the rejection reaction need not always occur. The second was the demonstration by Jacobson, Lorenz, and colleagues that mice could be protected against otherwise lethal exposure of total body irradiation by shielding the spleen or infusing marrow cells.

In the 1950s these initial studies were expanded by a number of investigators. But first, I must mention some other important personal events. In 1951, while doing postdoctoral work at Massachusetts Institute of Technology, Boston, Massachusetts I met George Santos, then an undergraduate, the beginning of a long and productive relationship. In 1959, I met Robert Good whose studies were to have a major impact on my own endeavors.

In 1955 I moved to the Mary Imogene Bassett Hospital in Cooperstown, New York, to join Joe Ferrebee and begin our studies of marrow transplantation in man and dog. Our efforts to achieve allogeneic marrow grafts in patients with advanced hematologic malignancies were largely unsuccessful except in a few patients fortunate in having an identical twin.

In the canine model, we found that dogs could be protected against several times the lethal dose of total body irradiation (TBI) if they were given an intravenous infusion of their own marrow that had been cryopreserved before irradiation. By laboriously collecting peripheral blood cells, we showed that dogs could be protected against lethal irradiation by infusion of these peripheral blood stem cells.

When dogs were given lethal irradiation and an infusion of marrow from another dog, even a littermate, almost all dogs died of what we now recognize as graft-

---

[a] Address for correspondence: Fred Hutchinson Cancer Research Center, 1124 Columbia Street, Seattle, WA 98104.

versus-host disease (GVHD) or graft rejection. However, some dogs survived with surprisingly few problems, indicating that marrow grafts might indeed be possible if the variables defining success or failure could be defined.

In 1963 Mrs. Thomas and I moved to Seattle, Washington, where we were joined by Bob Epstein, Rainer Storb, Dean Buckner, Alex Fefer, Paul Neiman, and over the years, a series of investigators who now make up the Seattle marrow transplant team.

By 1967 we had developed tissue typing sera for dogs which enabled us to show that we could get long-term survival of dogs given lethal irradiation and matched littermate marrow, especially if methotrexate was given for a few weeks postgrafting to ameliorate GVHD. These results made it feasible to return to marrow grafting in human patients using matched sibling marrow combined with short-term immunosuppression.

The development of marrow transplantation in animals and human patients was reviewed in detail in 1975, and references to the earlier work can be found in that article.[1] Dr. Storb's presentation summarizes the information gained from animal studies which continue to provide knowledge critical to improvement of human marrow transplantation.

THE MODERN ERA OF HUMAN MARROW TRANSPLANTATION

In December 1968, Bob Good and his team reported a successful marrow graft in a patient with severe combined immunologic deficiency disease using a matched sibling donor.[2] We did our first "modern" era transplant in March 1969 in a patient with the blastic phase of chronic myeloid leukemia whose donor was a matched sister. Our patient died of the complications of GVHD some months later, while Bob Good's patient is still alive and well. As the precision of human HLA typing improved, we found that the donors of both of these first patients were not HLA identical. Thus, we refer to those transplants as those using a "presumed" HLA-matched donor.

As more centers focused on marrow transplantation in the 1970s and 1980s, there were numerous failures and increasing numbers of successes. I will summarize some of the results of those years using the data from Seattle. There are, of course, many reports by other marrow transplant teams, and the Bone Marrow Transplant Registry has published numerous reports of combined data from many marrow transplant teams that do not include the Seattle data.[3]

Acute Lymphoid Leukemia

For acute lymphoid leukemia (ALL) in children, most but by no means all patients can be cured with combined chemotherapy. Dr. Gorin has provided an overview of the experience with marrow grafting for this disease. FIGURE 1 summarizes more than two decades of experience in Seattle. Of particular interest is the good disease-free survival in patients transplanted in the first remission because of poor prognostic indicators for long-term survival after chemotherapy.

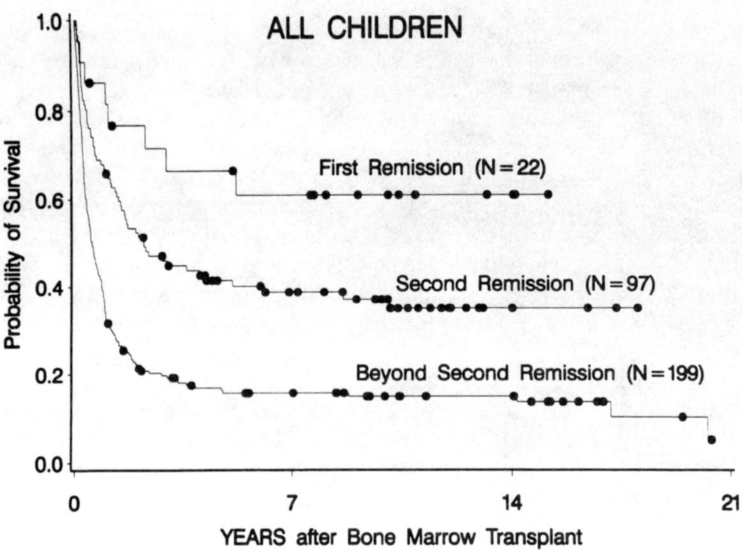

FIGURE 1. Kaplan-Meier product limit estimates of disease-free survival in children with acute lymphoid leukemia (ALL) given marrow grafts from HLA-identical siblings analyzed according to stage of disease. A summary of the experience in Seattle.

Acute Myeloid Leukemia

In acute myeloid leukemia (AML) in children or adults, slightly more than half the patients can achieve long-term disease-free survival if transplantation is performed during first remission, as Dr. Gorin indicated. In Seattle we carried out a study of intensive therapy and marrow grafting in adults with AML who received a marrow graft if an HLA-identical sibling was available and chemotherapy if not.[4] At publication, all patients had been followed up more than 5 years. Disease-free survival was 50% for marrow-grafted patients and 20% for chemotherapy recipients. Now, with all patients followed up more than 10 years, there have been no further failures in either group.

Chronic Myeloid Leukemia

The most interesting results have been achieved in chronic myeloid leukemia (CML), a disease not cured by chemotherapy. George Santos presented an overview of preparative regimens for marrow grafting. In Seattle, we studied patients with CML transplanted in the chronic phase who were randomized to receive a regimen of total body irradiation (TBI) and cyclophosphamide (CY), the regimen we had used since 1969, or busulfan (BU) with CY, the new regimen proposed by Santos and Tutschka. Postgrafting immunosuppression consisted of a short course of methotrexate and cyclosporine. In both arms of the study, long-term disease-free survival

PROTOCOL 428

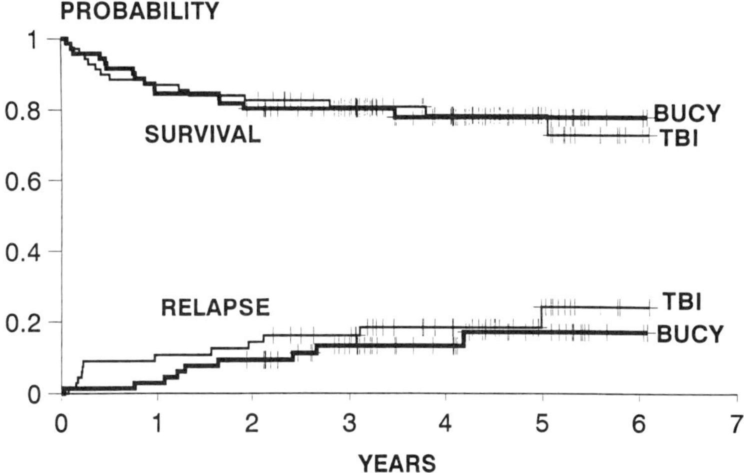

FIGURE 2. Kaplan-Meier product limit estimates of survival and relapse in patients with chronic myeloid leukemia (CML) randomized to a preparative regimen of busulfan (BU)-cyclophosphamide (CY) or CY and total body irradiation (TBI) and given a marrow graft from an HLA-identical sibling.

was achieved for approximately three fourths of the patients[5] (FIG. 2). Blume, Forman, and their colleagues reported on a regimen of etoposide and TBI which gives similar results.[6] Thus, there are three regimens that give excellent results in CML.

Nonmalignant and Genetic Diseases

Nonmalignant or genetic diseases can be treated successfully by an allogeneic marrow graft from a matched sibling. In patients with aplastic anemia[7] or thalassemia major[8] who have not had major complications of their disease, long-term survival after marrow grafting is better than 90%.

RESEARCH AND APPLICATION OF MARROW GRAFTING IN THE NEXT DECADE

Now let us turn to marrow grafting in the 1990s and beyond. Many aspects of the exciting on-going research studies are presented in this volume. It is possible to emphasize only some of the trends.

Autologous Marrow Transplantation

Perhaps most impressive is the rapidly growing use of autologous marrow grafts in almost every category of disease except aplastic anemia and genetic diseases.

Long-term disease-free survival is being achieved in leukemias, breast cancer, and multiple myeloma. Current research focuses on the assessment of various regimens and the determination of long-term results.

Peripheral Blood Hematopoietic Progenitors for Transplantation

As reported by Dr. Janssen, autologous marrow grafts are being carried out using peripheral blood stem cells. The development of continuous flow-centrifuges makes it possible to collect large numbers of peripheral blood nucleated cells. Mobilization of stem cells into the peripheral blood is facilitated by chemotherapy or preferably by administration of hematopoietic growth factors such as granulocyte-colony-stimulating factor (G-CSF). Preliminary results of allogeneic marrow grafts using peripheral blood stem cells show excellent engraftment without excessive GVHD, which had been feared because of the large number of T cells given with the stem cells. Peripheral blood cells generally give more rapid engraftment than does marrow, indicating that transplantation with these cells will probably replace the use of marrow.

Cord Blood Hematopoietic Progenitors for Transplantation

Dr. Broxmeyer reports the use of cord blood cells in marrow grafting. These hematopoietic stem cells are of great interest because they may induce less GVHD than do grafts of adult marrow. Cord blood cells are essentially a byproduct of normal pregnancy and are being cryopreserved to assemble banks of cells for transplantation.

Supportive Care

Major improvements in survival of marrow-grafted patients are occurring because of research in supportive care. Impressive is the reduction in mortality and morbidity from cytomegalovirus (CMV) disease through the use of ganciclovir.[9,10] Because of modern antibiotics, few patients die of bacterial disease. Control of fungal infections and prevention of venoocclusive disease of the liver are still major problems.

Hematopoietic Growth Factors

The use of hematopoietic growth factors has shortened the time to recovery of granulocytes, as summarized by Dr. Stewart. Early recovery of granulocytes has made possible earlier discharge from the hospital with consequent reduction in costs. There is as yet no evidence that G-CSF or granulocyte-macrophage colony-stimulating factor (GM-CSF) has reduced the incidence of infection. Many new cytokines and combinations of cytokines are currently under study.

Contamination of Marrow with Malignant Cells

A major problem in the application of intensive chemoirradiation and autologous marrow grafting in patients with leukemia or other malignancies is whether small numbers of malignant cells are present in the marrow but hidden among the large number of normal cells. Dr. Sharp summarizes the problems in detecting minimal residual disease. In autologous marrow from patients with leukemia in remission or patients with breast cancer, for example, these cells might bring about a recurrence of disease. Efforts to "purge" these cells by *in vitro* treatment with chemotherapeutic agents or antibodies are being studied. Although most patients with leukemia in remission are destined to have a relapse, many are cured by chemotherapy. A technique for detecting very small numbers of leukemic cells would make possible a decision about whether further treatment with marrow transplantation is necessary.

Minimal Residual Disease

The development of the polymerase chain reaction (PCR) to amplify and identify minute numbers of cells (less than 1 in 100,000) possessing a deletion, rearrangement, or translocation characteristic of the malignant cell provides the technique for detection of minimal residual disease. For example, in a recent study of patients who had a marrow transplant for CML, a negative PCR test for the 9 : 22 translocation 6-12 months after transplantation was a strong predictor of long-term disease-free survival.[11] On the other hand, a positive PCR result predicted almost certain relapse. These patients became candidates for a second transplant, treatment with interferon, or infusion of additional donor cells to create a graft-versus-leukemia effect.

Graft-versus-Host Disease and Tolerance

Several reports presented in this volume provide an excellent overview of the graft-versus-host reaction and its counterpart, tolerance. Graft-versus-host disease can range from absent to very mild to life-threatening, presumably due to unrecognized minor histocompatibility differences, even when the donor is an HLA-identical sibling. Prevention or treatment with immunosuppressive agents is usually effective, but some patients develop uncontrollable disease or progress to chronic GVHD. In contrast to patients receiving solid organ grafts, most marrow graft recipients can discontinue immunosuppressive treatment in a few months. They then demonstrate a state of "tolerance," that is, they have cells of donor origin living in the presence of cells and organs of the host. Many studies in progress are designed to evaluate the nature of the immunologic reactions between donor and host cells and particularly the nature of the tolerance that develops.

Dr. Starzl presents data on the remarkable demonstration that following solid organ grafts, donor immunologic cells can be found in small numbers throughout the organs of the recipient. These cells are presumed to play a major role in the tolerance to solid organ grafts and have led to attempts to facilitate solid organ grafts by infusion of additional donor marrow and/or monocyte-macrophage or dendritic cells.

In Vitro *Expansion of Hematopoietic Progenitor Cells*

With increasing knowledge of the nature of the stem cell, the characterization of the stem cell-microenvironmental cell interaction, and the availability of hematopoietic cytokines, it has become feasible to grow stem cells *in vitro*. Dr. Emerson summarizes these studies. Such cells obtained from small amounts of peripheral blood could be used for transplantation. Alternatively, by adjusting culture conditions, abnormal cells, such as leukemic cells, might die off, thus accomplishing a form of *in vitro* purging. Functional stem cells can currently be maintained in culture for a few months, but growth of these cells continues to be a formidable challenge.

Gene Transfer

The hematopoietic stem cell is in many ways an ideal candidate for gene therapy, as summarized by Dr. Chatterjee. There are many genetic diseases involving the stem cell, and many of the relevant genes have been cloned. Techniques for gene transfer have made it possible to begin studies of gene transfer in human patients. However, the problems of cloning some of the larger genes, efficient gene transfer, gene expression, and sustained gene expression represent major challenges. Many laboratories are working on this most exciting area of cell biology.

SUMMARY

Marrow grafting, now more appropriately called hematopoietic stem cell grafting, has come a long way from early bench studies and desperate bedside therapeutic attempts in terminal patients. Grafting of hematopoietic stem cells is now standard therapy for selected diseases and stages of disease, and increasing application on an outpatient basis is rapidly lowering the cost of the procedure. The combined efforts of the now many clinical marrow transplant teams and the interested basic science laboratories will undoubtedly make the coming decade an exciting and productive time for science and for the well-being of patients with otherwise incurable diseases.

REFERENCES

1. THOMAS, E. D., R. STORB, R. A. CLIFT, A. FEFER, F. L. JOHNSON, P. E. NEIMAN, K. G. LERNER, H. GLUCKSBERG & C. D. BUCKNER. 1975. Bone-marrow transplantation. N. Engl. J. Med. **292:** 832–843, 895–902.
2. GATTI, R. A., H. J. MEUWISSEN, H. D. ALLEN, R. HONG & R. A. GOOD. 1968. Immunological reconstitution of sex-linked lymphopenic immunological deficiency. Lancet **ii:** 1366–1369.
3. BORTIN, M. M., M. M. HOROWITZ, P. A. ROWLINGS, A. A. RIMM, K. A. SOBOCINSKI, M. J. ZHANG & R. P. GALE. 1993. 1993 Progress report from the International Bone Marrow Transplant Registry. Advisory Committee of the International Bone Marrow Transplant Registry. Bone Marrow Transplant. **12:** 97–104.
4. APPELBAUM, F. R., L. D. FISHER, E. D. THOMAS & AND THE SEATTLE MARROW TRANSPLANT TEAM. 1988. Chemotherapy v marrow transplantation for adults with acute nonlymphocytic leukemia: A five-year follow-up. Blood **72:** 179–184.
5. CLIFT, R. A., C. D. BUCKNER, E. D. THOMAS, W. I. BENSINGER, R. BOWDEN, E. BRYANT, H. J. DEEG, K. C. DONEY, L. D. FISHER, J. A. HANSEN, P. MARTIN, G. B. MCDONALD, J. E. SANDERS, G. SCHOCH, J. SINGER, R. STORB, K. M. SULLIVAN, R. P. WITHERSPOON & F. R. APPELBAUM. 1994. Marrow transplantation for chronic myeloid leukemia: A

randomized study comparing cyclophosphamide and total body irradiation with busulfan and cyclophosphamide. Blood **84:** 2036-2043.

6. SYNDER, D. S., R. S. NEGRIN, M. R. O'DONNELL, N. J. CHAO, M. D. AMYLON, G. D. LONG, A. P. NADEMANEE, A. S. STEIN, P. M. PARKER, E. P. SMITH, G. SOMLO, K. MARGOLIN, A. MOLINA, D. E. STEPAN, J. A. LIPSETT, R. T. HOPPE, M. L. SLOVAK, J. C. NILAND, A. C. DAGIS, R. M. WONG, S. J. FORMAN & K. G. BLUME. 1994. Fractionated total body irradiation and high dose etoposide as a preparatory regimen for bone marrow transplantation for 94 patients with chronic myelogenous leukemia. Blood **84:** 1672-1679.

7. STORB, R., W. LEISENRING, H. J. DEEG, C. ANASETTI, F. APPELBAUM, W. BENSINGER, C. D. BUCKNER, R. CLIFT, K. DONEY, J. HANSEN, P. MARTIN, J. SANDERS, P. STEWART, K. SULLIVAN, E. D. THOMAS & R. WITHERSPOON. 1994. Long-term follow-up of a randomized trial of graft-versus-host disease prevention by methotrexate/cyclosporine versus methotrexate alone in patients given marrow grafts for severe aplastic anemia (Letter). Blood **83:** 2749-2756.

8. BARONCIANI, D., M. GALIMBERTI, G. LUCARELLI, P. POLCHI, E. ANGELUCCI, C. GIARDINI, C. GIORGI & J. GAZIEV. 1993. Bone marrow transplantation in class 1 thalassemia patients. Bone Marrow Transplant. **12**(Suppl 1): 56-58.

9. SCHMIDT, G. M., D. A. HORAK, J. C. NILAND, S. R. DUNCAN, S. J. FORMAN & J. A. ZAIA. 1991. A randomized, controlled trial of prophylactic ganciclovir for cytomegalovirus pulmonary infection in recipients of allogeneic bone marrow transplants. N. Engl. J. Med. **324:** 1005-1011.

10. GOODRICH, J. M., R. A. BOWDEN, L. FISHER, C. KELLER, G. SCHOCH & J. D. MEYERS. 1993. Ganciclovir prophylaxis to prevent cytomegalovirus disease after allogeneic marrow transplant. Ann. Intern. Med. **118:** 173-178.

11. RADICH, J. P., G. GEHLY, T. GOOLEY, E. BRYANT, R. A. CLIFT, S. COLLINS, S. EDMANDS, J. KIRK, A. LEE, P. KESSLER, G. SCHOCH, C. D. BUCKNER, K. M. SULLIVAN, F. R. APPELBAUM & E. D. THOMAS. 1995. Polymerase chain reaction detection of the BCR-ABL fusion transcript after allogeneic marrow transplantation for chronic myeloid leukemia: Results and implications in 346 patients. Blood **85:** 2632-2698.

Characterization of Hematopoietic Stem Cells

G. FRITSCH,[a,b] M. STIMPFL,[a] M. KURZ,[c] A. LEITNER,[a]
D. PRINTZ,[a] P. BUCHINGER,[a] P. HOECKER,[c] AND
H. GADNER [a]

[a]Childrens' Cancer Research Institute (CCRI)
St. Anna Kinderspital
A-1090 Vienna, Austria

[c]Department of Transfusion Medicine
University of Vienna
A-1090 Vienna, Austria

For almost three decades, the clonogenic assay has been used for laboratory quantification and characterization of hematopoietic progenitor cells.[1] Ten years ago, the first monoclonal antibody (mAb) was described against a "stem cell"-specific antigen[2] which was later designated as CD34.[3] A variety of mAbs have since been developed against this epitope and are currently used mainly in flow cytometric (FACS) analysis. The latter method allows rapid determination of the amount of progenitor cells in transplants used to reconstitute hematopoiesis after myeloablative treatment of patients with malignancies. Although the number of CD34$^+$ cells required for successful transplantation has not yet been clearly defined, a threshold of 2×10^6 progenitor cells per kilogram of the recipient is today widely accepted for peripheral blood stem cells (PBSC).[4] On the other hand, bone marrow, which until recently was the only source of hematopoietic cells used for transplantation, has shown slower recovery after transplantation.[5,6] Recent studies have directly compared and characterized CD34$^+$ cells contained in these two cell sources as well as in cord blood (CB).[7-11] To add further information to this field of investigation, we summarize our data on differential CD34 FACS analysis. We present evidence that in terms of successful and rapid engraftment, peripheral blood (PB)- and CB-derived progenitor cells are probably superior, but at least equivalent to those obtained from bone marrow.

MATERIALS AND METHODS

Cell Sources. Cord blood samples obtained after normal full-term deliveries were handled within 12 hours after birth. Of all CB specimens analyzed,[12] only those for which the relevant set of FACS analyses was performed are considered ($n = 14$). Bone marrow samples ($n = 196$) were taken from healthy donors ($n = 46$) and from

[b]Address for correspondence: Gerhard Fritsch, PhD, CCRI, St. Anna Kinderspital, Kinderspitalgasse 6, A-1090 Vienna, Austria.

routine biopsies of patients in remission or after transplantation with no clinical signs of disease. Most patients were below 18 years of age. Peripheral blood specimens (n = 258) were taken from patients routinely analyzed for their recovery of CD34[+] cells after different treatment cycles with or without colony-stimulating factor support (G-CSF, GM-CSF). Samples were included in this evaluation only if no malignant cells that expressed the CD34 antigen were present, and when the amount of hemato-poietic progenitors was ≥0.1% of mononuclear cells. The products of leukaphereses aimed at the collection of PBSC for autologous transplantation were also included (Pher, n = 51). All analyzed cell samples had been density-separated by centrifugation on 1.077 g/cm^3 Ficoll-Paque (Pharmacia, Uppsala, Sweden) or Nycoprep (Nycomed, Oslo, Norway). Therefore, the results of flow cytometric analysis are expressed as a percentage of low-density mononuclear cells, the only exception being cells that had been positively selected for hematopoietic progenitors using biotin/streptavidin affinity separation (Ceprate SC, CellPro Inc., Bothell, Washington). In the latter samples, the proportions refer to the nucleated cells. Our analyses include such separations from bone marrow (BMsel, n = 2), cord blood (CBsel, n = 5), and peripheral blood (Psel, n = 18).

Immunologic Cell Staining. A detailed description of cell preparation and cell surface staining of the ingredients for the clonogenic assay and of the types of colonies grown is given elsewhere.[8] The mAbs relevant to the present communication recognized CD34 (HPCA2, Becton Dickinson, Sunnyvale, California), CD45RA (2H4, Coulter, Krefeld, Germany), CD19 (HD37, Dakopatts, Glostrup, Denmark), CD7 (3A1, Coulter), and glycophorin A (GPA, clone D2.10, Immunotech, Marseille, France). To minimize unspecific staining, cell staining was preceded by a 20-minute incubation of mononuclear cells (at 1 × 10^7/ml of IMDM/2% fetal bovine serum) in an equal volume of an unspecific mouse mAb (MOPC21, Sigma, St. Louis, Missouri, diluted at 1 mg/ml).

Data Acquisition and Analysis on FACS. All data were acquired on a FACSStar Plus (Becton Dickinson) with an argon ion laser (Coherent, Palo Alto, California) tuned to an excitation wavelength of 488 nm. Acquisition software included a FACStar Plus and Lysis II (both from Becton Dickinson). Each cell was characterized by its forward (FSC) and 90-degree scattering (SSC) properties and by three fluorescence signals (FL1, FL2, and FL3) even if only two-color staining was performed. Between 10,000 and 30,000 events were stored in list-mode files. To analyze the data, we employed predominantly PAINT-A-GATE software (Becton Dickinson) which facili-tates the characterization of CD34[+] cells as well as the recognition of false-positive events or nonspecific staining.

RESULTS

Evaluation of FACS Data

The PAINT-A-GATE software was routinely used to analyze stored list-mode file data. This software allows the analyzed cell sample to be depicted in six dotplots with different combinations of the five acquired parameters (FSC, SSC, FL1, FL2, and FL3) in the x and y axes as shown elsewhere.[8,13] The CD34[+] cells were quantified in the CD34 versus SSC dotplot. In contrast to other cell sources, it was a typical feature of many bone marrow samples that the CD34$^+$ and CD34$^-$ cell fractions were connected by a cell population of intermediate fluorescence intensity. Two-color analysis revealed that the latter cells represented CD10- and CD19-positive B-cell progenitors which were also positive for the CD45RA epitope, as determined in three-color stains (not shown). These early B cells, at concentrations of >0.5% of the CD34$^+$ cells, were only found in bone marrow, but not among the mononuclear cells prepared from peripheral or cord blood. Remarkably, their amount varied considerably between 0% and >80% of the CD34$^+$ mononuclear cells (see below).

Differential CD34 FACS Analysis in Bone Marrow, Peripheral Blood, and Cord Blood Low-Density Mononuclear Cells

The foregoing observations as well as reports in the literature about more rapid engraftment after transplantation of blood-derived compared to bone marrow-derived progenitor cells[5,6,10] prompted us to summarize our data on differential FACS analysis of CD34$^+$ cells contained in the three cell sources, bone marrow, peripheral blood, and cord blood. As detailed in TABLE 1, the highest percentage of CD34$^+$ mononuclear cells was found in bone marrow (mean = 5.66%, median = 4.5%, n = 196). In the 258 peripheral blood and 14 cord blood specimens analyzed, the mean/median proportions of CD34$^+$ mononuclear cells were 1.9%/0.7% and 1.7%/0.7%. B-cell progenitors, as defined by their coexpression of CD34 and CD19, were detected only in bone marrow (mean 2.2%, median 1.0% of mononuclear cells), whereas in peripheral and cord blood, the percentage of these cells was below the detection limit (<0.05%).

For easier comparison of the data, the CD34 subpopulations were also expressed as a percentage of CD34$^+$ mononuclear cells (TABLE 1, right). This preparation revealed a mean content ($\pm$ SD) of 29.97% ($\pm$24.31) B-cell progenitors in bone marrow (median 28.7%, range 0-83.3%). The mean amounts of the more differentiated, CD19$^-$ myeloid precursors, as defined by their expression of the CD45RA antigen, were 43.62% ($\pm$ 21.16) of the CD34$^+$ cells in bone marrow (median 40%, range 0-100%) compared with 41.76% ($\pm$17.46) in peripheral blood (median 42.86%, range 0-89%) and with 23.34 ($\pm$17.2) in cord blood (median 24.5%, range 0-50%).

The proportions of CD34$^+$ mononuclear cells in apheresis products (Pher) were always similar to those in analyzed peripheral blood samples drawn before leukaphereses. Among 51 Pher specimens analyzed, the mean CD34 content was 1.47% ($\pm$2.0) of the density-separated mononuclear cells (median 0.8%, range 0.15-12.5%, TABLE 1). Positive selection of CD34$^+$ cells (see Materials and Methods) was performed with density-separated cord blood (n = 5, CBsel) using the small scale lab column. The large column, for clinical use, was employed for buffy prepared from bone marrow (n = 2) and for apheresis products (n = 18). The CD34$^+$ cells were enriched to a purity median of 72% (49-86%) for cord blood and 86% (32-93%) for peripheral blood (PBsel, TABLE 1). In the two selections from bone marrow (BMsel), purity was 50% and 52%. Because of this enrichment, minor subpopulations of CD34$^+$ cells became visible in the FACS analysis: CD34$^+$ cells from all cell sources coexpressed GPA (median 0.15%, range 0-1.8%) and CD7 (median 0.25%, range 0-1.2%). The proportion of CD38$^-$ cells ranged from 0.7-4% of the CD34$^+$ cells (median 1.2%). Among the cord blood-derived CD34$^+$ cells, the amount of CD19$^+$ cells ranged from 0-3.4% (median 0.97%), and the peripheral blood-derived progenitors contained between 0 and 1.2% of these early B cells (median 0%). This was in striking contrast to the two bone marrow sources in which 27% and 66% of stem cells were of B-cell lineage (TABLE 1).

The foregoing data are summarized in two graphs: Columns in FIGURE 1a represent the mean proportions of CD34$^+$ cells expressed as a percentage of mononuclear cells or nucleated cells analyzed. The same data were used in FIGURE 1b in which the bars show the subpopulations of all CD34$^+$ cells (=100%). These relative values differentiate between CD34$^+$ cells of earlier myeloid lineage (CD34$^+$/CD45RA$^-$), of more differentiated myeloid lineage (coexpression of CD34 and CD45RA), and of B-cell lineage (coexpression of CD34 and CD19). As the success of transplantation is unlikely to depend on the amount of B-cell progenitors infused, it can logically be concluded from these data (FIG. 1b, TABLE 1) that bone marrow transplantation requires more CD34$^+$ cells than does transplantation of peripheral blood or even cord blood progenitors. Our results show that if successful and rapid engraftment depends on the amount of myeloid CD34$^+$ cells transplanted, the mean number of stem cells required is 1.4- (for all myeloid cells) or 2.2-fold (for earlier CD45RA$^-$ myeloid cells) higher for bone marrow than for peripheral blood. However, due to the high degree of variation, these factors can be lower, but also much higher, and they will have to be determined individually.

Suggested Combinations of mAbs to Characterize CD34$^+$ Cells in Two-Color Stains

The great amount of mAbs available allows multiple antibody combinations. However, routine laboratory FACS analysis should provide clear-cut results without major expenses in time and sources. In our experience, clear results are obtained with CD34 versus GPA (for contaminating erythroid cells), CD34 versus CD2 or CD7 (for coexpression of T-cell antigens), CD34 versus CD10 or CD19 (for coexpression of B-cell antigens), and CD34 versus CD45RA[13] (to differentiate between CD45RA$^-$ "earlier" myeloid and CD45RA$^+$ lymphoid and more differentiated myeloid progenitors). CD33 was not a helpful marker in discriminating between states of myeloid differentiation.[14] In addition, CD34$^+$/CD33$^-$ B-cell progenitors may complicate interpretation of the data. Other combinations, although of scientific interest, are more difficult to interpret. Some of them are CD34 versus the differentiation marker HLA-DR and CD34 versus CDw90 (Thy-1) or CD38.

DISCUSSION

Hematopoiesis originates in bone marrow during postnatal life. It was therefore surprising that patients transplanted with peripheral blood-derived stem cells showed more rapid hematopoietic reconstitution than did those who received bone marrow cells.[5,6] Several groups have since been looking for differences among these three cell sources, especially with regard to CD34 subpopulations.[7-11] This raises a question

TABLE 1. Summary of Data Obtained by Differential Flow Cytometric CD34 Analysis of Bone Marrow (BM), Blood (PB), Apheresis Products (Pher), and Cord Blood (CB), with or without Positive Selection of CD34$^+$ Cells (sel)[a]

	CD34 in % MNC				CD34 Subpopulations		
Original Material	Total CD34	Earlier Myeloids	Committed Myeloids	13-Precursors	Earlier Myeloids	Committed Myeloids	13-Precursors
BM (n = 196)							
Mean ± SD	5.66 ± 4.6	1.20 ± 0.095	2.24 ± 2.1	2.21 ± 2.86	26.51 ± 16.67	43.62 ± 21.16	29.97 ± 24.31
Median	4.5	1.0	1.5	1.0	21.7	40	28.7
Range	0.1–25.5	0–4.7	0–11.3	0–16.8	0–71.7	0–100	0–83.3
PB (n = 250)							
Mean ± SD	1.91 ± 2.58	1.03 ± 1.37	0.88 ± 1.47	0	58.24 ± 17.46	41.76 ± 17.46	0
Median	0.7	0.4	0.3	0	57.14	42.86	0
Range	0.05–18	0.02–8.1	0–14	—	11.1–100	0–89	—
Pher (n = 51)							
Mean ± SD	1.47 ± 2.01	0.86 ± 0.99	0.61 ± 1.06	0	63.45 ± 14.67	36.55 ± 14.67	0
Median	0.8	0.5	0.3	0	65.63	34.38	0
Range	0.15–12.5	0.1–6	0–6.5	—	33–100	0–67	—
CB (n = 4)							
Mean ± SD	1.68 ± 2.64	1.3 ± 2.02	0.38 ± 0.65	0	76.66 ± 17.2	23.34 ± 17.2	0
Median	0.7	0.5	0.2	0	75.48	24.52	0
Range	0.1–10.4	0.1–7.9	0–2.5	—	50–100	0–50	—

TABLE 1. (*Continued*)

Selected Cells	CD34 in % NC				CD34 Subpopulations		
	Total CD34	Earlier Myeloids	Committed Myeloids	B-Precursors	Earlier Myeloids	Committed Myeloids	B-Precursors
BM sel (*n* = 2)							
Mean ± SD	51.0 ± 1.41	12.25 ± 8.84	15.25 ± 6.01	23.5 ± 13.44	23.79 ± 16.67	29.75 ± 10.96	46.46 ± 27.63
Median	51	12.25	15.25	23.5	23.79	29.75	46.46
Range	50–52	6–18.5	11–19.5	14–33	12–35.6	22–37.5	27–66
PB sel (*n* = 18)							
Mean ± SD	78.89 ± 16.89	54.24 ± 15.64	24.58 ± 11.77	0.07 ± 0.16	68.86 ± 12.79	31.01 ± 12.75	0.12 ± 0.29
Median	86	57.5	22	0	71.33	28.67	0
Range	32–93	22–76	8.8–50.7	0–0.6	38.5–82.8	17.2–61.1	0–1.2
CB sel (*n* = 5)							
Mean ± SD	68.8 ± 15.51	55.2 ± 16.72	12.7 ± 5.97	0.9 ± 1.09	79.38 ± 11.35	19.32 ± 10.67	1.3 ± 1.42
Median	72	52	13.3	0.7	80	16.63	0.97
Range	49–86	32–77	5–20.3	0–2.7	65.3–91.2	8.8–32.7	0–3.4

[a] Values are expressed as a percentage of the mononuclear (MNC) or nucleated cells (NC) analyzed (*left part*) or as proportions of all CD34[+] cells (*right part*) and refer to the graphs shown in FIGURE 1.

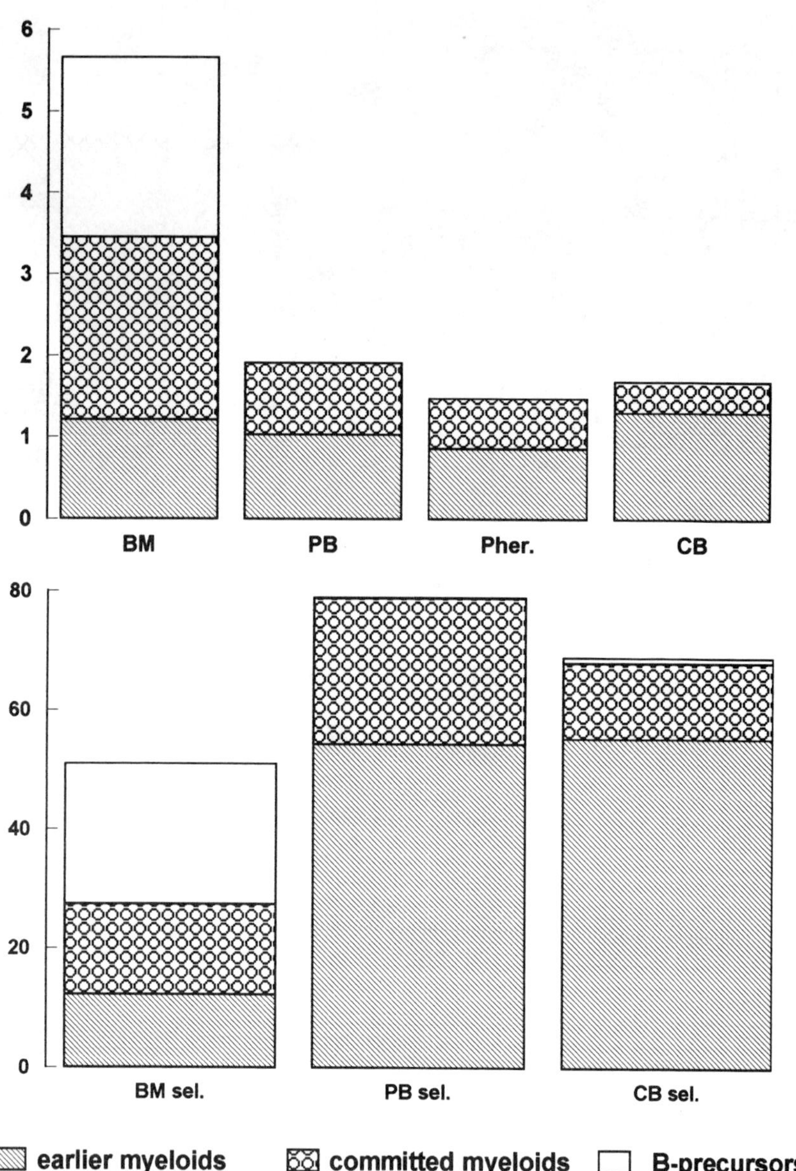

FIGURE 1a and b. Mean distributions of CD34 subpopulations in different sources of hematopoietic progenitor cells, as summarized in TABLE 1. Results are given in percentage of low-density mononuclear cells analyzed (**a**) and in percentage of all CD34[+] cells contained in the respective sources (**b**). The latter graph illustrates that if transplantations are based on the amount of stem cells infused per kilogram of the recipient, more CD34[+] cells will be required for transplantation of bone marrow than of peripheral or cord blood.

100%
80%
60%
40%
20%
0%
BM
PB
Pher.
CB
100%
80%
60%
40%
20%
0%
BM sel.
PB sel.
CB sel.
earlier myeloids
committed myeloids
B-precursors

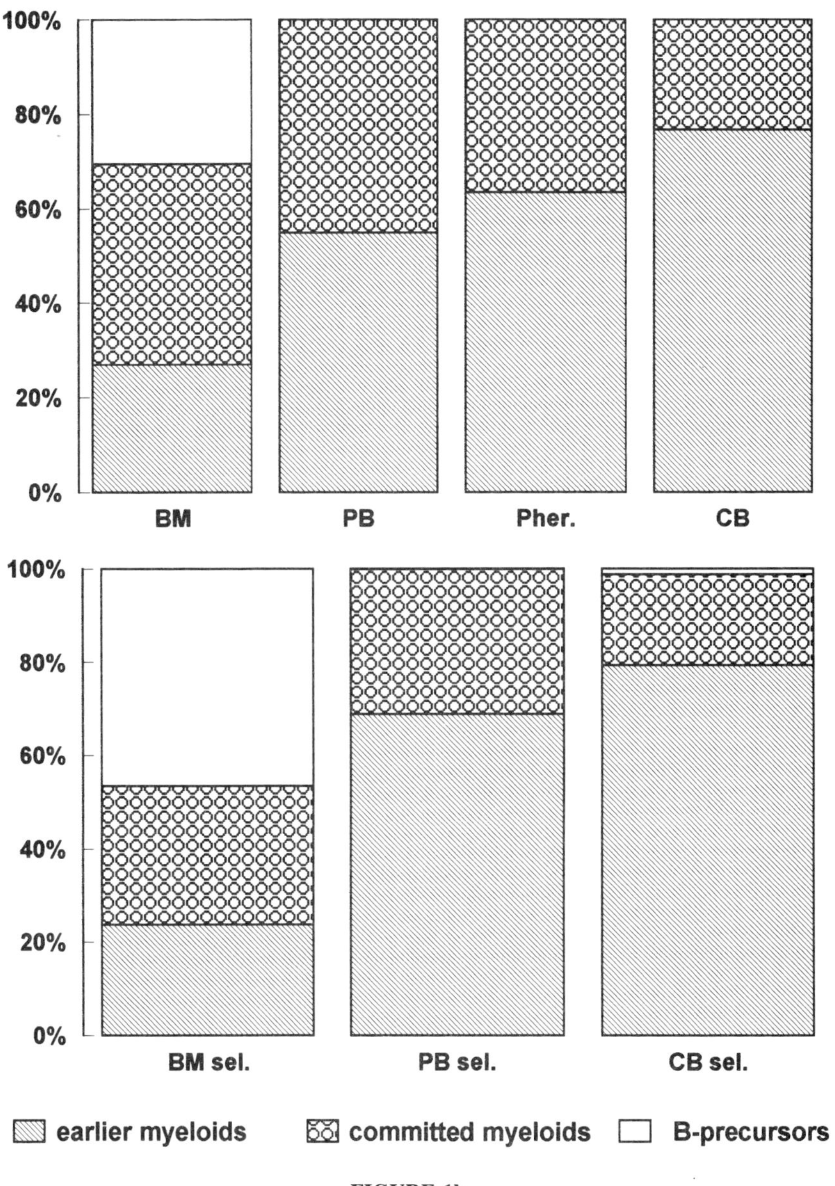

FIGURE 1b.

about the value of flow cytometric quantification or characterization of stem cells. Despite considerable worldwide efforts,[16,17] the respective methods have not yet been standardized among different laboratories, including the clones of mAbs and their combinations used for cell staining, cell preparation procedures, the way (and software) to evaluate FACS data and exclude false-positive events, and so forth.

The data summarized in this communication clearly show that we were unable to detect true B-cell progenitors in 323 analyzed low-density cell fractions prepared from samples of peripheral blood, cord blood, or leukapheresis products. This is in sharp contrast to bone marrow where distinct CD34[+]/CD19[+] cell populations were found in many cell samples, and it indicates that B-cell precursors are obviously not mobilized from the bone marrow to the bloodstream. Confirmation of the latter came from simultaneous analyses of bone marrow and peripheral blood samples from patients (data not shown). B-cell progenitors were also not detected in 190 peripheral blood samples of healthy volunteers stimulated with G-CSF or GM-CSF (5 μg/kg/ day) for 5 days.[18] This was also true for CD34[+] cells in the DNA synthesis (S/G$_2$M) phase which were found in bone marrow but not in peripheral blood or cord blood (Leitner *et al.*, submitted).

Positive selection of CD34[+] cells resulted in a mean 10-fold enrichment for the two bone marrow preparations and >40-fold for peripheral and cord blood. Only these highly enriched populations allowed the detection of minor CD34 subpopulations. Coexpression of the erythroid lineage marker GPA and of the T-cell marker CD7 ranged between 0 and 1.8% of CD34[+] cells, and proportions of up to 3.8% (for cord blood) and 1.2% (for peripheral blood) of the CD19[+] B-cell progenitors were detected. Similar or only slightly higher values were recently reported by others.[9,10] Measures to quantify transplantations were originally the amount of nucleated cells infused per kilogram of the recipient[15] or the number of myeloid clonogenic cells (CFU) determined in semisolid culture assays.[1,19] The production of monoclonal antibodies against the CD34 epitope[2] allowed more rapid detection and thus the quantification of CD34[+] cells by flow cytometric analysis (FACS). An amount of 2×10^6 stem cells per kilogram is generally accepted for autologous transplantation in patients after myeloablative treatment and results in timely reconstitution.[4] However, this threshold was determined using blood-derived progenitor cells. As just shown, it may be much higher if bone marrow cells are used as they can contain considerable proportions of B-lineage cells, but also of more differentiated myeloid precursors. Transplantations should therefore not be decided on the basis of single-color flow cytometric analysis (enumeration of CD34[+] cells) but on differential stains, as suggested.

SUMMARY

On the basis of density-separated mononuclear cells isolated from bone marrow, peripheral blood, and cord blood, we have repeatedly shown good correlation between two-color flow cytometric (FACS) CD34 analysis and colony formation in the clonogenic assay. We have analyzed the distributions of CD34 subpopulations in these three stem cell sources using patients' and donors' bone marrow biopsies ($n = 196$), cord blood samples from full-term deliveries ($n = 14$), and peripheral blood from patients mobilized by chemotherapy and/or cytokine treatment ($n = 258$). Irrespective of absolute cell counts, the mean ($\pm$SD) proportions of CD34$^+$ cells were clearly higher in bone marrow (5.6 $\pm$ 4.6% of mononuclear cells) than in peripheral blood (1.9 $\pm$ 2.6) and cord blood (1.7 $\pm$ 2.6). However, two-color FACS analyses revealed significant differences among these cell sources with regard to their distribution of CD34 subpopulations: B-cell progenitors coexpressing CD34 and CD19, at considerable concentrations of >0.5%, were only found in bone marrow (mean 30 $\pm$ 24.3% of CD34$^+$ mononuclear cells, median 28.7%, minimum 0%, maximum 83.3%). In addition, CD34$^+$ cells in S/G$_2$M phase were never detected in peripheral blood or cord blood, but only in bone marrow at a concentration of 10-15% of CD34$^+$ mononuclear cells. On the other hand, the proportions of relatively immature myeloid progenitors, as characterized by not expressing CD45RA and by higher clonogenic capacity, were significantly higher in cord blood (76.7 $\pm$ 17.2) and peripheral blood (58.2 $\pm$ 17.5) than in bone marrow (26.4 $\pm$ 16.7). These data were confirmed by analysis of apheresis products and of progenitors positively selected from different cell sources, and they may explain why, in autologous transplantations of analogous amounts of CD34$^+$ cells, peripheral blood is superior to bone marrow.

We conclude from our results that *if* successful transplantation and timely recovery depend on the number of CD34$^+$ cells transplanted, the mean amount of stem cells required is 1.4- (for myeloid cells) or 2.2-fold (for early myeloid cells) higher for bone marrow than for peripheral blood.

REFERENCES

1. BRADLEY, T. R. & D. METCALF. 1966. The growth of mouse bone marrow cells in vitro. Aust. J. Exp. Biol. Med. Sci. **44:** 286-299.
2. CIVIN, C. I., L. C. STRAUSS, C. BROVALL, M. J. FACKLER, J. F. SCHWARTZ & J. H. SHAPER. 1984. Antigenic analysis of hematopoiesis. III. A hematopoietic cell surface antigen defined by a monoclonal antibody raised against KG-Ia cells. J. Immunol. **133:** 157-161.
3. HOGG, N. & M. A. HORTON. 1987. Myeloid antigens: New and previously defined clusters. *In* Leukocyte Typing. III. White Cell Differentiation Antigens. A. J. McMichael *et al.,* Eds.: 576-602. Oxford University Press. Cambridge.
4. NEGRIN, R. S., C. R. KUSNIERZ-GLAZ, B. J. STILL, K. G. BLUME & S. STROBER. 1994. Minimum number of mobilized peripheral blood CD34$^+$ cells required for rapid trilineage engraftment (abstr.). Bone Marrow Transplant. **14**(Suppl 3): S87.
5. ELIAS, A. D., L. AYASH, K. C. ANDERSON, M. HUNT, C. WHEELER, G. SCHWARTZ, I. TEPLER, R. MAZANET, C. LYNCH, S. PAP, J. PALAEZ, E. REICH, J. CRITCHLOW, G. DEMETRI, J. BIBBO, L. SCHNIPPER, J. D. GRIFFIN, E. FREI & K. H. ANTMAN. 1992. Mobilization of peripheral blood progenitor cells by chemotherapy and granulocyte-macrophage colony-stimulating factor for hematologic support after high-dose intensification for breast cancer. Blood **79:** 3036-3044.
6. SHERIDAN, W. P., C. G. BEGLEY, C. A. JUTTNER, J. SZER, L. B. TO, D. MAHER, K. M. MCGRATH, G. MORSTYN & R. M. FOX. 1992. Effect of peripheral-blood progenitor cells mobilized by filgrastim (G-CSF) on platelet recovery after high-dose chemotherapy. Lancet **339:** 640-644.
7. BENDER, J. G., K. L. UNVERZAGT, D. E. WALKER, W. LEE, D. E. VAN EPPS, D. H. SMITH, C. C. STEWART & L. B. TO. 1991. Identification and comparison of CD34$^+$ cells and their subpopulations from normal peripheral blood and bone marrow using multi color flow cytometry. Blood **77:**2591-2596.
8. FRITSCH, G., P. BUCHINGER & D. PRINTZ. 1993. Use of flow cytometric CD34 analysis to quantify hematopoietic progenitor cells. Leukemia Lymphoma **10:** 443-451.

9. STEEN, R., G. E. TJONNFJORD & T. EGELAND. 1994. Comparison of the phenotype and clonogenicity of normal CD34⁺ cells from umbilical cord blood, granulocyte colony-stimulating factor-mobilized peripheral blood, and adult human bone marrow. J. Hematother. **3:** 253–262.

10. TO, L. B., D. N. HAYLOCK, T. DOWSE, P. J. SIMMONS, S. TRIMBOLI, L. K. ASHMAN & C. A. JUTTNER. 1994. A comparative study of the phenotype and proliferative capacity of peripheral blood (PB) CD34⁺ cells mobilized by four different protocols and those of steady-phase PB and bone marrow CD34⁺ cells. Blood **84:** 2930–2939.

11. PETTENGELL, R., T. LUFT, R. HENSCHLER, J. M. HOWS, T. M. DEXTER, D. RYDER & N. G. TESTA. 1994. Direct comparison by limiting dilution analysis of long-term culture-initiating cells in human bone marrow, umbilical cord blood, and blood stem cells. Blood **84:** 3653–3659.

12. FRITSCH, G., M. STIMPFL, P. BUCHINGER, D. PRINTZ, G. SLIUTZ, T. WAGNER, H. AGIS, P. VALENT & H. GADNER. 1994. Does cord blood contain enough stem cells for transplantation? J. Hematother. **3:** 291–298.

13. FRITSCH, G., P. BUCHINGER, D. PRINTZ, F. M. FINK, G. MANN, C. PETERS, T. WAGNER, A. ADLER & H. GADNER. 1993. Rapid discrimination of early CD34⁺ myeloid progenitors using CD45-RA analysis. Blood **81:** 2301–2309.

14. FRITSCH, G., P. BUCHINGER, D. PRINTZ, M. D. DWORZAK, D. STRUNK, H. AGIS, G. SLIUTZ, A. WILFING, U. SCHULZ & H. GADNER. 1994. Is CD33 a differentiation marker? Prog. Clin. Biol. Res. **389:** 377–382.

15. THOMAS, E. D. & R. STORB. 1970. Technique for human marrow grafting. Blood **36:** 507–515.

16. SOVALAT, H., E. WUNDER, A. TIENHAARA, T. OLOFSSON, G. FRITSCH, F. SILVESTRI & S. SERKE. 1993. Commentary: Prospects for standardization of the stem cell determination within Europe. J. Hematother. **3:** 293–296.

17. COLLINS, N. H. & A. P. GEE. 1994. ISHAGE — Teacher's pet (Editorial). J. Hematother. **3:** 247–248.

18. FRITSCH, G., G. FISCHMEISTER, M. KURZ, H. STROBL, A. LEITNER, O. A. HAAS, P. BUCHINGER, P. PRINTZ, T. STROEBEL, C. SCHEINECKER, W. KNAPP & H. GADNER. 1994. In vivo comparison of G-CSF and GM-CSF: Clinical study in healthy adults. Bone Marrow Transplant. **14** (Suppl. 1): S11.

19. TAKAUE, Y. 1991. Peripheral blood stem cell autografts in children with acute lymphoblastic lymphoma: Updated experience. Leukemia Lymphoma **3:** 241–256.

Cytokines in Stem Cell Transplantation

F. MARC STEWART

Hematology-Oncology Division
Cancer Center
University of Massachusetts Medical Center
Worcester, Massachusetts 01655

Improvements in supportive care have diminished the morbidity and mortality of stem cell transplantation (marrow or peripheral blood).[1,2] Nevertheless, severe neutropenia predisposes patients to fever, systemic infections, mucositis, and, not infrequently, prolonged hospitalizations. Most patients experience fever, and infection accounts for over half the early causes of death. To shorten the duration of cytopenia and provide better patient care, hematopoietic growth factors (HGF) have been employed to (1) speed marrow recovery immediately after transplantation, (2) treat graft failure in those who fail to recover or who develop late marrow failure after transplantation, and (3) mobilize peripheral blood progenitor cells for apheresis collection and cryopreservation. Other potential applications of HGFs include progenitor cell expansion *ex vivo*, enhancement of immunomodulatory effects on tumors or infections, and cycling of stem cells to improve gene transfer for human gene therapy. Hematopoietic growth factors are a promising approach to improvement in patients who receive stem cell grafts.

MODIFICATIONS OF THE STEM/PROGENITOR CELL PRODUCT

Allogeneic and autologous bone marrow transplantations have served as the standard stem cell delivery system for hematopoietic reconstitution after ablative therapy. Innovative manipulations or modifications of these approaches to improve stem cell repopulation potential and to enhance regeneration of hematopoiesis *in vivo* have been tried. In stem cell transplantation, hematopoietic growth factors play a pivotal role in (1) enhancing neutrophil recovery, (2) mobilizing stem/progenitor cells into the peripheral blood, (3) "priming" peripheral blood stem/progenitor cells to renew hematopoiesis more quickly, and (4) expanding progenitor cells *ex vivo*. Hematopoietic growth factors have been used often with nonmyeloablative doses of chemotherapy to mobilize stem cells into the peripheral blood for collection and preservation and to "prime" these cells for more rapid hematologic recovery. Priming bone marrow before harvest with either chemotherapy or cytokines is a more recent concept with some appeal. TABLE 1 outlines various strategies to accelerate marrow recovery in stem cell transplantation.

TABLE 1. Strategies to Accelerate Marrow Recovery in Stem Cell Transplantation

Sources of Stem Cells for Autologous or Allogeneic Transplantation

Bone marrow
Bone marrow, primed

Peripheral blood
Peripheral blood, primed

Bone marrow plus peripheral blood

Use of Cytokines in Stem Cell Transplantation

Adjunctive use of cytokines after transplantation
Neoadjunctive use of cytokines (with or without chemotherapy) for priming
Ex vivo cytokines for progenitor cell expansion and/or gene therapy

GM-CSF OR G-CSF AFTER AUTOLOGOUS MARROW TRANSPLANTATION

Initially, phase I/II studies in both autologous and allogeneic stem cell transplantation suggested that granulocyte-colony-stimulating factor (G-CSF) or granulocyte-macrophage colony-stimulating factor (GM-CSF) could augment marrow recovery, decrease hospitalization time, reduce mucositis, reduce organ toxicity, and occasionally diminish blood product requirements, such as platelet transfusions, when compared to historical controls.[3-8] Although these studies suggested a therapeutic advantage for HGF, retrospective comparisons could have conferred selection bias favoring HGF treatment. Factors that theoretically could have prejudiced outcome include disease or disease status at transplantation, extent of prior therapy, varied conditioning regimens, discharge criteria, patient age, dose of marrow or peripheral blood stem cells (PBSC), marrow cellularity, and tumor involvement of marrow or blood. In allogeneic transplant recipients, posttransplant graft-versus-host disease prophylaxis regimens, infection prophylaxis measures for cytomegalovirus and other organisms, and the degree of donor-recipient mismatch could influence outcome independent of HGFs.

Prospective studies evaluating growth factors in stem cell autografts are summarized in TABLE 2. At first glance these studies offer some support for the use of growth factors in autologous marrow transplantation, because practically all show improved neutrophil recovery, but when their role is viewed more broadly in the context of other more tangible patient care endpoints and newer outpatient approaches to practice, the effects of HGF are less impressive. In particular, the studies have mixed results regarding the prevention of infection, the number of febrile days, and shortening hospitalization time.

Duration of hospital stay is perhaps the best indicator of direct patient benefit, because patients must be clinically stable or improving in order to be discharged. Unfortunately, many studies have vague criteria for discharge. When discharge criteria are specified (e.g., a neutrophil count of 1,000/mm^3 for 3 consecutive days before discharge), a "trial-associated delay" may occur.[9] Patients not treated with HGFs who are otherwise in stable condition and by *current practice standards* would be discharged much earlier are forced by trial guidelines to remain in the hospital. Patients who do not receive HGFs are most likely to experience an unnecessary delay in discharge. This "moving target" of standard care illustrates how HGF studies are plagued by problems common to other clinical studies. The time to develop, activate, accrue to, analyze, present, and publish a multicenter placebo-controlled HGF trial is lengthy. As these studies continue, advances in the field often make the beneficial results of such studies, when published, obsolete.

Several studies[10,11] have reported data to address cost effectiveness. A prospective controlled study of 24 patients reported by Gulati and Bennett[10] purported cost savings with GM-CSF. Patients were discharged when in clinically stable condition and when an absolute neutrophil count exceeded 1,000/mm³. One third the patients in the GM-CSF-treated group had to be readmitted 8-30 days after initial discharge, and these costs were not included in the analysis (only one patient in the control group was readmitted). Similar cost savings were not apparent in a parallel French study.[12] Furthermore, patients apparently may likely be discharged safely with much lower blood counts and that significant cost savings in this setting may no longer be attributable to HGFs. As just noted, these newer criteria for discharge or "outpatient" management practices eventually supersede the design of the earlier, prospective reports.[13]

In a large study, Nemunaitis *et al.* reported on 128 patients with non-Hodgkin's lymphoma, Hodgkin's disease, and acute lymphocytic leukemia who were randomized to receive rhGM-CSF[14] versus placebo after autografting.[15] Days to ANC >500/mm³, incidence of severe infection, days of intravenous antibiotics, and days of hospitalization were modestly improved by rhGM-CSF (TABLE 2). With a median followup of 36 months no long-term side effects such as increased relapse rates, leukemogenesis, or graft failure were noted.[16] Discharge criteria were not specified. Cost analysis showed a significant savings when HGFs were used after transplantation. Trial-associated delay may have contributed to the apparent cost savings. Furthermore, when readmissions were included in the overall analysis, significance was lost.[11]

We are only beginning to develop analytical techniques that permit accurate evaluation of cost effectiveness. Hematopoietic growth factors have been purported to shorten hospital stay and thus reduce costs. Frequently, not included in these analyses are some impacting factors: costs of outpatient facility, physician/nurses' time to manage patients in this setting (often without charge), home nursing costs, and cost of income lost to relatives who must provide more care at home for patients. Unless beds reserved for transplant recipients are completely and consistently filled, discharging patients a few days "earlier" impacts least on true hospital costs because the acuity of care required for patients at this point is very low. Hospital charges often fail to reflect differences in acuity.

Hematopoietic growth factor studies should identify endpoints that describe tangible patient benefits, that is, those relevant to patient comfort, patient survival, and cost of treatment. If the interpretation of these studies is ultimately in favor of using HGFs in stem cell transplantation, the results should be applied in the proper context, that is, positive effects of HGFs in good risk patients should not necessarily justify their use in poor risk patients who have poor survival despite excellent supportive care.

TABLE 2. GM-CSF or G-CSF after Autologous Bone Marrow Transplantation: Prospective, Controlled Trials[a]

Author	Disease	Cond.	HGF	Pts (n) (HGF/ placebo)	Days ANC to 500/mm^3 (HGF/ placebo)	Days Plts to Independence (HGF/ placebo)	Plt Trans- fusion (HGF/ placebo)	Antibiotic Days (HGF/ placebo)	Hospital Days/ Cost (HGF/ placebo)	Relapse	Survival	Side Effects of HGF
Nemunaitis[1,5,16]	NHL HD ALL	Cy/TBI	GM-CSF vs placebo	65/63	19/26 $p = 0.001$	26/29 p = NS	NA	24/27 $p = 0.009$	27/33 $p = 0.01$ (cost NA)	p = NS at 3 yr. med f/u	p = NS at 3 yr. med f/u	p = NS
Link[55]	ALL NHL	Cy/TBI others	GM-CSF vs placebo	39/40	15/28 $p = 0.0001$	NA	NA	p = NS	30/31 p = NS	p = NS	p = NS	↑ Cap leak syndrome
Gorin[56]	NHL	BEA M CBV	GM-CS	44/47	14/21 p =	p = NS	NA	p = NS	23/29 p =	p = NS	p = NS	grIII/ IV tox
Khwaja[57,58]	NHL		GM-CSF vs placebo	29/29	14/20 $p = 0.001$	25/19 p = NS	NA	11/10 p = NS	24/25 p = NS (cost NA)			
Advani[17]	NHL HD	CBV Cy/VP-16/TBI	GM-CSF vs placebo	36/33	12/16 $p = 0.02$	p = NS	p = NS	NA	p = NS (cost NA)	p = NS	p = NS	p = NS
Gulati[10]	HD	CBV Cy/VP-16/TBI	GM-CSF vs placebo	12/12	NA (ANC > 1,000: 17 vs 27 $p = 0.003$)	13/21 $p = 0.02$	7/11 p = NS	NA	32/40 p = 0.004 $39K vs $62K p = 0.005	p = NS	p = NS	Edema/ erythema in two pts

TABLE 2. (*Continued*)

Author	Disease	Cond.	HGF	Pts (n) (HGF/ placebo)	Days ANC to 500/mm³ (HGF/ placebo)	Days Plts to Independence (HGF/ placebo)	Plt Trans-fusion (HGF/ placebo)	Antibiotic Days (HGF/ placebo)	Hospital Days/ Cost (HGF/ placebo)	Relapse	Sur-vival	Side Effects of HGF
Gisselbrecht[59]	HD NHL MM ALL solid tumors	NA (added 70 allo-geneic BMTs)	G-CSF (escalating dosages) vs placebo)	127/118	14/20 $p = <$ 0.001	22/2 INS	36/32.5 $p =$ NS	15/19 $p = <$ 0.001	25/29 $p =$ NA	$p =$ NS at 100 days	$p =$ NS at 100 days	$p =$ NS
Blaise[60]	ALL	Cy/TBI melp h/Ar ac/TBI	G-CSF vs placebo	NA total = 20	10/13 $p = 0.01$ K-M analysis	NA	NA	11/16 $p =$ NS	24/>28 $p = 0.05$	NA	NA	$p =$ NS
Schmitz[61]	HD NHL	CBV BEA M	G-CSF (escalating dosages) vs placebo	36/18	13/20 $p = 0.0004$	NA	NA	$p =$ NS	$p =$ NS	$p =$ NS at 60 days	NA	NA
Stahel[62]	NHL	NA	G-CSF (escalating dosages) vs placebo	29/14	10/18 $p = 0.0001$	NA	$p =$ NS	$p =$ NS	$p =$ NS	NA	NA	NA

[a]For abbreviations, see footnote to Table 3.

MOBILIZATION OF STEM CELLS WITH GM-CSF OR G-CSF

Mobilized PBSC autografts ± HGFs are a suitable if not preferable alternative to autologous marrow transplantation or intensive chemotherapy with HGF alone.[17–19] Selected growth factors such as GM-CSF, G-CSF, erythropoietin, interleukin-3 (IL-3), stem cell factor, and others with or without chemotherapy augment the collection of committed progenitor cells by up to 100-fold or more. Because measurement of progenitor cells such as CFU-C, CFU-GEMM, or CD34+ cells has correlated with engraftment rates to some extent, it is reasonable to suppose that mobilization of PBSCs with HGFs could positively affect outcome in autotransplantation. Studies using mobilized PBSCs show striking improvement in neutrophil and platelet recovery compared to historical controls, although no direct, prospective comparative studies between autologous marrow and PBSC autografts have been reported. Several trials are underway.[20]

Huan et al.[20a] evaluated 14 patients with metastatic solid tumors who received autologous marrow and rhuGM-CSF after the first course of intensive therapy. Following recovery from the first transplant, 11 of the original 14 received the same conditioning regimen and PBSC, previously mobilized by chemotherapy and rhGM-CSF, and posttransplant rhGM-CSF (PBSCs plus rhuGM-CSF). Each patient served as his or her own control. No difference was noted between median times to neutrophil count $\geq 500/mm^3$ in PBSC plus rhuGM-CSF compared to autologous bone marrow plus rhuGM-CSF (17 versus 18 days). However, platelet recovery to $50,000/mm^3$ was improved in the group receiving PBSCs plus rhuGM-CSF (19 versus 24 days, $p = 0.045$). No significant differences in recovery times were seen at platelet levels of $20,000/mm^3$ or $100,000/mm^3$. Interestingly, in this limited study, a retrospective comparison of autologous marrow plus rhuGM-CSF with historical patients who received autologous bone marrow alone resulted only in a 3-day advantage for median neutrophil recovery times to $100/mm^3$, $500/mm^3$, and $1,000/mm^3$ for the former approach. Potential deleterious effects of the first transplant on the marrow microenvironment could have affected the outcome of the second transplant. In a recent report Faucher et al.[21] compared 54 patients who received either G-CSF primed PBSC with posttransplant G-CSF versus autologous BMT plus G-CSF or autologous BMT alone.[21] Selection to receive a particular treatment was based on availability of apheresis and G-CSF. Median days to neutrophil level of $500/mm^3$ were 10, 12, and 16, respectively. Although no difference was noted in the number of hospital days between patients treated with bone marrow alone or bone marrow plus G-CSF (20 vs. 20 days), shortened hospital stay (15 days) and improved cost effectiveness were noted with G-CSF primed PBSC plus G-CSF. In another retrospective review, Peters et al.[22] noted a significant reduction in severe neutropenia and improved cost effectiveness with G-CSF mobilized PBSC plus bone marrow and posttransplant G-CSF compared to bone marrow alone, bone marrow plus G-CSF or GM-CSF, or GM-CSF primed PBSC plus bone marrow and GM-CSF.[22] Interestingly, no improvement in cost effectiveness was noted when charges from patients receiving bone marrow alone or bone marrow plus HGFs were compared.[22]

Although other small studies support the hypothesis that HGF-mobilized PBSC transplants enhance neutrophil or platelet recovery and potentially decrease patient morbidity and cost,[23,24] others do not.[25,26] Catheter-related complications (infection, pneumothorax, etc.), apheresis time, and inconvenience of stem cell collection raise questions about the purported adavantages of PBSC collection over bone marrow harvesting. One study estimated that the cost of a single cytokine-mobilized leukopheresis for PBSC collection equaled the cost of 1 day of hospitalization for a febrile, neutropenic transplant patient. In patients with hypocellular marrow or in those who experience poor platelet recovery after stem cell mobilization with chemotherapy and HGF, delayed platelet recovery after transplantation was observed occasionally. Extended transfusion support[27] or back-up marrows were required in some cases.

The addition of GM-CSF or G-CSF after mobilized PBSC transplantation offers no substantial benefit. In one prospective, controlled trial Spitzer *et al.*[28] reported shortened hospital stay with the addition of G-CSF posttransplantation after primed PBSC transplantation (19 versus 21 days, $p = 0.0112$). In a critical analysis of this outcome, they attributed early discharge in the G-CSF treated group to physicians' ''comfort'' with rapidly rising leukocyte counts, hence negating any conclusion that posttransplant G-CSF offers substantial benefit after PBSC transplantation. A cost analysis was not performed in this study.

Hematopoietic growth factors may have detrimental effects. Cytokine mobilization of tumor cells may be possible, particularly when cytokines are used in conjunction with chemotherapy. Sensitive immunohistochemical staining or polymerase chain reaction has detected increased circulating tumor cells after mobilization procedures.[29] Timing of stem cell collection or stem cell selection[30] may minimize this risk.

The optimum use of HGFs in mobilizing blood stem cells for collection and in enhancing stem cell growth posttransplant remains to be defined, although evolving studies suggest that stem cell factor combined with other cytokines such as G-CSF may be a very effective mobilizer.

GM-CSF OR G-CSF AFTER ALLOGENEIC MARROW TRANSPLANTATION

Phase I/II studies of patients undergoing allogeneic marrow transplantation showed that rhGM-CSF could be administered safely to recipients without an obvious increase in graft-versus-host disease or relapse. Phase III studies are in progress or undergoing analysis.[31] Several published studies are summarized in TABLE 3. In all studies the benefit of rhGM-CSF on neutrophil recovery, platelet recovery, prevention of graft failure, and days of hospitalization was not substantial. Although no adverse effect of rhGM-CSF on relapse rates or graft-versus-host disease was noted, no improvement in overall survival was discerned either. Other toxicities such as fever and abnormalities in renal or hepatic function tests were reported in patients receiving rhGM-CSF compared to placebo.[32,33]

For patients with graft failure, postallogeneic or autologous transplantation rhuGM-CSF was used to restore granulopoiesis. In one study, graft failure was defined as failure to achieve a neutrophil count of $100/mm^3$ by day 28 or by day 21 in the presence of a life-threatening infection or a decline in neutrophils to $<500/mm^3$ for 1 week in patients who achieved initial engraftment.[34] Bierman *et al.*[35] presented a prospective, multiinstitutional study of 140 allogeneic and autologous bone marrow recipients with graft failure treated with rhuGM-CSF. When compared with 103

TABLE 3. GM-CSF or G-CSF after Allogeneic Bone Marrow Transplantation: Prospective, Controlled Trial[a]

Author	Disease	Cond.	HGF	Pts (n) (HGF/ placebo)	Days ANC to 500/mm³ (HGF/ placebo)	Days Plts to 50K/mm³ (HGF/ placebo)	Plt Transfusion (HGF/ placebo)	Antibiotic Days (HGF/ placebo)	Hospital Days/Cost (HGF/ placebo)	Relapse/ GVHD	Survival	HGF Side Effects
Powles[32]	AML CML ALL other	Bu/Cy Melph/ TBI Cy/TBI	GM-CSF vs placebo	20/20	13/16 p = NS	NA	27/19 p = NS	↑ in HGF grp due to HGF fevers	24/24 p = NS	p = NS p = NS	p = NS	↑ Renal hepatic fevers
DeWitte[33]	AML ALL CML MDS AA CLL MM	Cy/TBI others all T-depleted	GM-CSF vs placebo	34/34	15/19 p = NS	NA	7/6.7 p = NS	p = NS	42/43 p = NS	p = NS p = NS	p = NS	↑ Fever
Gisselbrecht[5,9]	NHL, HD, ALL, MM, solid tumor	Mixed	G-CSF vs placebo	36/34	14/20 p = 0.01	NA	p = NS	p = NS	p = NA	p = NS	p = NS	
Blaise[60]	ALL	Cy/TBI melph/ Ara-c/ TBI	G-CSF vs placebo	NA total = 24	15/17 p = NS	NA	NA	16/21 p = 0.05	p = NS	NA	NA	p = NS

[a]Abbreviations: NS = not significant; NA = not available; Plt = platelet; ANC = absolute neutrophil recovery; AML = acute myelogenous leukemia; CML = chronic myelogenous leukemia; ALL = acute lymphoblastic leukemia; MDS = myelodysplastic syndrome; AA = aplastic anemia; CLL = chronic lymphocytic leukemia; MM = multiple myeloma; Cy/TBI = high dose cyclophosphamide plus total body irradiation; Melph = high dose melphalan; CBV = high dose cyclophosphamide, BCNU, etoposide; HGF = hematopoietic growth factor(s); GM-CSF = granulocyte-macrophage colony-stimulating factor; G-CSF = granulocyte colony-stimulating factor.

historical controls, the GM-CSF-treated patients showed a survival advantage. Unfortunately, comparisons were not valid. Virtually all controls were patients with acute leukemia, whereas a significant number were patients with lymphoma and other patients in the GM-CSF arm. At the end of the presentation it was acknowledged that no survival difference was noted in leukemic patients treated with GM-CSF compared to the leukemic patient control group. Thus, contrary to their conclusions, there is a strong indication that the use of GM-CSF confers no survival advantage in patients with graft failure.

ERYTHROPOIETIN AFTER BONE MARROW TRANSPLANTATION

Some prospective, controlled trials evaluate the role of erythropoietin to minimize blood transfusions after both allogeneic and autologous stem cell transplantation.[36-38] Results generally show no advantage for erythropoietin given posttransplantation (TABLE 4). On subset analysis one study suggested a late benefit of erythropoietin use. No effects on other cell lines or other clinical outcomes were noted in these studies.

POTENTIAL FUTURE APPROACHES

Even highly selected patients apparently have an obligatory neutropenic period of 8 days regardless of treatment modulations such as HGFs.[19,22] Future approaches to this obligate period of neutropenia will focus on (1) new HGFs (factors with stimulatory or inhibitory properties) applied in conventional settings of PBSC or autologous bone marrow transplantation, (2) combinations of new or established HGFs for both mobilization of PBSC[39] and posttransplant therapy, (3) the combination of HGFs and prophylactic antibiotics, (4) expansion of progenitor cells *in vitro* with HGFs before transplantation, and (5) perhaps resurrection of granulocyte transfusions mobilized with HGFs from normal donors.

New Cytokines

Studies of the effects of IL-6 on platelet recovery after conventional chemotherapy are in progress.[40] The use of IL-6 in the treatment of delayed platelet reconstitution after transplantation or thrombocytopenia associated with chronic graft-versus-host disease has obvious potential applications. A potent stimulator of thrombopoiesis, IL-6 is particularly useful in generating numerous autologous platelet units to be frozen before transplantation, minimizing the risk of allosensitization with alternative donor products. ''Hybrid'' molecules of IL-3-GM-CSF (PIXY321) are currently undergoing phase I testing and provide the theoretic advantage of local synergy.[41] Interleukin-3 and stem cell factor or kit ligand, both early acting hematopoietic factors with multilineage effects, are undergoing phase I trials in humans.[41] In animal studies, erythropoietin increases peripheral blood myeloid and erythroid progenitors, and efforts are underway to evaluate its effects on PBSC mobilization in human autografts.

TABLE 4. Prospective, Controlled Trials Using Erythropoietin (EPO) in Stem Cell Transplantation

Author	BMT	HGF	Pts (n)	Reticulocytes	# Erythrocyte Transfusions (n)	Hosp/Cost
Link[37]	Autologous	EPO vs placebo	114	NS	NS	?/?
Klaesson[38]	Allogeneic	EPO vs placebo	50	NS	+	?/?
Link[37]					+ day 21–40	
				+ day 21–40	18.4 vs 18.5	
	Allogeneic	EPO vs placebo	215	p <0.05	p = 0.05	?/?
Chao[36]	Autologous	EPO + G-CSF vs G-CSF	35	NS	NS	?/?

Erythropoietin may have a role in pretransplant marrow harvesting of normal donors. M-CSF, which does not appear to enhance marrow recovery posttransplantation, is currently undergoing evaluation for treatment of resistant fungal infections in immunocompromised hosts and eventually may find a role in stem cell transplantation.

The number of cytokines active on the lymphohematopoietic system continues to grow with interleukins-12 and 13 recently added to the list. Interleukin-11 is an IL-6 "look-a-like"[42] and clearly has activity on early stem cells with a predilection for elevating platelet counts. Recently, basic fibroblast growth factor[43] and hepatocyte growth factor[44] were shown to act on early stem cells, although their *in vivo* activity has yet to be defined. Perhaps some of the most interesting agents are those that have selective inhibitory action against early stem cells. Transforming growth factor-beta (TGF-β),[45] macrophage inflammatory protein-1 alpha (MIP-1-α), a tetrapeptide (*N*-acetyl-ser-asp-lys-pro), and a pentapeptide (p-glu-glu-asp-cys-lys-) all can inhibit cycling of early stem cells and were shown to have *in vivo* activity.[46,47] Their possible use in protecting marrow from cycle active cytotoxic treatments is particularly intriguing, as is the observation that the tetrapeptide appears to block normal hematopoietic stem cells but not leukemia cells from entering the cell cycle. The tetrapeptide and pentapeptide have entered phase I clinical trials as myeloprotectants. Similarly, another intriguing animal model suggests that interleukin-1, known for its radioprotective effect on marrow cells, administered before lethal irradiation and allogeneic bone marrow transplantation, resulted in an early, transient increase in autologous peripheral neutrophils with accelerated engraftment of allogeneic marrow.[48] The potential role of these agents in the marrow transplant settings has yet to be defined.

Multifactor Combinations

After transplantation the sequential use of HGF combinations such as IL-3 or stem cell factor followed by GM-CSF or G-CSF theoretically mimics the *in vivo* progenitor cell differentiation and proliferative process.[49] Thus, progenitor cell compartments may be expanded more rapidly and efficiently. Before transplantation the expansion of a harvested population of committed stem cells *in vitro* may lead eventually to more rapid recovery when infused into ablated recipients. This approach was attempted by Naparstek *et al.*[50] in 20 patients undergoing T-cell depleted allogeneic marrow transplantation. Two thirds of the marrow was infused on the scheduled day of transplantation, while the remaining one third of the allograft was cultured with GM-CSF and IL-3. The "booster" marrow was infused on day 4, and platelet recovery was marginally enhanced compared to historical controls.

Lowry *et al.*[51] have shown that multifactor synergistic combinations of up to six growth factors *in vitro* generate increased numbers of progenitor cells. Brugger *et al.*[52] tested the combination of stem cell factor, erythropoietin, IL-1, IL-3, IL-6, and gamma-interferon to expand progenitor cells *ex vivo* after large scale mobilization of PBPC with chemotherapy and G-CSF.[52] The number of multilineage colonies increased 250-fold and the absolute number of CD34+ progenitors increased significantly.

New approaches to mobilization include the use of multifactor HGF combinations. Brugger *et al.*[39] showed that sequential administration of IL-3 and GM-CSF significantly increased the number of peripheral blood CFU-GM, CFU-GEMM, and BFU-E compared to GM-CSF alone. Preliminary testing of these approaches is underway.[53]

HGFs with Other Modalities

The use of HGFs in conjunction with prophylactic antibiotics or large quantities of HGF-mobilized granulocyte transfusions may be evaluated to decrease fever and infections and contribute to outpatient management of transplant recipients.[13,54]

SUMMARY

The use of cytokines in stem cell transplantation is still in the early stages of development. Efficacy has not been established consistently at the present time. When cytokines are employed in the treatment setting, they should be employed in a study setting evaluating whether there has been real patient benefit-palliation without compromise of therapeutic outcome or, preferably, a survival advantage. Cost effectiveness has not been established and, in any case it should not be a consideration until therapeutic efficacy has been established.

The determination of various biologic parameters on cells such as cytokine receptors may permit more precise use of HGFs. In some cases there probably are subsets of patients who are benefited, while there are subsets who are harmed. The challenge of the future is to define these subsets.

REFERENCES

1. THOMAS, E. D. & R. A. CLIFT. 1989. Indications for marrow transplantation in chronic myelocytic leukemia. Blood **73:** 861.
2. FREEDMAN, A. S., T. TAKVORIAN, K. C. ANDERSON, P. MAUCH, S. N. RABINOWE, K. BLAKE, B. YEAP, R. SOIFFER, F. CORAL & L. HEFLIN. 1990. Autologous bone marrow transplantation in B-cell non-Hodgkin's lymphoma: Very low treatment-related mortality in 100 patients in sensitive relapse. J. Clin. Oncol. **8:** 784.
3. BRANDT, S. J., W. P. PETERS, S. K. ATWATER, J. KURTZBERG, M. J. BOROWITZ, R. B. JONES, E. J. SHPALL, R. C. BAST, Jr., C. J. GILBERT & D. H. OETTE. 1988. Effect of recombinant human granulocyte-macrophage colony-stimulating factor on hematopoietic reconstitution after high-dose chemotherapy and autologous bone marrow transplantation. N. Engl. J. Med. **318:** 869.
4. DEVEREAUX, S., D. C. LINCH, J. G. GRIBBEN, A. McMILLAN, K. PATTERSON & A. H. GOLDSTONE. 1989. GM-CSF accelerates neutrophil recovery after autologous bone marrow transplantation for Hodgkin's disease. Bone Marrow Transplant. **4:** 49.
5. LAZARUS, H. M., J. ANDERSEN, M. G. CHEN, D. VARIAKOJIS, E. G. MANSOUR, D. OETTE, C. A. ARCE, M. M. OKEN & S. L. GERSON. 1991. Recombinant granulocyte-macrophage colony-stimulating factor after autologous bone marrow transplantation for relapsed non-Hodgkin's lymphoma: Blood and bone marrow progenitor growth studies. A phase II Eastern Cooperative Oncology Group Trial. Blood **78:** 830.
6. SHERIDAN, W. P., G. MORSTYN, M. WOLF, A. DODDS, J. LUSK, D. MAHER, J. E. LAYTON, M. D. GREEN, L. SOUZA & R. M. FOX. 1989. Granulocyte colony-stimulating factor and neutrophil recovery after high-dose chemotherapy and autologous bone marrow transplantation. Lancet **2:** 891.

7. NEMUNAITIS, J., C. D. BUCKNER, F. R. APPELBAUM, C. S. HIGANO, M. MORI, J. BIANCO, C. EPSTEIN, J. LIPANI et al. 1991. Phase I/II trial of recombinant human granulocyte-macrophage colony-stimulating factor following allogeneic bone marrow transplantation. Blood **77**: 2065.

8. NEMUNAITIS, J., C. ANASETTI, R. STORB, J. A. BIANCO, C. D. BUCKNER, N. ONETTO, P. MARTIN et al. 1992. Phase II trial of recombinant human granulocyte-macrophage colony-stimulating factor in patients undergoing allogeneic bone marrow transplantation from unrelated donors. Blood **79**: 2572.

9. LINCH, D. C., H. SCARFFE, S. PROCTOR, R. CHOPRA, P. R. A. TAYLOR, G. MORGENSTERN, D. CUNNINGHAM, A. K. BURNETT, J. C. CAWLEY, I. M. FRANKLIN, A. J. BELL, T. A. LISTER, R. E. MARCUS, A. C. NEWLAND, A. C. PARKER & A. YVER. 1993. Randomized vehicle-controlled dose-finding study of glycosylated recombinant human granulocyte colony-stimulating factor after bone marrow transplantation. Bone Marrow Transplant. **11**: 307.

10. GULATI, S. C. & C. L. BENNETT. 1992. Granulocyte-macrophage colony-stimulating factor (GM-CSF) as adjunct therapy in relapsed Hodgkin's disease (abstr.). Ann. Intern. Med. **116**: 177.

11. LUCE, B. R., J. W. SINGER, J. M. WESCHLER, C. D. BUCKNER, S. H. SHEINGOLD, K. SHANNON-DORCY, F. R. APPELBAUM & J. NEMUNAITIS. 1994. Recombinant human granulocyte-macrophage colony-stimulating factor after autologous bone marrow transplantation for lymphoid cancer. PharmacoEconomics **1**: 42.

12. BENNETT, C. L., J. L. ARMITAGE, S. LESAGE, S. C. GULATI, J. O. ARMITAGE & N. C. GORIN. 1994. Economic analyses of clinical trials in cancer: Are they helpful to policy makers? Stem Cells **12**: 424.

13. CRUMP, M., M. ROSS, J. VRENDENBURGH et al. 1992. Early toxicity after high-dose therapy and autologous bone marrow transplantation (ABMT) for breast cancer: Implications for outpatient management (abstr). Blood **80** (10 Suppl. 1): 272.

14. NEMUNAITIS, J., J. W. SINGER, C. D. BUCKNER, T. MORI, J. LAPONI, R. HILL, R. STORB, K. M. SULLIVAN, J. A. HANSEN & F. R. APPELBAUM. 1991. Long-term follow-up of patients who received recombinant human granulocyte-macrophage colony stimulating factor after autologous bone marrow transplantation for lymphoid malignancy. Bone Marrow Transplant. **7**: 49.

15. NEMUNAITIS, J., S. N. RABINOWE, J. W. SINGER, P. J. BIERMAN, J. M. VOSE, A. S. FREEDMAN, N. ONETTO, S. GILLIS, D. OETTE, N. GOLD et al. 1991. Recombinant granulocyte-macrophage colony-stimulating factor after autologous bone marrow transplantation for lymphoid cancer. N. Engl. J. Med. **324**: 1773.

16. RABINOWE, S. N., D. NEUBERG, P. J. BIERMAN, J. M. VOSE & J. NEMUNAITIS. 1993. Long-term follow-up phase III study of recombinant human granulocyte-macrophage colony-stimulating factor after autologous bone marrow transplantation for lymphoid malignancies. Blood **81**: 1903.

17. ADVANI, R., N. J. CHAO, S. J. HORNING, K. G. BLUME, D. K. AHN, K. R. LAMBORN, N. C. FLEMING, E. M. BONNEM & P. L. GREENBERG. 1992. Granulocyte-macrophage colony-stimulating factor (GM-CSF) as an adjunct to autologous hemopoietic stem cell transplantation for lymphoma. Ann. Intern. Med. **116**: 183.

18. CRUMP, M., M. ROSS, J. VREDENBURGH, B. MEISENBERG, K. DUKELOW & W. P. PETERS. 1992. Early toxicity after high-dose therapy and autologous bone marrow transplantation (ABMT) for breast cancer: Implications for outpatient management. Blood **80**: 70a.

19. CROWN, J., A. KRITZ, L. VAHDAT, L. REICH, M. MOORE, N. HAMILTON, J. SCHNEIDER, M. HARRISON, T. GILEWSKI, C. HUDIS, S. GULATI & L. NORTON. 1993. Rapid administration of multiple cycles of high-dose myelosuppressive chemotherapy in patients with metastatic breast cancer. J. Clin. Oncol. **11**: 1144.

20. JANSSEN, W. E., J. PERKINS, J. W. HIEMENZ, K. K. FIELDS, P. E. ZORSKY, O. F. BALLESTER, S. C. GOLDSTEIN, R. SMILEE, L. KRONISH & G. J. ELFENBEIN. 1994. Granulocyte recovery

is not different following auto-transplant with G-CSF primed bone marrow or G-CSF mobilized peripheral blood "stem cells." Blood **84**: 95a.

20a. HUAN, S., J. HESTER, G. SPITZER *et al.* 1992. Influence of mobilized peripheral blood cells on the hematopoietic recovery by autologous marrow and recombinant human granulocyte-macrophage colony-stimulating factor after high-dose cyclophosphamide, etoposide, and cisplatin. Blood **79**: 3388.

21. FAUCHER, C., A. G. LE CORROLLER, D. BLAISE, G. NOVAKOVITCH, P. MANONNI, J. P. MOATTI, D. MARANINCHI. 1994. Comparison of G-CSF-primed peripheral blood progenitor cells and bone marrow auto transplantation: Clinical assessment and cost-effectiveness. Bone Marrow Transplant. **14**: 895.

22. PETERS, W. P., G. ROSNER, M. ROSS, J. VREDENBURGH, B. MEISENBERG, C. GILBERT & J. KURTZBERG. 1993. Comparative effects of granulocyte-macrophage colony-stimulating factor (GM-CSF) and granulocyte colony-stimulating factor (G-CSF) on priming peripheral blood progenitor cells for use with autologous bone marrow after high-dose chemotherapy. Blood **81**: 1709.

23. BOLWELL, B., A. FISHLEDER, P. BAUCCO *et al.* 1992. G-CSF primed peripheral blood progenitor cells (PBPC) enhances neutrophil and platelet engraftment in autologous bone marrow transplantation (ABMT). Blood **80** (Suppl. 1): Abstr. 1350.

24. BLAISE, D., J. P. VERNANT, D. FIERE *et al.* 1992. A randomized, controlled, multicenter trial of recombinant human granulocyte colony stimulating factor (filgrastim) in patients treated by bone marrow transplantation (BMT) with total body irradiation (TBI) for acute lymphoblastic leukemia (ALL) or lymphoblastic lymphoma (LL). Blood **80** (Suppl. 1): Abstr. 982.

25. KOUIDES, P. A., J. KAUKEINEN, J. HEAL *et al.* 1992. The potential benefits of mobilized peripheral blood stem cells (PBSC) in autologous bone marrow transplantation may be offset by the risks of PBSC harvesting with chemotherapy-CSF mobilization. Blood **80**: 235a.

26. HOLLAND, H. K., M. R. MOORE, E. F. WINTON *et al.* 1992. Hematologic recovery after high-dose chemotherapy (HDC) for breast cancer (BrCa) with rhu-GF is similar between autologous bone marrow transplantation (ABMT) vs peripheral blood stem cells (PBSC) mobilization. Blood **80** (Suppl. 1): 274a.

27. KORBLING, M., R. HOLLE, R. HAAS, W. KNAUF, B. DORKEN, A. D. HO, R. KUSE, H. PRALLE, T. M. FLIEDNER & W. HUNSTEIN. 1990. Autologous blood stem-cell transplantation in patients with advanced Hodgkin's disease and prior radiation to the pelvic site. J. Clin. Oncol. **8**: 978.

28. SPITZER, G., D. R. ADKINS, V. SPENCER, F. R. DUNPHY, P. J. PETRUSKA, W. S. VELASQUEZ, C. E. BOWERS, N. KRONMUELLER, R. NIEMEYER & W. MCINTYRE. 1994. Randomized study of growth factors post-peripheral-blood stem-cell transplant: Neutrophil recovery is improved with modest clinical benefit. J. Clin. Oncol. **12**: 661.

29. PASSOS-COELHO, J. L., A. A. ROSS, T. J. MOSS, J. M. DAVIS, A. M. HUELSKAMP, S. J. NOGA, N. E. DAVIDSON & M. J. KENNEDY. 1995. Absence of breast cancer cells in a single-day peripheral blood progenitor cell collection after priming with cyclophosphamide and granulocyte-macrophage colony-stimulating factor. Blood **85**: 1138.

30. SHPALL, E. J., R. B. JONES, S. I. BEARMAN, W. A. FRANKLIN, P. G. ARCHER, T. CURIEL, M. BITTER, H. N. CLAMAN, S. M. STEMMER, M. PURDY, S. E. MYERS, L. HAMI, S. TAFFS, S. HEIMFELD, J. HALLAGAN & R. J. BERENSON. 1994. Transplantation of enriched CD34-positive autologous marrow into breast cancer patients following high-dose chemotherapy: Influence of CD34-positive peripheral-blood progenitors and growth factors on engraftment. J. Clin. Oncol. **12**: 28.

31. NEMUNAITIS, J., R. ASH, M. FREEDMAN *et al.* 1992. Phase III double blind trial of rhGM-CSF following allogeneic bone marrow transplant (BMT). Blood **80** (Suppl. 1): 331a.

32. POWLES, R., C. SMITH, S. MILAN, J. TRELEAVEN, J. MILLAR, T. MCELWAIN, E. GORDON-SMITH, S. MILLIKEN & C. TILEY. 1990. Human recombinant GM-CSF in allogeneic

bone-marrow transplantation for leukaemia: Double-blind, placebo-controlled trial. Lancet **336:** 1417.

33. DE WITTE, T., A. GRATWOHL, N. VAN DER LELY, A. BACIGALUPO, A. C. STERN, B. SPECK, A. SCHATTENBERG, C. NISSEN, E. GLUCKMAN & W. E. FIBBE. 1992. Recombinant human granulocyte-macrophage colony-stimulating factor accelerates neutrophil and monocytes recovery after allogeneic T-cell-depleted bone marrow transplantation. Blood **79:** 1359.

34. NEMUNAITIS, J., J. W. SINGER, C. D. BUCKNER, D. DURNAM, C. EPSTEIN, R. HILL, R. STORB, E. D. THOMAS & F. R. APPELBAUM. 1990. Use of recombinant human granulocyte-macrophage colony stimulating factor in graft failure after bone marrow transplantation. Blood **76:** 245.

35. BIERMAN, P., F. APPELBAUM, D. OETTE, S. BILLIS, J. ARMITAGE & J. NEMUNAITIS. 1992. Granulocyte-macrophage colony stimulating factor (GM-CSF) for engraftment failure following autologous or allogeneic bone marrow transplantation (abstr.). Blood **80:** 1065.

36. CHAO, N. J., J. R. SCHRIBER, G. D. LONG, R. S. NEGRIN, M. CATOLICO, B. W. BROWN, L. L. MILLER & K. G. BLUME. 1994. A randomized study of erythropoietin and granulocyte colony-stimulating factor (G-CSF) versus placebo and G-CSF for patients with Hodgkin's and non-Hodgkin's lymphoma undergoing autologous bone marrow transplantation. Blood **83:** 2823.

37. LINK, H., M. A. BOOGAERTS, A. A. FAUSER, S. SLAVIN, J. REIFFERS, N. C. GORIN, A. M. CARELLA, F. MANDELLI, S. BURDACH, A. FERRANT, W. LINKESCH, S. TURA, A. BACIGA-LUPO, F. SCHINDEL & H. HEINRICHS. 1994. A controlled trial of recombinant human erythropoietin after bone marrow transplantation. Blood **84:** 3327.

38. KLAESSON, S., O. RINGDEN, P. LJUNGMAN, B. LONNQVIST & L. WENNBERG. 1994. Reduced blood transfusions requirements after allogeneic bone marrow transplantation: Results of a randomized, double-blind study with high-dose erythropoietin. Bone Marrow Transplant. **13:** 397.

39. BRUGGER, W., K. BROSS, J. FRISCH, P. DERN, B. WEBER, R. MERTELSMANN & L. KANZ. 1992. Mobilization of peripheral blood progenitor cells by sequential administration of interleukin-3 and granulocyte-macrophage colony-stimulating factor following poly-chemotherapy with etoposide, ifosfamide, and cisplatin. Blood **79:** 1193.

40. SAMUELS, B., R. BUKOWSKI, M. GORDON, S. SAMUEL, R. ISAACS & G. DEMETRI. 1993. Phase I study of rhIL-6 with chemotherapy (CT) in advanced sarcoma. Proc. ASCO **12:** 948a.

41. MILLER, L., J. SMITH, II, W. URBA, B. GAUSE, J. JANIK *et al.* 1993. A phase I study of an IL-3/GM-CSF fusion protein (PIXY321) and high-dose carboplatin (CBDCA) in patients with advanced cancer. Proc. ASCO **12:** 353a.

42. MUSASHI, M., Y.-C. YANG, S. R. PAUL, S. C. CLARK, T. SUDA & M. OGAWA. 1991. Direct and synergistic effects of interleukin 11 on murine hemopoiesis in culture. Proc. Natl. Acad. Sci. USA **88:** 765.

43. WILSON, E. L., D. B. RIFKIN, F. KELLY, M. J. HANNOCKS & J. L. GABRILOVE. Basic fibroblast growth factor stimulates myelopoiesis in long-term human bone marrow cultures. Blood **77:** 954.

44. KMEECIK, T. E., J. R. KELLOR, E. ROSEN & G. F. VANDEWOUDE. 1992. Hepatocyte growth factor is a synergistic factor for the growth of hematopoietic progenitor cells. Blood **80:** 2454.

45. JACOBSEN, S. E. W., J. R. KELLER, F. W. RUSCETTI, P. KONDAIAH, A. B. ROBERTS & L. A. FALK. 1991. Bidirectional effects of transforming growth factor B (TGF-B) on colony-stimulating factor-induced human myelopoiesis in vitro: Differential effects of distinct TGF-B isoforms. Blood **78:** 2239.

46. BROXMEYER, H. E. 1992. Suppressor cytokines and regulation of myelopoiesis. Am. J. Pediatr. Hematol.-Oncol. **14:** 22.

47. BROXMEYER, H. E., L. BENNINGER, N. HAGUE, P. HENDRIE, S. COOPER, C. MANTEL, K. CARNETTA, S. VADHAN-RAJ, A. SARRIS & L. LU. 1993. Suppressive effects of the chemokine (macrophage inflammatory protein) family of cytokines on proliferation of normal and leukemia myeloid proliferation. *In* Guigon *et al.* (Eds.) Inserm Eurstext Library. In press.

48. TIBERGHIEN, P., V. LAITHIER, M. MABED, E. RACADOT, C. W. REYNOLDS *et al.* 1993. Interleukin-1 administration before lethal irradiation and allogeneic bone marrow transplantation: Early transient increase of peripheral granulocytes and successful engraftment with accelerated leukocyte, erythrocyte, and platelet recovery. Blood **81:** 1933.

49. FAY, J. W., H. LAZARUS, R. HERZIG, R. SAEZ, D. A. STEVENS, R. H. COLLINS, L. A. PINEIRO, B. W. COOPER, J. DiCESARE & M. CAMPION. 1994. Sequential administration of recombinant human interleukin-3 and granulocyte-macrophage colony-stimulating factor after autologous bone marrow transplantation for malignant lymphoma: A phase I/II multicenter study. Blood **84:** 2151.

50. NAPARSTEK, E., Y. HARDAN, M. BEN-SHAHAR, A. NAGLER, R. OR, M. MUMCUOGLU, L. WEISS, S. SAMUEL & S. SLAVIN. 1992. Enhanced granulocyte-macrophage colony-stimulating factor. Blood **80:** 1673.

51. LOWRY, P. A., K. M. ZSEBO, D. H. DEACON, C. E. EICHMAN & P. J. QUESENBERRY. 1991. Effects of rrSCF on multiple cytokine responsive HPP-CFC generated from sca+ lin-murine hematopoietis progenitors. Exp. Hematol. **19:** 994.

52. BRUGGER, W., W. MOCKLIN, S. HEIMFELD, R. J. BERENSON, R. MERTELSMANN & L. KANZ. 1993. Ex vivo expansion of enriched peripheral blood CD34 + progenitor cells by stem cell factor, interleukin-1B (IL-1B), IL-6, IL3, interferon-y, and erythropoietin. Blood **81:** 2579.

53. ATKINSON, K., A. BARTLETT, A. DODDS & M. RALLINGS. 1994. Lack of efficacy of a short ex vivo incubation of human allogeneic donor marrow with recombinant human GM-CSF prior to its infusion into the recipient. Bone Marrow Transplant. **14:** 573.

54. BENSINGER, W. J., T. H. PRICE, D. C. DALE, F. R. APPELBAUM, R. CLIFT, K. LILLEBY, B. WILIAMS, R. STORB, E. D. THOMAS & C. D. BUCKNER. 1993. The effects of daily recombinant human granulocyte colony-stimulating factor administration on normal granulocyte donors undergoing leukapheresis. Blood **81:** 1883.

55. LINK, H., M. A. BOOGAERTS, A. M. CARELLA, A. FERRANT, H. GADNER, N. C. GORIN, I. HARABACZ *et al.* 1992. A controlled trial of recombinant human granulocyte-macrophage colony-stimulating factor after total body irradiation, high-dose chemotherapy, and autologous bone marrow transplantation for acute lymphoblastic leukemia or malignant lymphoma. Blood **80:** 2188.

56. GORIN, N. C., B. COIFFIER, M. HAYAT, L. FOUILLARD, M. KUENTZ, M. FLESCH, P. COLOMBAT, P. BOIVIN, S. SLAVIN & T. PHILIP. 1992. Recombinant human granulocyte-macrophage colony-stimulating factor after high-dose chemotherapy and autologous bone marrow transplantation with unpurged and purged marrow in non-Hodgkin's lymphoma: A double-blind placebo-controlled trial. Blood **80:** 1149.

57. GORDON, B. G., K. L. SAVING, J. A. McCALLISTER, P. I. WARKENTIN, J. R. McCONNELL, W. M. ROBERTS, P. F. COCCIA & W. D. HAIRE. 1991. Cerebral infarction associated with protein C deficiency following allogeneic bone marrow transplantation. Bone Marrow Transplant. **8:** 323.

58. KÖPPLER, H., K. H. PFLÜGER & K. HAVEMANN. 1991. Hematopoietic reconstitution after high-dose chemotherapy and autologous nonfrozen bone marrow rescue. Ann. Hematol. **63:** 253.

59. GISSELBRECHT, C., H. G. PRENTICE, A. BACIGALUPO, P. BIRON, N. MILPIED, H. RUBIE, D. CUNNINGHAM, M. LEGROS, J. L. PICO, D. C. LINCH, A. K. BURNETT, J. H. SCARFFE, W. SIEGERT & A. YVER. 1994. Placebo-controlled phase III trial of lenograstim in bone-marrow transplantation. Lancet **343:** 696.

60. BLAISE, D., J. P. VERNANT, D. FIERE, E. GLULCKMAN, J. REIFFERS, J. L. HAROUSSEAU, D. SAINTY, D. FAUCHER, C. MARCEL & D. MARANINCHI. 1992. A randomized, controlled multicenter trial of recombinant human granulocyte colony stimulating factor (filgrastim) in patients treated by bone marrow transplantation (BMT) with total body irradiation (TBI) for acute lymphoblastic leukemia (ALL) or lymphoblastic lymphoma (LL). Blood **80:** 248a.

61. SCHMITZ, N., P. DREGER, A. R. ZANDER, G. EHNINGER, H. WANDT, A. A. FAUSER, H. J. KOLB, A. ZUMSPREKEL, A. MARTIN & T. HECHT. 1995. Results of a randomised, controlled, multicentre study of recombinant human granulocyte colony-stimulating factor (filgrastim) in patients with Hodgkin's disease and non-Hodgkin's lymphoma undergoing autologous bone marrow transplantation. Bone Marrow Transplant **15:** 261.

62. STAHEL, R. A., L. M. JOST, T. CERNY, G. PICHERT, H. HONEGGER, A. TOBLER, E. JACKY, M. FEY & E. PLATZER. 1994. Randomized study of recombinant human granulocyte colony-stimulating factor after high-dose chemotherapy and autologous bone marrow transplantation for high-risk lymphoid malignancies. J. Clin. Oncol. **12:** 1931.

Biology of Bone Marrow Stroma

BRIAN R. CLARK AND ARMAND KEATING[a]

University of Toronto Autologous Blood and Marrow Transplant
Program
The Toronto Hospital
Toronto, Ontario, Canada

The bone marrow stromal microenvironment is a complex network of cells and extracellular matrix which maintains the hematopoietic system throughout the life of the individual.[1] A study of the organization of the components of this functional structure and its interaction with hematopoietic progenitor cells has provided insights into the developmental regulation of the blood system and has led to the identification of numerous cytokines of potential clinical significance.[2] Recent studies have focused on the complex interaction of cytokine combinations in stroma-free cultures. Further advances in this field, however, are more likely after a reappraisal of the hematopoietic microenvironment and its influence on the self-renewal and differentiation of hematopoietic stem cells. In this review we examine the biology of bone marrow stroma and its role in the regulation of hematopoiesis.

THE HEMATOPOIETIC MICROENVIRONMENT

Normal hematopoiesis occurs in the cavities of bones within a net-like structure of interconnected reticular cells. Hematopoietic cells are found in the spaces between the marrow vasculature and are closely associated with this reticular cell network.[1,3–5] Some of the cells, adventitial reticular cells, are in contact with the abluminal surface of the vascular endothelium. In conjunction with basement membrane extracellular matrix and vascular endothelium, the adventitial cells contribute to trilaminar regions of interface between peripheral blood and bone marrow.[3,6] When examined in situ, human marrow reticular cells are positive for alkaline phosphatase, a marker for nonhematopoietic mesenchymal cells. Unfortunately, analysis of the marrow microenvironment *in vivo* is hampered by the diffuse nature of the structure and by technical limitations. The application of computerized image analysis has recently provided a means of visualizing sequential marrow sections three dimensionally and reveals continuous cords of developing erythroid cells with associated macrophages beside the marrow-draining sinuses.[7] Despite these technical advances, the most fruitful approach to analysis of the hematopoietic microenvironment results from a study of the adherent layer of long-term bone marrow cultures.

[a] Address for correspondence: Dr. Armand Keating, The Toronto Hospital, General Division, MLW 2-036, 200 Elizabeth Street, Toronto, Ontario M5G 2C4, Canada.

THE HEMATOPOIETIC MICROENVIRONMENT IN LONG-TERM MARROW CULTURES

The human long-term marrow culture (LTMC) system, adapted from the murine model developed by Dexter and colleagues,[8,9] provides a means of studying the differentiation of early hematopoietic precursors and their interaction with stromal elements. Several groups demonstrated long-term production of committed progenitors (CFU-GM and BFU-E) up to 20 weeks after culture initiation[10,11] and also the differentiation of early precursors to the more committed colony-forming cells.[11,12] An essential feature of the cultures is the presence of an adherent layer composed of flat angulated mesenchymal cells lacking hematopoietic characteristics. Early studies indicate that in the absence of this layer hematopoiesis in the cultures declines rapidly.[9] Although the cultures lack the organized three-dimensional structure of the reticular network in bone marrow, detailed electron microscopy (EM) studies show that the LTMC adherent cells are multilayered and surrounded by a rich extracellular matrix.[13] These data suggest that the stromal cell layer in LTMC is a relatively close *in vitro* counterpart to the hematopoietic microenvironment. Because of the accessibility of this layer, much of the recent research on the microenvironment has involved dissection of its cellular and extracellular components.

Cellular Components of the Microenvironment

In contrast to the stromal layer in murine LTMC, most cells comprising the adherent layer of human cultures are nonhematopoietic. This population expresses interstitial and basal lamina collagen types, laminin, vimentin, muscle actins including smooth muscle actin, CD10,[1,14,15] and Stro-1[16] and lacks the CD45 and Mac-1 determinants.[17] A minority of cells are positive for Factor VIII-associated antigen,[15] suggesting an endothelial origin. Hematopoietic cells make up less than 30% of the cellular component of the layer and consist of macrophages, granulocytic cells at various stages of differentiation, and early progenitors as well as lymphocytes of B and T lineage.[1,17]

Examination of granulopoietic foci by light microscopy shows that granulocytes are commonly associated with macrophages in phase-dark structures.[13] Electron microscopy of these granulopoietic foci shows that the cells appear phase-dark due to the presence of a thin overlying cell termed the ''blanket cell.'' The juxtaposition of the blanket cell with the hematopoietic cells imparts a ''cobblestone'' appearance to this region of the adherent layer. Cobblestone regions are observed in active cultures and are totally devoid of erythroid development. This suggests that a cobblestone area contains a microenvironment restricted to supporting granulocytic development. These *in vitro* cobblestone regions are thought to be analogous to *in vivo* associations of granulocytic precursors and macrophages observed in bone marrow sections.[18] Limited erythropoiesis occurs in LTMCs and is associated with isolated clusters of macrophages and erythroblasts termed erythroblastic islands. Time-lapse video microscopy of erythroblastic islands shows that the erythroblasts undergo enucleation with remarkable synchrony.[19]

Macrophages may play an important role in supporting both erythropoiesis and granulopoiesis because they can produce a range of hematopoietic growth factors[20,21] and phagocytose nuclei shed by erythroblasts.[19] These data indicate that macrophages have an important role in the microenvironment. Many investigators, however, have focused on stromal cells, functionally defined as capable of supporting hematopoiesis and lacking hematopoietic determinants (for example, CD45 and Mac-1). To study this population in detail, several approaches can be undertaken. For example, permanent cell lines can be generated. In contrast to murine cells, human stromal cells do not readily form spontaneous lines; they require transformation with agents such as SV40 or transfection with SV40 large T antigen. This approach has yielded interesting data,[22] but it may not reflect the situation *in vivo*. Another approach that generates a phenotypically homogeneous population is the serial passage of cells comprising the adherent layer of LTMC to yield nontransformed stromal cells with a widely differing capacity to support hematopoiesis.[23] The cells are selected by virtue of their high proliferative capacity and most have limited ability to support hematopoiesis. Cloning of stromal cells present in the primary adherent layer is usually unsuccessful, suggesting that additional cytokines or microenvironmental cell interactions are required. Nonetheless, stromal cells isolated by various strategies have led to the identification of several important hematopoietic cytokines including interleukin-7 (IL-7), IL-8, IL-11, and stem cell factor.[24]

Little is known regarding the proliferation and regulation of stromal cells themselves. In early studies we showed that stromal cells in human LTMC express functional PDGF and EGF receptors.[25] Interesting studies by Simmons and Tork-Storb[16,26] have identified some characteristics of stromal precursors. These workers showed that stromal progenitors express the Stro-1 antigen, are CD34(+), glycophorin A(-), HLA-DR low, and CD10(-). The presence of CD34 on the stromal precursor population has implications regarding the use of grafts positively selected for cells carrying this antigen. Factors influencing the regulation and differentiation of stromal precursors remain to be established.

Extracellular Matrix of the Microenvironment

In the adherent layers of LTMC at least, the abundant extracellular matrix consists of basal lamina and interstitial collagen types, fibronectin as well as proteoglycans.[1,27] We previously showed that collagen types I, III, IV, and V were well represented.[1,15] In addition, chondroitin sulfate-containing proteoglycans are a major component of biosynthetic products from stromal cells and appear to coat the layer.[28] Radionuclide pulse-labeling studies indicate that in addition to chondroitin sulfate, dermatan sulfate and hyaluronic acid are also produced.[28]

STROMAL REGULATION OF HEMATOPOIESIS

Additional evidence that stromal cells influence the regulation of hematopoiesis comes from the work of Eaves and colleagues[29] who showed that progenitor cells undergo increased cell cycling after media changes. In contrast, progenitors cultured in the absence of stromal layers exposed to media changes undergo continuous cycling. Further evidence supporting the regulatory role of stroma in restricting cell cycling is based on the effect of hematopoietic cytokines added to LTMC. Neither sustained enhancement nor depletion of progenitor cell numbers is observed in response to GM-CSF.[30]

The ability of stroma to support primitive cells was further addressed in culture systems that used pre-established irradiated LTMC layers from allogeneic donors.[31] These studies were extended to provide a means of quantifying high primitive progenitors by employing a murine stromal cell line capable of supporting human hematopoiesis seeded by limiting dilution with human hematopoietic cells.[32,33]

STROMAL-PROGENITOR CELL INTERACTIONS

Hematopoietic cells can be shown to interact with cellular and extracellular matrix components of the microenvironment. In addition to cytokine-mediated mechanisms, two levels of interaction are possible: cell-cell contact and effects of the extracellular matrix. Cell-cell interactions involve adhesion of hematopoietic precursors to stromal cells via members of the integrin family of adhesion molecules.[27] Several studies indicate that adhesion of granulocyte-macrophage progenitors to stroma is inhibited by antibodies blocking the function of integrins containing the $\alpha 4$ chain.[34,35] The stromal ligand for $\alpha 4$ integrins may be fibronectin or the VCAM-1 molecule.[27,34]

The adhesion of progenitor cells to cellular and/or extracellular matrix elements of the microenvironment will facilitate interaction with a range of growth regulatory molecules (cytokines and inhibitors) that are on the cell surface (e.g., SCF or M-CSF) or are localized to the extracellular matrix.[27,36-39] Many cytokines have specific binding sites for matrix components including glycosaminoglycan side chains of complex proteoglycans. Although the importance of matrix-bound factors, such as GM-CSF, in mediating granulopoiesis was suggested almost a decade ago,[37,38] a surprisingly small amount of work has since been done in this area. A recent study demonstrated punctate staining with antibodies to GM-CSF in the stromal layer.[39] These data support the notion that matrix-bound cytokines may generate large variations in local cytokine concentrations, perhaps giving rise to discrete microenvironments within the stroma.[40]

Glycosaminoglycans in the stromal extracellular matrix may also be substrates for progenitor cell adhesion molecules. The adhesion of cells from a murine lymphoid line to a permanent bone marrow derived adherent line is inhibited by antibodies to CD44.[41] CD44 is a cell surface adhesion molecule that binds hyaluronic acid.

THE ORIGIN OF STROMAL CELLS AFTER BONE MARROW TRANSPLANTATION

Most studies examining the marrow stroma after bone marrow transplantation indicate that the stroma is of host origin.[42-46] In contrast, Keating and colleagues[15] showed that the stromal cells from LTMC generated from patients undergoing allogeneic marrow transplantation became progressively donor-derived after a marrow transplant. Several murine studies support the contention of a donor origin for marrow stroma after a transplant.[47-49] These conflicting results may be explained by differences in culture conditions, by different definitions of marrow stromal cells, or by different doses of mature marrow stromal and/or stromal precursor cells in the graft.

Further studies specifically examining engraftment of stromal cells were conducted by Greenberger, Anklesaria, and colleagues.[50] Anklesaria *et al.*[51] showed that cloned, transformed murine stromal cells could engraft and influence hematopoiesis *in vivo*. Wu and Keating[52] recently investigated the possibility that a nontransformed phenotypically homogeneous population of murine marrow stromal cells could engraft in transplant recipients. Lethally irradiated animals were transplanted with hematopoietic cells coinfused with nontransformed passaged marrow stromal cells. The stromal cells lacked the macrophage determinants Mac-1 and F4/80, but they expressed collagen types I and IV. The cells were transfected with a marker gene, and at 6–8 weeks after transplantation, marked stromal cells were obtained from two of five recipients. In related experiments, male donor stromal cells were identified in the passaged stromal cells derived from LTMC of female transplant recipients by southern analysis and in situ hybridization using a probe for Y chromosome-specific sequences. Approximately one third of the passaged stromal cells from the transplant recipients were of donor origin.

STROMA IN CELL THERAPY

The data just described strongly suggest that marrow stromal cells are capable of engraftment and may provide a novel means of cell therapy. A particularly exciting prospect is to use marrow stromal cells as vehicles for gene delivery. In earlier studies we showed that stromal cells are attractive targets for gene transfer by electroporation, especially if the transgene is transcribed from the human immediate early cytomegalovirus promoter.[53] Recently, we demonstrated successful electrotransfection of human stromal cells with human factor IX cDNA and the production of functional FIX protein for at least 3 weeks *in vitro*.[54] Our observations suggest that engineered marrow stromal cells may provide a novel and suitable approach to the gene therapy of single gene disorders in which the recombinant protein need not be stringently regulated.

Clinical data are already available to suggest the feasibility of stromal transplants. Patients with chronic or acute myeloid leukemia received autologous marrow transplants of long-term marrow culture cells that may contain as many as 3×10^8 mature stromal cells.[55,56] The infusion of these cultured cells is well tolerated.[56] Furthermore, a phase I study of stromal cell infusion was recently reported by Lazarus and colleagues.[57] Thirteen patients with inactive hematologic malignancies received infusions of escalating doses of autologous mesenchymal progenitor cells with osteoid features. No side effects were attributable to the infusions.

SUMMARY

The marrow microenvironment is a complex, three-dimensional structure composed of many cell types and abundant extracellular matrix. Much of the data are derived from analysis of the adherent layer of murine and, especially, human long-term marrow cultures. An essential feature of this *in vitro* counterpart to the marrow microenvironment is the presence of flat angulated cells functionally defined as marrow stromal cells with the following phenotype: type IV collagen(+), laminin(+), vimentin(+), CD10(+), muscle actin(+), Stro-1(+), and negative for CD45, Mac-1, and HLA-DR. Stromal precursors are Stro-1(+) and CD34(+).

Regulation of hematopoietic precursors by the microenvironment occurs by elaboration of regulatory molecules such as hematopoietic cytokines, by cell-cell contact via adhesion molecules such as $\alpha4\beta1$ integrin, and by interactions with components of the extracellular matrix as in the case of the glycosaminoglycan hyaluronic acid with cell-associated CD44.

Although little about the regulation of stromal cell development itself is known, several studies indicate the transplantability of marrow stromal cells under specific conditions. These developments suggest a potential role of stromal cells in cell therapy. Transfected stromal cells may serve as suitable vehicles for gene delivery to correct single gene disorders in which the product of the target gene does not require stringent regulation as, for example, in the correction of Factor VIII and Factor IX deficiency. Further studies are warranted to investigate marrow stromal cell physiology and regulation to better understand hematopoiesis and to explore the possible use of stroma in therapy.

REFERENCES

1. SINGER, J. W., A. KEATING & T. H. WIGHT. 1985. The human hematopoietic microenvironment. *In* Advances in Haematology. V. Hoffbrand, Ed. **4:** 1–24. Churchill Livingstone. London.

2. LORD, B. I. & T. M. DEXTER. (Eds). 1992. Growth factors in haemopoiesis. *In* Balliere's Clinical Haematology, vol. 5.

3. TAVASSOLI, M. & A. FRIEDENSTEIN. 1983. Hemopoietic stromal microenvironment. Am. J. Hematol. **15:** 195–203.

4. WEISS, L. & L.-T. CHEN. 1975. The organisation of hematopoietic cords and vascular sinuses in the bone marrow. Blood Cells **1:** 617–638.

5. LICHTMAN, M. D. 1984. The relationship of stromal cells to hemopoietic cells in marrow. *In* Long Term Bone Marrow Culture. D. G. Wright & J. S. Greenberger, Eds.: 57–96. Alan R. Liss. New York.

6. LICHTMAN, M. D. 1981. The ultrastructure of the hemopoietic environment of the marrow: A review. Exp. Hematol. **9:** 391–410.

7. NAITO, K., N. TAMAHASHI, T. CHIBA *et al.* 1992. The microvasculature of the human bone marrow correlated with the distribution of hematopoietic cells. A computer-assisted three-dimensional reconstruction study. Tohoku. J. Exp. Med. **166:** 439–450.

8. DEXTER, T. M., T. D. ALLEN & L. G. LAJTHA. 1977. Conditions controlling the proliferation of haemopoietic stem cells *in vitro*. J. Cell. Physiol. **91:** 335–344.

9. DEXTER, T. M. 1982. Stromal cell associated haemopoiesis. J. Cell. Physiol. (Suppl. 1): 87–94.

10. GARTNER, S. M. & H. S. KAPLAN. 1980. Long-term culture of human bone marrow cells. Proc. Natl. Acad. Sci. USA **77:** 4756–4761.

11. KEATING, A., J. POWELL, M. TAKAHASHI & J. W. SINGER. 1984. The generation of human long-term marrow cultures from marrow depleted of Ia(HLA-DR) positive cells. Blood **64:** 1159–1162.

12. COLOUMBEL, L., A. C. EAVES & C. J. EAVES. 1983. Enzymatic treatment of long-term marrow cultures reveals the preferential location of primitive hemopoietic progenitors in the adherent layer. Blood **62:** 291–297.

13. ALLEN, T. D., T. M. DEXTER & P. J. SIMMONS. 1990. Marrow biology and stem cells. *In* Hematology, Colony Stimulating Factors: Molecular and Cellular Biology. T. M. Dexter, J. M. Garland & N. G. Testa, Eds. Vol. IX.: 1–38. Dekker. New York.

14. KEATING, A., C. K. WHALEN & J. W. SINGER. 1983. Cultured marrow stromal cells express common acute lymphoblastic leukemia antigen (CALLA): Implications for marrow transplantation. Br. J. Haematol. **55:** 623-628.

15. KEATING, A., J. W. SINGER, P. D. KILLEN *et al.* 1982. Donor origin of the in vitro haematopoietic microenvironment after marrow transplantation in man. Nature **298:** 280-283.

16. SIMMONS, P. J. & B. TOROK-STORB. 1991. Identification of stromal cell precursors in human bone marrow by a novel monoclonal antibody STRO-1. Blood **78:** 55-62.

17. BERNEMAN, Z. N., Z. Z. CHEN, D. VAN BOCKSTAELE D. *et al.* 1989. The nature of the adherent hemopoietic cells in human long-term bone marrow cultures (HLTBMCs): Presence of lymphocytes and plasma cells next to the myelomonocytic population. Leukemia **3:** 648-661.

18. WESTEN, H. & D. F. BAINTON. 1979. Association of alkaline-phosphatase-positive reticulum cells in bone marrow with granulocytic precursors. J. Exp. Med. **150:** 919.

19. ALLEN, T. D. 1987. Time lapse video microscopy using an animation control unit. J. Microsc. **147:** 129-135.

20. GORDON, S., I. FRASER, D. NATH *et al.* 1992. Macrophages in tissues and *in vitro.* Curr. Opin. Immunol. **4:** 25-32.

21. TEMELES, D. S., H. E. MCGRATH, E. L. KITTLER *et al.* 1993. Cytokine expression from bone marrow derived macrophages. Exp. Hematol. **21:** 388-393.

22. SINGER, J. W., P. CHARBOND, A. KEATING, J. NEMUNAITIS, G. RAUGI, T. N. WIGHT, J. LOPES, J. ROTH, L. DOW & P. J. FIALKOW. 1987. Simian virus-40 transformed adherent cells from human long-term marrow cultures: Clone cells produced with "stromal" and hematopoietic characteristics. Blood **70:** 464-474.

23. KEATING, A., K. JUST-MITCHELL, P. TOOR, M. KLEIN & J. SODEK. 1986. Passaged human marrow stromal cells: A unique cell population. Exp. Hematol. **14:** 426.

24. KINCADE, P. W. 1992. Cell interaction molecules and cytokines which participate in B lymphopoiesis. : 575-598.

25. ROSENFIELD, M., A. KEATING D. BOWEN-POPE, J. W. SINGER & R. ROSS. 1985. Responsiveness of the *in vitro* hematopoietic microenvironment to platelet-derived growth factor. Leuk. Res. **9:** 427-434.

26. SIMMONS, P. J. & B. TOROK-STORB. 1991. CD34 expression by stromal precursors in normal adult bone marrow. Blood **78:** 2848-2853.

27. CLARK, B. R., J. T. GALLAGHER & T. M. DEXTER. 1992. Cell adhesion in the stromal regulation of haemopoiesis. *In* Growth Factors in Haemopoiesis. B. I. Lord & T. M. Dexter, Eds. Ballière's Clinical Haematology **5:** 619-652.

28. WIGHT, T. N., M. G. KINSELLA, A. KEATING & J. W. SINGER. 1986. Proteoglycans in human long-term bone marrow cultures: Biochemical and ultrastructural analyses. Blood **67:** 1333-1343.

29. CASHMAN, J., A. C. EAVES & C. J. EEAVES. 1985. Regulated proliferation of primitive hematopoietic progenitor cells in long-term human marrow cultures. Blood **66:** 1002-1005.

30. COUTINHO, L. H., A. WILL, J. RADFORD, R. SCIRO, N. G. TESTA & T. M. DEXTER. 1990. Effects of recombinant human granulocyte colony-stimulating factor, human granulocyte-macrophage-CSF and Gibbon interleukin-3 on hematopoiesis in human long-term bone marrow culture. Blood **75:** 2118-2129.

31. TAKAHASHI, M., A. KEATING & J. W. SINGER. 1985. A functional defect in irradiated adherent layers from chronic myelogenous leukemia long-term marrow cultures. Exp. Hematol. **13:** 926-931.

32. SUTHERLAND, H. J., C. J. EAVES, A. C. EAVES, W. DRAGOWSKA & P. M. LANSDORP. 1989. Characterisation and partial purification of human marrow cells capable of initiating long-term hematopoiesis *in vitro.* Blood **74:** 1563.

33. SUTHERLAND, H. J., P. M. LANSDORP, D. H. HENKLEMAN, A. C. EAVES & C. J. EAVES. 1990. Functional characterisation of individual human hematopoietic stem cells cultured

at limiting dilution on supportive marrow stromal layer. Proc. Natl. Acad. Sci. USA **87:** 3584.

34. SIMMONS, P. J., B. MASINOVSKY, B. M. LONGENECKER. *et al.* 1992. Vascular cell adhesion molecule-1 expression by bone marrow stromal cells mediates the binding of hematopoietic progenitor cells. Blood **80:** 388–395.

35. TEIXIDO, J., M. E. HEMLER, J. S. GREENBERGER & P. ANKLESARIA. 1992. Role of beta 1 and beta 2 integrins in the adhesion of human CD34hi stem cells to bone marrow stroma. J. Clin. Invest. **90:** 358–367.

36. NATHAN, C. & M. SPORN. 1991. Cytokines in context. J. Cell Biol. **113:** 981.

37. GORDON, M. Y., C. R. DOWDING & G. P. RILEY. 1987. Compartmentalisation of a haemopoietic growth factor (GM-CSF) by glycosaminoglycans in the bone marrow environment. Nature **326:** 403–405.

38. ROBERTS, R. A., J. T. GALLAGHER, E. SPOONCER & T. M. DEXTER. 1988. Heparan sulphate-bound growth factors: A mechanism for stromal cell-mediated haemopoiesis. Nature **332:** 376–378.

39. DE WYNTER, E., T. ALLEN, L. COUTINHO, D. FLAVELL, S. U. FLAVELL & T. M. DEXTER. 1993. Localisation of granulocyte macrophage colony-stimulating factor in human long-term marrow cultures. Biological and immunocytochemical characterisation. J. Cell Sci. **106:** 761–769.

40. KEATING, A. & M. Y. GORDON. 1988. Hierarchical organisation of haematopoietic microenvirononemnts. Leukemia **2:** 766–769.

41. MIYAKE, K., K. L. MEDINA, S. I. HAYASHI *et al.* 1990. Monoclonal antibodies to PgP-1/CD44 block lympho-hemopoiesis in long-term bone marrow cultures. J. Exp. Med. **171:** 477–488.

42. FRIEDENSTEIN, A. J., A. A. IVANOV-SMOLENSKI, R. K. CHAJLAKJAN *et al.* 1978. Origin of bone marrow stromal mechanocytes in radiochimeras and heterotopic transplants. Exp. Hematol. **60:** 440–444.

43. BENTLEY, S. A., T. KNUTSEN & J. WHANG-PENG. 1982. The origin of the hematopoietic microenvironment in continuous bone marrow culture. Exp. Hematol. **10:** 367–372.

44. LAVER, J., S. C. JHANWAR, R. J. O'REILLY & H. CASTRO-MALASPINA. 1987. Host origin of human hematopoietic microenvironment following allogeneic bone marrow transplantation. Blood **70:** 1966–1968.

45. AGEMATSU, K. & Y. NAKAHORI. 1991. Recipient origin of bone marrow-derived fibroblastic stromal cells during all periods following bone marrow transplantation. Br. J. Haematol. **79:** 359–365.

46. SIMMONS, P. J., D. PRZEIPIORKA, E. D. THOMAS & B. TOROK-STORB. 1987. Host origin of marrow stromal cells following allogeneic bone marrow transplantation. Nature **328:** 429.

47. PIERSMA, A. H., R. E. PLOEMACHER & K. G. BROCKBANK. 1983. Transplantation of bone marrow fibroblastoid stromal cells in mice via the intravenous route. Br. J. Haematol. **54:** 285–290.

48. MARSHALL, M. J., N. W. NISBET & S. EAVEN. 1984. Donor origin of the *in vitro* hematopoietic microenvironment after marrow transplantation in mice. Experientia **45:** 385–386.

49. VAN ZANT, G., B. P. HOLLAND, P. W. ELDRIDGE & J. J. CHEN. 1990. Genotype-restricted growth and aging patterns in hematopoietic stem cell populations of allophenic mice. J. Exp. Med. **171:** 1547–1565.

50. ANKLESARIA, P., K. KASE, J. GLOWACKI *et al.* 1987. Engraftment of a clonal bone marrow stromal cell line *in vivo* stimulates hematopoietic recovery from total body irradiation. Proc. Natl. Acad. Sci. USA **84:** 7681–7685.

51. ANKLESARIA, P., T. J. FITZGERALD, K. KASE, A. OHARA & J. S. GREENBERGER. 1989. Improved hematopoiesis in anemic SI/SI^d mice by splenectomy and therapeutic transplantation of a hematopoietic microenvironment. Blood **74:** 1144–1151.

52. WU, D. D. & A. KEATING. 1991. Engraftment of donor derived bone marrow stromal cells. Exp. Hematol. **19:** 485.

53. KEATING, A., W. HORSFALL, R. HAWLEY & F. TONEGUZZO. 1990. Effect of different
     promoters on expression of genes introduced into hematopoietic and marrow stromal
     cells by electroporation. Exp. Hematol. **18:** 99–102.
54. FOUILLARD, L. & A. KEATING. 1993. Expression of factor IX cDNA introduced into human
     marrow stromal cells by electroporation. Exp. Hematol. **21:** 550.
55. CHANG, J., L. COUTINHO, G. MOGENSTERN *et al.* 1986. Reconstitution of hematopoietic
     system with autologous marrow taken during relapse of acute myeloblastic leukemia
     and grown in long-term culture. Lancet **I:** 294–295.
56. BARNETT, J. M., C. J. EAVES, G. PHILLIPS *et al.* 1989. Successful autografting in chronic
     myeloid leukemia after maintenance of marrow in culture. Bone Marrow Transplant.
     4: 345–351.
57. LAZARUS, H. L., S. E. HAYNESWORTH, S. L. GERSON & A. I. CAPLAN. 1992. Marrow
     derived stromal progenitors (mesenchymal stem cells): A phase I clinical trial. Blood
     80 (Suppl. 1): 934.

Strategies for Efficient Gene Transfer into Hematopoietic Cells

The Use of Adeno-Associated Virus Vectors in Gene Therapy

SASWATI CHATTERJEE,[a,b] DI LU,[a]
GREG PODSAKOFF,[a,d] AND K. K. WONG, Jr. [c]

[a]*Division of Pediatrics*
and
[c]*Department of Hematology and Bone Marrow Transplantation*
City of Hope National Medical Center
Duarte, California 91010

Over the last 30 years, bone marrow transplantation has become accepted as standard curative therapy for many pathophysiologic conditions[1] including metabolic diseases, immunodeficiencies,[2] and malignancies.[3] Thus, reconstitution of the hematopoietic system with normal allogeneic cells capable of providing long-term engraftment with disease-free, physiologically functional cells has been used to treat various inherited diseases including severe combined immunodeficiency disease, Wiskott-Aldrich syndrome, various hemoglobinopathies, and lysosomal storage disorders. However, difficulties in acquisition of histocompatible marrow cells for transplantation and onset of graft-versus-host disease in partially matched and even fully matched allografts have led to a continued search for better therapeutic strategies. Meanwhile, delineation of the genetic bases of many inherited diseases and the subsequent isolation of appropriate wild-type genes promoted the feasibility of correction at the DNA level. To this end, much effort has focused on the development of both identification of genetic correction strategies as well as efficient methods of gene delivery to appropriate target cells.

Cells of the hematopoietic system readily lend themselves to *ex vivo* gene therapy. Bone marrow cells provide an accessible source of lineage-committed progenitor cells and, importantly, pluripotent hematopoietic stem cells potentially capable of both self-renewal and multilineage reconstitution of the entire hematopoietic system with gene-modified cells. The ability to provide long-term correction of inherited diseases through the genetic modification of *stem* cells is attractive. Whereas bone marrow, cytokine-mobilized peripheral blood, and umbilical cord blood have been identified as sources of hematopoietic stem and progenitor cells, the precise identification and purification of pluripotent stem cells have remained elusive. Recent studies demonstrated that cell populations exhibiting high levels of cell surface expression

---

[b]To whom correspondence should be addressed.

[d]Present address: Avigen Inc, Alameda, CA 94502.

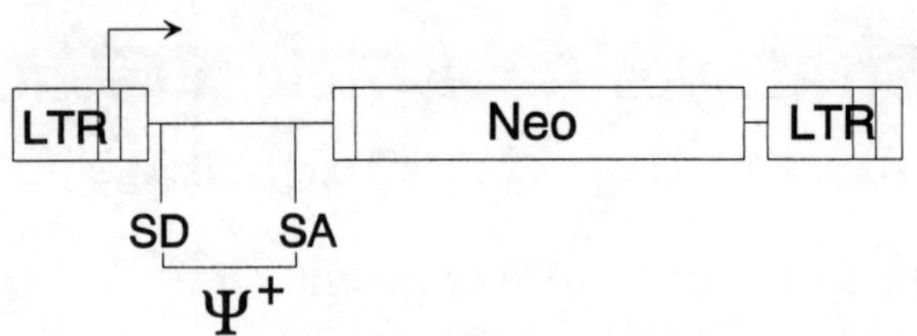

FIGURE 1. Map of a retroviral vector encoding transgene expression under long terminal repeat (LTR) control and a selectable marker under control of a second promoter.

of the CD34 differentiation antigen, exhibiting low expression of thy 1 antigen, and lacking lineage-specific differentiation markers contain primitive cells capable of giving rise to cells of both lymphoid and myeloid lineages in SCID mice repopulated with human cells.[4]

Primitive cells capable of multilineage differentiation are largely quiescent cells, only a few cells being in an active cell cycle at any given time.[5] As with other pluripotent stem cells, hematopoietic stem cell division is associated with both differentiation along lineage pathways as well as self-renewal. Therefore, for permanent gene therapy of the hematopoietic system, gene transfer into self-renewing pluripotential stem cells is highly desirable to ensure the continued presence of the transgene in terminally differentiated progeny, while maintaining a pool of genetically modified progenitor cells. For effective stem cell gene therapy, permanent integration of transgenes into the stem cell genome must be achieved to ensure transmittal to progeny. Of the currently available gene transfer systems only two offer the possibility of stable transgene integration. These include viral vectors based on retroviruses and adeno-associated viruses (AAV). Other gene transfer methods, including adenovirus vectors and liposome-based DNA delivery methods, do not result in transgene integration at high frequencies. Thus, the major use of these systems may lie in gene therapy strategies requiring transient transgene expression. For stem cell gene therapy, we shall focus on integrating vectors.

VIRAL VECTORS

Retroviral Vectors

Retroviral vectors based on murine leukemia virus (MLV) have been studied extensively for their capacity to transfer gene into hematopoietic progenitor cells.[6] Vectors are constructed replacing viral genes with heterologous open reading frames downstream of the retroviral long terminal repeats (LTR) (FIG. 1). Retention of the packaging signal assures efficient packaging of genomic viral RNA into core particles. The vectors are packaged in producer cell lines that are permanently transformed with both retroviral gag, pol, and env genes and vector sequences.[7] Derivation of producer lines requires the presence of a selectable marker in the vector, which aids in clonal selection of producer lines. Infectious retroviruses are produced by budding from plasma membrane into the tissue culture supernatant. Transductions or gene transfers are performed by adding vector-containing supernatant to target cells or by coculturing target cells with producer cells. Transgene expression is controlled by either the retroviral LTR or an internal promoter. Some retroviral constructs with tRNA promoters driving expression of short biologically active RNA molecules have also been reported. To avoid promoter interference and increase expression, these have been placed within the LTRs.

Gene therapy strategies using retroviral vectors are being developed for the hematopoietic system for a variety of diseases including AIDS, Gaucher's diseases, and adenosine deaminase deficiency as well as for genetic marking of cells during cancer therapy. Retroviral vector biology is well defined and currently represents the most utilized viral vector system in clinical trials. However, retroviral vectors require active cell division[8] and nuclear membrane breakdown for efficient transduction.[9] Thus, although gene transfer into cytokine- or chemotherapy-stimulated progenitor cells has been accomplished with retroviruses, efficient gene transfer frequencies into unmanipulated primitive stem cells has remained elusive. Cytokine stimulation of primitive stem cells either by the addition of exogenous cytokines[10] or by growth on stromal cell layers[11] has now become standard procedure for retroviral transduction. However, cytokines that stimulate stem cells to proliferate without concomitant differentiation have yet to be identified. Cytokine combinations used to date all result in the loss of self-renewal capacity and in lineage commitment[5] of primitive hematopoietic stem cells. Thus, cytokine-facilitated gene transfer and cell preparative procedures for retrovirus-mediated gene therapy may not be ideally suited for long-term stem cell transduction. These limitations may be reflected in low retroviral gene transfer frequencies into hematopoietic stem cells *in vivo* in large animal models with transduction frequencies <5% in canine and simian models and <1% in actual human clinical trials.[5,12,13]

Additionally, retroviral vector-encoded transgenes are prone to silencing, possibly because of mechanisms including methylation of CpG sequences in the MLV LTRs[14] which act as a promoter element directing transgene expression. Thus, in addition to low transduction frequencies, sustained gene expression of retroviral-encoded transgenes has been problematic. Hence, the continued search for other novel vectors for use in stem cell gene therapy is compelling.

Adeno-Associated Virus-Based Vectors

Adeno-associated virus (AAV) is a nonpathogenic, replication-defective human parvovirus with a single-stranded DNA genome of 4.7 kb in length. The AAV genome is flanked at either end by palindromic inverted terminal repeats (ITR).[15] Coinfection with a helper virus, such as herpes simplex virus or adenovirus, is necessary for productive infection. In the absence of helper virus coinfection, wild-type AAV integrates in a site-specific fashion via the ITRs into the q-ter13.2-13.4 of the human chromosome 19.[16] Latent wild-type AAV infections have been stably maintained in tissue culture for over 100 serial passages in the absence of selective pressure, attesting to the stability of AAV genomic integration.[17]

Vectors based on AAV have been constructed by replacing endogenous viral genes with genes of interest under transcriptional control of a variety of promoters

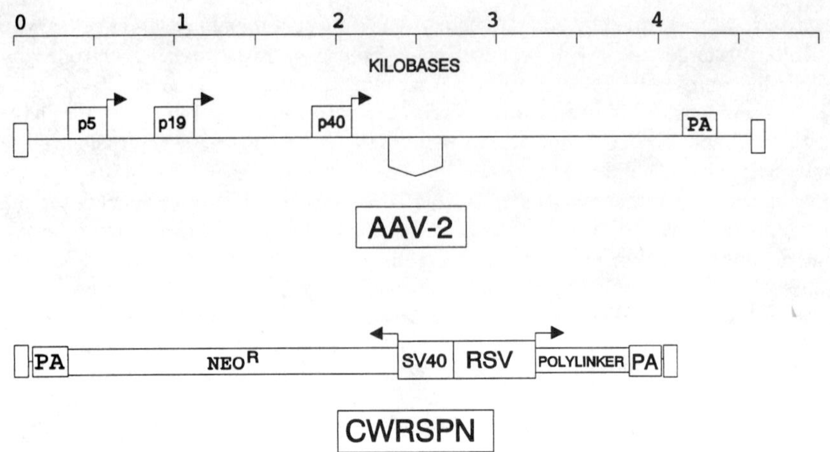

FIGURE 2. Maps of wild-type adeno-associated virus (AAV-2) and an AAV vector (CWRSPN). The AAV genome map shows locations of the promoters driving *rep* (*p5* and *p19*) and *cap* gene expression (p40). CWRSPN is an AAV vector encoding two gene cassettes, an RSV LTR driving the gene of interest and an SV40 early promoter driving the Neo gene. Each expression unit in the vector uses a separate polyadenylation signal. *Arrows* show direction of transcription. The kilobase scale indicates approximate size of genes.

and using separate termination and polyadenylation signals (FIG. 2). Promoters shown to be active in AAV vectors include the Rous sarcoma virus LTR, the SV40 early promoter, the cytomegalovirus immediate early promoter, and the murine leukemia virus LTR.[18–24] Multiple genes, each under separate transcriptional control, are functional in AAV vectors. RNA polymerase II- and III-dependent promoters are active in single and multigene constructs.[25] A major limitation of AAV vector constructs is the size of the vector genome. Adeno-associated viral vectors efficiently encapsidate up to 5 kb of single-stranded DNA.

Most AAV vector packaging procedures reported to date involve the transfection of the vector plasmid along with another plasmid providing AAV rep (DNA replication) and cap (virion proteins) genes into helper virus-infected cells. Cell-associated recombinant vectors are harvested 48–72 hours after transfection. Cells are lysed and processed to release virions, and after heat inactivation of helper virus, the crude cell lysates serve as a source of transducing vector.[20] Like wild-type AAV, AAV vectors are resistant to various treatments including certain lipid solvents and heating to 56°C for up to 10–16 hours. These properties may be used to further purify virions away from helper viruses. Adeno-associated viral vectors may also be further purified on isopycnic cesium chloride gradients in which wild-type AAV bands at a density of 1.41. The density of vectors depends on the size of the genome.

Adeno-associated viral vectors have a wide host range and tissue tropism and, like the wild-type virus, integrate into host chromosomal DNA. We recently used viral vectors based on the AAV, to efficiently confer intracellular resistance to human immunodeficiency virus (HIV-1) and herpes simplex virus (HSV-1).[21,22] To further develop AAV vector systems for gene therapy of HIV infection[21] and oncogenesis,[23] we are investigating AAV-mediated gene transfer into human hematopoietic progenitor cells.

Adeno-Associated Viral Transduction of Nondividing Cells

To initially define the biology of AAV-mediated gene transfer, we tested the ability of an AAV vector to efficiently introduce transgenes into nonproliferating cell populations.[26] Cells were induced into a nonproliferative state by treatment with DNA synthesis inhibitors or by contact inhibition induced by confluence and serum starvation. Cells in logarithmic growth or DNA synthesis arrest were transduced with vCWR : Beta Gal, an AAV-based vector encoding β-galactosidase under Rous sarcoma virus LTR promoter control. Under each condition tested, vCWR : βGal expression in nondividing cells was at least equivalent to that in actively proliferating cells, suggesting that mechanisms for virus attachment, nuclear transport, virion uncoating, and perhaps limited second-strand synthesis of AAV vector were present in nondividing cells. Southern hybridization analysis of vector sequences from cells transduced while in DNA synthetic arrest and expanded after release of block confirmed the ultimate integration of the vector genome into cellular chromosomal DNA.

Unlike the findings of Alexander *et al.*,[27] in which the induction of DNA damage was required for efficient AAV transduction of nondividing human diploid fibroblasts, our results and those of others indicate that transduction efficiencies ranging from 50-100% are observed in a reproducible fashion in unmanipulated cells. Furthermore, our results were recently confirmed by Flotte *et al.*[28] who also showed sustained gene expression in nondividing respiratory epithelial cells and Kaplitt *et al.*[29] who reported stable AAV-mediated gene transfer and long-term transgene expression in neurons of adult rats, a cell population known to primarily be nondividing. Thus, these findings suggest the utility of AAV-based vectors for gene transfer into quiescent cell populations such as terminally differentiated blood cells and pluripotent stem cells.

Adeno-Associated Virus Transduction of CD34+ Hematopoietic Progenitor Cells

Recently, we tested AAV-mediated gene transfer into a panel of human marrow-derived CD34+ hematopoietic progenitor cells, using vectors encoding either placental alkaline phosphatase or neomycin phosphotransferase genes under the control of several viral and cellular promoters. Transduction was evaluated by integration of vector sequences into chromosomal DNA and analysis of transgene expression. FIGURE 3 shows transduction CD34 cells assessed 7 days after transduction with CWR : βGal. In other experiments, Southern hybridization analysis of transduced CD34 cell DNA revealed the presence of integrated vector sequences in chromosomal DNA, indicating stable transduction. From 80-90% of CD34 cells in suspension cultures and 50-95% of myeloid colonies differentiating *in vitro* from transduced CD34 cells demonstrated specific transgene expression in cells from different donors regardless of the transgene or selective pressure. Comparisons of CD34 transduction either before or after cytokine stimulation revealed similar gene transfer frequencies.

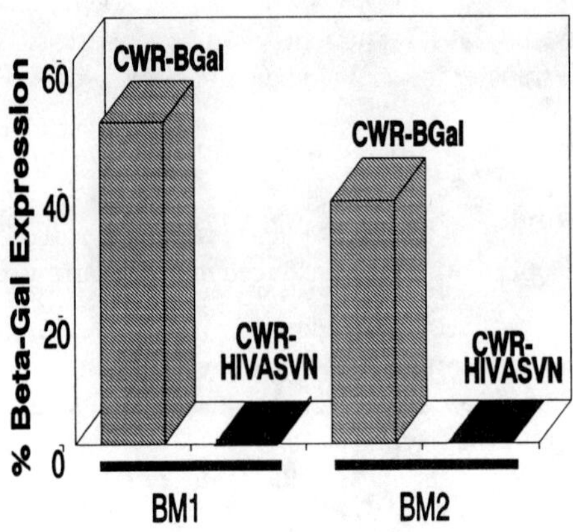

FIGURE 3. Transduction of CD34 cells with CWR-βGal, an AAV vector encoding the beta-galactosidase gene under RSV LTR control. Shown is beta-galactosidase expression in CD34 cells 7 days posttransduction as assessed by histochemical stain. CWR-HIVASVN-transduced cells serve as negative controls. BM1 and BM2 represent cells obtained from two different marrow samples.

These results suggested that AAV-mediated gene transfer into primary human hematopoietic progenitor cells is stable and highly efficient. Recently other groups also demonstrated efficient AAV transduction of cord blood hematopoietic progenitor cells by assaying for the Neo transgene and by PCR analyses.[29] Wild-type AAV infection and transduction of non-human primate CD34 cells was demonstrated by PCR analysis.[30] Adeno-associated virus transduction of Fanconi anemia complementation group C into peripheral blood CD34 cells was shown by clonogenic assays and RNA PCR analysis.[31] Miller *et al.*[32] described AAV transduction of the gamma globin gene into human erythroid colony-forming cells. By contrast to the findings of Halbert *et al.,*[34] our results and those of others suggest that AAV vectors transduce primary human cells at high efficiencies.

Adeno-Associated Virus Transduction of Primitive Hematopoietic Precursor Cells

The lack of assay systems to directly test self-renewing, multilineage, pluripotential human stem cells *in vitro* has impeded attempts to analyze gene transfer into this important cell population. However, long-term marrow cultures in which a microenvironment capable of supporting hematopoiesis for up to 8 weeks has been described.[34] In this culture system, the committed, late progenitor cells die out in the first 3 weeks of culture, whereas clonogenic cells surviving longer than 5 weeks exhibit a primitive phenotype.[35] These cells show good correlation with long-term marrow repopulating activity and represent the most primitive hematopoietic progenitor cell currently assayable *in vitro*.[36] On analyzing gene transfer into this population of cells, we found both the stable transduction of hematopoietic cells in long-term cultures and efficient AAV-mediated gene transfer into primitive marrow-derived precursor cells capable of initiating long-term cultures (LTC-IC). Human marrow mononuclear cells (MNC) and CD34+ hematopoietic progenitor cells were transduced with either vCWRHIVaSVN, an AAV vector encoding antisense sequences to the HIV-1 LTR,[21] or vCWRAP, an AAV vector encoding the human placental alkaline phosphatase gene, at culture initiation in the *absence* of selective pressure. Analyses of vector sequences by quantitative amplification methods and transgene expression at both the protein and the RNA level suggested that significant proportion of primitive human hematopoietic progenitor cells were transduced by AAV even in the *absence* of selective pressure.[37]

As the best available assay of stem cell function to date is long-term multilineage hematopoietic reconstitution, we tested the ability of AAV-transduced murine marrow cells to engraft lethally irradiated mice. Early results demonstrated that mice transplanted with AAV-transduced marrow cells showed evidence of long-term, multilineage reconstitution.[38] Transgene expression cells were detected in peripheral blood and hematopoietic organs at >6 months posttransplantation. These findings suggest that AAV-mediated gene transfer into primary hematopoietic progenitor cells is highly efficient and may provide the basis for novel modes of *ex vivo* gene therapy.

CONTROVERSIES AND CHALLENGES IN ADENO-ASSOCIATED VIRUS GENE THERAPY

Do the Data Show True Viral Transduction?

As most transduction studies with AAV vectors have been performed with crude vector preparations consisting mainly of cell lysate, the question arises as to whether reported results represent true viral transduction or a manifestation of direct transfer of transgene-encoded proteins to target cells. Several lines of evidence, to be summarized, indicate that results obtained by us and others are representative of true viral AAV transduction. Transcription of transgene-encoded RNA has been detected for extended periods after transduction.[21] Extended *in vitro* and *in vivo* expression of vector-encoded transgene in the absence of selective pressure has been observed as already described herein. In addition to our murine transplantation studies, Flotte *et al.*[40] also reported long-term *in vivo* expression of an AAV-vector encoded cystic fibrosis transmembrane conductance regulatory gene in rabbit airway epithelial cells. It is highly unlikely that protein transfer could result in such extended detection.

The kinetics of transgene expression after 293 cell transduction with vCWRAP, encoding the thermostable placental alkaline phosphatase gene (PLAP), are consistent with gene transfer and not protein transfer. FIGURE 4 shows that PLAP expression increases from 5% at 24 hours to 80% at 72 hours after transduction with vCWRAP. For direct protein transfer rather than transduction, greatest PLAP activity would be detected immediately after transduction and would show a subsequent decline as cells divide. However, the kinetics of transgene expression demonstrate a gradual increase with time, consistent with entry of recombinant virus into the cell, followed by second DNA strand synthesis before transcription and translation. Lastly, similar results are obtained with preparations of recombinant AAV vectors purified through isopycnic gradients, suggesting that transgene expression is definitively due to transduction with an encapsidated viral vector.

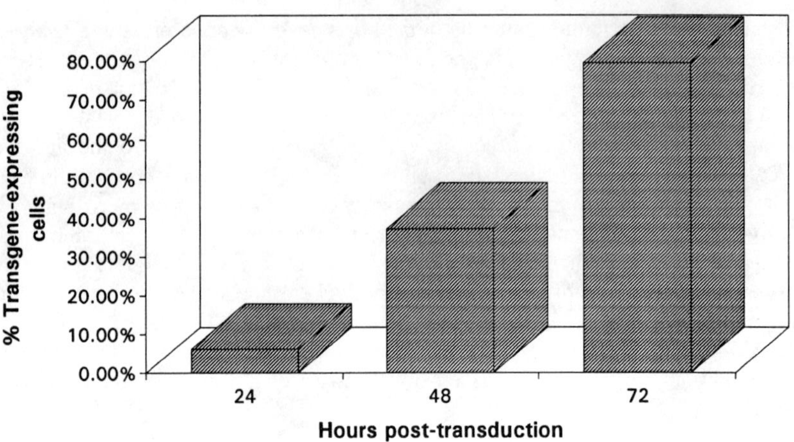

FIGURE 4. Kinetics of transgene expression. Parallel samples of 293 cells were transduced with CWRAP, an AAV vector encoding the thermostable alkaline phosphatase gene and processed for transgene expression at 24, 48, and 72 hours post-transduction. Alkaline phosphatase activity was assessed by histochemical stain.

Adeno-Associated Viral Vector Integration

Do Adeno-Associated Viral Vectors Integrate into Genomic DNA?

Wild-type AAV integrates into cellular genomic DNA upon infection in the absence of helper virus. This integration is targeted to a region defined as AAVS1 which maps to q13.2-13.4 of human chromosome 19. The mechanism of site-specific integration is at least partially mediated by AAV-encoded *rep* proteins. However, because wild-type free AAV vectors do not have detectable *rep* proteins, site specificity of integration is probably lost. However, some controversy exists in the literature on the ability of AAV vectors to integrate. Flotte *et al.*[28] report that sustained transduction occurs in the absence of detectable vector integration. However, our data suggest that AAV vector integration is indeed detectable.[26] Early after transduction, a large fraction of cells show transgene expression. As integration is unnecessary for transgene expression, a portion of transduced cells may carry episomal, double-stranded copies of the vector, some of which may eventually be lost. The exact proportion of cells that will exhibit long-term transduction and vector integration is currently unclear as is the time of vector integration. Although we and others have shown transduction of nondividing cells and we have shown *eventual* vector integration, we do not know if integration occurred with the cells still in a nondividing state or after initiation of DNA synthesis and mitosis. The cellular conditions that permit AAV vector integration are currently being investigated.

Analysis of the role of specific AAV vector sequences along with packaging and purification techniques should help clarify some of these issues. Adeno-associated viral vectors derived by various groups currently retain differing amounts of wild-type sequences. In some families of vectors, sequences have been altered by the addition of linkers. The role of such modifications to the fate of the vector genomes within the cell is currently unknown. Additionally, varying methods of packaging AAV vectors are used by different laboratories. Conceivably, the amounts of *rep* or other proteins necessary for integration may vary in different preparations. This area will no doubt be explored further as AAV vectors move closer to the arena of clinical trials.

Is Site-Specific Vector Integration Necessary?

Wild-type AAV infection is nonpathogenic and usually associated with site-specific virus integration. However, as AAV vectors may not exhibit site-specific integration, the possible effects of random AAV vector integration are being investigated. Random integration introduced the possibility of insertional mutagenesis and oncogene activation. However, retroviral vectors that have been extensively used for gene therapy also integrate randomly. No deleterious effects of wild-type free retrovirus transduction have yet been noted in human trials. Thus, random integration of AAV vectors, at worst, would be comparable to that of retroviruses.

Scale-Up of Clinical Grade Recombinant Adeno-Associated Viral Vector Production

Large scale production of recombinant AAV vectors is a major impediment to their widespread use. Currently used vector packaging methods are expensive and labor intensive. DNA transfection into helper virus-infected cells and purification of vectors from crude cell lysates and away from helper viruses is time consuming. These procedures also are prone to batch-to-batch variability, which is undesirable for regulatory purposes. Complete separation from pathogenic helper viruses is mandatory before use in humans. The derivation of AAV vector packaging lines that provide AAV gene *rep* and *cap* gene functions has been approached by several groups with variable success. Cellular toxicity of AAV rep protein expression has been problematic. Much effort from both academic and biotechnology sectors is currently focused on large scale vector production to allow the generation of sufficient quantities of helper virus-free and wild-type AAV-free clinical grade vectors to initiate human gene therapy trials.

CONCLUSIONS

Adeno-associated viral vectors are rapidly emerging as promising human gene therapy by virtue of their high transduction frequencies in primary cells and their ability to transduce nondividing cells and primitive hematopoietic progenitor cells. Transcription of transgenes from AAV vectors is efficient and sustained. These properties render AAV vectors as good candidates for therapeutic gene transfer in the treatment of hereditary diseases,[31,32] in antiviral approaches to diseases such as AIDS,[21] as antioncogene strategies,[23] and in marking studies to detect minimal residual disease in stem cell transplants. As applications for human gene therapy expand, the particular biologic properties of each vector system may be exploited for use in specific situations. The high efficiency of AAV-mediated gene transfer into primary human cells makes it imperative to focus on areas of controversy and challenge, as just outlined.

REFERENCES

1. FORMAN, S. J., K. G. BLUME & E. D. THOMAS, Eds. 1994. Bone Marrow Transplantation. Blackwell Scientific Publications. Cambridge, MA.
2. BLAESE, R. M. 1993. Development of gene therapy for immunodeficiency: adenosine deaminase deficiency. Pediatr. Res. **33:** S49.
3. BRENNER, M. K., D. R. RILL, M. S. HOLLADAY, H. E. HESLOP, R. C. MOEN, M. BUSCHLE, R. A. KRANCE, V. M. SANTANA, W. F. ANDERSON & J. N. IHLE. 1993. Gene marking to determine whether autologous marrow infusion restores long-term haemopoiesis in cancer patients. Lancet **342:** 1134–1137.
4. BAUM, C. M., I. L. WEISSMAN, A. S. TSUKAMOTO, A. M. BUCKLE & B. PEAULT. 1992. Isolation of a candidate human hematopoietic stem-cell population. Proc. Natl. Acad. Sci. USA **89:** 2804–2808.
5. OGAWA, M. 1993. Differentiation and proliferation of hematopoietic stem cells. Blood **81:** 2844–2853.
6. MILLER, A. D., D. G. MILLER, J. V. GARCIA & C. M. LYNCH. 1993. Use of retroviral vectors for gene transfer and expression. Methods Enzymol. **217:** 581–599.
7. MILLER, A.D. 1990. Retrovirus packaging cells. Human Gene Therapy **1:** 5–14.
8. MILLER, D. G., M. A. ADAM & A. D. MILLER. 1990. Gene transfer by retrovirus vectors occurs only in cells that are actively replicating at the time of infection. Mol. Cell Biol. **10:** 4239–4242.
9. ROE, T. Y., T. C. REYNOLDS, G. YU & P. O. BROWN. 1993. Integration of murine leukemia virus DNA depends on mitosis. EMBO J. **12:** 2099–2108.
10. LUSKEY, B. D., M. ROSENBLATT, K. ZSEBO & D. A. WILLIAMS. 1992. Stem cell factor, interleukin-3, and interleukin-6 promote retroviral-mediated gene transfer into murine hematopoietic stem cells. Blood **80:** 396–402.
11. NOLTA, J. A., G. M. CROOKS, R. W. OVERELL, D. E. WILLIAMS & D. B. KOHN. 1992. Retroviral vector-mediated gene transfer into primitive human hematopoietic progenitor cells: Effects of mast cell growth factor (MGF) combined with other cytokines. Exp. Hematol. **20:** 1065–1071.
12. CARTER, R. B., A. C. ABRAMS-OGG, J. E. DICK, S. A. KRUTH, V. E. VALLI, S. KAMEL-REID & I. D. DUBE. 1992. Autologous transplantation of canine long-term marrow culture cells genetically marked by retroviral vectors. Blood **79:** 356.
13. KANTOFF, P. W., A. P. GILLIO, J. R. McKACHLIN, C. BORDIGNON, M. A. EGLITIS, N. A. KERNAN, R. C. MOEN, D. B. KOHN, S.-F. YU, E. KARSON, S. KARLSSON, J. A. ZWIEBEL, E. GILBOA, R. M. BLAESE, A. NIENHUIS, R. J. O'REILLY & W. F. ANDERSON. 1987. Expression of human adenosine deaminase in nonhuman primates after retrovirus-mediated gene transfer. J. Exp. Med. **166:** 219–234.
14. CHALLITA, P.-M. & D. B. KOHN. 1994. Lack of expression from a retroviral vector after transduction of murine hematopoietic stem cells is associated with methylation *in vivo*. Proc. Natl. Acad. Sci. USA **91:** 2567–2571.
15. BERNS, K. I. & R. A. BOHENZKY. 1987. Adeno-associated viruses: An update. Adv. Virus Res. **32:** 243–306.
16. KOTIN, R. M., M. SINISCALCO, R. J. SAMULSKI, X. D. ZHU, L. HUNTER, C. A. LAUGHLIN, S. MCLAUGHLIN, N. MUZYCZKA, M. ROCCHI & K. I. BERNS. 1990. Site-specific integration by adeno-associated virus. Proc. Natl. Acad. Sci. USA **87:** 2211–2215.
17. BERNS, K., T. PINKERTON, G. F. THOMAS & M. N. HOGGAN. 1975. Detection of adeno-associated virus (AAV)-specific nucleotide sequences in DNA isolated from latently infected Detroit 6 cells. Virology **68:** 556–560.

18. MUZYCZKA, N. 1992. Use of AAV as a general transduction vector for mammalian cells. Curr. Top. Microbiol. Immunol. **158:** 97-129.

19. LEBKOWSKI, J. S., M. M. MCNALLY, T. B. OKARMA & L.B. LERCH. 1988. Adeno-associated virus: A vector system for efficient introduction and integration of DNA into a variety of mammalian cell types. Mol. Cell Biol. **8:** 3988-3996.

20. CHATTERJEE, S. & K. K. WONG. 1993. Adeno-associated virus vectors for the delivery of antisense RNA. Methods (Methods in Enzymol.) **5:** 51-59.

21. CHATTERJEE, S., P. R. JOHNSON & K. K. WONG. 1992. Dual target inhibition of HIV-1 in vitro with an adeno-associated virus-based antisense vector. Science **258:** 1485-1488.

22. WONG, K. K., JR., J. A. ROSE & S. CHATTERJEE. 1991. Restriction of HSV-1 production in cell lines transduced with an antisense viral vector targeting the HSV-1 ICP4 gene. *In* Vaccine 91. F. Brown, R. Chanock, H. Ginsberg & R. Lerner, Eds.: 183-189. Cold Spring Harbor, NY.

23. LU, D., S. CHATTERJEE, D. BRAR & K. K. WONG, JR. 1994. High efficiency *in vitro* cleavage of transcripts arising from the major transforming genes of human papillomavirus type 16 mediated by ribozymes transcribed from an adeno-associated virus-based vector. Cancer Gene Therapy. **1:** 267-277.

24. BRAR, D., K. K. WONG, JR., P. PERMANA & S. CHATTERJEE. 1994. Promoter interactions in adeno-associated virus vectors encoding multiple gene cassettes: Potential use in anti-oncogene vector design. Cancer Gene Therapy **1:** 321.

25. CHATTERJEE, S. & K. K. WONG. 1993. Adeno-associated viral vectors for the delivery of antisense RNA. Methods (Methods in Enzymol.) **5:** 51-59.

26. PODSAKOFF, G., K. K. WONG, JR. & S. CHATTERJEE. 1994. Stable and efficient gene transfer into non-dividing cells by adeno-associated virus (AAV)-based vectors. J. Virol. **68:** 5656-5666.

27. ALEXANDER, I. E., D. W. RUSSELL & A. D. MILLER. 1994. DNA-damaging agents greatly increase the transduction of nondividing cells by adeno-associated virus vectors. J. Virol. **68:** 8282-8287.

28. FLOTTE, T. R., S. A. AFIONE & P. L. ZEITLIN. 1994. Adeno-associated virus vector gene expression occurs in nondividing cells in the absence of vector DNA integration. Am. J. Respir. Cell Mol. Biol. **11:** 517-521.

29. KAPLITT, M. G., P. LEONE, R. J. SAMULSKI, X. XIAO, D. W. PFAFF, K. L. O'MALLEY & M. J. DURING. 1994. Long-term gene expression and phenotypic correction using adeno-associated virus vectors in the mammalian brain. Nature Genet. **8:** 148-153.

30. ZHOU, S. Z., S. COOPER, L. Y. KANG, L. RUGGIERI, S. HEIMFELD, A. SRIVASTAVA & H. E. BROXMEYER. 1994. Adeno-associated virus 2-mediated high efficiency gene transfer into immature and mature subsets of hematopoietic progenitor cells in human umbilical cord blood. J. Exp. Med. **179:** 1867-1875.

31. GOODMAN, S., X. XIAO, R. E. DONAHUE, A. MOULTON, J. MILLER, C. WALSH, N. S. YOUNG, R. J. SAMULSKI & A. W. NIENHUIS. 1994. Recombinant adeno-associated virus-mediated gene transfer into hematopoietic progenitor cells. Blood **84:** 1492-1500.

32. WALSH, C. E., A. W. NIENHUIS, R. J. SAMULSKI, M. G. BROWN, J. L. MILLER, N. S. YOUNG & J. M. LIU. 1994. Phenotypic correction of Fanconi anemia in human hematopoietic cells with a recombinant adeno-associated virus vector. J. Clin. Invest. **94:** 1440-1448.

33. MILLER, J. L., R. E. DONAHUE, S. E. SELLERS, R. J. SAMULSKI, N. S. YOUNG & A. W. NIENHUIS. 1994. Recombinant adeno-associated virus (rAAV)-mediated expression of a human gamma-globin gene in human progenitor-derived erythroid cells. Proc. Natl. Acad. Sci. USA **91:** 10183-10187.

34. HALBERT, C. L., I. E. ALEXANDER, G. M. WOLGAMOT & A. D. MILLER. 1995. Adeno-associated virus vectors transduce primary cells much less efficiently than immortalized cells. J. Virol. **69:** 1473-1479.

35. DEXTER, T. M., T. D. ALLEN & L. G. LAJTHA. 1977. Conditions controlling the proliferation of haemopoietic stem cells *in vitro*. J. Cell. Physiol. **91:** 335-344.

36. SUTHERLAND, J. H., P. M. LANSDORP, D. H. KENKELMAN, A. C. EAVES & C. J. EAVES. 1990. Functional characterization of individual human hematopoietic stem cells cultured at limiting dilution on supportive marrow stromal layers. Proc. Natl. Acad. Sci. USA **87:** 3584-3588.

37. SUTHERLAND, H. J., C. J. EAVES, P. M. LANSDORP, J. D. THACKER & D. E. HOGGE. 1991. Differential regulation of primitive human hematopoietic cells in long-term cultures maintained on genetically engineered murine stromal cells. Blood **78:** 666-672.

38. LU, D., K. K. WONG, JR., G. PODSAKOFF & S. CHATTERJEE. 1994. Stable and efficient adeno-associated virus-mediated gene transfer into primitive human marrow-derived hematopoietic cells in long term culture. Blood. **84** (Suppl. 1): 360a.

39. PODSAKOFF, G., E. A. SHAUGHNESSY, D. LU, K. K. WONG, JR. & S. CHATTERJEE. 1994. Long term in vivo reconstitution with murine marrow cells transduced with an adeno-associated virus vector. Blood **84** (Suppl.): 256a.

40. FLOTTE, T. R., S. A. AFIONE, C. CONRAD, S. A. MCGRATH, R. SOLOW, H. OKA, P. L. ZEITLIN, W. B. GUGGINO & B. J. CARTER. 1993. Stable in vivo expression of the cystic fibrosis transmembrane conductance regulator with an adeno-associated virus vector. Proc. Natl. Acad. Sci. USA **90:** 10613.

Purification and Expansion of Human Hematopoietic Stem/ Progenitor Cells

CURT I. CIVIN[a] AND DONALD SMALL

Oncology Center
The Johns Hopkins University School of Medicine
Baltimore, Maryland 21287-5001

My10 was the first CD34 antibody[1] and prototype for the CD34 antibody cluster of the International Leukocyte Differentiation Workshops, now including dozens of antibodies against various epitopes of the CD34 antigen.[2-6] The IgG_1 My10 monoclonal antibody is the product of a hybridoma, generated from a mouse immunized with the KG1a myeloid leukemia cell line. My10 was selected as part of a strategy seeking antibodies that specifically recognize small subsets of human marrow cells, but not mature blood or lymphoid cell types. My10 labels KG1a cells intensely, but with a large series of marrow aspirates from healthy adult human donors, My10 specifically detected an average of only 1.5% of low density mononuclear cells.[7,8] My10 labeling of blood cell types was indistinguishable from staining with an irrelevant isotope control immunoglobulin.[9]

My10$^+$ marrow cells were immunoaffinity purified from normal human marrow aspirate cell samples. The My10$^+$ cell population was remarkably enriched in morphologic blast cells, in contrast to the My10$^-$ cell fraction, which contained predominantly recognizable precursor cells at diverse maturation stages of the hematopoietic lineages. Some of the My10$^+$ cells had morphologic features suggesting erythroid commitment, and others had granulocytic, monocytic, megakaryocytic, or lymphoid features. However, most of the My10$^+$ cells did not have lineage-specific morphologic features and could only be classified morphologically as blast or young cells.

Immunoaffinity-purified My10$^+$ marrow and cord blood cells are 10-100-fold enriched in colony-forming units (CFU), whereas My10$^-$ cells are depleted. The My10$^+$ cells include erythroid as well as monocytic and granulocytic colony-forming cells and are particularly enriched in the earliest types of colony-forming cells such as CFU-mix and CFU-blast.[10] A number of laboratories have confirmed that the CD34$^+$ cell population contains essentially all of the hematopoietic colony-forming cells in normal marrow and other hematopoietic stem cell sources. An exception is that a fraction of the most mature unipotent CFU, such as CFU-E and CFU-G, can immunopurify into the My10$^-$ cell fraction. Taken together, this suggests that CD34 at high levels is expressed on the earliest hematopoietic cells and decreases to undetectable levels at about the stage that maturing hematopoietic cells lose the

[a] Address for correspondence: Oncology 3-109, Johns Hopkins Hospital, 600 N. Wolfe St., Baltimore, MD 21287-5001.

capacity to form colonies *in vitro*.[10] The CD34[+] cell population also includes immature lymphoid cells, including all cells expressing terminal deoxynucleotidyl transferase, which is taken to mark the stage at which lymphoid cells rearrange their immunoglobulin or T-cell receptor genes. In analogy to its selective expression on early myeloid and erythroid progenitor cells, CD34 expression falls to undetectable levels on lymphoid cells at the stage marked by the disappearance of nuclear terminal deoxynucleotidyl transferase.

Multicolor flow cytometry was used to define more precisely the cell membrane expression of CD34 on lymphohematopoietic cells. These studies found no detectable CD34[+] cells in cell surface marker-defined mature blood T, B, or NK lymphoid cells. Similarly, blood granulocytes, monocytes, platelets, and red blood cells were shown to be CD34[-]. Among marrow cells, only a small fraction consisting of the earliest cells of each lymphohematopoietic lineage express CD34. For example, early CD34[+] B cells expressing CD19 and CD10 coexpress CD34, whereas later CD20[+] B cells are CD34[-].

The work of many laboratories and three International Leukocyte Differentiation Workshops now confirms that CD34 is expressed selectively on early human hematopoietic cells, but not on cells of the human lymphohematopoietic system beyond the aforementioned early stages of maturation.[6] The cellular expression of human CD34 has been determined by multiple immunologic methods with dozens of CD34 antibodies identifying a range of epitopes on the CD34 antigen and was confirmed using molecular probes.[2,3,6] In addition, recent work to date with probes for murine CD34 mRNA and protein indicates that CD34 expression in mouse follows the same pattern. Thus, CD34 was the first marker to enable identification and purification of hematopoietic progenitor cells, and potentially lymphohematopoietic stem cells, by means of a single reagent.

All CD34 monoclonal antibodies recognize a CD34 protein with electrophoretic mobility corresponding to ~105-115 kD.[2,3] The CD34 transmembrane protein has a relatively short intracellular tail. CD34 is phosphorylated on intracellular serines by protein kinase C, suggesting a role for CD34 in signal transduction. The main portion of the CD34 protein is extracellular and is heavily *N*- and *O*-glycosylated. Extensive terminal sialic acids confer a high negative charge to the molecule and affect its electrophoretic mobility.[11] Indeed, the CD34 cDNA encodes a polypeptide of only ~40 kD. The CD34 cDNA sequence on chromosome 1q32 is unique, with no strong homologies to know genes; however, there are homologies of certain short domains with domains in cellular adhesins.[12-18] Also, broad structural similarities exist between CD34 and sialomucins, especially CD43/leukosialin.[19,20]

Binding of antibodies to CD34 neither down-modulates CD34 expression (even using polyclonal anti-CD34 antibodies or cross-linking of CD34 monoclonals with secondary antibodies) nor affects the proliferation or differentiation of CD34[+] cells.[19] It is unlikely that CD34 is a conventional growth factor receptor. Outside the hematopoietic system, CD34 is expressed only on endothelial cells and embryonic fibroblasts.[21,22] A role for CD34 in endothelial cell adhesion was suggested by electron microscopic studies which localized CD34 to intercellular junctions between human endothelial cells.[23] In mouse, endothelial cell CD34 appears to be a ligand for L-selectin and is involved in the selective binding of lymphocytes to high endothelial venules.[24] Because all endothelial cells express CD34, this observation further suggests that glycosylation variants (glycoforms) of the CD34 molecule exist and that specific CD34 glycoforms may play a role in adhesion of various cell types to endothelium. In addition, it can be speculated that CD34 glycoforms on stem and progenitor cells may govern "homing" of these cells to endothelia or "stroma." Binding of stem and progenitor cells to "nurse cells" via CD34 may transmit intercellular signals between these cells, conceivably involving protein kinase C-mediated CD34 phosphorylation (see above). It will be very interesting to learn the functional effects of overexpression versus knock-out of cellular CD34 expression *in vitro* and *in vivo*.

Incomplete understanding of the physiological role of the CD34 phosphoglycoprotein has not hampered its use as a marker for the identification and purification of early lymphohematopoietic stem progenitor cells. CD34 is widely used in leukemia cell subclassification[25–28] and in progenitor cell estimation for timing of blood progenitor cell harvesting and quality control of *ex vivo* hematopoietic graft processing.[29,30] Several lines of evidence strongly suggest that lymphohematopoietic stem cells, in addition to progenitor cells, express CD34. First, because endothelial and lymphohematopoietic cells are derived embryologically from a common stem cell,[31] expression of CD34 on endothelial cells as well as lymphohematopoietic progenitors would be consistent with an intermediate CD34$^+$ cell, the lymphohematopoietic stem cell. Second, CD34$^+$ cells from subhuman primate marrow can generate hematopoiesis in lethally irradiated animals, whereas CD34$^-$ marrow cells fail to engraft.[32] Third, CD34$^+$ cells generate human hematopoiesis long-term in the human-fetal sheep chimera model.[33] Fourth and most important, purified human CD34$^+$ cell autografts provide prompt engraftment in myeloablated patients with bone marrow transplants.[34–36] Thus, the CD34$^+$ cell population must at least contain long-lived multipotent progenitor cells. Indeed, positive selection of CD34$^+$ autografts by several methods is used in dozens of clinical trials for autologous transplantation of patients with CD34$^-$ tumors and in several gene therapy trials. Current clinical trials using CD34$^+$ cell autografts in bone marrow transplantation should allow determination of whether the CD34$^+$ cell allografts, as opposed to residual host stem cells, provide long-term multilineage lymphohematopoiesis in humans and thus satisfy conclusively the most stringent definition of stem cells.[37] This will be supplemented by studies in mouse models, given the availability of polyclonal and monoclonal antibodies against murine CD34.[38]

Immunopurification of CD34$^+$ cells is now the first step in most research laboratory stem cell purification strategies. Several approaches are available for further purification of human lymphohematopoietic stem cells, taking advantage of markers that subdivide the CD34$^+$ cell population. It is often helpful to use negative immunoaffinity selection to deplete residual mature CD34$^-$ cells that "contaminate" any imperfect CD34$^+$ cell-selected preparation. Panels of CD monoclonal antibodies against "lineage" antigens expressed on mature cells but not on stem cells have been used for this purpose.[39,40] Certain of these antibodies, such as CD19, have the additional benefit of removing a non-stem cell subset of the CD34$^+$ cell population (i.e., the CD34$^+$/CD19$^+$ early B lymphoid cell). Care must be taken to use antibodies that were conclusively shown not to bind to stem cells, as by prompt and sustained engraftment after human transplantation of negatively selected cells.

The most useful single target for purification of the earliest component of the CD34$^+$ cell population is CD38. It was noted serendipitously that CD38 is expressed on most CD34[+] cells, but not on about 1-10%. This tiny population of CD34[+]/CD38[−] cells does not contain cells expressing lineage antigens and is enriched in multipotent progenitor cells.[41,42] Our preliminary results indicate that isolated human CD34[+]/CD38[−] cells transfer retransplantable multilineage human hematopoietic cells in the human-sheep chimera model. CD34[+]/CD38[−] cells have a frequency of ~1:10,000 in human marrow, approaching the estimated frequency of the stem cell.[43] Other markers, such as Thy-1, subdivide the CD34[+]/CD38[−] cell population and therefore may enable further stem cell purification.[39] Based on the selective expression of the FLK2/FLT3/STK1 receptor[44,45] and the restricted action of its ligand (FLT3 ligand) on progenitor cells,[46–48] monoclonal antibodies against STK1 may permit positive selection of stem cells from the CD34[+] cell population.[45] Human bone marrow (or stem cell) transplantation will remain the ultimate means of proving that a population contains human lymphohematopoietic stem cells. Nevertheless, stem cell purification will be greatly aided by the advent of feasible laboratory assays that can provide at least a preliminary measure (ideally a quantitative measure) of human stem cells. The human-immunodeficient mouse assay may apparently meet this need, but stem cell quantification in this assay will be difficult.[49–51]

Available recombinant human hematopoietic growth factors stimulate extensive expansion of isolated CD34[+] cells in 1-2 week *ex vivo* cultures. However, the expanded cells are mainly committed myeloid and erythroid precursor cells. Such preparations of expanded cells might possibly be useful in clinical transplantation for shortening time to a protective neutrophil count.[52] In some systems, human progenitor cells are reported to also be amplified to some degree, but frequencies of the earliest progenitor cells, and inferentially stem cells, appear to decline with time in most, if not all, of these expansion systems.[53] A further deficit is the absence of lymphoid cells in these systems.

Perfusion culture systems engineered to support lymphohematopoiesis are needed to provide expanded stem and progenitor cells for patients, but further understanding of the cell and molecular biology of stem and progenitor cells will also be necessary. To this end, we have begun to identify, then clone, sequence, and determine the physiological roles of novel genes expressed in human stem and progenitor cells. STK1, the human homolog of the FLK2/FLT3 receptor tyrosine kinase,[45] was the first new molecule identified in this search. We hope to find additional molecules that regulate survival, proliferation, and differentiation of lymphohematopoietic stem and progenitor cells in diseased as well as in normal subjects.

SUMMARY

CD34 monoclonal antibodies bind selectively to the most immature 1.5% of low-density human bone marrow mononuclear cells, including terminal deoxynucleotidyl transferase-positive lymphoid precursor cells, all types of *in vitro* assayed hematopoietic progenitor cells, and lymphohematopoietic stem cells capable of reconstituting myeloablated humans in clinical transplantation. Positive selection of highly enriched CD34[+] stem and progenitor cells is widely used in research and is now being investigated in many applications of autologous and allogeneic clinical transplantation. More highly purified stem cells are also desired in research and may have clinical use. Immunoaffinity isolation of CD34[+] cell subsets using antibodies against CD38 permits 10-100-fold further purification of stem cells. It will be valuable to be able to expand stem and progenitor cells from small marrow and blood samples. We are now identifying the genes expressed in stem and progenitor cells to eventually allow the control of stem and progenitor cell survival, proliferation, and differentiation.

REFERENCES

1. CIVIN, C. I., L. C. STRAUSS, C. BROVALL, M. J. FACKLER, J. F. SCHWARTZ & J. H. SHAPER. 1984. Antigenic analysis of hematopoiesis. III. A hematopoietic progenitor cell surface antigen defined by a monoclonal antibody raised against KG-1a cells. J. Immunol. **133:** 157-165.

2. GREAVES, M. F., I. TITLEY, S. M. COLMAN, H.-J. BUHRING, L. CAMPOS, G. L. CASTOLDI, F. GARRIDO, G. GAUDERNACK, J.-P. GIRARD, J. INGLES-ESTEVE, R. INVERNIZZI, W. KNAPP, P. M. LANSDORP, F. LANZA, H. MERLE-BERAL, C. PARRACIVINI, K. RAZAK, F. RUIZ-CABELLO, T. A. SPRINGER, C. E. VAN DER SHOOT & D. R. SUTHERLAND. 1995. M10 CD34 Cluster Workshop Report. *In* Leukocyte Typing. V. White Cell Differentiation Antigens. S. F. Schlossman, L. Boumsell, W. Gilks, J. M. Harlan, T. Kishimoto, C. Morimoto, J. Ritz, S. Shaw, R. Silverstein, T. Springer, T. F. Tedder & R. F. Todd. Vol 1: 840-846. Oxford University Press. New York. In press.

3. CIVIN, C. I., T. M. TRISCHMANN, M. J. FACKLER, I. D. BERNSTEIN, H. J. BUEHRING, L. CAMPOS, M. F. GREAVES, M. KAMOUN, D. R. KATZ, P. M. LANSDORP, A. T. LOOK, B. SEED, D. R. SUTHERLAND, R. W. TINDLE & B. UCHANSKA-ZIEGLER. 1989. Report on the CD34 Cluster Workshop. *In* Leukocyte Typing IV. W. Knapp, B. Dorken, W. R. Gilks, E. P. Rieber, R. E. Schmidt, H. Stein & A. E. G. von dem Borne.: 818-825. Oxford University Press.

4. ANDREWS, R. G., J. W. SINGER & I. D. BERNSTEIN. 1986. Monoclonal antibody 12-8 recognizes a 115-kd molecular present on both unipotent and multipotent hematopoietic colony-forming cells and their precursors. Blood **67:** 842-845.

5. KATZ, R., R. W. TINDLE, D. R. SUTHERLAND & M. D. GREAVES. 1985. Identification of a membrane glycoprotein associated with hemopoietic progenitor cells. Leuk. Res. **9:** 191-198.

6. CIVIN, C. I. 1995. Purification and expansion of human hematopoietic stem cells. *In* Leucocyte Typing. V. White Cell Differentiation Antigens. S. F. Schlossman, L. Boumsell, W. Gilks, J. M. Harlan, T. Kishimoto, C. Morimoto, J. Ritz, S. Shaw, R. Silverstein, T. Springer, T. F. Tedder & R. F. Todd. Vol 1: 869-871. Oxford University Press. New York. In press.

7. LOKEN, M. R., V. O. SHAH, K. L. DATTILIO & C. I. CIVIN. 1987. Flow cytometric analyses of human bone marrow. II. Normal B lymphocyte development. Blood **70:** 1316-1324.

8. LOKEN, M. R., V. O. SHAH, K. DATTILIO & C. I. CIVIN. 1987. Flow cytometric analysis of human bone marrow. I. Normal erythroid development. Blood **69:** 255-263.

9. CIVIN, C. I., M. L. BANQUERIGO, L. C. STRAUSS & M. R. LOKEN. 1987. Antigenic analysis of hematopoiesis VI. Flow cytometric characterization of My-10 positive progenitor cells in normal human bone marrow. Exp. Hematol. **15:** 10-17.

10. STRAUSS, L., S. ROWLEY, S. LA RUSSA, R. STUART & C. CIVIN. 1986. Antigenic analysis of hematopoiesis. V. Characterization of My-10 antigen expression by normal lympho-hematopoietic progenitor cells. Exp. Hematol. **14:** 878-886.

11. FACKLER, M. J., C. I. CIVIN, D. R. SUTHERLAND, M. A. BAKER & W. S. MAY. 1990. Activated protein kinase C directly phosphorylates the CD34 antigen on hematopoietic cells. J. Biol. Chem. **265:** 11056-11061.

12. BROWN, J., M. F. GREAVES & H. V. MOLGAARD. 1991. The gene encoding the stem cell antigen CD34 is conserved in mouse and expressed in haemopoietic progenitor cell lines, brain, and embryonic fibroblasts. Int. Immunol. **3:** 175-184.

13. SIMMONS, D. L., A. B. SATTERTHWAITE, D. G. TENEN & B. SEED. 1992. Molecular cloning of a cDNA encoding CD34, a sialomucin of human hematopoietic stem cells. J. Immunol. **148:** 267–271.

14. NAKAMURA, Y., H. KOMANO & H. NAKAUCHI. 1993. Two alternative forms of cDNA encoding CD34. Exp. Hematol. **21:** 236–243.

15. SUDA, J., T. SUDO, M. ITO, N. OHNO, Y. YAMAGUCHI & T. SUDA. 1992. Two types of murine CD34 mRNA generated by alternative splicing. Blood **79:** 2288–2295.

16. SATTERTHWAITE, A., T. BURN, M. LEBEAU & D. TENEN. 1992. Structure of the gene encoding CD34, a human hematopoietic stem cell antigen. Genomics **12:** 788–794.

17. HE, X., V. ANTAO, J. BASILA MARX & B. DAVIS. 1992. Isolation and molecular characterization of the human CD34 gene. Blood **79:** 2296.

18. MELOTTI, P. & B. CALABRETTA. 1994. Ets-2 and c-myb act independently in regulating expression of the hematopoietic stem cell antigen CD34. J. Biol. Chem. **269:** 25303–25309.

19. FACKLER, M. J., C. I. CIVIN & W. S. MAY. 1992. Up-regulation of surface CD34 is associated with protein kinase C-mediated hyperphosphorylation of CD34. J Biol Chem. **267:** 17540–17546.

20. DELIA, D., M. LAMPAGHANI, M. RESNATI, E. DEJANA, A. AIELLO, E. FONTANELLA, D. SOLIGO, M. PEIROTTI & M. GREAVES. 1993. CD34 expressions is regulated reciprocally with adhesion molecules in vascular endothelial cells in vitro. Blood **81:** 1001–1008.

21. BESCHORNER, W. E., C. I. CIVIN & L. C. STRAUSS. 1985. Localization of hematopoietic progenitor cells in tissue with the anti-My-10 monoclonal antibody. Am J Pathol. **119:** 1–4.

22. FINA, L., H. V. MOLGAARD, D. ROBERTSON, N. J. BRADLEY, P. MONAGHAN, D. DELIA, D. R. SUTHERLAND, M. A. BAKER & M. F. GREAVES. 1990. Expression of the CD34 gene in vascular endothelial cells. Blood **75:** 2417–2426.

23. GREAVES, M. F., J. BROWN, H. V. MOLGAARD, N. K. SPURR, D. ROBERTSDON, D. DELIA & D. R. SUTHERLAND. 1992. Molecular features of CD34: A hemopoietic progenitor cell-associated molecule. Leukemia **6:** 31–36.

24. BAUMHUETER, S., M. S. SINGER, W. HENZEL, S. HEMMERICH, M. RENZ, S. D. ROSEN & L. A. LASKY. 1993. Binding of L-selection to the vascular sialomucin CD34. Science **262:** 436–438.

25. BOROWITZ, M. J., J. J. SHUSTER, C. I. CIVIN, A. J. CARROLL, A. T. LOOK, F. G. BEHM, V. J. LAND, D. J. PULLEN & W. M. CRIST. 1990. Prognostic significance of CD34 expression in childhood B-precursor acute lymphocytic leukemia: A Pediatric Oncology Group study. J. Clin. Oncol. **8:** 1389–1398.

26. PUI, C. H., F. G. BEHM & W. M. CRIST. 1993. Clinical and biologic relevance of immunologic marker studies in childhood acute lymphoblastic leukemia. Blood **82:** 343–362.

27. VAUGHAN, W. P., C. I. CIVIN, D. D. WEISENBURGER, J. E. KARP, M. L. GRAHAM, W. G. SANGER, H. L. GRIERSON, S. S. JOSHI & P. J. BURKE. 1988. Acute leukemia expressing the normal human hematopoietic stem cell membrane glycoprotein CD 34 (MY10). Leukemia **2:** 661–666.

28. HURWITZ, C. A., M. R. LOKEN, M. L. GRAHAM, J. E. KARP, M. J. BOROWITZ, D. J. PULLEN & C. I. CIVIN. 1988. Asynchronous antigen expression in B lineage acute lymphoblastic leukemia. Blood **72:** 299–307.

29. SIENA, S., M. BREGNI, B. BRANDO, N. BELLIS, F. RAVAGNANI, L. GANDOLA, A. C. STERN, P. M. LANDSDORP, G. BONADONNA & A. M. GIANNI. 1991. Flow cytometry for clinical estimation of circulating hematopoietic progenitors for autologous transplantation in cancer patients. Blood **77:** 400–409.

30. TRISCHMANN, T. M., K. G. SCHEPERS & C. I. CIVIN. 1993. Measurement of CD34$^+$ cells in bone marrow by flow cytometry. J. Hematother. **2:** 305–313.

31. HUANG, S. & L. W. M. M. TERSTAPPEN. 1992. Formation of hematopoietic microenvironment and hematopoietic stem cells from single human bone marrow stem cells. Nature **360:** 745-749.

32. BERENSON, R. J., R. G. ANDREWS, W. I. BENSINGER, D. F. KALAMASZ, G. KNITTER & I. D. BERNSTEIN. 1988. Antigen CD34$^+$ marrow cells engraft lethally irradiated baboons. Am. Soc. Clin. Invest. **81:** 951-955.

33. SROUR, E. F., E. D. ZANJANI, K. CORNETTA, C. M. TRAYCOFF, A. W. FLAKE, M. HEDRICK, J. E. BRANDT, T. LEEMHUIS & R. HOFFMAN. 1993. Persistence of human multilineage, self-renewing lymphohematopoietic stem cells in chimeric sheep. Blood **82:** 3333-3342.

34. BERENSON, R. J., W. I. BENSINGER, R. S. HILL, R. G. ANDREWS, J. GARCIA-LOPEZ, D. F. KALAMASZ, B. J. STILL, G. SPITZER, C. D. BUCKNER, I. D. BERNSTEIN *et al.* 1991. Engraftment after infusion of CD34$^+$ marrow cells in patients with breast cancer or neuroblastoma. Blood **77:** 1717-1722.

35. SHPALL, E. J., R. B. JONES, C. JOHNSTON, L. HAMI, S. STEMMER, M. L. AFFRONTI, T. CURIEL & R. J. BERENSON. 1992. Purified CD34 positive (+) marrow progenitor cells provide effective reconstitution for breast cancer (Ca) and non-Hodgkin's lymphoma (NHL) patients receiving high dose chemotherapy with autologous bone marrow support (HDC/ABMS): Recombinant granulocyte colony stimulating factor (G-CSF) accelerates hematopoietic recovery. J. Clin. Oncol. **11:** 59-63.

36. SHPALL, E. J., R. B. JONES, M. H. PURDY, W. A. FRANKLIN, S. HEIMFELD & R. J. BERENSON. 1994. Transplantation of CD34$^+$ marrow and/or peripheral blood progenitor cells (PBPCs) into patients with breast cancer or non-Hodgkin's lymphoma following high dose chemotherapy. Exp. Hematol. **22:** 774-779.

37. JONES, R. J., J. E. WAGNER, P. CELANO, M. S. ZICHA & S. J. SHARKIS. 1990. Separation of pluripotent haematopoietic stem cells from spleen colony-forming cells. Nature **347:** 188-189.

38. KRAUSE, D., T. ITO, M. FACKLER, M. COLLECTOR, S. SHARKIS & W. MAY. 1994. Characterization of murine CD34, a marker for hematopoietic progenitor and stem cells. Blood **84:** 691-701.

39. BAUM, C. M., I. L. WEISSMAN, A. S. TSUKAMOTO, A. M. BUCKLE & B. PEAULT. 1992. Isolation of a candidate human hematopoietic stem-cell population. Proc. Natl. Acad. Sci. USA **89:** 2804-2808.

40. SPRANGRUDE, G. J., S. HEIMFELD & I. L. WEISSMAN. 1988. Purification and characterization of mouse hematopoietic stem cells. Science **241:** 58-62.

41. TERSTAPPEN, L. W. M. M., S. HUANG, M. SAFFORD, P. M. LANSDORP & M. R. LOKEN. 1991. Sequential generations of hematopoietic colonies derived from single nonlineage-committed CD34^{pl} CD38$^-$ progenitor cells. Blood **77:** 1218-1227.

42. TERSTAPPEN, L., D. GANDOUR, S. HUANG, F. LUND-JOHANSEN, K. MANION, M. NGUYEN, R. MICKAELS, J. OLWEUS & S. TOPKER. 1993. Assessment of hematopoietic cell differentiation by multidimensional flow cytometry. J. Hematother. **2:** 431-447.

43. CIVIN, C. I., M. J. LEE & M. HEDRICK. 1993. Purified CD34$^+$/lineage/38-cells contain hematopoietic stem cells. Blood **82:** 180a.

44. MATTHEWS, W., C. T. JORDAN, G. W. WIEGAND, D. PARDOLL & I. R. LEMISCHKA. 1991. A receptor tyrosine kinase specific to hematopoietic stem and progenitor cell-enriched populations. Cell **65:** 1143-1152.

45. SMALL, D., M. LEVENSTEIN, E. KIM, C. CAROW, S. AMIN, P. ROCKWELL, L. WITTE, C. BURROW, M. Z. RATAJCZAK, A. M. GEWIRTZ & C. I. CIVIN. 1994. STK-1, the human homolog of FLK2/FLT3, is selectively expressed in CD34$^+$ human bone marrow cells and is involved in the proliferation of early progenitor/stem cells. Proc. Natl. Acad. Sci. USA **91:** 459-463.

46. LYMAN, S. D., L. JAMES, T. VANDEN BOS, P. DE VRIES, K. BRASEL, B. GLINIAK, L. T. HOLLINGSWORTH, K. S. PICHA, H. J. MCKENNA, R. R. SPLETT, F. A. FLETCHER, E. MARASKOVSKY, T. FARRAH, D. FOXWORTHE, D. E. WILLIAMS & M. P. BECKMANN.

1993. Molecular cloning of a ligand for the flt3/flk-2 tyrosine kinase receptor: A proliferative factor for primitive hematopoietic cells. Cell **75:** 1157-1167.

47. LYMAN, S. D., L. JAMES, J. ZAPPONE, P. R. SLEATH, M. P. BECKMANN & T. BIRD. 1993. Characterization of the protein encoded by the flt3 (flk2) receptor-like tyrosine kinase gene. Oncogene **8:** 815-822.

48. LYMAN, S. D., L. JAMES, S. S. ESCOBAR, K. BRASEL, H. DOWNEY, K. D. STOCKING, M. P. BECKMANN & P. DE VRIES. 1994. Alternative splicing of murine and human FLT3 ligand mRNAs regulates production of cell bound and soluble forms of the protein. Exp. Hematol. **22:** 753-758.

49. LAPIDOT, T., C. SIRARD & J. VORMOOR. 1994. A cell initiating human acute myeloid leukaemia after transplantation into SCID mice. Nature **367:** 645-648.

50. LAPIDOT, T., F. PFLUMIO, M. DOEDENS, B. MURDOCH, D. E. WILLIAMS & J. E. DICK. 1992. Cytokine stimulation of multilineage hematopoiesis from immature human cells engrafted in SCID mice. Science **255:** 1137-1141.

51. CASHMAN, J. D., T. LAPIDOT, L. SCHULTZ, P. LANSDORP, C. J. EAVES & J. DICK. 1994. Presence of CD34⁺THY-1⁺ cells and LTC-IC in SCID mice repopulated with normal human marrow cells. Exp. Hematol. **22:** 838-843.

52. HAYLOCK, D. N., L. B. TO, T. L. DOWSE, C. A. JUTTNER & P. J. SIMMONS. 1992. Ex vivo expansion and maturation of peripheral blood CD34⁺ cells into the myeloid lineage. Blood **80:** 1405-1412.

53. CAUX, C., C. FACRE, S. SAELAND, V. DUVERT, P. MANNONI, I. DURAND, J. P. AUBRY & J. E. DE VRIES. 1989. Sequential loss of CD34 and class II MHC antigens on purified cord blood hematopoietic progenitors cultured with IL-3: Characterization of CD34⁻, HLA-DR⁺ cells. Blood **74:** 1287-1294.

The Potential for Clinical *Ex Vivo* Hematopoiesis

STEPHEN G. EMERSON

Departments of Medicine and Pediatrics
and
Division of Hematology-Oncology
Cancer Center Associate Director for Clinical Research
The University of Pennsylvania
Philadelphia, Pennsylvania 19104

The ability to expand *ex vivo* hematopoietic stem and progenitor cells at will would greatly improve our ability to care for patients, providing a nonlimiting source of hematopoietic cells for the support of compromised patients and perhaps a vehicle for delivering genetic therapies as well. Two distinctive approaches to hematopoietic cell expansion have been taken, with distinctive underlying theories: expansion of CD34 selected cells in liquid culture and perfusion-based expansion of native or selected cells.

HIGH DOSE CYTOKINE EXPANSION OF ENRICHED PROGENITOR CELLS

In the first approach, enriched progenitor cells are cultured in liquid in the presence of large doses of multiple hematopoietic growth factors (HGFa). Thus, the original cell population is first subjected to $CD34^+$ cell selection, and the selected cells are then placed in a 37°C CO_2 incubator for 7-14 days in the presence of high concentrations of interleukin-3 (IL-3), steel factor, IL-6, and sometimes erythropoietin, granulocyte-macrophage colony-stimulating factor (GM-CSF), G-CSF, and even gamma interferon (γ-IFN) as well.

This approach, particularly when practiced with mobilized peripheral blood cells or umbilical cord blood cells, results in significant expansion of precursor and progenitor cells. However, true stem cells apparently are not expanded by these procedures (at least not with bone marrow and peripheral blood) and may likely be lost.

From the clinician's perspective, this approach could be valuable as long as stem cells are not themselves required. In autologous support scenarios in which the patient has not received stem cell toxins during myeloablation, these cells could offer clinical benefit even if stem cells are depleted or lost during culture. However, one would realistically need to feel comfortable that essentially all such patients would have sufficient stem cell pools after myeloablation to present them with the risk of graft failure if no stem cells were reinfused.

Although in the United States this approach has yet to be attempted, studies to test these hypotheses are now underway in Europe. If they are successful, similar studies will undoubtedly occur in the United States, pending collaboration between the many corporate interests controlling the multiple HGFs required for these expansions.

All investigators, however, have found that this approach requires both (1) high doses of multiple cytokines (the more the better), and (2) up-front enrichment of hematopoietic progenitor cells. These requirements raise their own questions. Evidence strongly suggests that high dose cytokines themselves drive early hematopoietic cells out of the stem cell pool, thus reducing the number of long-term repopulating cells. Thus, if these cells are clinically important, the techniques required for late progenitor expansion may promote an increased incidence of late graft failure.

Progenitor cell purification, on the other hand, as it is currently practiced, has little intrinsic benefit. Therefore, progenitor cell enrichment requires an extra, costly step that results in obligate stem and progenitor cell losses as well. In fact, current CD34$^+$ selection techniques only recover 30-50% of clonogenic cells in CD34$^+$ fractions. Motivation for stem and progenitor cell selection comes from two issues distinct from hematopoietic cell expansion: tumor cell contamination and reduction of target cell numbers for gene therapy.

Tumor Cell Contamination. In theory, tumor cell contamination of hematopoietic support grafts should contribute significantly to patient relapse. Therefore, if purified hematopoietic cells could be infused, this source of patient relapse would be eliminated, resulting in patient benefit.

The first efforts at this approach used negative immunoselection (e.g., anti-CD10 for pre-B ALL and *in vitro* chemotherapy (e.g., 4-hydroperoxycytoxan for acute myelogenous leukemia.) Negative selection, however, requires a different technique for each disease and requires that all tumor cells bear the target molecular or sensitivity.

Positive selection, that is, isolating hematopoietic cells directly, has the appeal of being useful in any clinical condition as long as the contaminating tumor cells do not share the characteristic with hematopoietic cells that is being used for selection. To date, the widest studied approach has been positive selection with CD34, the antigen expressed on progenitor and stem cells. At this time, several positives have been achieved. Investigators have demonstrated that: (1) bone marrow and peripheral blood mononuclear cell preparations enriched in CD34$^+$ cells smoothly engraft in autologous and allogeneic transplant settings; (2) reduction in tumor cell contamination of 2+ logs has been achieved in samples contaminated by breast cancer and myeloma cells; (3) CD34+ transplants require very few cells, allowing space savings in blood banks; and (4) CD34+ enrichment can easily be achieved by solid phase immunoabsorption technologies using either beads, columns, or plates.

However, using the technologies that have been widely exploited thus far, neither perfect tumor cell purging nor decreased posttransplant toxicity has been observed. Therefore, it is not clear what clinical benefits would be conferred by using CD34+ selected cells, even though feasible and intellectually satisfying.

Interestingly, although it might have been predicted that CD34+ cells not containing many precursors would provide inferior myeloprotection in the early posttransplant period, this has not yet been observed. This could be true because either (1) precursors contribute little or nothing, even early on; or (2) currently employed CD34+ selection techniques are imperfect, leaving 5-20% precursor and mature cells.

In the near future, the "envelope" of stem cell selection for autologous marrow transplantation will likely be pushed, using highly sophisticated ultra-fast cell sorters in true stem cell preparations that are operationally free (>5 logs) of tumor cells. The time to engraftment in these patients will be carefully observed. If successful, patient survival compared with survival of those undergoing standard autologous bone marrow transplants (ABMTs) will be the key endpoint to evaluate.

Stem Cell Gene Therapy. For permanent correction of disease by hematopoietic cell gene transfer, the most primitive stem cells must be transduced. Because current stem cell transduction techniques are imperfect, the efficiency of stem cell transduction could be improved by stem cell selection before infection. The number of non-target cells would be reduced, thereby effectively increasing the efficiency of the infection. Thus far, however, there is only a little evidence that the barrier to high efficiency stem cell transduction is related to stem cell purity.

PERFUSION-BASED HEMATOPOIETIC CELL EXPANSION

Perfusion-based hematopoietic expansions simply attempt to recreate and augment the hematopoietic physiology that occurs during transplant engraftment. This approach, pioneered by Koller, Palsson, and colleagues, allows for the maintenance and modest amplification of the earliest hematopoietic cells that can be assayed *in vitro* and is in contrast to static cultures of progenitor cells in high dose HGFs in which these cells decay.

Preliminary studies of *ex vivo* perfusion-expanded hematopoietic cells suggest that these cells are well tolerated and that patients who receive these cells in conjunction with standard ABMT have extremely low rates of fever and infection, low blood product utilization, and early hospital discharge. FDA-certified IDE trials of perfusion culture systems for hematopoietic support are currently being established and conducted in the United States.

Perfusion-based hematopoietic expansions can be conducted with a variety of hematopoietic populations, but work best when conducted on a hematopoietic stromal layer which can derived from the initial cell population itself. These perfusion expansion cultures can be performed with highly selected or purged cells and so can be combined with stem cell selection technologies if desired.

One particular ramification of this approach is that it may encourage gene transfer into primitive stem cells by encouraging stem cell division in the perfusion cultures. If so, combination perfusion expansion infection cultures could be a very attractive approach to hematopoietic cell gene therapy.

POTENTIAL CLINICAL USES FOR *EX VIVO* EXPANDED HEMATOPOIETIC CELLS

With full command over hematopoietic cell expansion and differentiation, a wide array of clinical applications can be envisioned (TABLE 1). At the most basic level, *ex vivo* expanded myeloid cells could be used in hematopoietically compromised patients in a variety of settings now seen commonly in clinical hematology/oncology including high dose chemotherapy and autologous and allogeneic bone marrow transplantation. During transplantation, *ex vivo* expansion could be employed both to reduce the morbidity of the induced nadirs and to eliminate the need for operative

TABLE 1. Potential Clinical Application of *Ex Vivo* Expanded Hematopoietic Cells

Myelopoietic Support of Hematopoietically Compromised Host
    Autologous bone marrow transplantation
    Allogeneic bone marrow transplantation
    Non-transplant nadir rescue
    Umbilical cord blood transplantation

***Ex Vivo* Education/Modification of Stem Cells and Derivative Cells**
    T-cell depletion of stem cell grafts for allogeneic bone marrow transplantation
    Active purging of tumor cells from stem cell autographs *in vitro*
    Adoptive immunotherapy via T cells generated and educated *ex vivo*
    Permanent genetic modification of stem cells

harvests or leukephereses. For autologous applications, *ex vivo* cultures and expansions could theoretically be employed for directed tumor purging, both passive purging in culture and active, specific antitumor therapeutics.

A direct extension of myeloid expansion of adult cells is to use *ex vivo* expanded umbilical cord blood cells for hematopoietic support. This approach is intriguing for several reasons. First, fetal and umbilical cord hematopoietic cells clearly have increased proliferative capacity, and fetal and umbilical cord stem cells may have increased capacity for true self-renewal. Second, it is possible, although not yet evident, that lymphoid cells derived from umbilical stem cells may cause less graft-versus-host disease in the allogeneic setting than do postnatally derived lymphoid cells. Third, cord blood cells are truly a wasted resource waiting for medical application, because they are simply discarded at the present time. *Ex vivo* expansion will be very important in the general applicability of umbilical cord blood to routinely provide sufficient numbers of hematopoietic cells for large recipients, whether umbilical cord blood is used either as a large matched-unrelated donor bank or as long-term autologous hematopoietic "insurance."

The ability to control hematopoietic expansion beyond the myeloid lineage could have wider and more sophisticated applications. *Ex vivo* lymphoid expansion from prolymphocytes could allow *ex vivo* education of donor T cells to anti-tumor activity, providing a more sustained and effective approach to adoptive immunotherapy, such as LAK cell therapy. One can envision the simultaneous expansion of myeloid and lymphoid cells before reinfusion, thereby providing both myeloid support and direct, expanded antitumor activities.

Finally, the ability to control and amplify pluripotent stem cell self-renewal and expansion will provide a major boon to stem cell gene therapeutics. For both retroviral and adenovirus-based vectors, stem cell division appears to be a major rate-limiting step to stem cell transduction. The ability to regulate stem cell division *ex vivo* would permit increased levels of stem cell transduction, thus allowing diverse applications of stem cell modification.

CURRENT STATUS OF *EX VIVO* HEMATOPOIETIC EXPANSION: WHAT WE KNOW, WHAT WE DON'T KNOW, AND WHAT WE NEED TO FIND OUT

In summary, we now have only partial knowledge of the biology and applicability of *ex vivo* hematopoiesis in clinical practice. However, we have learned some things, and as a community we are well positioned to ask the proper questions to carefully answer the critical outstanding questions. To summarize our current understanding, we know that hematopoietic cells can be cultured *ex vivo,* resulting in expansion of precursor, progenitors, and long-term culture initiating cells. We know that maintenance of primitive cells is best supported by the presence of an adherent stromal layer, which functions best when it is perfused. These conclusions have been uniformly supported by data with LTCIC expansion, *in vitro* retroviral gene transfer, and *in vivo* persistence of transferred genes. We know that the output of mature cells in a perfusion expansion culture can be widely manipulated by cytokine modulation. Finally, we know that *ex vivo* expanded cells can be reinfused, no obvious complications being observed in the initial patients.

These advances, however, still leave us in need of answers to many critical questions including: Which patients will benefit, in an augmentation setting, from infused *ex vivo* expanded cells: those with ABMT? AlloBMT? PSCT? Nontransplant nadir reduction? Do *ex vivo* expanded cells contain truly permanent repopulating stem cells suitable for allogeneic bone marrow transplantation (6 months? 2 years? >>?). Does permanent reconstitution following autologous transplantation require LTCIC or are progenitors sufficient? Ever? Sometimes? Always? What is the *in vitro* and *in vivo* physiology of bone marrow-derived T cells? Why do umbilical cord blood cell grafts take slowly? Can *ex vivo* expanded umbilical cord blood cells circumvent this problem or will this problem be accentuated in *ex vivo* expanded grafts?

CLINICAL *EX VIVO* EXPANSION: THE IMMEDIATE FUTURE

Given these developments and opportunities, the next 2-3 years will clearly see an explosion in studies of *ex vivo* expanded hematopoietic cells. Autologous bone marrow transplantation augmentation and replacement, allogeneic bone marrow transplantation augmentation and replacement, and high dose chemotherapy support will likely be the initial applications. Expansion of umbilical cord blood hematopoietic cells both to reduce the required amount of umbilical cord blood cells needed for pediatric transplants and to permit adult engraftment will likely follow shortly. Simultaneous genetic modification and expansion of stem cells will also be explored in great detail. Overall, this promises to be an extremely exciting time in clinically applied hematopoiesis research, one in which major clinical benefits will likely result from our increasing ability to gain true control over the fate of hematopoietic stem cells *ex vivo.*

REFERENCES

1. HOLZER, H., J. BIEHL, P. ANTIN, *et al.* 1983. Quantal and proliferative cell cycles: How lineages generate cell diversity and maintain fidelity. Prog. Clin. Biol. Res. **134:** 213–227.

2. BENTLEY, S. A. 1982. Bone marrow connective tissue and the haemopoietic microenvironment. Br. J. Haematol. **50:** 1-6.
3. EMERSON, S. G., Y. C. YANG, S. C. CLARK & M. L. LONG. 1988. Human recombinant granulocyte-macrophage colony stimulating factor and interleukin 3 have overlapping but distinct hematopoietic activities. J. Clin. Invest. **82:** 1282-1287.
4. LEARY, A. G., K. IKEBUCHI, Y. HIRAI et al. 1988. Synergism between interleukin-6 and interleukin-3 in supporting proliferation of human hematopoietic stem cells: Comparison with interleukin-1 alpha. Blood **71:** 1759-1763.
5. TAICHMAN, R. S. & S. G. EMERSON. 1994. Human osteoblasts support hematopoiesis through the production of granulocyte colony stimulating factor. J. Exp. Med. **179:** 1677-1682.
6. GUBA, S. C., C. I. SARTOR, L. R. GOTTSCHALK, J. YE-HU, L. C. XIAO, T. MULLIGAN & S. G. EMERSON. Bone marrow stromal cells secrete IL-6 and GM-CSF in the absence of inflammatory stimuli: Demonstration by serum-free bioassay, ELISA, and reverse transcriptase polymerase chain reaction. Blood **80:** 1190-1198.
7. KESSINGER, A. & J. O. ARMITAGE. 1991. The evolving role of autologous peripheral stem cell transplantation following high-dose therapy for malignancies [editorial]. Blood **77:** 211.
8. HAYLOCK, D. N., L. B. TO, T. L. DOWSE, C. A. JUTTNER & P. J. SIMMONS. 1992. Ex vivo expansion and maturation of peripheral blood CD34$^+$ cells into the myeloid lineage. Blood **80:** 1405-1412.
9. SROUR, E. F., J. E. BRANDT, R. A. BRIDDELL, S. GRIGSBY, T. LEEMHUIS, & R. HOFFMAN. 1993. Long-term generation and expansion of human primitive hematopoietic progenitor cells in vitro. Blood **81:** 661-669.
10. COUTINHO, L. H., A. WILL, J. RADFORD, R. SCHIRO, N. TESTA & T. M. DEXTER. 1990. Blood **75:** 2118-2129.
11. CALDWELL, J., B. LOCEY, M. F. CLARKE, S. G. EMERSON & B. O. PALSSON. 1991. The influence of culture conditions on genetically engineered NIH-3T3 cells. Biotech. Prog. **7:** 1-8.
12. CALDWELL, J., B. LOCEY, B. O. PALSSON & S. G. EMERSON. 1991. The influence of culture perfusion conditions on normal human bone marrow stromal cell metabolism. J. Cell Physiol. **147:** 344-353.
13. SCHWARTZ, R., B. O. PALSSON & S. G. EMERSON. 1991. Rapid medium and serum exchange increases the longevity and productivity of human bone marrow cultures. Proc. Natl. Acad. Sci. USA **88:** 6760-6764.
14. SCHWARTZ, R., S. G. EMERSON, M. F. CLARKE & B. O. PALSSON. 1991. In vitro myelopoiesis stimulated by rapid medium exchange and supplementation with hematopoietic growth factors. Blood **78:** 3155-3161.
15. PALSSON, B. O., S.-H. PAEK, R. M. SCHWARTZ, M. PALSSON, G.-M. LEE, S. SILVER & S. G. EMERSON. 1993. Expansion of human bone marrow progenitor cells in a high cell density continuous perfusion system. Bio/Technology **11:** 368-361.
16. KOLLER, M. R., S. G. EMERSON & B. O. PALSSON. 1993. Large-scale expansion of human hematopoietic stem and progenitor cells from bone marrow mononuclear cells in continuous perfusion culture. Blood **82:** 378-384.
17. SILVER, S. M., P. T. ADAMS, R. J. HUTCHINSON, J. W. DOUVILLE, L. A. PAUL, M. F. CLARKE, B. O. PALSSON & S. G. EMERSON. 1993. Phase I evaluation of ex vivo expanded hematopoietic cells produced by perfusion cultures in autologous bone marrow transplantation. Blood **82** (Suppl. 1): 297a.

Cord Blood Transplantation and the Potential for Gene Therapy

Gene Transduction Using a Recombinant Adeno-Associated Viral Vector[a]

HAL E. BROXMEYER,[b-e] SCOTT COOPER,[b,d]
MARYSE ETIENNE-JULAN,[b,d] XU-SHAN WANG,[c]
SELVARANGAN PONNAZHAGAN,[c]
STEPHEN BRAUN,[b,d] LI LU,[b,d] AND
ARUN SRIVASTAVA [b-d]

*Departments of [b]Medicine (Hematology/Oncology)
[c]Microbiology/Immunology
and
[d]Walther Oncology Center
Indianapolis, Indiana 46202-5121*

Hematopoietic stem and progenitor cells from different tissue sources, including adult bone marrow, growth-factor mobilized adult peripheral blood, and umbilical cord/placental blood collected at the birth of a child have been used for transplantation.[1-6] These transplants were done to repopulate the hematopoietic system of individuals whose blood cells were compromised by disease or by chemotherapy/irradiation treatment to cure a disease. Cord blood is a rich source of hematopoietic stem and progenitor cells, especially of the more immature/primitive subsets of these cells.[7-14] The first successful cord blood transplant was performed in October 1988 for a male with Fanconi anemia using HLA-matched cells from his sister.[15] Now more than 6 years have passed since the transplant. The recipient's blood system is essentially completely repopulated with his sister's cells and he is cured of the hematologic manifestations of Fanconi anemia. Since this initial transplantation performed on the basis of a prior biological assessment of the proliferation of stem/progenitor cells in cord blood,[7] over 60 cord blood transplantations have been per-

[a] The work shown and cited from the authors' laboratories was supported by U.S. Public Health Service grants RO1 HL46549, R37 CA36464, RO1 HL49202, RO1 HL54037, and a project in PO1 HL53586 from the National Institutes of Health (NIH) and the National Cancer Institute to H.E.B., by R29 AI26323, RO1 HL48342, and projects in P50 DK49218 and PO1 HL53586 from the NIH, by an Established Investigator award from the American Heart Association to A.S., and by grants from the Phi Beta Psi Sorority to A.S. and L.L. M.E.J. was supported in part by a grant from the Association de Recherche sur le Cancer, France. S.B. was supported by NIH training program T32 DK07519 to H.E.B.

[e] Address for correspondence: Hal E. Broxmeyer, Ph.D., Walther Oncology Center, Indiana University School of Medicine, 975 West Walnut Street, IB 501, Indianapolis, IN 46202-5121.

formed using complete HLA-matched or, less frequently, 1-, 2-, or 3-HLA antigen disparate sibling cord blood cells.[15–30] This information was obtained through a newly established international cord blood transplant registry.[17,29,31] Transplantations have been done for: Fanconi anemia, aplastic anemia, β-thalassemia, severe combined immunodeficiency, x-linked lymphoproliferative disease, Hurler's syndrome, Hunter's syndrome, Wiskott-Aldrich Syndrome, acute and chronic myelogenous leukemia, acute lymphocytic leukemia, juvenile chronic myelogenous leukemia, myelodysplasia, and neuroblastoma. Of the first 50 evaluated transplants in which HLA-matched or 1-antigen mismatched cord blood was used, the survival of recipients after 1.5 years was about 70%, of which 54% was disease-free survival.[17] Since the initial reports of successful cord blood transplants, banks have been established to store cord blood frozen in cryopreserved form for potential use in autologous and allogeneic transplantation.[32–36] Presently, more than 35 frozen cord blood specimens from such banks, which were unrelated to the recipient and either HLA-matched or 1- to 3-HLA-antigen mismatched, have been used for transplantation. Thirty-five of these unrelated samples came from the cord blood bank directed by Dr. Pablo Rubinstein at the New York Blood Center. Most recipients of unrelated cord blood engrafted. No published reports of these unrelated cord blood transplants currently exist. All related and most unrelated transplants were performed in children. The weight of the heaviest recipient thus far transplanted and engrafted with cord blood is about 70 kg. One 40-kg child with acute lymphoblastic leukemia underwent transplantation at the Indiana University School of Medicine directed by Drs. David Emanuel and Franklin Smith with unrelated cord blood cells from the New York Blood Center's cord blood bank. Of interest and clinical relevance is the limited graft-versus-host disease noted in related and unrelated cord blood transplants. This may reflect the low immune reactivity of cord blood T lymphocytes[37–39] and natural killer cells.[40]

Primitive progenitors in cord blood have phenotypically been characterized as being $CD34^{3+}$,[11] $CD34^{+}CD45RA^{lo}CD71^{lo}$,[12] $CD34^{+}CD38^{-}$,[13] $CD34^{+}thy1^{+}$,[41] and $CD34^{+}HLA-DR^{+}$.[42,43] Functionally these cells are slowly cycling,[42–45] but very sensitive when stimulated to proliferate.[7–14] They have high proliferative and replating capacity[7–14,46] and can be greatly expanded *ex vivo*.[8,10,12,13,42,43,45,47–52] Stem/progenitor cells from human cord blood also can extensively engraft the marrow of sublethally irradiated mice with severe combined immunodeficiency disease.[53,54]

Many questions remain regarding umbilical cord blood hematopoietic stem and progenitor cells and their use in transplantation. These questions, which have been discussed elsewhere,[55] include: the use of cord blood for transplantation of adults, the potential uniqueness of stem and progenitor cells in cord blood, the possibility of *ex vivo* expansion of long-term marrow repopulating cells in cord blood, the immunologic reactivity of cord blood cells, the separation of cord blood stem and progenitor cells for use in transplantation, the banking of cord blood cells in a cryopreserved form, and the use of these cells for gene transduction and possible gene therapy to treat genetic or other disorders. This latter possibility forms the basis for our experiments with the use of adeno-associated viral (AAV) vectors to place new genetic material into stem/progenitor cells from human cord blood.

Both retroviral[56–61] and AAV[62,63] vectors have been used to place genes into more mature subsets of stem cells and immature and mature subsets of progenitor cells

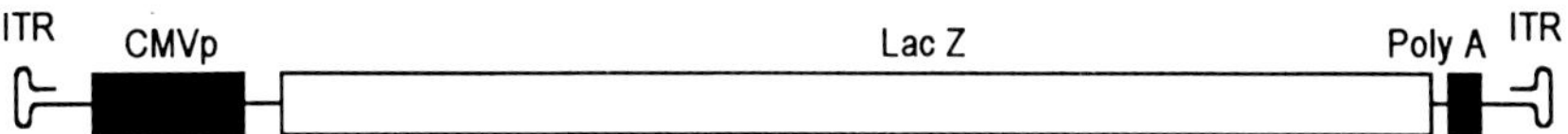

vCMVp-Lac Z

FIGURE 1. Schematic representation of recombinant adeno-associated viral vector containing the *lacZ* gene under the control of a cytomegalovirus (CMV) promoter (p). The *lacZ* gene contained a nuclear localization factor. ITR = inverted terminal repeat.

from cord blood. The present study involves the use of a recombinant AAV vector containing the CMV promoter-driven β-galactasidase (*lacZ*) gene to demonstrate efficient transduction and expression of the β-galactasidase gene in immature subsets of myeloid progenitor cells from cord blood.

MATERIALS AND METHODS

Cells and Cell Separation. Cells were obtained from normal human umbilical cord blood scheduled to be discarded after delivery of the infant and after the prior need for samples for clinical study had been satisfied. Low-density cells were obtained after density cut using Ficoll-Hypaque (density, 1.077 g/cm^3; Pharmacia Piscataway, New Jersey. CD34^{3+} cells were obtained after sorting nonadherent low-density T-lymphocyte-depleted cells on a FACS Star Plus Cell Sorter (Becton-Dickinson, San Jose, California.)[57] This population was >98% pure for cells expressing the CD34 antigen. CD3^{3+} cells included 20% of CD34 antigen-expressing cells with highest density distribution of CD34 antigens. This fraction is richest in stem/progenitor cells.[11]

Vector and Transduction Procedure. A diagram of the recombinant AAV vector used, vCMVp-LacZ, is shown in Figure 1. This vector was prepared in a manner similar to that used for a vector containing the neo-phosphotransferase sequence,[62] except that expression of LacZ was driven by the cytomegalovirus (CMV) promoter. Freshly isolated low-density or CD34^{3+} cord blood cells were either mock-infected or infected with vCMVp-LacZ virions at a multiplicity-of-infection of 1 as described elsewhere for other viral vectors before washing the cells twice and plating them in semisolid culture medium for assessment of progenitor cells.[62]

Colony Assays and Detection of β-gal$^+$ Cells. Low-density (2.5 × 10^4/ml) or CD34^{3+} (200/ml) cells were plated in 1% methylcellulose culture medium with 30% fetal bovine serum (Hyclone, Logan, Utah) in the presence of 1 U/ml recombinant human (rhu) erythropoietin (Epo; purchased from Amgen, Thousand Oaks, California), 100 U/ml rhu granulocyte-macrophage colony-stimulating factor (GM-CSF), 100 U/ml rhu interleukin (IL)-3, and 50 ng/ml rhu steel factor (SLF) for assessment of immature subsets of granulocyte-macrophage (CFU-GM) and multipotential (CFU-GEMM) progenitor cells and in the presence of these concentrations of Epo, GM-CSF, and IL-3 for assessment of more mature subsets of CFU-GM and BFU-E.[8] GM-CSF, IL-3, and SLF were kind gifts from Immunex Corp, Seattle, Washington.

TABLE 1. Transduction of Immature Subsets of Cord Blood Myeloid Progenitor Cells with a Recombinant Adeno-Associated Viral (AAV)-LacZ Vector[a]

| | β-Gal+ Colonies (%) | |
Cells	CFU-GM	CFU-GEMN
Mock-infected	5 ± 2 (1–9)[b]	10 ± 2 (4–14)
vCMVp-LacZ-infected	28 ± 12[c] (7–59)	53 ± 5[c] (45–67)

[a] Low-density or CD34^{3+} cord blood cells were either mock infected or infected with the recombinant AAV-LacZ virions. Cells were treated and plated as described in Materials and Methods. Colonies containing β-galactosidase-expressing cells were assessed after 14 days of incubation for cells from four separate experiments (two using low-density cells and two using CD34^{3+} cells with over 1,000 colonies evaluated). Although the *lacZ* gene contained a nuclear localization factor, no attempts were made to distinguish nuclear from cytoplasmic staining in these experiments. Results are expressed as mean ± 1 SEM.

[b] Range of percentages of β-gal+ colonies.

[c] Significant difference from mock-treated cells by Student's *t* test, $p < 0.001$.

We previously demonstrated[8] and it has been substantiated[10] that in the presence of SLF (also called stem cell factor) with other colony-stimulating factors, CFU-GEMM but not BFU-E colonies can be detected in cord blood. Thus, results are shown for CFU-GM and CFU-GEMM when cord blood is stimulated with Epo, GM-CSF, IL-3, and SLF. Colonies were scored after 14 days of incubation in 5% CO_2 and lowered (5%) O_2. Twenty-four hours before scoring the colonies, a 0.1-ml solution containing 150 μg X-galactoside was added to all 1-ml plates.

RESULTS AND DISCUSSION

To evaluate the expression of new genetic material transduced into myeloid progenitor cells from cord blood, we used a recombinant AAV vector containing the *LacZ* gene under the control of the CMV promoter. As shown in TABLE 1, we detected expression of β-galactosidase in the progeny (cells within colonies) of immature subsets of CFU-GM and CFU-GEMM incubated with the vCMVp-LacZ AAV vector and then stimulated to proliferate in semisolid culture medium in the presence of the combination of Epo, GM-CSF, IL-3, and SLF. The results shown are averages from four separate experiments in which either low-density ($n = 2$) or CD34^{3+} ($n = 2$) cells were transduced. Some background staining of colonies derived from mock-treated cells was detected, but the percentage of β-gal+ colonies deriving from the lacZ-containing vector-infected cells was significantly higher and many times greater than that of the mock-infected cells. It is not clear what caused the background staining, but this may represent endogenous expression of proteins that can act on the X-gal substrate. The background level of β-gal+ colonies varied from 1–14%, making it clear that the true expression potential of such transduced cells cannot be assessed without an appropriate control. Examples of positive transduced and negative control colonies are shown in FIGURE 2a–d. As seen in FIGURE 2e–h, expression of β-gal was also seen in colonies deriving from more mature subsets of CFU-GM and BFU-E transduced with the *lacZ* gene and stimulated to form colonies with Epo, GM-CSF, and IL-3. Variability was noted between colonies in the percentage of β-gal⁺ cells per colony. It is currently not clear if gene expression occurs in only a portion of transduced cells. Actual transduction efficiency determination awaits analysis by polymerase chain reaction amplification of the DNA of the transduced gene from colony cells.

The use of recombinant AAV vectors to efficiently transduce cord blood stem/progenitors with genes does not appear to require preincubation of the cells with growth factors[62] as is necessary for high efficiency transduction of these cells with retroviral vectors.[59] Because preincubation of stem/progenitor cells with growth factors could possibly cause differentiation of the earliest cells, those with long-term marrow-repopulating ability that would be desirable to transduce, the use of AAV vectors in some circumstances may be more advantageous than that of retroviral vectors. The lack of the need for growth factor preincubation for efficient transduction with AAV vectors of slow or noncycling cells, such as those found in cord blood,[40–45] does not mean that cell division is not necessary for integration of the gene. Integration of new genetic material may still require cell division which can occur in response to growth factors after the preincubation phase in which cells are exposed to viral vectors.

For gene transduction with recombinant AAV vectors to be of use in gene therapy, it is important to know if expression of the introduced gene is still high after expansion of the transduced cell population *in vivo* or *ex vivo*. In this context, we expanded immature subsets of cord blood CFU-GM and CFU-GEMM, after 7 days in suspension culture with a combination of growth factors, by greater than 60- and 6-fold, respectively, with maintenance of high level expression of the *lacZ* gene introduced by the recombinant AAV-LacZ vector (unpublished data). Although more experimentation is needed in this area, the results suggest that long-term expression of genes introduced by recombinant AAV vectors may be possible. Unfortunately, without a quantitative assay for human stem cells with long-term marrow-repopulating capacity,[64] we do not yet know the transduction efficiency of this cell type and whether this cell is expanded, maintained, or lost after efforts at *ex vivo* expansion of these rare but important cells.

In the future it may be possible to enhance *ex vivo* expansion of stem and progenitor cells by placing genes into these cells for cytokines or receptors for cytokines. Moreover, recent preliminary studies using retroviral vectors suggest that stem/progenitor cells purified from cryopreserved cord blood could be transduced with high efficiency and expanded *ex vivo* with stable integration and expression of the introduced gene.[65] Also, transduced cells could be frozen and recovered with the thawed cells expressing the introduced gene.[66] The latter reports[65,66] suggest that it may be possible to alter stem and progenitor cells by introducing new genetic material either before or after banking these cells in a cryopreserved state.

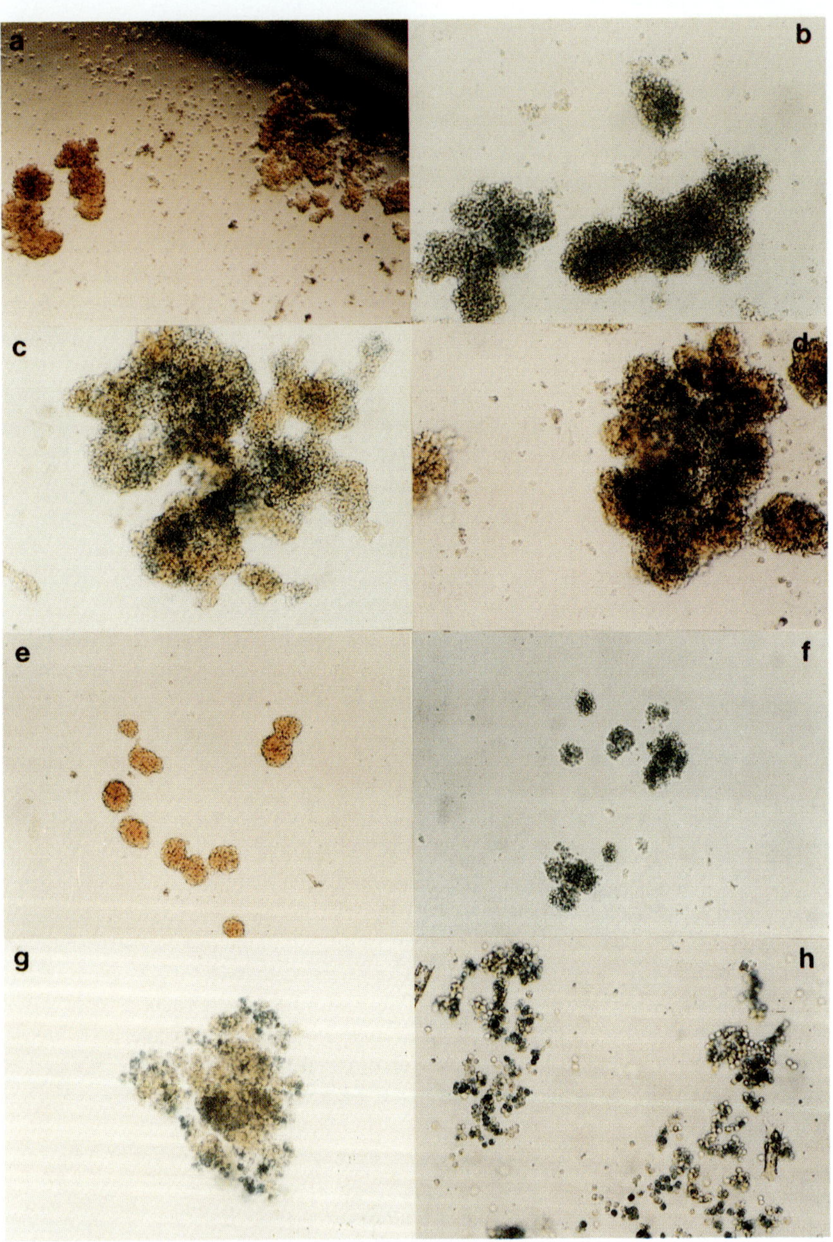

FIGURE 2. Examples of expression of the β-galactosidase gene in cells of colonies derived from multipotential (CFU-GEMM) (**b–d**) and erythroid (BFU-E) (**f** and **g**) and granulocyte-macrophage (CFU-GM) (**h**) progenitor cells from CD34^{3+} cord blood cells transduced with the recombinant adeno-associated viral (AAV) LacZ vector. Magnification × 40. The CFU-GEMM colonies were photographed after 14 days of incubation of cells grown in the presence of Epo, IL-3, GM-CSF, and SLF, whereas BFU-E and CFU-GM colonies were photographed after growth of cells in the presence of Epo, IL-3, and GM-CSF. Panels **a** and **e**, respectively, show CFU-GEMM and BFU-E colonies derived from mock-infected cells, which did not stain.

SUMMARY

Cord blood, which contains a high frequency of immature stem/progenitor cells with extensive proliferative and replating capacity *in vitro* was used as a clinical source of transplantable stem and progenitor cells. These cells can be efficiently transduced with new genetic material by using AAV or retroviral vectors. Using a recombinant AAV vector, high level expression of the *lacZ* gene under a CMV promoter was demonstrated in immature subsets of cord blood progenitor cells.

REFERENCES

1. BROXMEYER, H. E. 1995. Cord blood as an alternative source for stem and progenitor cell transplantation. Current Opin. Pediatr. **7:** 47-55.
2. BROXMEYER, H. E. 1994. Clinical and biological aspects of human umbilical cord blood transplantation for disease. *In* Hemopoietic Growth Factors, Oncogenes and Cytokines in Clinical Hematology. E. Cacciola, A. B. Deisseroth & R. Giustolisi, Eds.: 284-298. Basel. Karger.
3. BROXMEYER, H. E., L. LU, J. GADDY, L. RUGGIERI, A. SRIVASTAVA & G. RISDON. 1994. Human umbilical cord blood transplantation: The immunology, expansion, and therapeutic applications of hematopoietic stem and progenitor cells. *In* Hematopoietic Stem Cells: Biology and Therapeutic Applications. D. J. Levitt & R. Mertelsmann, Eds.: 297-317. Marcel Dekker Publishers. New York.
4. BROXMEYER, H. E. 1994. Cord blood stem cells. *In* Scientific Basis of Transfusion Medicine: Implications for Clinical Practice. K. C. Anderson & P. M. Ness, Eds.: 499-506. W. B. Saunders Co. Philadelphia.
5. LU, L., R. N. SHEN & H. E. BROXMEYER. 1995. Stem cells from bone marrow, umbilical cord blood and peripheral blood for clinical application: Current status and future application. Crit. Rev. Oncol/Hematol. In press.
6. THOMAS, E. D. 1991. Frontiers in bone marrow transplantation. Blood Cells **17:** 259-267.
7. BROXMEYER, H. E., G. W. DOUGLAS, G. HANGOC, S. COOPER, J. BARD, D. ENGLISH, M. ARNY, L. THOMAS & E. A. BOYSE. 1989. Human umbilical cord blood as a potential source of transplantable hematopoietic stem/progenitor cells. Proc. Natl. Acad. Sci. USA **86:** 3828-3832.
8. BROXMEYER, H. E., G. HANGOC, S. COOPER, R. C. RIBEIRO, V. GRAVES, M. YODER, J. WAGNER, S. VADHAN-RAJ, L. BENNINGER, P. RUBINSTEIN & E. R. BROUN. 1992. Growth characteristics and expansion of human umbilical cord blood and estimation of its potential for transplantation in adults. Proc. Natl. Acad. Sci. USA **89:** 4109-4113.
9. HOWS, J. M., B. A. BRADLEY, J. C. W. MARSH, T. LUFT, L. COUTINHO, N. G. TESTA & T. M. DEXTER. 1992. Growth of human umbilical-cord blood in long term haematopoietic cultures. Lancet **340:** 73-76.
10. MIGLIACCIO, G., A. R. MIGLIACCIO, M. L. DRUZIN, P. J. V. GIARDINA, K. M. ZSEBO & J. W. ADAMSON. 1992. Long-term generation of colony-forming cells in liquid culture of CD34$^+$ cord blood cells in the presence of recombinant human stem cell factor. Blood **79:** 2620-2627.
11. LU, L., M. XIAO, R. N. SHEN, S. GRIGSBY & H. E. BROXMEYER. 1993. Enrichment, characterization, and responsiveness of single primitive CD34^{+++} human umbilical cord blood hematopoietic progenitors with high proliferative and replating potential. Blood **81:** 41-48.
12. LANSDORP, P. M., W. DRAGOWSKA & H. MAYANI. 1993. Ontogeny-related changes in proliferative potential of human hematopoietic cells. J. Exp. Med. **178:** 787-791.
13. CARDOSO, A. A., M. L. LI, P. BATARD, A. HATZFELD, E. L. BROWN, J. P. LEVESQUE, H. SOOKDEO, B. PANTERNE, P. SANSILVESTRI, S. C. CLARK & J. HATZFELD. 1993. Release

from quiescence of CD34$^+$ CD38$^-$ human umbilical cord blood cells reveals their potentiality to engraft adults. Proc. Natl. Acad. Sci. USA **90:** 8707–8711.

14. CAROW, C., G. HANGOC & H. E. BROXMEYER. 1993. Human multipotential progenitor cells (CFU-GEMM) have extensive replating capacity for secondary CFU-GEMM: An effect enhanced by cord blood plasma. Blood **81:** 942–949.

15. GLUCKMAN, E., H. E. BROXMEYER, A. D. AUERBACH, H. S. FRIEDMAN, G. W. DOUGLAS, A. DEVERGIE, H. ESPEROU, D. THIERRY, G. SOCIE, P. LEHN, S. COOPER, D. ENGLISH, J. KURTZBERG, J. BARD & E. A. BOYSE. 1989. Hematopoietic reconstitution in a patient with Fanconi's anemia by means of umbilical-cord blood from an HLA-identical sibling. N. Engl. J. Med. **321:** 1174–1178.

16. WAGNER, J. E., H. E. BROXMEYER, R. L. BYRD, B. ZEHNBAUER, B. SCHMECKPEPER, N. SHAH, C. GRIFFIN, P. D. EMANUEL, K. S. ZUCKERMAN, S. COOPER, C. CAROW, W. BIAS & G. W. SANTOS. 1992. Transplantation of umbilical cord blood after myeloablative therapy: Analysis of engraftment. Blood **79:** 1874–1881.

17. WAGNER, J. E., N. A. KERNAN, H. E. BROXMEYER & E. GLUCKMAN. 1994. Transplantation of umbilical cord blood in 50 patients: Analysis of the registry data (abstr.) Blood **84**(Suppl 1): 395a.

18. KOHLI-KUMAR, M., N. T. SHAHIDI, H. E. BROXMEYER, M. MASTERSON, C. DELAAT, J. SAMBRANO, C. MORRIS, A. D. AUERBACH & R. E. HARRIS. 1993. Haematopoietic stem/ progenitor cell transplant in Fanconi anaemia using HLA-matched sibling umbilical cord blood cells. Br. J. Haematol. **85:** 419–422.

19. BOGDANIC, V., D. NEMET, A. KASTELAN, V. LATIN, M. PETROVECKI, L. BRKLJACIC-SURLAKOVIC, V. KERHIN-BRKLJACIC, I. AURER, J. KONJA, M. MRSIC, S. KALENIC & B. LABAR. 1992. Umbilical cord blood transplantation in a patient with Philadelphia chromosome-positive chronic myeloid leukemia. Transplantation **56:** 477–479.

20. VOWELS, M. R., R. LAM-PO-TANG, V. BERDOUKAS, D. FORD, D. THIERRY, D. PURTILO & E. GLUCKMAN. 1993. Brief Report: Correction of x-linked lymphoproliferative disease by transplantation of cord-blood stem cells. N. Engl. J. Med. **329:** 1623–1625.

21. VOWELS, M. R., K. TIEDEMANN, R. LAM-PO-TANG & D. P. TUCKER. 1994. Use of granulocyte-macrophage colony stimulating factor in two children treated with cord blood transplantation. Blood Cells **20:** 249–255.

22. PAHWA, R. N., A. FLEISCHER, S. THAN & R. A. GOOD. 1994. Successful hematopoietic reconstitution with transplantation of erythrocyte-depleted allogeneic human umbilical cord blood cells in a child with leukemia. Proc. Natl. Acad. Sci. USA **91:** 4485–4488.

23. PAHWA, R. N., A. FLEISCHER, S. SHIH, D. UCKAN, S. DURHAM, P. GAROFALO, G. KARAYALCIN, A. SHENDE, A. REDNER, C. PALEY, R. A. GOOD & P. LANZKOWSKY. 1994. Erythrocyte-depleted allogeneic human umbilical cord blood transplantation. Blood Cells **20:** 267–274.

24. KERNAN, N. A., M. L. SCHROEDER, D. CIAVARELLA, R. A. PRETI, P. RUBINSTEIN & R. J. O'REILLY. 1994. Umbilical cord blood infusion in a patient for correction of Wiskott Aldrich Syndrome. Blood Cells **20:** 245–248.

25. ISSARAGRISIL, S. 1994. Cord blood transplantation in thalassemia. Blood Cells **20:** 259–263.

26. KURTZBERG, J., M. GRAHAM, J. CASEY, J. OLSEN, C. STEVENS & P. RUBINSTEIN. 1994. The use of umbilical cord blood in mismatched related and unrelated hemopoietic stem cell transplantation. Blood Cells **20:** 275–284.

27. VILMER, E., E. QUELVENNEC, E. PLOUVIER, E. DENAMUR, P. ROHRLICH, J. ELION & G. STERKERS. 1994. HLA mismatched cord blood transplantation immunological studies. Blood Cells **20:** 235–241.

28. VILMER, E., G. STERKERS, C. RAHIMY, E. DENAMUR, J. ELION, A. BROYART, B. LESCOEUR, J. M.TIERCY, J. GEROTA & J. BLOT. 1992. HLA mismatched cord blood transplantation in a patient with advanced leukemia. Transplantation **53:** 1128–1134.

29. WAGNER, J. E., N. A. KERNAN, M. STEINBACH, H. E. BROXMEYER & E. GLUCKMAN. 1995. Allogeneic sibling umbilical cord blood transplantation in forty-four children with malignant and non-malignant diseases. Lancet **346:** 214–219.

30. ISSARAGRISIL, S., S. VISUTHISAKCHAI, V. SUVATTE, V. S. TANPHAICHITR, D. CHANDANAYINGYONG, T. SCHREINER, S. KANOKPONGSAKDI, N. SIRITARARATKUL & A. PIANKIJAGUM. 1995. Transplantation of cord blood stem cells into a patient with severe thalassemia. N. Engl. J. Med. **332:** 367-369.

31. GLUCKMAN, E., J. WAGNER, J. HOWS, N. KERNAN, B. BRADLEY & H. E. BROXMEYER. 1993. Cord blood banking for hematopoietic stem cell transplantation: An international cord blood transplant registry. Bone Marrow Transplant. **11:** 199-200.

32. RUBINSTEIN, P., R. E. ROSENFIELD, J. W. ADAMSON & C. E. STEVENS. 1993. Stored placental blood for unrelated bone marrow reconstitution. Blood **81:** 1679-1690.

33. RUBINSTEIN, P., P. E. TAYLOR, A. SCARADAVOU, J. W. ADAMSON, G. MIGLIACCIO, D. EMANUEL, R. L. BERKOWITZ, E. ALVAREZ & C. E. STEVENS. 1994. Unrelated placental blood for bone marrow reconstitution: Organization of the placental blood program. Blood Cells **20:** 587-600.

34. GLUCKMAN, E. 1994. European organisation for cord blood banking. Blood Cells **20:** 601-608.

35. McCULLOUGH, J., M. E. CLAY, S. FAUTSCH, H. NOREEN, M. SEGALL, E. PERRY & D. STRONCEK. 1994. Proposed policies and procedures for the establishment of a cord blood bank. Blood Cells **20:** 609-626.

36. VAN ROOD, J. J. 1994. Commentary: Cord blood banking for bone marrow reconstitution: A need for standardization and international cooperation. Blood Cells **20:** 627-629.

37. RISDON, G., J. GADDY, F. B. STEHMAN & H. E. BROXMEYER. 1994. Proliferative and cytotoxic responses of human cord blood T lymphocytes following allogeneic stimulation. Cell. Immunol. **154:** 14-24.

38. RISDON, G., J. GADDY & H. E. BROXMEYER. 1994. Allogeneic responses of human umbilical cord blood. Blood Cells **20:** 566-572.

39. RISDON, G., J. GADDY, M. HORIE & H. E. BROXMEYER. 1995. Alloantigen priming induces a state of unresponsiveness in human cord blood T cells. Proc. Natl. Acad. Sci. USA **92:** 2413-2417.

40. GADDY, J., G. RISDON & H. E. BROXMEYER. 1995. Cord blood natural killer cells are functionally and phenotypically immature but readily respond to IL-2 and IL-12. J. Interferon and Cytokine Res. **15:** 527-536.

41. MAYANI, H. & P. M. LANSDORP. 1994. Thy-1 expression is linked to functional properties of primitive hematopoietic progenitor cells from human umbilical cord blood. Blood **83:** 2410-2417.

42. TRAYCOFF, C. M., M. R. ABBOUD, J. LAVER, J. E. BRANDT, R. HOFFMAN, P. LAW, L. ISHIZAWA & E. F. SROUR. 1994. Evaluation of the in vitro behavior of phenotypically defined populations of umbilical cord blood hematopoietic progenitor cells. Exp. Hematol. **22:** 215-222.

43. TRAYCOFF, C. M., M. R. ABBOUD, J. LAVER, D. W. CLAPP, R. HOFFMAN, P. LAW & E. F. SROUR. 1994. Human umbilical cord blood hematopoietic progenitor cells: Are they the same as their adult bone marrow counterparts? Blood Cells **20:** 382-391.

44. LU, L., M. XIAO, S. GRIGSBY, W. X. WANG, W. WU, R. N. SHEN & H. E. BROXMEYER. 1993. Comparative effects of suppressive cytokines on isolated single CD34^{+++} stem/progenitor cells from human bone marrow and umbilical cord blood plated with and without serum. Exp. Hematol. **31:** 1442-1446.

45. MOORE, M. A. S. & I. HOSKINS. 1994. Ex vivo expansion of cord blood derived stem cells and progenitors. Blood Cells **20:** 468-481.

46. NAKAHOTA, T. & M. OGAWA. 1982. Hematopoietic colony forming cells in umbilical cord blood with extensive capability to generate mono- and multipotential hematopoietic progenitors. J. Clin. Invest. **70:** 1324-1328.

47. RUGGIERI, L., S. HEIMFELD & H. E. BROXMEYER. 1994. Cytokine-dependent ex vivo expansion of early subsets of CD34$^+$ cord blood myeloid progenitors is enhanced by cord blood plasma, but expansion of the more mature subsets of progenitors is favored. Blood Cells **20:** 436-454.

48. XIAO, M., H. E. BROXMEYER, M. HORIE, S. GRIGSBY & L. LU. 1994. Extensive proliferative capacity of single isolated CD34^{+++} human cord blood cells in suspension culture. Blood Cells **20:** 455–467.

49. VAN ZANT, G., S. A. RUMMEL, M. R. KOLLER, D. B. LARSON, I. DRUBACHEVSKY, M. PALSSON & S. G. EMERSON. 1994. Expansion in bioreactors of human progenitor populations from cord blood and mobilized peripheral blood. Blood Cells **20:** 482–491.

50. HEIMFELD, S., D. F. KALAMASZ, B. L. FOGARTY, R. FEI, Z. N. TSUI, H. M. JONES & R. J. BERENSON. 1994. Isolation and ex vivo expansion of CD34$^+$ cells from cord blood using dextran sedimentation and avidin column selection. Blood Cells **20:** 397–403.

51. VAN EPPS, D. E., J. BENDER, W. LEE, M. SCHILLING, A. SMITH, S. SMITH, K. UNVERZAGT, P. LAW & J. BURGESS. 1994. Harvesting, characterization and culture of CD34$^+$ cells from human bone marrow, peripheral blood and cord blood. Blood Cells **20:** 411–423.

52. LEBKOWSKI, J. S., L. SCHAIN, M. HALL, M. WYSOCKI, B. DADEY & W. BIDDLE. 1994. Rapid isolation and serum-free expansion of human CD34$^+$ cells. Blood Cells **20:** 404–410.

53. VORMOOR, J., T. LAPIDOT, F. PFLUMIO, G. RISDON, B. PATTERSON, H. E. BROXMEYER & J. E. DICK. 1994. Immature human cord blood progenitors engraft and proliferate to high levels in severe combined immunodeficient mice. Blood **83:** 2489–2497.

54. ORAZI, A., S. E. BRAUN & H. E. BROXMEYER. 1994. Immunohistochemistry represents a useful tool to study human cell engraftment in SCID mice transplantation models. Blood Cells **20:** 323–330.

55. BROXMEYER, H. E. 1995. Questions to be answered regarding umbilical cord blood hematopoietic stem and progenitor cells and their role in transplantation. Transfusion. **35:** 694–702.

56. MORITZ, T., D. C. KELLER & D. A. WILLIAMS. 1993. Human cord blood cells as targets for gene transfer: Potential use in genetic therapies of severe combined immunodeficiency disease. J. Exp. Med. **178:** 529–536.

57. LU, L., M. XIAO, D. W. CLAPP, Z. H. LI & H. E. BROXMEYER. 1993. High efficiency retroviral ediated gene transduction into single isolated immature and replatable CD34^{+++} hematopoietic stem/progenitor cells from human umbilical cord blood. J. Exp. Med. **178:** 2089–2096.

58. LU, L., M. XIAO, D. W. CLAPP, Z. H. LI & H. E. BROXMEYER. 1994. Stable integration of retrovirally transduced genes into human umbilical cord blood high-proliferative potential colony forming cells (HPP-CFC) as assessed after multiple HPP-CFC colony replatings in vitro. Blood Cells **20:** 525–530.

59. SHI, Y. J., R. N. SHEN, L. LU & H. BROXMEYER. 1994. Comparative analysis of retroviral-mediated gene transduction into CD34$^+$ cord blood hematopoietic progenitors in the presence and absence of growth factors. Blood Cells **20:** 517–524.

60. HANLEY, M. E., J. A. NOLTA, R. PARKMAN & D. B. KOHN. 1994. Umbilical cord blood cell transduction by retroviral vectors: Pre-clinical studies to optimize gene transfer. Blood Cells **20:** 539–546.

61. WILLIAMS, D. A. & T. MORITZ. 1994. Umbilical cord blood stem cells as targets for genetic modification: New therapeutic approaches to somatic gene therapy. Blood Cells **20:** 504–516.

62. ZHOU, S. Z., S. COOPER, L. Y. KANG, L. RUGGIERI, S. HEIMFELD, A. SRIVASTAVA & H. E. BROXMEYER. 1994. Adeno-associated virus 2-mediated high efficiency gene transfer into immature and mature subsets of hematopoietic progenitor cells in human umbilical cord blood. J. Exp. Med. **179:** 1867–1875.

63. SRIVASTAVA, A. 1994. Parvovirus-based vectors for human gene therapy. Blood Cells **20:** 531–538.

64. BROXMEYER, H. E. 1994. Consequences of human stem cells taking up residence in sheep. J. Clin. Invest. **93:** 919.

65. Lu, L., Y. Ge, Z. H. Li, B. Freie, D. W. Clapp & H. E. Broxmeyer. 1995. CD34^{+++} stem/progenitor cells purified from cryopreserved normal cord blood can be transduced with high efficiency by a retroviral vector and expanded ex vivo with stable integration and expression of Fanconi anemia complement c gene. Cell Transplant. **4:** in press

66. Li, Z. H., H. E. Broxmeyer & L. Lu. 1995. Cryopreserved cord blood myeloid progenitor cells can serve as targets for retroviral-mediated gene transduction and gene-transduced progenitors can be cryopreserved and recovered. Leukemia. In press.

Mobilization of Peripheral Blood Stem Cells for Autologous Transplantation

Methods, Mechanisms, and Role in Accelerating Hematopoietic Recovery

WILLIAM EARL JANSSEN[a]

University of South Florida
Departments of Internal Medicine and Pathology/Lab Medicine
at the H. Lee Moffitt Cancer Center
Tampa, Florida 33612

SOURCES OF STEM CELLS

Transplantation of hematopoietic progenitor cells to correct aplasia due either to pathologic processes or to high dose cytotoxic therapy in the treatment of neoplastic disease has been used as a therapeutic modality since the late 1950s.[1] Traditionally, bone marrow has been the source of transplanted material both for allogeneic and subsequently for autologous transplants. In recent years, however, alternative sources of hematopoietic progenitors for transplant have been receiving increasing attention. Transplants have been carried out in animal models and/or humans, using yolk sac cells, fetal liver cells,[2] umbilical cord and placenta derived cells,[3] and peripheral blood derived cells.[1,4] Of these alternative hematopoietic cell sources, peripheral blood stem cells (PBSC) have received the most attention.[5,6]

PERIPHERAL BLOOD STEM CELLS FOR AUTOLOGOUS TRANSPLANTATION

The earliest attempts to employ PBSC for autologous transplant were in chronic myelogenous leukemia (CML). The patient's blood cell count was allowed to rise, typically as high as 100,000 WBC/μl, and the patient was leukopheresed. The collected cells were stored in liquid nitrogen, and when the patient entered blast crisis, they were treated with total body irradiation and high doses of chemotherapy and reinfused with their stored cells, with the intent of restoring the chronic phase of the disease. Although this restored most patients to a chronic phase state, most of these second

[a] Address for correspondence: Dr. William E. Janssen, Bone Marrow Transplant Program, H. Lee Moffitt Cancer Center, University of South Florida, 12902 Magnolia Drive, Tampa, FL 33612.

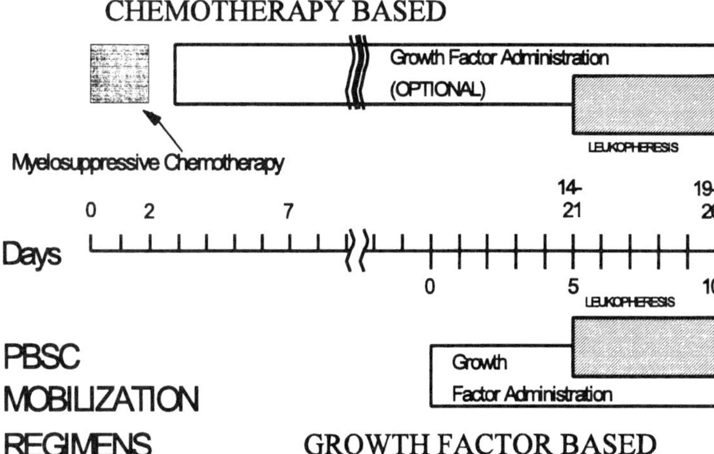

FIGURE 1. Schematic comparison of chemotherapy-based versus growth factor-based peripheral blood stem cell (PBSC) mobilization regimens.

chronic phases were very short-lived.[7] At about the same time, however, there was a report of a patient with CML who had blood cells leukopheresed following chemotherapy and was successfully transplanted with them.[8] More recently, PBSC have been employed to rescue individuals who have neoplastic diseases with primary sites outside of the bone marrow from the myeloablative effects of high dose radiochemotherapy.[9–13] Studies have also been reported in which PBSC were used in the treatment of leukemias and myeloma.[14–17]

The absolute number of circulating hematopoietic stem cells relative to the number of hematopoietic stem cells in the bone marrow of adults is difficult to determine. However, based on relative numbers of CD34 positive cells and granulocyte-macrophage colony-forming cells (CFU-GMs) it is estimated that it would take the hematopoietic cell content of 100 liters of normal blood to equal that of 1 liter of normal bone marrow, a routine-sized harvest. Although apheresis technology allows the *ex vivo* separation of leukocytes from the blood and thus the effective concentration of PBSC, it can still take up to greater than 20 apheresis procedures to collect adequate numbers of cells for transplant from unmobilized blood.[9]

PERIPHERAL BLOOD STEM CELL

To reduce the number of apheresis procedures necessary to collect sufficient PBSC for transplant, a variety of methods have been employed to *mobilize* them. Mobilization regimens may be loosely categorized into one of two groups, represented schematically in FIGURE 1. In the first group, referred to as chemotherapy-induced mobilization, the patient from whom stem cells are to be collected is treated with myelosuppressive chemotherapy. Phereses are performed during leukocyte recovery

TABLE 1. Summary Comparison of a Representative Sample of Chemotherapy-Based Peripheral Blood Stem Cell Mobilization Techniques

Investigator (ref.)	Drugs Employed	Growth Factors	Outcomes
Siena et al.[20]	Cyclophosphamide	GM-CSF	Elevated CD34+
			Rapid engraftment
To et al.[21]		None	Elevated CFU-GM
To et al.[19]	Daunarubicin, Ara-C, 6-Thioguanine (for AML patients)	None	Elevated CFU-GM
Elias et al.[27]	Doxirubicin, 5-FU, MTX	GM-CSF	Rapid engraftment
Brugger et al.[25]	Etoposide, ifosfamide, cis-platin	GM-CSF ± IL-3	Elevated CD34+ Elevated CFU-GM
Shimazaki et al.[24]	ARA-C + etoposide or aclarubicin	G-CSF	
Teshima et al.[23]	Standard therapy for disease	G-CSF	Elevated CFU-GM with G-CSF

Abbreviations: AML = acute myelogenous leukemia; 5-Fu = 5-fluorouracil; MTX = methotrexate.

from chemotherapy, during which period circulating progenitor cells were shown to be more numerous.[18,19] In some of these regimens, hematopoietic growth factors are administered during the postchemotherapy period. The second group, growth factor induced mobilization, consists of regimens in which the patient is administered hematopoietic growth factors without any immediately preceding chemotherapy.

The most commonly reported method of mobilization is the administration of myelosuppressive chemotherapy with PBSC collection during the postchemotherapy leukocyte recovery. It has long been known that following administration of chemotherapeutic agents which are myelosuppressive, the circulating white blood cell count will reach a nadir and then will rapidly recover, frequently overshooting normal levels for a short while. During this recovery phase, the number of circulating hematopoietic stem cells is elevated to well above normal levels.[20–27] To take advantage of this phenomenon for the collection of PBSC, the patient is treated with chemotherapy (TABLE 1), the WBC reach a nadir, and once the circulating leukocyte count passes a minimum necessary for effective leukopheresis, PBSC are collected. In most regimens, hematopoietic growth factors (G-CSF, G-CSF, or interleukin [IL-3]) are given to the patients following the administration of chemotherapy to hasten WBC recovery and to boost the number of circulating hematopoietic cells. Notably, although there have been reports of chemotherapeutic regimens that fail to mobilize PBSC,[21] in all cases wherein hematopoietic growth factors have been administered postcytotoxic therapy, irrespective of the chemotherapy employed, PBSC mobilization has been effective.[20,22–25,27]

Peripheral blood stem cell mobilization facilitated by giving hematopoietic growth factors, notably G-CSF[28–31] or GM-CSF[31,32] but also including IL-3,[25] to patients without

TABLE 2. Summary Comparison of a Representative Sample of Growth Factor-Based Peripheral Blood Stem Cell Mobilization Techniques

Investigator (ref.)	Growth Factors	Usage	Outcomes
Sheridan et al.[28]	G-CSF	PBSC alone	Rapid platelet recovery
Chao et al.[29]			Rapid platelet and neutrophil recovery
Bensinger et al.[30]			Rapid neutrophil recovery
Peters et al.[31]	G-CSF or GM-CSF	With autologous bone marrow	Rapid neutrophil recovery Fewer platelet transfusions
Bishop et al.[32]	GM-CSF	PBSC alone	Rapid neutrophil recovery

any preceding chemotherapy has also been reported. These treatments have increased the number of circulating CD34 antigen-expressing cells,[29] the number of CFU-GMs,[28] or both.[31] When growth factors are used to mobilize PBSC (TABLE 2), growth factor administration is carried out for a set number of days preceding PBSC collection. Daily PBSC apheresis procedures are carried out while growth factor administration continues (FIG. 1). Growth factor administration is generally continued through the last day of PBSC collection. Mobilization which is effected by growth factor administration has two key advantages over chemotherapy-stimulated PBSC mobilization. First, there is substantially less time from initiation of mobilization to completion of PBSC collection (FIG. 1) Second, because the time between initiation of mobilization and initiation of collection is not variable, as with chemotherapy-based mobilization (FIG. 1), it is easier to coordinate the stem cell freezing laboratory, the pheresis team, and all other aspects of the autologous transplant process. These advantages may be offset by the potential for tumor reduction concomitant with mobilizing chemotherapy.

ADVANTAGES OF MOBILIZED PERIPHERAL BLOOD STEM CELLS

Multiple advantages associated with the use of hematopoietic stem cells derived from the circulation have been described. Most obvious is the reduction in exposure to operating rooms and anesthesia. Of greater consequence is the ability to collect PBSC when bone marrow cannot be collected, as when the patient's bone marrow is hypocellular, fibrotic, or infiltrated with tumor. It has also been proposed that PBSC collection is safer than marrow harvesting for autologous transplant. This latter suggestion ignores the risks of myelosuppressive chemotherapy when chemotherapy mobilization is employed and the risks associated with placement of indwelling venous access catheters, which are essential for efficient PBSC collection.

In considering disease-infiltrated marrow, it may be hypothesized that peripheral blood stem cell collection represents a form of *in vivo* marrow purging. In general, neoplastic cells can best colonize in the presence of a solid substrate to which they may adhere. Bone marrow, the structure of which is sponge-like, provides such a substrate. Conversely, circulating cells are nonadherent. It may be speculated then, albeit simplistically, that tumor cells may move through peripheral circulation, but they are unlikely to colonize there. Hypothetically, the probability of collecting a tumor cell in a milliliter of blood may be expected to be less than the probability of collecting one in a milliliter of bone marrow. One report has shown data that are consistent with this hypothesis.[33] Other reports have indicated, however, that tumor cells may be found in circulating blood, and their concentration may be increased by the same treatments that mobilize hematopoietic progenitors.[34-36]

It may also be hypothesized that non-stem cells, such as mature lymphocytes, lymphokine-activated killer cells, and natural killer cells, which are collected and reinfused with peripheral blood stem cells,[37,38] may have the beneficial effect of preventing disease recurrence.

In a recent report lymphoma patients who had disease-infiltrated bone marrow were transplanted with PBSC and experienced a significantly better 3-year disease-free survival than did a concurrent group of patients with disease-free marrow who were transplanted with unpurged autologous bone marrow.[39] A related report indicated that the superior survival from the PBSC transplant was limited to patients with better-risk disease at the time of transplant.[40] Either of the foregoing hypotheses would be supported by these findings. Conversely, our group compared disease-free survival in breast cancer patients transplanted with either autologous bone marrow or PBSC and found no difference.[41] These findings are not necessarily contradictory in that the patients in the first study were good risk patients with lymphoma, whereas the patients in our study were poor risk patients with breast cancer.

ACCELERATED HEMATOLOGIC RECOVERY (EARLY ENGRAFTMENT) WITH PERIPHERAL BLOOD STEM CELLS

The most cited advantage of PBSC over bone marrow for autologous stem cell rescue is a shortened period of aplasia following return of the cells to the high dose therapy treated patient.[42-45] This accelerated early engraftment was reported both with PBSC used as a single product.[26,28,29,46] and with PBSC infused concomitantly with autologous bone marrow.[31] The acceleration has been reported in both the granulocytic and the thrombocytic lineages. Since opportunistic infections and bleeding complications are frequent causes of bone marrow transplant morbidity and mortality, a reduction in the aplastic period following stem cell infusion would be a great clinical advantage. This phenomenon, however, is not universally reported. Reports of PBSC transplant in which the PBSC were not mobilized have not included data indicating accelerated engraftment[9] even when PBSC were transplanted concomitantly with bone marrow.[47]

All of the mobilization methods just described involve stimulation of hematopoietic stem cells either by administration of exogenous cytokines or as part of the natural process of recovery from cytotoxic insult. By contrast, bone marrow for autotransplant is generally collected when the stem cells are likely to be quiescent. Therefore, the observed reductions in post-stem cell transplant aplasia could hypothetically be explained by the activated state of key hematopoietic progenitor populations. If this is true, then similar reductions in post-stem cell transplant aplasia could be

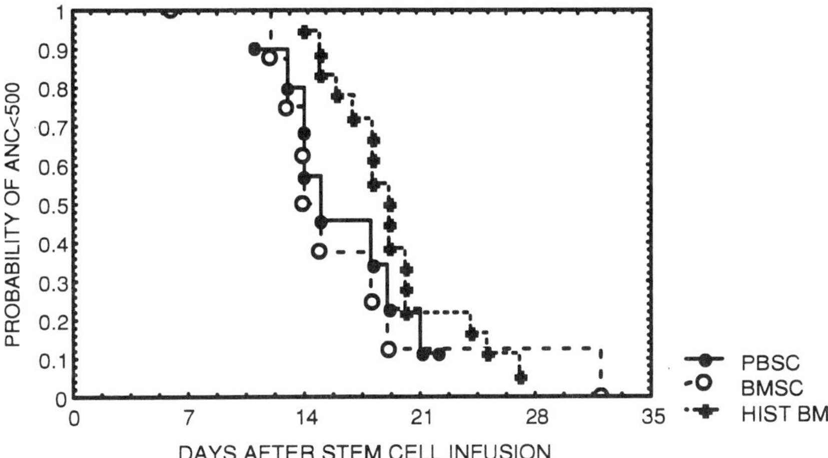

FIGURE 2. Period of aplasia after stem cell transplant with either marrow- or blood-derived cells. Patients received 5 days of G-CSF after which marrow was harvested on day 6 and PBSC were collected on days 7-10. Administration of G-CSF was continued through the penultimate day of collection. Patients were treated with high dose ICE chemotherapy (see text) and by randomization received either marrow- or blood-derived stem cell product. PBSC = patients infused with peripheral blood stem cells collected with G-CSF mobilization. BMSC = patients infused with bone marrow stem cells collected after G-CSF priming. HIST BM = historic control of patients transplanted with resting bone marrow.

expected by treating individuals with hematopoietic growth factor(s) prior to bone marrow harvesting. We have tested this hypothesis with a clinical trial in which both bone marrow and PBSC are harvested in all patients concomitant with G-CSF administration. Following high dose chemotherapy, patients randomly receive one product or the other, and the posttransplant aplasia is monitored. Although the results are preliminary, we found no difference in the period of post stem cell infusion neutropenia between the blood- (median days to achieve absolute neutrophil recovery [ANC > 500] is 14) or marrow- (median days to achieve ANC >500 is also 14) derived stem cell products, although the rate of neutrophil recovery with primed bone marrow is accelerated relative to historic controls (median days to achieve ANC >500 is 19)[48,49] (FIG. 2). These data suggest that the priming/mobilization of blood-borne hematopoietic cells may have greater influence on their potential for early engraftment than does the anatomic compartment from which they are derived. Accordingly, it is desirable to know if one mobilization regimen is superior to others in the rate of engraftment obtained when the derivative cells are transplanted.

PERIPHERAL BLOOD STEM CELL MOBILIZATION METHODS

Little data have been reported providing a direct comparison of different mobilization regimens. Whether one mobilization method is more effective than others in

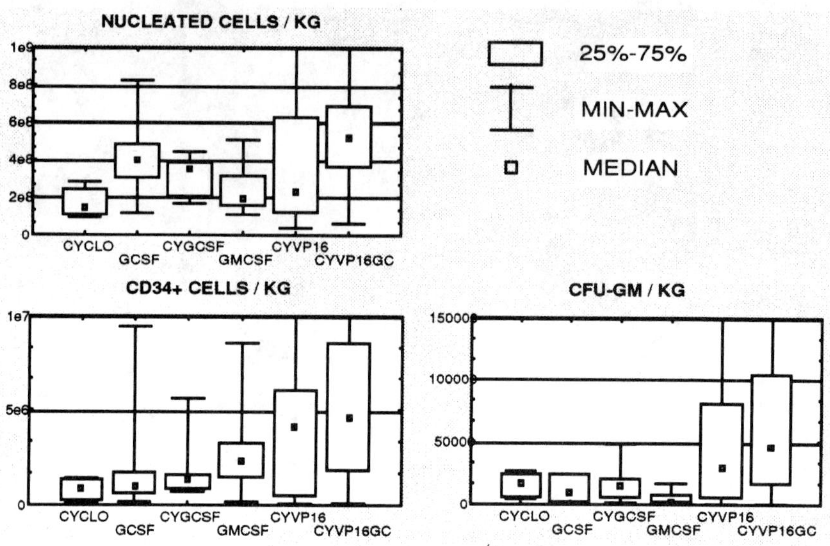

FIGURE 3. Numbers of cells collected, by type, as a function of the PBSC mobilization regimen employed. CYCLO = cyclophosphamide, 50 mg/kg/day × 2 days; collect PBSC after WBC recovery past 1,000/mm³. GCSF = G-CSF 16 μg/kg/day × 5 days; collect PBSC × 4 days. CYGCSF = cyclophosphamide, 50 mg/kg/day × 2 days followed by G-CSF 5 mg/kg/ day; collect PBSC after WBC recovery >1,000/mm³. GMCSF = GM-CSF 10 μg/kg/day × 5 days; collect PBSC × 4 days. CYVP16 = cyclophosphamide administered with etoposide; collect PBSC after WBC recovery >1,000/mm³. CYVP16GC = cyclophosphamide and etoposide followed by G-CSF 5 μg/kg/day.

increasing the number of circulating hematopoietic progenitors or in producing stem cells that accelerate engraftment cannot be deduced from the current literature. However, the use of chemotherapy combined with growth factors appears to provide superior mobilization to chemotherapy alone[23,50] and may be superior to growth factors used singly as well.[51] In fact, the addition of G-CSF to chemotherapy regimens, including chemotherapy regimens that are reported as nonmobilizing,[21,24] improves the overall yield of stem cells collected.

We compared several mobilization regimens within our own patient population and observed that both total nucleated cell yield and specific subset yield are affected by the regimen employed[51] (Fig. 3). Specifically, we examined PBSC mobilization following cyclophosphamide chemotherapy with or without the addition of etoposide and with or without subsequent G-CSF growth factor administration. We also examined growth factor mobilization with either GM-CSF or G-CSF. In comparing total cell collections from each of these mobilization methods, we found that total nucleated cells, total CFU-GMs, and total CD34⁺ cells collected were greatest after cyclophosphamide and etoposide administration, with subsequent G-CSF (CYVP16GC). These collections were greater than the sum of collections following cyclophosphamide and G-CSF (CYG) or after cyclophosphamide and etoposide but without subsequent G-CSF (CYVP1G).

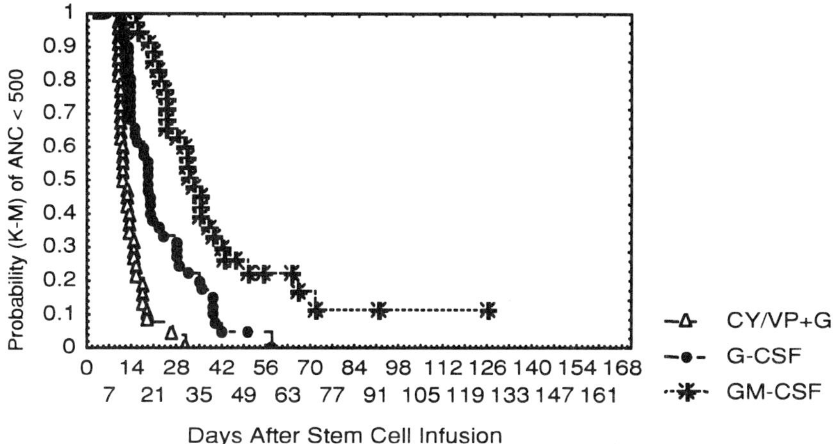

FIGURE 4. Comparison of engraftment following transplant with PBSC mobilized using different schema. CY/VP + G = cyclophosphamide with etoposide plus G-CSF following chemotherapy; G-CSF for 5 days prior to harvesting; GM-CSF = GM-CSF for 5 days before harvesting.

We also observed statistically significant changes in the rate of early engraftment following transplant of different stem cell products (Fig. 4). Of particular interest was the observation that PBSC mobilized with GM-CSF produced dramatically *slower* neutrophil recovery following transplantation than did PBSC mobilized with G-CSF, even though the number of collected CD34[+] cells was not statistically different.[52] This latter result appears to conflict with a report from the University of Nebraska, wherein GM-CSF-mobilized PBSC produced rapid posttransplant engraftment.[32] It must be noted, however, that in our study, growth factor administration was carried out for 5 days prior to PBSC harvesting, whereas in the Nebraska study PBSC harvesting commenced within a day of initiating GM-CSF administration. That prolonged administration of GM-CSF may "burn out" the pool of granulocyte-macrophage progenitors is supported by data presented by Peters *et al.*[31] which showed reduced CFU-GM capture after 12 days of GM-CSF mobilization than after 8 days.

ARE HEMATOPOIETIC STEM CELLS REALLY MOBILIZED, AND HOW?

It is an article of faith that PBSC collected following mobilization migrate into the circulation from the bone marrow; there is no demonstrable evidence. It is not entirely impossible that the increased hematopoietic progenitor population in the blood following PBSC mobilization may result from expansion of an extramedullary hematopoietic cell pool.

The data just presented, which show very different products and different engraftment potentials from different mobilization methods (chemotherapy ± growth

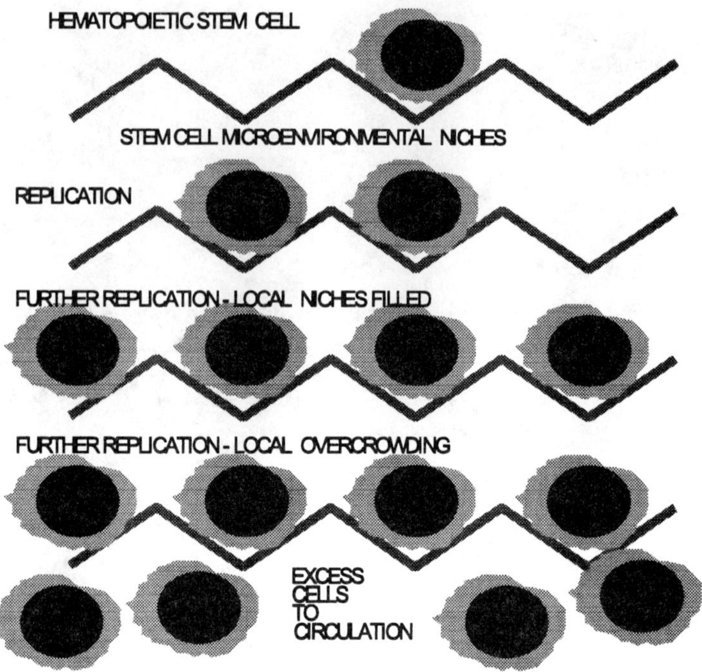

FIGURE 5. Overcrowding model of PBSC mobilization. Local islands of hematopoietic cells are stimulated to divide. After limited division cycles, all available niches are filled and new daughter cells must exit to the circulation and seek empty niches in other marrow spaces.

factors vs growth factors alone), different mobilization agents (cyclophosphamide vs other drugs or cyclophosphamide in combination, GM-CSF vs G-CSF), and different mobilization schedules (short vs long GM-CSF administration), suggest that more than one mobilization mechanism may be active. Although not an exhaustive list, three possible mechanisms are (1) random release modulated by local adhesive affinity, (2) overcrowding of the marrow niches, and (3) chemotaxis/chemokinesis.

The local release model postulates that hematopoietic stem cells are normally held captive in the marrow microenvironment by adhesion molecules. Random release of cells from the marrow to the blood occurs albeit at a low level due to the binding affinity of the adhesion molecules. Mobilization causes modulation of these molecules by reducing either their number or the affinity of their binding, thus increasing the rate of release of stem cells into circulation and consequently increasing the number of stem cells in circulation.

The overcrowding model (FIG. 5) postulates that the density of stem cells in the marrow is limited by available niches. If the stem cells are stimulated to divide, as would be the case following myelosuppressive chemotherapy, the earliest produced daughter cells may have available niches adjacent to the original cell. As subsequent daughter cells would not have available niches, they would be forced into circulation

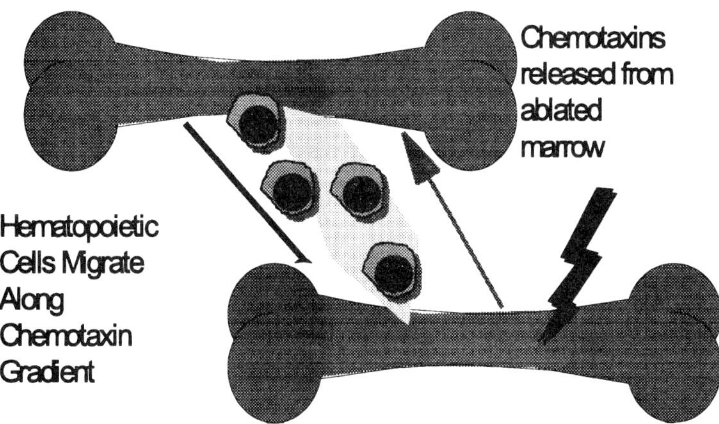

FIGURE 6. Chemotaxis model of PBSC mobilization. Regions of marrow that have been rendered hypocellular by radiochemotherapy release chemotaxins into circulation. Hematopoietic cells migrate from local surviving islands of hematopoiesis in response to chemotaxins, moving through circulation in an attempt to migrate to chemotaxin source.

to seek niches in other marrow spaces. This fairly simple model is consistent with observed mobilization following chemotherapy.

The chemotaxis/chemokinesis model (FIG. 6) postulates that stromal elements in ablated areas of marrow will release chemotaxins to recruit new stem cells to the area. Stem cells in still populated islands of hematopoiesis detect the chemotaxins and migrate through the circulation seeking the chemotaxin source. This model is consistent with the rapid disappearance of hematopoietic cells from blood following stem cell transplantation.

CONCLUSIONS

Although the mechanism of PBSC mobilization or whether, in fact, mobilization is occurring at all is unclear, it is clear that manipulation of the total hematopoietic pool of cells by chemotherapy insult or administration of growth factors will result in an increase in circulating hematopoietic progenitors that are capable of repopulating a myeloablated host. It is equally clear that not all of the regimens for PBSC mobilization produce the same results, whether measured by hematopoietic cell collections or by rate of engraftment following PBSC transplant.

What is not clear and remains to be elucidated through systematic study is what factors are critical in determining the quantity and quality of hematopoietic progenitors that are circulating following mobilization. Possible factors include the extent of myelosuppression, relative toxicity of mobilizing chemotherapy to hematopoietic stromal elements, range of action of hematopoietic growth factors employed, underlying neoplastic disease, invasion of bone marrow by the underlying disease, amount of previous radiation and chemotherapy the patient has been subjected to, the age and gender of the patient, and other active medical interventions that may be on-going at the time of PBSC mobilization. Finally, it is unclear that the benefits associated with PBSC transplantation actually require the use of PBSC. It is possible that through appropriate *in vivo* or *ex vivo* treatments, hematopoietic cells derived from marrow might be induced to possess the same qualities.

Much effort, both at the bench and at the bedside, will be required before we can definitely address these issues. Until they are addressed, the clinician who is setting out to mobilize and collect PBSC for transplant must approach the activity with caution and with awareness of the factors that may determine the outcome of his or her efforts.

REFERENCES

1. THOMAS, E. D. 1994. Stem cell transplantation: Past, present and future. Stem Cells **12:** 539–544.
2. IKUTA, K. & Y. KOMAGATA. 1995. Developmental potential of fetal hematopoietic stem cells. *In* Hematopoietic Stem Cells: Biology and Therapeutic Applications. D. Levitt & R. Mertelsmann. Eds.: 69–83. Marcel Dekker, Inc. New York.
3. BROXMEYER, H. E., L. LU, J. GADDY, L. RUGGIERI, A. SRIVASTAVA & G. RISDON. 1995. Human umbilical cord blood transplantation: The immunology, expansion, and thera-peutic applications of hematopoietic stem and progenitor cells. *In* Hematopoietic Stem Cells: Biology and Therapeutic Applications. D. Levitt & R. Mertelsmann, Eds.: 297–317. Marcel Dekker, Inc. New York.
4. CHARBORD, P. 1994. Hemopoietic stem cells: Analysis of some parameters critical for engraftment. Stem Cells **12:** 545–562.
5. JUTTNER, C. A., W. E. FIBBE, J. NEMUNAITIS, L. KANZ & A. M. GIANNI. 1994. Blood cell transplantation: Report from an International Consensus Meeting. Bone Marrow Transplant. **14:** 689–693.
6. RUSSELL, N. H. & A. E. HUNTER. 1994. Peripheral blood stem cells for allogeneic transplantation [editorial]. Bone Marrow Transplant. **13:** 353–355.
7. GOLDMAN, J. M. 1979. Autografting cryopreserved buffy coat cells for chronic granulocytic leukemia in transformation. Exp. Hematol. **7** (Suppl. 5): 389.
8. KORBLING, M., P. BURKE, H. BRAINE, G. ELFENBEIN, G. SANTOS & H. KAIZER. 1981. Successful engraftment of blood derived normal hemopoietic stem cells in chronic myelogenous leukemia. Exp. Hematol. **9:** 684–690.
9. KESSINGER, A., J. O. ARMITAGE, J. D. LANDMARK, D. M. SMITH & D. D. WEISENBURGER. 1988. Autologous peripheral hematopoietic stem cell transplantation restores hemato-poietic function following marrow ablative therapy. Blood **71:** 723–727.
10. BARR, R. D. & J. A. MCBRIDE. 1982. Hemopoietic engraftment with peripheral blood cells in the treatment of malignant disease. Br. J. Haematol. **51:** 181–187.
11. KORBLING, M., B. DORKEN, A. D. HO et al. 1986. Autologous transplantation of blood-derived hemopoietic stem cells after myeloablative therapy in a patient with Burkitt's lymphoma. Blood **67:** 529–532.
12. LASKY, L. C., D. D. HURD, J. A. SMITH & R. HAAKE. 1989. Peripheral blood stem cell collection and use in Hodgkin's disease. Comparison with marrow in autologous transplantation. Transfusion **29:** 323–327.
13. WILLIAMS, S. F., J. M. BITRAN, J. M. RICHARDS et al. 1990. Peripheral blood-derived stem cell collections for use in autologous transplantation after high dose chemotherapy: An alternative approach. Bone Marrow Transplant. **5:** 129–133.
14. MEHTA, J., R. L. POWLES, V. SHEPHERD, M. DAINTON, J. TRELEAVEN. 1993. Transplantation of autologous peripheral blood stem cells mobilized using GM-CSF for acute leukemia with myelofibrosis. Leukemia & Lymphoma **11:** 157–158.

15. OSSENKOPPELE, G. J., A. R. JONKHOFF, P. C. HUIJGENS, J. J. NAUTA, K. G. VAN DER HEM, A. M. DRAGER & M. M. LANGENHUIJSEN. 1994. Peripheral blood progenitors mobilised by G-CSF (filgrastim) and reinfused as unprocessed autologous whole blood shorten the pancytopenic period following high-dose melphalan in multiple myeloma. Bone Marrow Transplant. **13:** 37-41.

16. PETTENGELL, R., G. R. MORGENSTERN, P. J. WOLL, J. CHANG, M. ROWLANDS, R. YOUNG, J. A. RADFORD, J. H. SCARFFE, N. G. TESTA & D. CROWTHER. 1993. Peripheral blood progenitor cell transplantation in lymphoma and leukemia using a single apheresis. Blood **82:** 3770-3777.

17. SASAKI, A., M. TSUKAGUCHI, M. HIRAI, H. OHIRA, Y. NAKAO, T. YAMANE, K. PARK, T. IM & N. TATSUMI. 1994. Transplantation of allogeneic peripheral blood stem cells after myeloablative treatment of a patient in blastic crisis of chronic myelocytic leukemia. Am. J. Hematol. **47:** 45-49.

18. RICHMAN, C. M., R. S. WEINER & R. A. YANKEE. 1976. Increase in circulating stem cells following chemotherapy in man. Blood **47:** 1031-1039.

19. TO, L. B., D. N. HAYLOCK, R. J. KIMBER & C. A. JUTTNER. 1984. High levels of circulating haemopoietic stem cells in very early remission from acute non-lymphoblastic leukaemia and their collection and cryopreservation. Br. J. Haematol. **58:** 399-410.

20. SIENA, S., M. BREGNI, B. BRANDO *et al.* 1989. Circulation of CD34⁺ hematopoietic stem cells in the peripheral blood of high-dose cyclophosphamide-treated patients: Enhancement by intravenous recombinant human granulocyte-macrophage colony-stimulating factor. Blood **74:** 1905-1914.

21. TO, L. B., K. M. SHEPPERD, D. N. HAYLOCK *et al.* 1990. Single high doses of cyclophosphamide enable the collection of high numbers of hemopoietic stem cells from the peripheral blood. Exp. Hematol. **18:** 442-447.

22. BREGNI, M., S. SIENA, M. MAGNI *et al.* 1991. Circulating hemopoietic progenitors mobilized by cancer chemotherapy and by rhGM-CSF in the treatment of high-grade non-Hodgkin's lymphoma. Leukemia **5** (suppl. 1): 123-127.

23. TESHIMA, T., M. HARADA, Y. TAKAMATSU *et al.* 1992. Cytotoxic drug and cytotoxic drug/G-CSF mobilization of peripheral blood stem cells and their use for autografting. Bone Marrow Transplant. **10:** 215-220.

24. SHIMAZAKI, C., N. OKU, E. ASHIHARA *et al.* 1992. Collection of peripheral blood stem cells mobilized by high-dose Ara-C plus VP-16 or aclarubicin followed by recombinant human granulocyte-colony stimulating factor. Bone Marrow Transplant. **10:** 341-346.

25. BRUGGER, W., K. BROSS, J. FRISCH, P. DEM, B. WEBER, R. MERTELSMANN & L. KANZ. 1992. Mobilization of peripheral blood progenitor cells by sequential administration of interleukin-3 and granulocyte-macrophage colony-stimulating-factor following polychemotherapy with etoposide, ifosfamide and cisplatin. Blood **79:** 1193-1200.

26. TO, L. B., M. M. ROBERTS, D. N. HAYLOCK *et al.* 1992. Comparison of haematological recovery times and supportive care requirements of autologous recovery phase peripheral blood stem cell transplants, autologous bone marrow transplants and allogeneic bone marrow transplants. Bone Marrow Transplant. **9:** 277-284.

27. ELIAS, A. D., L. AYASH, K. C. ANDERSON *et al.* 1992. Mobilization of peripheral blood progenitor cells by chemotherapy and granulocyte-macrophage colony-stimulating-factor for hematologic support after high-dose intensification for breast cancer. Blood **79:** 3036-3044.

28. SHERIDAN, W. P., C. G. BEGLEY, C. A. JUTTNER *et al.* 1992. Effect of peripheral-blood progenitor cells mobilised by filgrastim (G-CSF) on platelet recovery after high-dose chemotherapy. Lancet **339:** 640-644.

29. CHAO, N. J., J. R. SCHRIBER, K. GRIMES *et al.* 1993. Granulocyte colony-stimulating factor "mobilized" peripheral blood progenitor cells accelerate granulocyte and platelet recovery after high-dose chemotherapy. Blood **81:** 2031-2035.

30. BENSINGER, W., J. SINGER, F. APPELBAUM *et al.* 1993. Autologous transplantation with peripheral blood mononuclear cells collected after administration of recombinant granulocyte stimulating factor. Blood **81**: 3158-3163.

31. PETERS, W. P., G. ROSNER, M. ROSS *et al.* 1993. Comparative effects of granulocyte-macrophage colony-stimulating factor (GM-CSF) and granulocyte colony-stimulating factor (G-CSF) on priming peripheral blood progenitor cells for use with autologous bone marrow after high-dose chemotherapy. Blood **81**: 1709-1719.

32. BISHOP, M. R., J. R. ANDERSON, J. D. JACKSON, P. J. BIERMAN, E. C. REED, J. M. VOSE, J. O. ARMITAGE, P. I. WARKENTIN & A. KESSINGER. 1994. High-dose therapy and peripheral blood progenitor cell transplantation: Effects of recombinant human granulocyte-macrophage colony-stimulating factor on the autograft. Blood **83**: 610-616.

33. NAGASU, M., S. AIZAWA, H. HOJO, A. TSUDA, M. YAGUCHI, M. NAKANO & K. TOYAMA. 1992. Detecting of the minimal residual disease contaminated in peripheral blood stem cell transplantation in the B-cell malignant lymphoma patients [see comments]. Am. J. Hematol. **41**: 107-112.

34. MOSS, T. J., D. G. SANDERS, L. C. LASKY & B. BOSTROM. 1990. Contamination of peripheral blood stem cell harvests by circulating neuroblastoma cells. Blood **76**: 1879-1883.

35. BRUGGER, W., K. J. BROSS, M. GLATT, F. WEBER, R. MERTELSMANN & L. KANZ. 1994. Mobilization of tumor cells and hematopoietic progenitor cells into peripheral blood of patients with solid tumors [see comments]. Blood **83**: 636-640.

36. VORA, A. J., C. H. TOH, J. PEEL & M. GREAVES. 1994. Use of granulocyte colony-stimulating factor (G-CSF) for mobilizing peripheral blood stem cells: Risk of mobilizing clonal myeloma cells in patients with bone marrow infiltration. Br. J. Haematol. **86**: 180-182.

37. NEUBAUER, M. A., M. C. BENYUNES, J. A. THOMPSON, W. I. BENSINGER, C. G. LINDGREN, C. D. BUCKNER & A. FEFER. 1994. Lymphokine-activated killer (LAK) precursor cell activity is present in infused peripheral blood stem cells and in the blood after autologous peripheral blood stem cell transplantation. Bone Marrow Transplant. **13**: 311-316.

38. VERBIK, D. J., J. D. JACKSON, S. J. PIRRUCCELLO, K. D. PATIL, A. KESSINGER & S. S. JOSHI. 1995. Functional and phenotypic characterization of human peripheral blood stem cell harvests: A comparative analysis of cells from consecutive collections. Blood **85**: 1964-1970.

39. VOSE, J. M., P. J. BIERMAN, J. R. ANDERSON *et al.* 1992. High-dose chemotherapy with hematopoietic stem cell rescue for non-Hodgkin's lymphoma (NHL): Evaluation of event-free survival based on histologic subtype and rescue product (abstr.). Proc. Ann. Am. Soc. Clin. Oncol. **11**: A1080.

40. VOSE, J. M., J. R. ANDERSON, A. KESSINGER, P. J. BIERMAN, P. COCCIA, E. C. REED, B. GORDON & J. O. ARMITAGE. 1993. High-dose chemotherapy and autologous hematopoietic stem-cell transplantation for aggressive non-Hodgkin's lymphoma. J. Clin. Oncol. **11**: 1846-1851.

41. AGALIOTIS, D. P., K. K. FIELDS, O. F. BALLESTER, J. W. HIEMENZ, P. E. ZORSKY, W. E. JANSSEN, J. B. PERKINS & L. D. PACH. 1993. Event free survival in patients with metastatic breast cancer undergoing high dose chemotherapy and autologous bone marrow or peripheral blood stem cell transplantation (abstr.). Exp. Hematol. **21**: 1130.

42. HENON, P. R. 1993. Peripheral blood stem cell transplantations: Past, present and future [Review]. Stem Cells **11**: 154-172.

43. HOGGE, D. E., H. J. SUTHERLAND, P. M. LANSDORP, G. L. PHILLIPS & C. J. EAVES. 1993. The elusive peripheral blood hemopoietic stem cells [Review]. Semin. Hematol. **30**: 82-89; discussion 90-91.

44. GOLDMAN, J. 1995. Peripheral blood stem cells for allografting. Blood **85**: 1413-1415.

45. HENON, P. R. 1995. Autologous blood stem-cell versus bone marrow transplantation: Comparison of cost-effectiveness and of clinical benefits. *In* Hematopoietic Stem Cells:

Biology and Therapeutic Applications. D. Levitt & R. Mertelsmann, Eds.: 421–434. Marcel Dekker, Inc. New York.

46. BRUGGER, W., R. BIRKEN, H. BERTZ, T. HECHT, K. PRESSLER, J. FRISCH, G. SCHULZ, R. MERTELSMANN & L. KANZ. 1993. Peripheral blood progenitor cells mobilized by chemotherapy plus granulocyte-colony stimulating factor accelerate both neutrophil and platelet recovery after high-dose VP16, ifosfamide and cisplatin. Br. J. Haematol. **84:** 402–407.

47. LOBO, F., A. KESSINGER, J. D. LANDMARK, D. M. SMITH, D. D. WEISENBURGER, R. S. WIGTON & J. O. ARMITAGE. 1991. Addition of peripheral blood stem cells collected without mobilization techniques to transplanted autologous bone marrow did not hasten marrow recovery following myeloablative therapy. Bone Marrow Transplant. **8:** 389–392.

48. JANSSEN, W. E., J. W. HIEMENZ, K. K. FIELDS, P. E. ZORSKY, O. F. BALLESTER, S. C. GOLDSTEIN, R. SMILEE, L. KRONISH & G. J. ELFENBEIN. 1994. Peripheral blood "stem cells" do not always produce faster engraftment that bone marrow in autotransplantation (abstr.) Exp. Hematol. **22:** 765.

49. JANSSEN, W. E., J. PERKINS, J. W. HIEMENZ, K. K. FIELDS, P. E. ZORSKY, O. F. BALLESTER, S. C. GOLDSTEIN, R. SMILEE, L. KRONISH & G. J. ELFENBEIN. 1994. Granulocyte recovery is ALLESTER, S. C. GOLDSTEIN, R. SMILEE, L. KRONISH & G. J. ELFENBEIN. 1994. Granulocyte recovery is not different following auto-transplant with G-CSF primed bone marrow or G-CSF mobilized peripheral blood "stem cells" (abstr.). Blood **84:** 95a.

50. TO, L. B., D. N. HAYLOCK, T. DOWSE, P. J. SIMMONS, S. TRIMBOLI, L. K. ASHMAN & C. A. JUTTNER. 1994. A comparative study of the phenotype and proliferative capacity of peripheral blood (PB) CD34$^+$ cells mobilized by four different protocols and those of steady-phase PB and bone marrow CD34$^+$ cells. Blood **84:** 2930–2939.

51. JANSSEN, W. E., R. SMILEE, R. CARTER, D. RAHN, M. CAIRO, J. H. HIEMENZ, P. E. FIELDS, O. BALLESTER, J. PERKINS, L. KRONISH & G. J. ELFENBEIN. 1994. Mobilization of peripheral blood stem cells: Comparing cyclophosphamide and growth factor based regimens. Prog. Clin. Biol. Res. **389:** 429–439.

52. JANSSEN, W. E., G. J. ELFENBEIN, K. K. FIELDS, J. W. HIEMENZ, P. E. ZORSKY, O. F. BALLESTER, S. C. GOLDSTEIN, R. C. SMILEE, L. KRONISH, B. BEACH & G. LEPARC. 1995. Comparison of cell collections and rates of posttransplant granulocyte recovery when G-CSF and GM-CSF are used as mobilizers of peripheral blood stem cells for autotransplantation. *In* Autologous Marrow and Blood Transplantation. Proceedings of the Seventh International Symposium, Arlington, Texas. K. A. Dicke & A. Keating, Eds.: 527–539. The Cancer Treatment Research and Educational Institute, Arlington, Texas.

Prevention and Treatment of Graft-versus-Host Disease

NELSON J. CHAO[a] AND PAUL G. SCHLEGEL

Bone Marrow Transplant Division
Department of Medicine
Stanford University Medical Center
Stanford, California 94305

The area of prophylaxis for acute graft-versus-host disease (GVHD) began with the studies by Uphoff[1] who demonstrated that the use of aminopterin in mice receiving allogeneic bone marrow transplantation (BMT) decreased the incidence of acute GVHD. However, synthesis of the experimental observations on GVHD did not occur until the classic paper by Billingham[2] in 1966 which details the requirements for the development of GVHD:

1. The graft must contain immunologically competent cells;
2. The host must possess important transplantation isoantigens that are lacking in the graft donor, so that the host appears foreign to it and is therefore capable of stimulating it antigenically;
3. The host itself must be incapable of mounting an effective immunological reaction against the graft, at least for sufficient time for the latter to manifest its immunological capabilities − i.e., the graft must have some security of tenure.

The description of GVHD in Billingham's original article is an excellent historical review of the field to that point. This description still holds true today, even though the second postulate needs to be modified to address the phenomenon of autologous GVHD. In that setting, the autologous cells that are normally deleted are not and therefore recognize self-antigens and cause the disease. Moreover, GVHD occurs not only in the setting of BMT, but also after allografting of solid organs as well as allogeneic blood transfusions.

Early work in humans by the Seattle group[3] demonstrated that the single agent methotrexate was effective in preventing GVHD in approximately 50-60% of patients (rates of GVHD are for those presenting with grade II-IV acute GVHD).[3] Cyclosporine alone was also effective in decreasing the rate of GVHD to approximately 30-60% when compared to methotrexate. Other regimens for prophylaxis included: antithymocyte globulin/methotrexate/prednisone,[4] methotrexate/prednisone,[5] cyclosporine/prednisone,[6] and cyclosporine/methotrexate.[7,8] The most commonly used

[a] Address for correspondence: Nelson J. Chao, Stanford University Medical Center, 300 Pasteur Drive, H-1353, Stanford, CA 94305.

regimen is currently cyclosporine and a short course of methotrexate, as developed by the Seattle group.

With the continued growth of allogeneic BMT and the expansion into mismatched related and matched unrelated donors, the importance of improved prophylaxis and therapy in GVHD is apparent. These approaches are reviewed and newer maneuvers are discussed.

PATHOPHYSIOLOGY

Recognition of allogeneic differences by competent immunologic cells is a central tenet of GVHD. When siblings are matched at the major histocompatibility complex (MHC), the cause of GVHD is ascribed to minor histocompatibility differences. These minor histocompatibility differences are now known to be peptide differences between host and donor. Alloreactive T cells recognize these peptidic differences presented on the same MHC molecules (because siblings are genotypically identical) and will cause a graft-versus-host reaction which can lead to GVHD. The pathophysiology of this disease was reviewed.[9] The first step is that the T-cell recognize the peptide as foreign. The second step is the need for a costimulatory signal. This second signal is crucial in that it will determine if peptide recognition will lead to activation of an immunologic reaction, partial activation, or a shut down of response (anergy).[10] If the reaction leads to activation, then interleukin-2 (IL-2) is secreted and the IL-2 receptor is upregulated. This IL-2 secretion leads to clonal expansion and proliferation. T cells and monocytes release cytokine (e.g., IL-1, IL-2, tumor neurosis factor-alpha [TNF-α] and gamma-interferon [IFN-γ]) to recruit other T cells or other effector cells (e.g., natural killer [NK] cells). These cytokines set off a ''cytokine storm'' cascade of further activation and tissue damage, leading to more cytokine release.[11] Therefore, these cytokines may contribute to tissue damage by recruiting effector cells or directly damaging tissues.

CLINICAL MANIFESTATIONS

The classic manifestations of GVHD are found in three primary organs: skin, liver, and gastrointestinal tract.

Skin

The first, and most common, clinical manifestation of acute GVHD is a maculopapular skin rash usually occurring at or near the time of white blood cell engraftment. In the early stages this rash may be pruritic, involving the nape of the neck, the ears and shoulders as well as the palms of the hands and soles of the feet. It can also be described as a sunburn. From these initial areas of presentation, the rash may spread to the whole integument and become confluent. In severe GVHD, the maculopapular rash forms bullous lesions with epidermal necrolysis. The progression of GVHD can be clinically defined in four stages, depending on the extent of involvement of each

TABLE 1. Graft-versus-Host Disease Grading of Individual Organ Systems[a]

Organ	Grade	Description
Skin	+1	Maculopapular eruption over <25% of body area
	+2	Maculopapular eruption over 25–50% of body area
	+3	Generalized erythroderma
	+4	Generalized erythroderma with bullous formation and often with desquamation
Liver	+1	Bilirubin 2.0–3.0 mg/dl; SGOT 150–750 IU
	+2	Bilirubin 3.1–6.0 mg/dl
	+3	Bilirubin 6.1–15.0 mg/dl
	+4	Bilirubin >15.0 mg/dl
Gut	+1	Diarrhea >30 ml/kg or >500 ml/day
	+2	Diarrhea >60 ml/kg or τ1,000 ml/day
	+3	Diarrhea >90 ml/kg or >1,500 ml/day
	+4	Diarrhea >90 ml/kg or >2,000 ml/day or severe abdominal pain with or without ileus

[a] Adapted from Glucksberg et al.[13]

organ (TABLE 1). Each of the three organs can have a specific stage of disease, which results in an overall grade of GVHD (TABLE 2).

Liver

The second organ most commonly involved by acute GVHD is the liver. Rarely, patients will have moderate to severe liver GVHD without evidence of cutaneous disease. Liver involvement is manifested by abnormal liver function test results and is difficult to treat effectively. The earliest and most common abnormality is a rise in conjugated bilirubin and alkaline phosphatase. This reflects the pathology associated with liver GVHD, that is, damage to the bile canaliculi leading to cholestasis. Biopsy is the most definitive method of diagnosing GVHD of the liver. Unfortunately, it may not be feasible primarily because of acute bleeding which can be significant early after BMT. Newer approaches, such as the transjugular approach, may be better

TABLE 2. Overall Grade of Acute Graft-versus-Host Disease

Grade	Skin	Liver		Gut	ECOG Performance
I	+1–+2	0		0	0
II	+1–+3	+1	and/or	+1	0–1
III	+2–+3	+2–+4	and/or	+2–+3	2–3
IV	+2–+4	+2–+4	and/or	+2–+4	3–4

suited for biopsy if an adequate amount of tissue is obtained. Primary histologic findings are bile duct atypia and degeneration leading occasionally to severe cholestasis.

Gastrointestinal Tract

The third main organ system to be affected by GVHD is the gut. Gut GVHD is often the most severe, is difficult to treat, and is characterized by diarrhea and abdominal cramping. Diarrhea can be so voluminous that it becomes difficult to maintain an adequate fluid balance in some patients. The crampy abdominal pain associated with severe GVHD can also be difficult to treat. Severe ileus may be associated with GVHD or with increased narcotic use to control the physical discomfort. The diarrhea in some patients can be in excess of 10 Liters per day (TABLE 1). It may be watery initially, reflecting primarily a salt and water reabsorption defect in the distal small bowel and colon, but it frequently becomes bloody so that transfusion requirements can be significant. It is not unusual for patients to need 2 units of packed red blood cells nearly daily to keep the hematocrit in the 30% range. The stages of gut GVHD are usually graded by the volume of diarrhea. In severe gut GVHD, whole areas may be denuded, with total loss of epithelium similar to that observed in the skin. Rectal biopsy is usually helpful in diagnosing gut GVHD. Colonoscopy or upper endoscopy is usually also performed. However, infectious agents, most notoriously cytomegalovirus, may mimic the clinical as well as histologic features of acute GVHD in the gut. Selective staining for such pathogens should be pursued to rule out an infectious agent as the cause of gastrointestinal symptoms.

Hematolymphoid Organ

Although the hematolymphoid organ is not commonly considered to be involved in acute GVHD, the ravages of GVHD are expressed in this organ system. In the early studies of GVHD, it was recognized that the brunt of the graft-versus-host reaction occurred in host lymphoid organs. As a consequence, the host's immune competence was affected, leading to frequent and possibly fatal infectious complications. A profound drop in immunoglobulins was often observed. GVHD may also affect hematopoiesis, leading to a reduction in hematopoietic cells. Although there was not a clear decrease in peripheral blood counts in murine models, the number of hematopoietic precursors remained low. In humans, following BMT, the effect of GVHD on the hematopoietic system is usually not dramatic. However, persistent thrombocytopenia is a frequent manifestation of GVHD. Moreover, the presence of active GVHD not only may be immunosuppressive but also may decrease responsiveness to active immunization. One study suggests that immune responses to polio vaccination resulted in less protection in patients who had graft-versus-host disease.

PROPHYLAXIS

The major emphasis in controlling GVHD lies in prophylaxis, because of the difficulty in controlling the disease once it occurs. The most common form of prophylaxis is pharmacologic. Beginning in 1976, investigators at the City of Hope designed and implemented a series of sequential trials for the prophylaxis of acute GVHD. Each trial was aimed at decreasing the incidence of grades II–IV acute GVHD. A prospective randomized study carried out between January 1983 and December 1985 comparing the combination of methotrexate and prednisone with that of cyclosporine and prednisone demonstrated a significant reduction in acute GVHD, from 47% in patients receiving methotrexate and prednisone to 28% in those receiving cyclosporine and prednisone (p <0.05). The incidence of chronic GVHD was significantly higher in the group receiving cyclosporine and prednisone. Disease-free survival between these two treatment arms was not statistically significant.

In 1986 these investigators modified the combination of cyclosporine and predni-sone by increasing the dose and staring prednisone on day +7, as described by the Ohio State group. When this change was tested in a phase II trial, the incidence of grade II–IV acute GVHD decreased to 12%. This observation led to a second random-ized study to determine if the addition of three doses of methotrexate to the combina-tion of cyclosporine could further decrease the incidence of acute GVHD. The reasons for this particular schema were (1) three rather than the conventional four doses of methotrexate were used because many were unable to receive the fourth dose of methotrexate, and (2) prednisone was used in combination with cyclosporine and methotrexate because prednisone is the most effective drug in the treatment of acute GVHD.

During the 5-year period between December 1986 and December 1991, 150 patients were enrolled. This uniform group of patients consisted of those with acute leukemia in first complete remission, chronic myelogenous leukemia in first chronic phase, or lymphoblastic lymphoma in first complete remission. All patients received a uniform preparative regimen consisting of fractionated total body irradiation (1,320 cGy) and etoposide (60 mg/kg). Patients received a genotypically major histocompati-bility complex (MHC)-matched bone marrow graft and were randomized to receive either cyclosporine and prednisone or cyclosporine, methotrexate, and prednisone. The dosing schema for this regimen is shown in TABLE 3.

Patients were well balanced in terms of disease, age, donor recipient gender, and parity status of the donor (if female). Seventy-six patients were randomized to receive cyclosporine, methotrexate, and prednisone and 73 patients received cyclosporine and prednisone. One patient died on day +19 and was not evaluable for GVHD but was included in the survival analysis. Median follow-up for the two groups was 25 and 20 months, respectively. The median number of days to sustain engraftment to 500 granulocytes/μl was 19 for those receiving the three-drug regimen and 13 for the two-drug regimen (p <0.001). The median time to sustained platelet engraftment >25,000/μl was 23 days in those receiving the three drugs and 18 days for those receiving cyclosporine and prednisone (p = 0.003). Twenty-two patients on the three-drug regimen died compared to 26 patients on the two-drug regimen. There was no statistically significant difference in any cause of mortality. Five relapses occurred with the three-drug regimen compared to seven relapses with the two-drug regimen. The overall actuarial incidence of grade II–IV acute GVHD was 9% in those receiving three drugs and 23% in those receiving the two-drug regimen.[12] The overall incidence of chronic GVHD was 57% with the three-drug regimen and 60% with the two-drug regimen. However, analysis of the Karnofsky status revealed that both groups enjoyed

TABLE 3. Dosing Schema

Day	Cyclosporine	Prednisone	Methotrexate
−2	5 mg/kg iv qd		—
+1	5 mg/kg iv qd		15 mg/m^2 iv
+	5 mg^g iv qd		10 mg/m^2 iv
+4	3 mg/kg iv qd	−	
+6	3 mg/kg iv qd	−	10 mg/m^2 iv
+7	3 mg/kg iv qd	0.5 mg/kg iv qc	
+15	3.75 mg/kg iv qd	1.0 mg/kg pv qd	
+29	3.75 mg/kg iv qd	0.8 mg/kg po qd	
+36	10 mg/kg po qd	0.8 mg/kg po qd	
+43	10 mg/kg po qd	0.5 mg/kg po qd	
+57	10 mg/kg po qd	0.2 mg/kg po qd	
+84	8 mg/kg po qd	0.2 mg/kg po qd	
+98	6 mg/kg po qd	0.2 mg/kg po qd	
+120	4 mg/kg po qd	0.1 mg/kg po qd	
+180	Off	Off	

a median Karnofsky performance score of 90 (range 60-100). The actuarial recurrence rate of leukemia was 13% for the three-drug regimen and 16% for the two-drug regimen. Disease-free survival at 3 years was 64% for those receiving cyclosporine, methotrexate, and prednisone and 59% for those receiving cyclosporine and prednisone (p = NS).

These improved results with cyclosporine, methotrexate, and prednisone led to our third on-going prospective randomized study comparing cyclosporine, methotrexate, and prednisone to the cyclosporine and methotrexate regimen developed by the Seattle group. This trial involves two institutions, Stanford University and the City of Hope National Medical Center. Patients eligible for this study are those with acute leukemia in first or second remission or early relapse or with chronic myelogenous leukemia in first chronic phase or accelerated phase, with genotypically HLA identical donors. Patients are randomized to receive the preparative regimen consisting of fractionated total body irradiation and cyclophosphamide versus fractionated total body irradiation and etoposide. This trial will determine the contribution of this three-drug regimen compared to the most commonly used GVHD prophylaxis regimen.

Recently, other agents have reached clinical trials. Tests with FK506 in phase I/II trials suggest that it may have the same efficacy as cyclosporine. Monoclonal antibodies have also been used. A monoclonal antibody conjugated to ricin A chain and directed against CD5 (a T-cell marker) has been tested clinically. Another monoclonal antibody directed against the IL-2 receptor (HAT) has also been used recently. A large phase III trial with this monoclonal antibody for use in prophylaxis following allogeneic matched unrelated donor BMT has just been completed. Another interesting approach has been the use of a soluble IL-1 receptor or an IL-1 receptor antagonist. Although these studies are promising, larger trials are necessary for a more definitive result.

T-CELL DEPLETION

Since T cells are the effector cells in GVHD, attempts to remove T cells would logically result in a lower incidence of the disease. Although this is true, unfortunately most T-cell depletion techniques are also associated with a higher relapse rate and lack of engraftment. The higher relapse rate is due to removal of the T cells that are responsible for the graft-versus-leukemia effect. More selective T-cell depletion or less stringent depletion may partially circumvent these problems. However, the various methods used for lymphocyte depletion and the addition of other pharmacologic immunosuppressive drugs make comparison of the data difficult. The most common approaches to T-cell depletion has been the use of monoclonal antibodies targeting all T cells or specific T-cell subsets. Other approaches use physical separation density gradients or mechanical separation such as elutriation.

TREATMENT

Unfortunately, once moderate to severe GVHD occurs, treatment options are limited. The first line of therapy following failure of GVHD prophylaxis has been the use of glucocorticoids (steroids). Patients with mild to moderate GVHD respond; however, patients with severe GVHD do poorly. Of note, successful therapy of acute GVHD did not affect the risk of leukemic relapse. The Seattle group also reported a retrospective analysis of therapy for acute GVHD in patients in whom primary treatment failed. Four hundred twenty-seven patients were identified. Most patients (75%) had a rash, with liver dysfunction being the second most common manifestation (59%) and gut dysfunction the third (53% of patients). Secondary treatment consisted of glucocorticoids in most patients ($n = 249$), cyclosporine ($n = 80$), antithymocyte globulin ($n = 214$), or monoclonal antibody ($n = 19$). Most of these patients received single treatment; however, 37 received a combination of these single agents. Improvement or resolution of GVHD in the respective organs was seen in 45% of patients with skin disease, 25% with liver disease, and 35% with gut disease. Forty percent of patients showed some response to treatment. The highest complete response rate was seen when GVHD recurred during the taper phase of primary glucocorticoid treatment. Increasing the dose of glucocorticoids allowed for a second complete response. Severe dysfunction in the skin, liver, or gut at the beginning of treatment was associated with a lower incidence of response or improved outcome. Although increasing the dose of glucocorticoids represents the most effective therapy or strategy when GVHD recurs during the taper phase of primary treatment, unfortunately less than half the patients showed durable overall improvement. These results suggest that the potential efficacy of immunosuppressive agents can be assessed meaningfully in patients who have not responded adequately to primary treatment and that more effective treatments are needed.

Antithymocyte globulin (ATG) has also been used with mixed results. Patients treated with ATG experienced only a few incomplete responses in the gastrointestinal tract and liver. Untoward effects of ATG included hemolytic anemia, severe thrombocytopenia, neutropenia, fever, chills, polyarthritis, myalgias, nausea, vomiting, urticaria, and serum sickness.

Monoclonal antibody OKT3 was first shown to be effective in the treatment of rejection in renal transplant recipients. Because treatment with monoclonal antibody OKT3 specific for the CD3 complex instead of the T-cell antigen receptor can reverse or cure rejection of human renal allografts, use of OKT3 has been attempted in the treatment of GVHD. A pilot trial in eight allogeneic recipients with grade II or IV acute GVHD showed response in six patients, especially those with minimal disease. A second study of 10 patients with grade III-IV acute GVHD that was resistant to cyclosporine, methylprednisolone, and OKT3 induced complete responses in five and partial responses in four patients; however, acute GVHD recurred frequently. The efficacy of anti-CD3 antibodies in the treatment of patients with GVHD, however, has not been established. The dose-limiting side effect results from T-cell activation induced by some anti-CD3 antibodies *in vivo*. This has discouraged further use of this monoclonal antibody. A different approach was used in a phase I/II study with the anti-CD3 antibody BC3. This anti-CD3 antibody is not capable of cross-linking CD3 with Fc receptors on accessory cells. Thus, it is unable to induce T-cell proliferation. BC3 is a murine IgG 2b which reacts with the CD3 complex but does not interact well with Fc receptors on human monocytes. Therefore, BC3 does not activate proliferation of T lymphocytes. Seventeen patients were enrolled in this study and five patients achieved complete resolution of GVHD. Eight patients had partial improvement, two patients had no change, and two patients had progression. Of note, 8 of the 13 patients had sustained responses. Of interest, the administration of this nonmitogenic anti-CD3 antibody did not depend on depletion of circulating T cells. Thus, the mechanism of action of this antibody is related to some form of immunosuppression through modulation of T-cell function. Unfortunately, the use of OKT3 or anti-CD3 monoclonal antibodies results in a lymphoproliferative syndrome from polyclonal proliferation of B cells infected with the Epstein-Barr virus. This is frequently a fatal complication of the immunodeficiency state after transplantation. Clearly, further clinical trials will be necessary to establish the importance of these newer agents in the treatment of acute GVHD.

Another approach has been the use of anti-IL-2 receptor monoclonal antibody (B-B10, CD25) to treat patients with steroid-resistant grade II-IV acute GVHD. In a multicenter pilot trial, no complete responses were observed; however, eight patients achieved a good partial response. Of interest, gut lesions responded best, followed by skin and liver. Graft-versus-host disease recurred when treatment was discontinued. Three patients are alive following treatment with this monoclonal antibody. In another trial, full response of organ involvement was achieved in 22 patients (68.7%); unfortunately this study did not state whether these responses were durable. A follow-up study of 58 patients suggested that 26 of 58 (44.8%) were alive between 240 and 900 days after GVHD treatment with B-B10. Although the response rate was gratifying, the GVHD recurrence rate remained high at 41%. However, those who responded to treatment with B-B10 had a significant survival advantage.

Another method of treatment of severe acute GVHD has been a monoclonal antibody against tumor necrosis factor alpha (TNF-α). A monoclonal anti-TNF-α termed B-C7 has been used to treat patients with grade III-IV acute GVHD. Eighteen patients responded, 21% with a complete response and 61% with improvement. However, active GVHD appeared rapidly in eight patients. Only 22% of the patients were alive following treatment with anti-TNF. Clearly more patients will need to be treated to extend these observations. This pilot study suggests that a monoclonal anti-TNF-α antibody may be of benefit to some patients with severe refractory acute GVHD, but it is ineffective in preventing recurrent GVHD in most patients.

Another approach has been to use Xomazyme (anti-CD5 conjugated to ricin A chain). Thirty-four patients with moderate to severe steroid-resistant acute GVHD were treated with Xomazyme. Seventy-two percent had a response in at least one organ and another 16% had stable disease. However, GVHD recurrence was frequent. Major difficulties with murine monoclonal antibody include febrile reactions, fluctuations in blood count, and, most importantly, B-cell lymphoproliferative disorders which may lead to death in many patients. Flu-like symptoms including fever, tremors, lethargy, anorexia, myalgias, and arthralgias were observed with ricin-A immunoconjugants.

FUTURE APPROACHES

New Pharmacologic Agents

As mentioned earlier, FK506 has been approved for liver transplantation and appears to be effective for GVHD prophylaxis. Trials of its use in combination with methotrexate are ongoing. With our continued improvement in understanding of the mechanisms of GVHD, a more rational approach to pharmacologic agents may be possible. Therefore, newer drugs such as rapamycin, which appears to act synergistically with cyclosporine, will need to be tested but hold considerable promise. Other drugs that may proceed to phase I/II trials include the mycophenolic acid leflunomide. Yet other drugs are being pursued in animal models.

Immunomodulation

Another approach that appears promising is the use of monoclonal antibodies as prophylaxis, before cytokines are released. A phase III study of the HAT antibody has already been completed and the results are being analyzed. The use of soluble IL-1 receptor or IL-1 receptor antagonist showed significant promise in early trials. This specific blockade of early cytokine release may be critical in preventing amplification of the graft-versus-host reaction leading to GVHD. Other approaches include monoclonal antibodies or CTLA4Ig to induce anergy and therefore prevent GVHD. An extreme form of T-cell depletion is the use of purified stem cells. Current approaches suggest that if pure stem cells could be transplanted without an increased risk of graft rejection, GVHD should not occur. This approach is being pursued using highly selected CD34⁺ cells, cord blood cells, or fetal liver cells. It is too early to know if these approaches will be successful.

Ultraviolet Therapy

Another interesting approach is to use ultraviolet B or PUVA irradiation of donor marrow in the prevention of GVHD. PUVA has been used in therapy for GVHD with some success. Another related approach is the use of extracorporeal photopheresis in the therapy for GVHD. We have observed that this method has produced excellent responses in skin GVHD, but the response in other organs is less exciting.

SUMMARY

Graft-versus-host disease remains a formidable barrier in allogeneic bone marrow transplantation. Studies have shown that effective prophylaxis results in improved overall survival for patients following allogeneic bone marrow transplantation. Various methods to prevent GVHD have been devised over the years including drug therapy, monoclonal antibodies, and T-cell depletion. Many of these prophylaxis regimens have been successful in improving the outcome in patients, with some regimens resulting in only a 9% incidence of acute GVHD in selected patients. Yet, GVHD remains an important problem for those patients in whom prophylaxis fails. Therapy for GVHD has relied on drugs and monoclonal antibodies, and the results of therapy for severe GVHD have been unsatisfactory. As immunologic understanding of the afferent and efferent phases of GVHD continues to be elucidated, more targeted therapy will be introduced and hopefully will result in better outcomes.

REFERENCES

1. UPHOFF, D. 1958. Alteration of homograft reaction by a-methopterin in lethally irradiated mice treated with homologous marrow. Proc. Soc. Exp. Biol. Med. **99:** 651.
2. BILLINGHAM, R. 1966. The biology of graft-versus-host reaction. Harvey Lecture. 21.
3. STORB, R., H. J. DEEG, V. FAREWELL *et al.* 1986. Marrow transplantation for severe aplastic anemia: Methotrexate alone compared with a combination of methotrexate and cyclosporine for prevention of acute graft-versus-host disease. Blood **68:** 119.
4. RAMSAY, N. K. C., J. KERSEY, L. L. ROBISON *et al.* 1982. A randomized study of the prevention of acute graft-versus-host disease. N. Engl. J. Med. **306:** 392.
5. FORMAN, S. J., K. G. BLUME, R. A. KRANCE *et al.* 1987. A prospective randomized study of acute graft-v-host disease in 107 patients with leukemia: Methotrexate/prednisone v cyclosporin a/prednisone. Transpant. Proc. **19:** 2905.
6. TUTSCHKA, P. J., E. A. COPELAN, J. P. KLEIN *et al.* 1987. Bone marrow transplantation for leukemia following a new busulfan and cyclophosphamide regimen. Blood **70:** 1382.
7. STORB, R., H. J. DEEG, J. WHITEHEAD *et al.* 1986. Methotrexate and cyclosporine compared with cyclosporine alone for prophylaxis of acute graft-versus-host disease after marrow transplantation for leukemia. N. Engl. J. Med. **314:** 729.
8. STORB, R., H. J. DEEG, M. PEPE *et al.* 1989. Methotrexate and cyclosporine versus cyclosporine alone for prophylaxis of graft-versus-host disease in patients given HLA-identical marrow grafts for leukemia: Long-term follow-up of a controlled trial. Blood **73:** 1729.
9. CHAO, N. J. 1992. Graft-versus-host disease following allogeneic bone marrow transplantation. Current Opinion Immunol. **4:** 571.
10. GUINAN, E. C., J. G. GRIBBEN, V. A. BOUSSIOTIS *et al.* 1994. Pivotal role of the B7 : CD28 pathway in transplantation tolerance and tumor immunity. Blood **84:** 3261.
11. FERRARA, J. L. M. 1992. Advances in GVHD: Novel lymphocyte subsets and cytokine dysregulation. Bone Marrow Transplant. **10** (suppl): 10.

12. CHAO, N. J., G. M. SCHMIDT, J. C. NILAND *et al.* 1993. Cyclosporine, methotrexate, and prednisone compared with cyclosporine and prednisone for prophylaxis of acute graft-versus-host disease. N. Engl. J. Med. **327:** 1225.

13. GLUCKSBERG, H., R. STORB, A. FEFER *et al.* 1974. Clinical manifestations of graft-versus-host disease in human recipients of marrow from HLA-matched sibling donors. Transplantation **18:** 295.

T-Cell Subsets and Their Cytokine Profiles in Transplantation and Tolerance

HERVÉ GROUX, MATTHIEU ROULEAU,
ROSA BACCHETTA, AND
MARIA-GRAZIA RONCAROLO

*DNAX Research Institute of Molecular and Cellular Biology
Human Immunology Department
901 California Avenue
Palo Alto, California 94304-1104*

The body is armed with a variety of immune mechanisms for attacking invading pathogens. Although T cells have long been known as essential components of this arsenal, a major conceptual advance in our knowledge about mechanisms of immunity has resulted from the establishment of the Th1/Th2 paradigm of helper (or CD4[+]) T cells, a model of T-cell specialization originally proposed by Mosmann and Coffman[1] in the mid-1980s. Although more complex than originally envisioned, this theory is based on a simple dichotomy: following stimulation, T cells differentiate into one or two major subsets of CD4[+] T cells. These T-cell subsets, Th1 and Th2, are defined on the basis of their cytokine repertoire. Furthermore, the distinct cytokine profile of each subset dictates its function in the immune response. The Th1 subset is characterized by the production of gamma-interferon (IFN-γ) and interleukin-2 (IL-2), cytokines that favor cell-mediated immune responses such as delayed type hypersensitivity and T-cell cytotoxicity. By contrast, Th2 cells secrete IL-4, IL-5, IL-6, and IL-10, which regulate humoral immunity. Generally, naïve T helper cells (CD4[+] CD45RA[+]) first progress to a Th0 phenotype, a subset of T helper cells capable of producing both Th1 and Th2 cytokines. Following repeated stimulation with specific antigens, Th0 cells differentiate further into either Th1 or Th2 cells. The resulting CD4[+] T-cell subset remains predominant throughout that particular immune episode, in part through the production of at least four cross-regulatory cytokines, IFN-γ, IL-12, IL-4, and IL-10.

The characteristics of a pathogen or the host defense that determine whether the Th1 or the Th2 pathway will dominate in a given immune response are currently unknown. However, both *in vitro* and *in vivo* studies have shown that the presence or absence of certain cytokines during primary stimulation of naive Th0 cells plays a pivotal role in the differentiation of T helper cells.[2-4]

Studies of naturally susceptible and resistant mouse strains infected with the protozoan *Leishmania major* have demonstrated that resistant mice develop a Th1 response, whereas the Th2 response predominates in susceptible mice.[5] The cytokine profile in the microenvironment during early stages of immune stimulation tips the balance towards either the Th1 or the Th2 subset in the ensuing immune response to *Leishmania* infection.[3] Indeed, treatment of resistant mice with anti-IFN-γ monoclonal antibodies (mAb) leads to Th2 cell differentiation and progressive infection,[4] whereas anti-IL-4 mAb treatment of susceptible mice promotes Th1 cell development and resistance to disease.[5] Similar observations were made in studies employing fungal[6] and bacterial[7,8] pathogens, underscoring the universal nature of the phenomenon in the murine immune response.

In humans, most alloreactive or PHA-induced CD4$^+$ T-cell clones derived from the peripheral blood of healthy donors have a Th0 phenotype and do not fit into the Th1 or Th2 subsets.[9] Therefore, this classification into Th1 and Th2 cells was judged invalid for human T cells. Recently, however, several studies found that CD4$^+$ T-cell clones exhibiting Th1- or Th2-like profiles can be isolated from tissues or peripheral blood of patients with different diseases.[10,11] For example, most allergen-specific T-cell clones derived from atopic donors have a Th2-like phenotype and produce relatively high levels of IL-4 and IL-5, but limited amounts of IFN-γ and IL-2. By contrast, all T-cell clones specific for bacterial antigens produce large amounts of IL-2 and IFN-γ, whereas only a proportion of these clones secrete low levels of IL-4 and/or IL-5.

T-CELL SUBSETS ASSOCIATED WITH GRAFT-VERSUS-HOST DISEASE OR TOLERANCE

Despite significant progress in the last 10 years, graft-versus-host disease (GVHD) remains the major barrier in effective allogeneic transplantation.[12,13] This disease is due to an immune response of both CD4$^+$ and CD8$^+$ donor T cells towards host tissues. Although donor-derived T cells in the transplanted cell suspension play a major role in this immune reaction, proinflammatory cytokines produced by these T cells as well as the accessory cells clearly contribute to the induction and maintenance of this process. We can speculate that the balance between allograft rejection/GVHD and tolerance is due to selective activation of either Th1- or Th2-type cells, respectively.

Sequential analysis of allografts undergoing rejection indicates that IL-2 and IFN-γ expression preceded and accompanied graft rejection.[14] IFN-γ is believed to recruit macrophages at the site of the graft and to induce their activation. In addition, IFN-γ enhances cytotoxic T lymphocyte activation and increases MHC antigen expression by the graft, whereas IL-2 promotes CD4$^+$ and CD8$^+$ T-cell expansion and activation of these cells. On the basis of these and other observations, it was concluded that these two Th1 cytokines induce and enhance the cellular proinflammatory immune response. However, recent experiments using IL-2-deficient mice demonstrated that these mice can readily reject allografts, indicating that IL-2 secretion is not absolutely required for mounting allogeneic immune responses *in vivo*.[15]

In vivo studies examining the pattern of cytokine expression during tolerance induction indicated a dramatic decrease in the expression of Th1 cytokines, such as IL-2 and IFN-γ, whereas increased levels of IL-4 transcripts were observed.[16] These results suggested that during the induction of tolerance, a "Th2 cytokine program" is induced, whereas a "Th1 program" is silenced. However, no direct proof currently exists that Th2 cytokines mediate allograft tolerance. In addition, in most of these studies cytokine profiles during allograft rejection or tolerance induction were analyzed by *in situ* hybridization techniques, by polymerase chain reaction (PCR) analysis of fresh tissues, or by measuring cytokine production by *in vitro* activated cells obtained from infiltrated tissues. Although these techniques provide information about the cytokines present in the rejected or tolerated organs, they may not reflect the cytokine profiles of alloantigen-specific CD4[+] T cells.

To address this question, we analyzed the cytokine production profiles of donor- or host-derived T-cell clones specific for HLA-antigens expressed by the host or the donor cells, respectively. These T-cell clones were obtained in two different experimental models: SCID patients in whom complete tolerance was achieved after HLA-mismatched fetal liver or bone marrow stem cell transplantation and SCID-hu mice reconstituted with human fetal liver and fetal thymus and subsequently engrafted with an allogeneic HLA-mismatched fetal pancreas.

SCID PATIENTS AS A MODEL FOR STUDYING TRANSPLANTATION TOLERANCE

SCID encompasses congenital disorders characterized by abnormal lymphoid development. Although different genetic defects can be responsible for the disease, infants with SCID share a profound impairment of both cellular and humoral immune functions. SCID patients can be successfully transplanted with hematopoietic stem cells derived from HLA-mismatched donors and therefore may serve as a model to investigate the mechanisms of induction and maintenance of tolerance after allogeneic transplantation. After immunologic reconstitution, these children developed a split chimerism in which T cells were donor-derived, whereas B cells and monocytes were of host origin. Despite HLA incompatibility between donor-derived T cells and host cells, tolerance towards donor and host was established after transplantation. These patients had no sign of GVHD even in the absence of any immunosuppressive treatment. In addition, the donor-derived T cells were unresponsive to the host HLA in a primary mixed lymphocyte reaction. However, clonal analysis of T cells from different transplanted patients showed that many of these CD4[+] and CD8[+] T-cell clones were specific for class I or class II HLA molecules expressed by the host, indicating that host-reactive T cells are not deleted from the repertoire, but that they are not operational *in vivo*.[9,17–19]

Cytokine Profiles of Host-Reactive T Cells Isolated from Transplanted SCID Patients

Host-Reactive T-Cell Clones Fail to Produce Interleukin-4

To define the cytokine production profiles of both CD4[+] and CD8[+] host-reactive T-cell clones, we studied their lymphokine production after stimulation with specific HLA-antigens or polyclonal activators.[9,17,18] CD8[+] T-cell clones isolated from normal donors and CD8[+] host-reactive T-cell clones isolated from SCID patients transplanted with HLA-mismatched fetal liver stem cells produce IL-2, IL-5, and high levels of IFN-γ and GM-CSF after antigen stimulation. However, all host-reactive CD8[+] T-cell clones from SCID patients in contrast to those from normal donors fail to produce IL-4 after antigen-specific or polyclonal stimulation, indicating that this is a specific property of host-reactive T-cell clones isolated from SCID patients reconstituted with fetal liver stem cells.

CD8[+] T-cell clones that were specifically cytotoxic for the HLA antigens encoded by the mismatched haplotype of the host were also isolated from SCID patients transplanted with haploidentical bone marrow cells.[17] These CD8[+] host-reactive T-cell clones did not secrete IL-2, IL-4, or IL-5 after optimal activation by host-specific antigens presented by host-derived Epstein-Barr virus-transformed B-cell lines (EBV-LCL), whereas IL-10, IFN-γ, and GM-CSF were only detectable at very low levels. After polyclonal activation these clones secreted levels of IL-10, IFN-γ, and GM-CSF that were in the same range as those produced by T-cell clones isolated from normal donors. Production of IL-4 and IL-5 was not observed, and only low levels of IL-2 secretion were detected after polyclonal activation. The reason for the lower cytokine production by CD8[+] host-reactive T-cell clones in patients transplanted with bone marrow cells than in patients transplanted with fetal tissues[9,18] is not clear. One possibility is that the patients transplanted with fetal liver stem cells do not require immunosuppressive treatment after transplantation, because the fetal liver cell suspensions are devoid of mature T cells capable of provoking GVHD. Therefore, the use of posttransplant immunosuppression could account for the differences in cytokine production patterns in host-reactive T-cell clones obtained from these two types of patients.

CD4[+] host-reactive T-cell clones produced variable levels of IL-5, IFN-γ, and GM-CSF, but like the CD8[+] host-reactive T-cell clones, they did not secrete IL-4 after stimulation with host-derived EBV-LCL or polyclonal activation. In addition, cytokine production was considerably lower than that in the supernatants of CD4[+] T-cell clones isolated from normal donors. However, cytokine production was normal when CD4[+] host-reactive T-cell clones were polyclonally activated with concanavalin A,12-0-tetradecanoyl-phorbol-13-acetate (TPA) plus anti-CD3 mAb, or TPA plus Ca[2+] ionophore. The lack of IL-4 production in all CD4[+] and CD8[+] host-reactive T-cell clones from these patients indicates that this is a specific property of host-reactive T cells. These clones did produce IL-5 and therefore differ from classic Th1 cells which fail to produce both IL-4 and IL-5. This specific lack of IL-4 production may have important consequences for the growth requirement and function of these cells *in vivo*.

Host-Reactive T-Cell Clones and Monocytes of Host Origin Produce High Levels of Interleukin-10

CD4[+] host-reactive T-cell clones generally displayed a low proliferative capacity and produced low levels of IL-2 after specific activation with host HLA-antigens.[18-20] By contrast, they produced high levels of IL-10, particularly in one patient.[20] These high levels of IL-10 were only observed after antigen-specific stimulation and represent a specific property of host-reactive clones. Alloreactive T-cell clones specific for third-party alloantigens, isolated from the same patient, produced levels of IL-10 that were comparable to those detected in the supernatants of alloreactive T-cell clones isolated from normal donors, but considerably lower than those produced by host-reactive T-cell clones. In addition, blocking experiments using neutralizing anti-IL-10 mAb showed that the high levels of endogenously produced IL-10 could suppress the proliferative responses of host-reactive T-cell clones.[20]

In addition to the high levels of IL-10 protein production by host-reactive T-cell clones, high levels of IL-10 mRNA were detected by semiquantitative PCR analysis of freshly isolated peripheral blood mononuclear cells from transplanted SCID patients. Cell fractionation studies indicated that in addition to donor-derived T cells, monocytes of host origin constitutively expressed high levels of IL-10 mRNA *in vivo*. This *in vivo* IL-10 production seems to be of biologic relevance, because HLA-DR expression on monocytes of one of these patients was significantly lower than that of monocytes derived from healthy individuals, a finding that is consistent with the notion that IL-10 downregulates class II MHC expression on monocytes.[20]

Collectively, these data indicate that host-reactive T-cell clones with a specific cytokine profile, which does not fit the classic Th1/Th2 classification, could be isolated from transplanted SCID patients. The most important features of these clones are that they lack IL-4 secretion, they produce low levels of IL-2, but they secrete high levels of IL-10, which in part may be responsible for the low proliferative responses of these clones *in vitro* (see below). This information, together with the high level of *in vivo* IL-10 production in SCID patients in whom tolerance has been achieved after HLA-incompatible transplantation, suggested that IL-10 may play an important role in establishing and maintaining transplantation tolerance and in preventing GVHD.

THE EFFECTS OF INTERLEUKIN-10 ON ALLOGENEIC RESPONSES *IN VITRO*

Interleukin-10 is produced by a variety of cells including T lymphocytes and monocytes.[21] It is primarily described as a Th2 cell type product in mice, but in humans IL-10 is produced by Th0, Th1, and Th2 cells. However, the levels of IL-10 production by Th2 cells are generally higher than those produced by Th0 or Th1 subsets.[22] IL-10 has been noted to reduce antigen-specific activation of human T cells, first by directly inhibiting IL-2 secretion by T cells, but also by inhibiting the antigen-presenting and accessory function of monocytes/macrophages and dendritic cells.[23,24] Similar to its inhibitory effects on T-cell proliferation in response to a soluble antigen, IL-10 strongly reduces the proliferation of human alloreactive cells in classic mixed lymphocyte reaction.[25] The levels of cytokines produced in a mixed lymphocyte reaction were significantly reduced in the presence of exogenous IL-10. The amounts of IL-2, IFN-γ, tumor necrosis factor-α (TNF-α), and GM-CSF were reduced two- to threefold.[25] IL-10 also inhibited the generation of allo-specific cytotoxic T cells in a primary mixed lymphocyte reaction and strongly suppressed the proliferative responses of CD4[+] allogeneic T-cell clones. Along with reduced proliferation, reduced levels of IL-2, IL-5, GM-CSF, and IFN-γ production by these T-cell clones were also observed.[25]

In addition, we recently demonstrated that stimulation of CD4[+] T cells with allogeneic monocytes in the presence of IL-10 (100 U/ml) rendered these cells unresponsive to further activation with the same allogeneic cells, whereas CD4$^+$ T cells activated in the absence of IL-10 proliferated vigorously after a secondary stimulation. This induction of anergy was antigen-specific, because the anergized cell population proliferated normally in response to third-party allogeneic monocytes. In addition, the proliferative responses to polyclonal activators, such as anti-CD3 mAb, were normal. When stimulated through their T-cell receptor, these anergized cells failed to secrete IL-2, IL-4, IL-5, IL-10, GM-CSF, IFN-γ, and TNF-α, whereas antigen-specific stimulation of CD4$^+$ T cells, activated without IL-10, resulted in the production of all of these cytokines except IL-4 (H. Groux *et al.*, unpublished data).

Taken together, these results support the hypothesis that IL-10 may be a key cytokine in the mechanisms that lead to tolerance induction. Furthermore, they indicate that IL-10 may have therapeutic potential in preventing or limiting GVHD.

SCID-HU MICE AS A MODEL FOR STUDYING ALLOGRAFT REJECTION

To analyze the different T-cell subsets involved in human allograft rejection and their cytokine production profiles, we established a model of allograft rejection in SCID-hu mice. On the basis of our studies showing that the allogeneic repertoire is normal in SCID-hu mice reconstituted with human fetal liver and fetal thymus,[26,27] we predicted that human T cells and accessory cells in the human thymus would migrate to the allograft and mount an immune response against the allogeneic tissue. Fetal human pancreas was chosen as an allogeneic tissue source, because it engrafts and matures normally in SCID mice and its macroscopic and microscopic structure can easily be recognized by standard histologic techniques.

SCID mice were reconstituted with human fetal liver and fetal thymus of one donor, 3-4 months before transplantation of the fetal pancreas from a different donor. After 4-10 weeks, mice were sacrificed and the pancreases were analyzed by histology and immunolabeling. In addition, the infiltrating T cells were isolated and characterized.

Histological analysis performed 10 weeks after transplantation revealed massive infiltration of leukocytes with tissue destruction of pancreas β-islet cells. Immunolabeling of these infiltrating cells with CD45 mAbs showed that they were predominantly of human origin, with low levels of Ly5$^+$ mouse cells. Moreover, immunolabeling with anti-CD45RO mAb revealed that most infiltrating T cells were activated and had a memory phenotype, whereas circulating human cells in SCID-hu mice were naive cells, expressing the CD45RA molecule. Among the human cells, monocytes, T cells, and some plasma cells were detected. The presence of human T cells was further confirmed by staining with anti-CD3, anti-CD4, and anti-CD8 mAb. Most human infiltrating T cells were CD4$^+$ T helper cells. Interestingly, this massive infiltration of cells was accompanied by high expression of MHC class II molecules on epithelial cells of the pancreatic grafts.

To confirm that the infiltrating T cells were of thymic origin and were not derived from the pancreas donor, we constructed SCID mice using an HLA-A2$^+$, HLA-A3$^-$, and HLA-B7$^-$ fetal liver and thymus donor and a fetal pancreas expressing HLA-A3 and HLA-B7 molecules, but not HLA-A2. Using HLA-B7 or HLA-A2-specific mAb, we showed that all infiltrating cells were HLA-A2 positive and therefore of thymic origin.

Extensive clonal analysis of T cells infiltrating the rejected pancreas indicated that most T-cell clones were HLA-A2⁺, confirming their thymic origin. Most T-cell clones were CD4⁺, but various CD8⁺ T-cell clones were also isolated. To analyze the specificity of these clones we used EBV-LCL derived from either the thymus donor or the fetal pancreas donor and HLA-matched EBV-LCL isolated from normal donors.

Many CD8⁺ T-cell clones isolated from rejected pancreas displayed cytotoxic activity against EBV-LCL, or T-cell blasts derived from the pancreas donor and not against EBV-LCL, or T-cell blasts derived from the thymus donor, indicating that CD8⁺ T cells infiltrating the pancreas are specifically directed against HLA class I antigens expressed on pancreatic cells. These cytotoxic T cells may be responsible for the tissue destruction observed.

Similarly, many CD4⁺ T-cell clones isolated from the infiltrated pancreas proliferated vigorously when activated with pancreatic donor-derived EBV-LCL, whereas no significant proliferation was observed in response to EBV-LCL derived from thymus donor. Therefore, these CD4⁺ T cell are specific for the HLA class II antigens expressed on pancreas cells and may also be involved in the rejection process. Preliminary results showed that all pancreas-specific CD4⁺ T-cell clones display a Th2-type cytokine profile, secreting high amounts of IL-4, IL-5, and GM-CSF, with variable amounts of IL-10 and TNF-α and very low levels of IL-2 and IFN-γ (M. Rouleau *et al.*, unpublished data).

These data were unexpected because, as discussed, graft rejection is thought to be associated with secretion of just Th1 cytokines IL-2 and IFN-γ. However, we may have analyzed a late phase of the rejection process and the cytokine profile may be different at earlier time points. On the other hand, most data involving the role of IFN-γ and IL-2 in the rejection process in humans have been generated by analyzing proteins or transcripts for these cytokines *in situ* in the rejected allograft, whereas in our study cytokine profiles of the alloantigen-specific T cells were analyzed selectively.

Collectively, our studies indicate that host-reactive T cells, which cannot be classified as Th1/Th2 cells but which have a unique cytokine profile, are present in transplanted SCID patients in whom tolerance is achieved. On the other hand, chronic rejection of an allotransplant in an SCID-hu mouse model may be associated with transplant-specific T cells with a Th2 phenotype. In addition, these results lead us to conclude that although the Th1/Th2 paradigm has been extremely useful in understanding the CD4⁺ T-cell activation program, events other than or in addition to a switch between Th1/Th2 cells must be critical to tolerance induction versus rejection.

REFERENCES

1. MOSMANN, T. R. & R. L. COFFMAN. 1987. Immunol. Today **8:** 223–237.
2. SHER, A. & R. L. COFFMAN. 1991. Ann. Rev. Immunol. **10:** 385–391.
3. SCOTT, P. 1991. J. Immunol. **147:** 3149–3155.
4. HEINZEL, F. P., M. D. SADICK, B. J. HOLADAY, R. L. COFFMAN & R. M. LOCKSLEY. 1989. J. Exp. Med. **169:** 59–72.

5. LOCKSLEY, R. M. & P. SCOTT. 1991. Immunol. Today **12:** A58-A61.
6. ROMANI, L., A. MENCACCI, U. GROHMANN, S. MOCCI, P. MOSCI, P. PUCCETTI & F. BISTONI. 1992. J. Exp. Med. **176:** 19-25.
7. HAAK-FRENDSCHO, M., J. F. BROWN, Y. IIZAWA, R. D. WAGNER & C. J. CZUPRYNSKI. 1992. J. Immunol. **148:** 3978-3985.
8. HSIEH, C. S., S. E. MACATONIA, C. S. TRIPP, S. F. WOLF, A. O'GARRA & K. M. MURPHY. 1993. Science **260:** 547-549.
9. BACCHETTA, R., R. DE WAAL MALEFIJT, H. YSSEL, J. ABRAMS, J. E. DE VRIES, H. SPITS & M. G. RONCAROLO. 1990. J. Immunol. **144:** 902-908.
10. MAGGI, E., P. BISWAS, G. DEL PRETE, P. PARRONCHI, D. MACCHIA, C. SIMONELLI, L. EMMI, M. DE CARLI, A. TIRI & M. RICCI. 1991. J. Immunol. **146:** 1169-1174.
11. WIERENGA, E. A., M. SNOEK, C. DE GROOT, I. CHRETIEN, J. D. BOS, H. M. JANSEN & M. L. KAPSENBERG. 1990. J. Immunol. **144:** 4651-4656.
12. PARKMAN, R. 1991. Immunodef. Rev. **2:** 253-259.
13. FERRARA, J. L. M. & H. J. DEEG. 1991. N. Engl. J. Med. **324:** 667-678.
14. DALLMAN, M. J., C. P. LARSEN & P. J. MORRIS. 1991. J. Exp. Med. **174:** 493-496.
15. SCHORLE, H., T. HOLTSCHKE, T. HUNIG, A. SCHIMPL & I. HORAK. 1991. Nature **352:** 621-624.
16. NICKERSON, P. W., D. N. RUSH, J. R. JEFFERY, D. POCHINCO & R. M. MCKENNA. 1993. Transplant. Proc. **25:** 984-989.
17. BACCHETTA, R., R. PARKMAN, M. MCMAHON, K. WEINBERG, M. BIGLER, J. E. DE VRIES & M. G. RONCAROLO. 1995. Blood **85:** 1944-1953.
18. BACCHETTA, R., B. A. VANDEKERCKHOVE, J. L. TOURAINE, M. BIGLER, S. MARTINO, L. GEBUHRER, J. E. DE VRIES, H. SPITS & M. G. RONCAROLO. 1993. J. Clin. Invest. **91:** 1067-1078.
19. RONCAROLO, M. G., H. YSSEL, J. L. TOURAINE, H. BETUEL, J. E. DE VRIES & H. SPITS 1988. J. Exp. Med. **167:** 1523-1534.
20. BACCHETTA, R., M. BIGLER, J. L. TOURAINE, R. PARKMAN, P. A. TOVO, J. ABRAMS, R. DE WAAL MALEFYT, J. E. DE VRIES & M. G. RONCAROLO. 1994. J. Exp. Med. **179:** 493-502.
21. MOORE, K. W., A. O'GARRA, R. DE WAAL MALEFYT, P. VIEIRA & T. R. MOSMANN. 1993. Ann. Rev. Immunol. **11:** 65-75.
22. YSSEL, H., R. DE WAAL MALEFYT, M. G. RONCAROLO, J. S. ABRAMS, R. LAHESMAA, H. SPITS & J. E. DE VRIES. 1992. J. Immunol. **149:** 2378-2384.
23. DE WAAL MALEFYT, R., H. YSSEL & J. E. DE VRIES. 1993. J. Immunol. **150:** 4754-4765.
24. DE WAAL MALEFYT, R., J. ABRAMS, B. BENNETT, C. G. FIGDOR & J. E. DE VRIES. 1991. J. Exp. Med. **174:** 1209-1220.
25. BEJARANO, M. T., R. DE WAAL MALEFYT, J. S. ABRAMS, M. BIGLER, R. BACCHETTA, J. E. DE VRIES & M. G. RONCAROLO. 1992. Int. Immunol. **4:** 1389-1397.
26. VANDEKERCKHOVE, B., J. F. KROWKA, J. M. MCCUNE, J. E. DE VRIES, H. SPITS & M. G. RONCAROLO. 1991. J. Immunol. **146:** 4173-4179.
27. VANDEKERCKHOVE, B., R. BACCALA, D. JONES, D. H. KONO, A. N. THEOFILOPOULOS & M. G. RONCAROLO. 1992. J. Exp. Med. **176:** 1619-1624.

Prevention of Graft-versus-Host Disease

Studies in a Canine Model[a]

RAINER STORB,[b] H. JOACHIM DEEG,
ROBERT RAFF, FRIEDRICH SCHUENING, CONG YU,
BRENDA M. SANDMAIER, AND
THEODORE GRAHAM

Clinical Research Division
Fred Hutchinson Cancer Research Center
and
Department of Medicine
University of Washington School of Medicine
Seattle, Washington 98104-2092

Prevention of graft-versus-host disease (GVHD) has been accomplished by histocompatibility matching of marrow donors and recipients, the use of immunosuppressive drugs after transplant, the placement of patients into a pathogene-poor environment, and *in vitro* manipulation of the graft. The role of histocompatibility typing has been well established by previous studies, and the usefulness of the protective environment has been described in mice and some human patients, particularly those transplanted for aplastic anemia.[1,2] The current report reviews the use of immunosuppressive drugs after transplant as it evolved in canine studies of marrow transplantation, and it addresses some of the problems encountered with the use of T-cell depletion from the marrow graft in that model.

It is important that the method of GVHD prevention used does not interfere with the acceptance of the marrow graft by the host or otherwise seriously impair the function of the transplant. This requirement has excluded a number of immunosuppressive agents from clinical use, as determined by results of canine studies. For example, cyclophosphamide,[3] cytosine arabinoside,[4] and procarbazine[4] were marrow toxic when given at doses that promised to be immunosuppressive, thereby causing death of animals from graft failure. When doses were lowered, engraftment was seen, but

[a]This work was supported by grants CA18221, CA31787, CA15704, DK42716, and HL36444 awarded by the National Institutes of Health, Department of Health and Human Services, Bethesda, Maryland. Support was also received from the Josef Steiner Krebsstiftung, Bern, Switzerland; Wyeth-Ayers, Princeton, New Jersey; Amgen Co., Thousand Oaks, California; Fujisawa Pharmaceutical Co., Deerfield, Illinois; Neurobiological Technologies, Inc., Richmond, California; and Cetus, Emeryville, California.

[b]Address for correspondence: Rainer Storb, MD, Fred Hutchinson Cancer Research Center, 1124 Columbia St., M318, Seattle, WA 98104-2092.

TABLE 1. Dogs Given 9.2 Gy Total Body Irradiation and DLA-Nonidentical Unrelated Hematopoietic Grafts (Single Agent Immunosuppression Is Given after Transplant)

Postgrafting Immunosuppression	No. of Dogs	Median Survival (days)	No. of Dogs Surviving >100 days
None	76	10	0
Cyclophosphamide	18	12	0
Procarbazine	6	9.5	0
Cytosine arabinoside	6	10	0
Corticotropin-releasing factor	8	15	0
15-Deoxyspergualin	5	19	0
6-Mercaptopurine	8	14.5	0
Azathioprine	2	20	0
Tacrolimus (FK506)	10	20	1
Succinylacetone	5	22	0
Cyclosporine	15	17	1
Methotrexate	51	21	9

GVHD occurred. Results with these agents are shown in TABLE 1. Other agents had nonmarrow toxicities. An example is succinylacetone which was immunosuppressive (TABLE 1) but had untoward neurological toxicities that resulted in irreversible cerebellar ataxia.[5]

Again, other drugs (TABLE 1) such as 6-mercaptopurine,[4] azathioprine,[4] cyclosporine,[6] tacrolimus (FK506),[7] deoxyspergualin,[8] and corticotropin-releasing factor[9] had good immunosuppressive properties in unrelated DLA-nonidentical recipients and resulted in significantly prolonged survival. However, none of the dogs so treated became a long-term survivor, indicating that these drugs were incapable of inducing stable graft-host tolerance. An exception to that rule was the antimetabolite methotrexate.[2,10] Not only did methotrexate prolong recipient survival, but also a small percentage of DLA-nonidentical unrelated and a large percentage of DLA-identical littermate recipients became long-term survivors, even though methotrexate was discontinued by day 100 (TABLE 1 and FIGS. 1 and 2). The exact mechanism by which graft-host tolerance ensued is as yet unknown, but previous studies point towards a role for specific suppressor cells. For methotrexate to be effective, it needed to be given for a prolonged period (approximately 3 months after transplant), whereas a shorter course was only marginally effective. The early results in dogs led to application of methotrexate in humans. As in the dog, long-term administration of methotrexate was better than short-term administration,[11] and it was possible to discontinue the drug in most marrow graft recipients after 3 months without the subsequent development of GVHD. These findings contrasted sharply with the more prolonged need for immunosuppressive drugs in patients undergoing transplants of solid organs. Nevertheless, despite methotrexate, acute GVHD was seen in approximately 35-60% of patients transplanted with marrow from HLA-identical sibling donors.[12] Given that

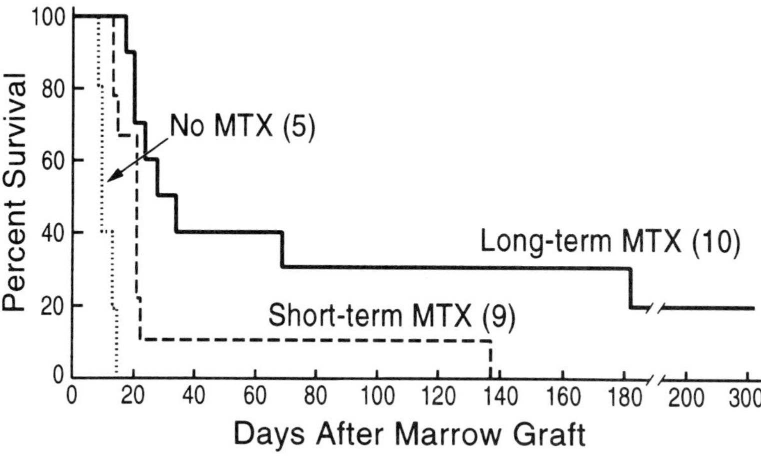

FIGURE 1. Survival of dogs given 9.2 Gy total body irradiation and hematopoietic grafts from DLA-nonidentical unrelated donors. Dogs received either no immunosuppression after transplant, a short course of methotrexate administered on days 1, 3, 6, and 11, or a long course of methotrexate administered on days 1, 3, 6, and 11 and then once weekly until day 102 after transplant.

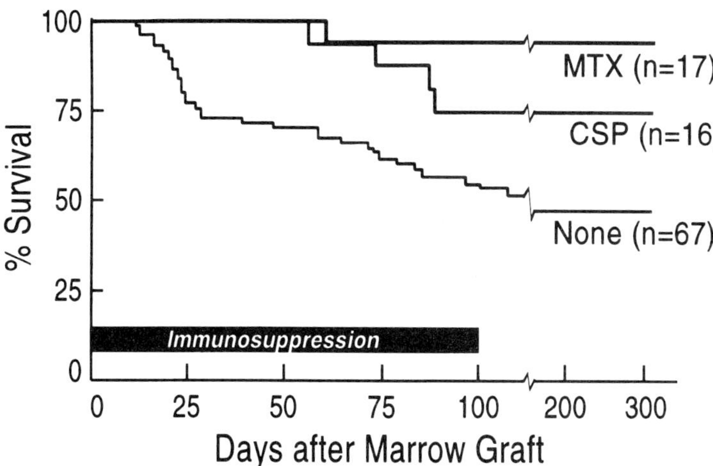

FIGURE 2. Survival of dogs given 9.2 Gy total body irradiation and hematopoietic grafts from genotypically DLA-identical littermates. Dogs received either no immunosuppression after transplant, intermittent methotrexate on days 1, 3, 6, and 11 and once weekly until day 102, or daily cyclosporine from day −1 to day 100 after transplant.

TABLE 2. Dogs Given 9.2 Gy Total Body Irradiation and DLA-Nonidentical Unrelated Hematopoietic Grafts (Combinations of Immunosuppression Are Given after Transplant)

Postgrafting Immunosuppression	No. of Dogs	Median Survival (days)	No. of Dogs Surviving >100 days
Methotrexate (MTX) + cyclophospha- mide (CY)	8	19.5	0
MTX + 6-mercaptopurine	8	36.5	1
Azathioprine + cyclosporine (CSP)	10	22	2
MTX + 6-mercaptopurine (high dose) + CY + methylprednisolone	8	40	1
MTX + 6-mercaptopurine (low dose) + CY + methylprednisolone	8	23	0
MTX + procarbazine	9	27	1
MTX + antithymocyte serum (ATS)	10	45.5	2
MTX + procarbazine + ATS	17	30	0

finding and given the 50% mortality associated with acute GVHD, the search for improved immunosuppressive drugs continues.

On the basis of the principles of additive and even synergistic effects observed with chemotherapeutic agents in the treatment of patients with malignancy, we explored combinations of immunosuppressive drugs for GVHD prevention. TABLE 2 summarizes early findings with methotrexate-containing combinations.[4] Although some regimens were remarkably effective in prolonging median survival of canine marrow graft recipients, none resulted in an increased percentage of long-term survivors over that with methotrexate alone. The combination of methotrexate and antithymocyte serum (ATS) was of interest.[13] In that regimen, ATS was administered only when methotrexate-treated dogs began showing early evidence of GVHD. This resulted in reversal of clinical signs and symptoms of GVHD in many dogs. This finding led to the application of antithymocyte globulin in the treatment of acute GVHD in patients in 1973, the first clinical study to show that acute GVHD could be reversed in some cases.[14]

Many drug combinations, particularly the quadruple combination of methotrexate, 6-mercaptopurine (high dose), cyclophosphamide, and methylprednisolone, were marrow suppressive,[4] and dogs died of infections rather than of GVHD. Because of these side effects, most of the early drug combinations studied did not find their way into clinical use.

In the late 1970s, cyclosporine, a T-cell activation blocker, became available for preclinical studies. TABLE 1 and FIGURE 2 show that cyclosporine[6] was as effective as methotrexate in GVHD prevention in dogs. Subsequent randomized clinical studies comparing methotrexate to cyclosporine for GVHD prevention in patients also showed the two drugs to be equivalent.[15] Further work in dogs indicated synergism between the two drugs when they were administered concurrently to prevent GVHD. Results

TABLE 3. Dogs Given 9.2 Gy Total Body Irradiation and DLA-Nonidentical Unrelated Marrow Grafts (Short Methotrexate Is Given Alone or Combined with Other Drugs)

Postgrafting Immunosuppression	No. of Dogs	Median Survival (days)	No. of Dogs Surviving >100 days
Methotrexate (MTX)	29	19	1
MTX + corticotropin-releasing factor	7	28	0
MTX + cyclosporine	17	100	8
MTX + tacrolimus	10	>150	5

TABLE 4. Dogs Given 9.2 Gy Total Body Irradiation and Hematopoietic Grafts from DLA-Haploidentical Littermates

Postgrafting Immunosuppression	No. of Dogs	Median Survival (days)	No. of Dogs Surviving >100 days
None	6	10.5	0
Methotrexate (MTX)	23	37	4
Succinylacetone	7	17	0
MTX + succinylacetone	5	42	0
MTX + cyclosporine	10	1,172	9
Trimetrexate + cyclosporine	10	150	6

of these studies are shown in TABLES 3 and 4 as well as in FIGURES 3 and 4. Long-term survival of DLA-nonidentical unrelated recipients was 35% compared to 6% with methotrexate and 0% with cyclosporine alone,[16] although 60% of surviving dogs had chronic GVHD. Even better results were seen when methotrexate and cyclosporine were combined and given to DLA-haploidentical littermate recipients.[17] Seventy percent of littermates showed event-free survival, and no chronic GVHD was seen. The combination of methotrexate and cyclosporine was subsequently compared to either drug alone in two randomized prospective clinical trials.[18,19] In both trials, significant reductions in the incidence of acute GVHD were found in patients given the drug combination. None of the patients given the drug combination had severe grade IV GVHD. As a result of improved GVHD prevention, transplant-related mortality decreased. Strong trends towards improved event-free survival were noted in patients transplanted for chronic myelocytic leukemia in chronic phase, aplastic anemia, and myelodysplasia. The two-drug combination is now widely used in clinical marrow transplantation. While remarkably effective in patients given genotypically HLA-identical marrow grafts, methotrexate/cyclosporine did not prevent the development of acute GVHD in most patients given either HLA-haploidentical related marrow

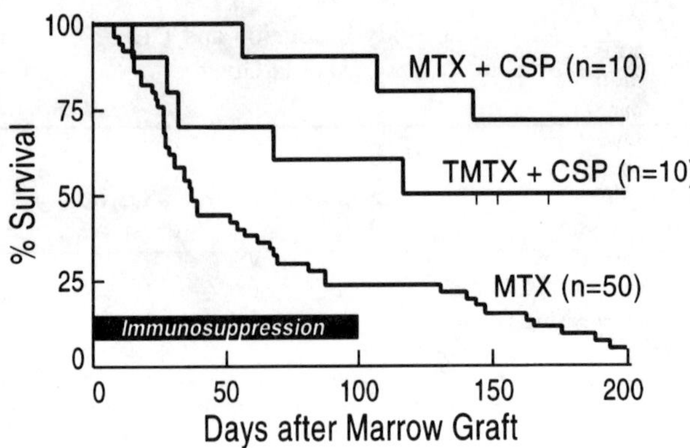

FIGURE 3. Survival of dogs given 9.2 Gy total body irradiation and hematopoietic grafts from DLA-haploidentical littermates. Dogs were given either intermittent methotrexate for the first 102 days, a short course of methotrexate (days 1, 3, 6, and 11) along with cyclosporine for the first 100 days after transplant, or a short course of trimetrexate (days 1, 3, 6, and 11) along with cyclosporine for the first 100 days.

grafts or grafts from unrelated donors, prompting continued research in the area of GVHD prevention.[20,21]

Accordingly, we investigated new immunosuppressive drugs either alone or in combination with other drugs. When cyclosporine was combined with azathioprine, no synergism was found[4]; in fact, survival of dogs was not lengthened over that with either drug alone (TABLE 2). Also, when succinylacetone was combined with methotrexate for use in recipients of DLA-haploidentical littermate marrow (TABLE 4), no synergism was found.[22] More recent work on FK506 (tacrolimus), a macrolide lactone isolated from *Streptomyces tsukubaensis* that blocks T-cell activation in a manner similar to that of cyclosporine, is summarized in TABLES 1 and 3 and FIGURE 4.[7] The work was carried out in DLA-nonidentical unrelated canine recipients and demonstrated synergism between the macrolide and methotrexate, with half of the dogs so treated becoming long-term survivors even though tacrolimus was discontinued by day 90 after transplantation. None of the long-term survivors had clinical evidence of chronic GVHD, a finding that may suggest differences between tacrolimus and cyclosporine. Results have encouraged clinical trials, and currently comparisons of methotrexate/tacrolimus to the standard methotrexate/cyclosporine regimen are underway in recipients of marrow grafts from HLA-identical siblings and from unrelated donors. Combining methotrexate with yet another immunosuppressive agent, corticotropin-releasing factor, suggested at best additive effects of the two drugs[9] (TABLE 3).

Previous studies of methotrexate had stressed the importance of giving the drug for a prolonged period after transplant (FIG. 1) before graft-host tolerance became established. Yet, when methotrexate is combined with cyclosporine clinically, the antimetabolite can often not be administered beyond day 11 because of cyclosporine-associated renal dysfunction. The problem arises because methotrexate is excreted through the kidneys. Administration of the drug in patients with renal insufficiency

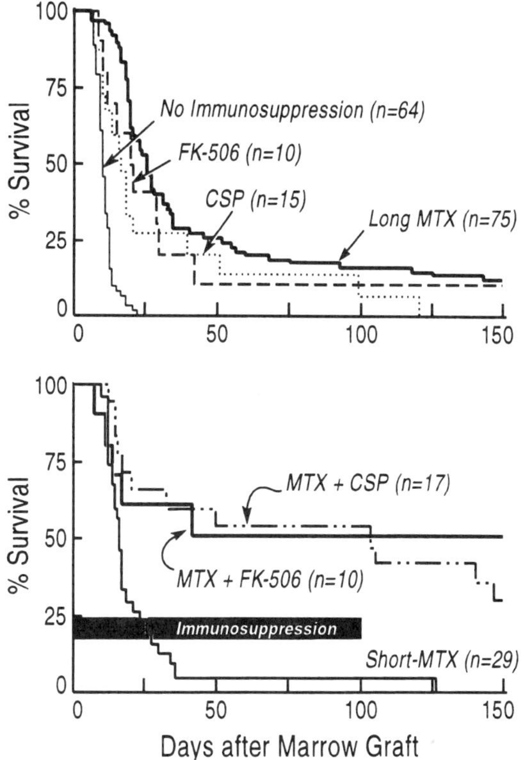

FIGURE 4. Survival of dogs given 9.2 Gy total body irradiation and hematopoietic grafts from DLA-nonidentical unrelated donors. The *upper panel* shows survival of dogs given no immunosuppression, cyclosporine for the first 100 days, intermittent methotrexate for the first 102 days, and FK506 (tacrolimus) for the first 90 days after transplant. The *lower panel* shows survival of dogs given either a short course of methotrexate (days 1, 3, 6, and 11), a short course of methotrexate combined with 100 days of cyclosporine, or a short course of methotrexate combined with 90 daily doses of FK506 (tacrolimus).

would entail the risk of methotrexate toxicity, and serious depression of marrow function might ensue. We therefore investigated a methotrexate-like antimetabolite, trimetrexate, which does not depend on renal excretion but rather is metabolized in the liver.[23] Results of a study in which trimetrexate was combined with cyclosporine to prevent GVHD after marrow grafts from DLA-haploidentical littermates are depicted in FIGURE 3. Survival of littermates given trimetrexate/cyclosporine was better than that of those given methotrexate alone and not significantly different from that obtained with methotrexate/cyclosporine. Results have prompted a pilot study in patients with advanced hematologic diseases given marrow grafts from family members who were HLA-haploidentical and mismatched for no more than one-HLA antigen on the nonshared haplotype.[24] In this study, timetrexate was administered on

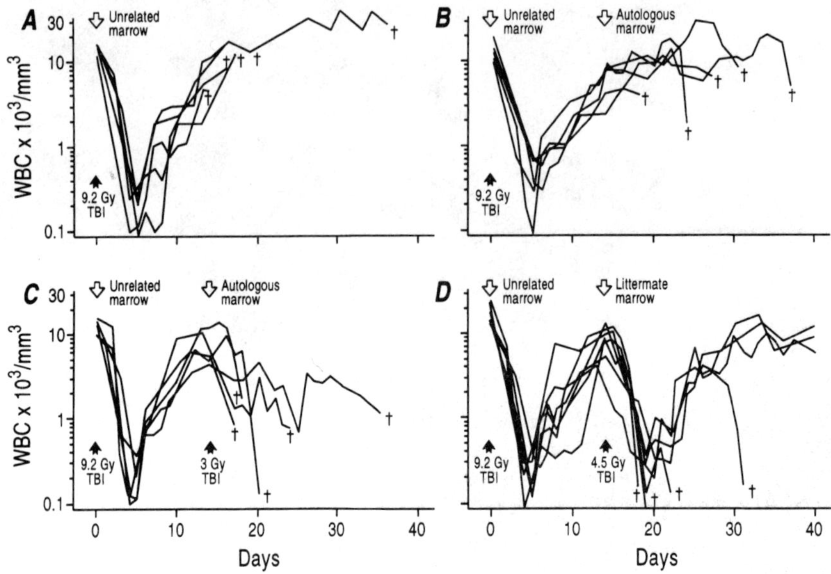

FIGURE 5. White blood cell changes in dogs given 9.2 Gy total body irradiation (TBI) followed by hematopoietic grafts from unrelated DLA-nonidentical donors. All dogs were given a short course of methotrexate (days 1, 3, 6, and 9) to delay the onset of acute GVHD. No other therapy was given to dogs in panel **A.** Dogs in panel **B** were given an autologous marrow infusion on day 14. Dogs in panel **C** received 3 Gy of TBI on day 14 followed by infusion of previously stored autologous marrow. Dogs in panel **D** were given 4.5 Gy of TBI on day 14 followed by hematopoietic grafts from DLA-identical littermates; all received additional methotrexate on days 1, 3, 6, and 11 and then once weekly following the second marrow transplant.

days 1, 3, 6, and 11 and then once weekly until day 39, spanning the time frame during which acute GVHD is usually observed. Results were encouraging, and a Phase II study is now in progress.

Yet another study in dogs involved the macrolide rapamycin (unpublished data). Results are summarized in TABLE 5. Although somewhat effective in delaying the onset of GVHD, major problems in dogs turned out to be diarrhea and weight loss as well as graft failure. The latter problem was also seen in earlier studies with cyclosporine and presumably resulted from blockage of the graft-enhancing effect of donor lymphocytes by the macrolide. In the cyclosporine studies, graft failure was overcome by the addition of methotrexate, presumably because the antimetabolite suppressed those surviving host immune cells which were responsible for graft rejection. Because of the severity of gastrointestinal toxicity with rapamycin, further investigation of this drug in dogs was suspended; however, because of encouraging findings in the rodent model, rapamycin is now being explored in the clinic.

In another study we evaluated whether GVHD, once established, could be reversed by subsequent transplantation of either previously stored autologous marrow or mar-

TABLE 5. Survival of Dogs Given 9.2 Gy Total Body Irradiation and Either Autologous Marrow Grafts or Grafts from DLA-Nonidentical Unrelated Donors along with Postgrafting Immunosuppression with Rapamycin

Source of Marrow	Dog No.	Rapamycin Regimen (mg/kg/day) days 0–24	Engraftment	Marrow Cellularity	GVHD	Survival (days)	Cause of Death
Autologous	D229	0.05 iv	No	20%	NA	9	GI toxicity, septicemia
	D279	0.05 iv	No	<5%	NA	6	GI toxicity, pneumonia
	D334	0.1 sc	Yes	100%	NA	74	Euthanized[a]
	D430	0.1 sc	Yes	100%	NA	67	Euthanized[a]
	D413	0.2 sc	Yes	40%	NA	29	GI toxicity, septicemia
DLA-nonidentical unrelated	D524	0.1 sc	No	<5%	No	8	Pneumonia
	D509	0.1 sc	Yes	NL	Transient	>150	Alive
	D453	0.1 sc	Yes	0%	No	15	Graft failure
	D455	0.1 sc	Yes	40%	Yes	26	GVHD skin, gut, liver
	D460	0.1 sc	Yes	>5%	Yes	17	GVHD skin, gut
	D545	0.1 sc	No	0%	No	20	GI toxicity, graft failure

[a] Euthanized at end of study.

Abbreviations: iv = intravenously; sc = subcutaneously; NA = not applicable; GI = gastrointestinal; NL = normal.

row from a littermate that was DLA-identical to the recipient.[25] The study was undertaken because of the potential usefulness of GVHD in eradicating residual malignant cells, as in patients transplanted for advanced leukemia (graft-versus-leukemia effect). After the graft-versus-leukemia effect had taken place, but before GVHD became fatal, the histoincompatible graft was displaced by a second transplant of cells that were either genetically identical to the recipient (autologous) or closely related (DLA-identical littermate). Hematological changes in dogs from these studies are summarized in FIGURE 5. All were given DLA-nonidentical unrelated hematopoietic grafts followed by GVHD prevention with four doses of methotrexate on days 1, 3, 6, and 9. Engraftment was prompt. All five dogs given no further therapy died with acute GVHD between 16 and 39 days after transplant (panel A). Similarly, all five dogs given an autologous marrow infusion on day 14 died with acute GVHD between days 19 and 37 (panel B). They showed no evidence of surviving cells of host type upon cytogenetic examination of marrow. Therefore, in an attempt at tilting the advantage towards the autologous marrow graft, the next five dogs received a second dose of total body irradiation (3 Gy) on day 14 followed by infusion of autologous marrow (panel C). As a consequence of the second dose of total body irradiation, blood counts began to fall. In all five dogs, GVHD persisted and there was no evidence of autologous engraftment. Dogs died between days 18 and 35. Therefore, in a fourth experiment seven dogs were given a dose of 4.5 Gy of total body irradiation on day 14 (panel D). This was followed by grafts of marrow from the recipients' DLA-identical littermates. Dogs continued to receive methotrexate following the second transplant. Three of the seven died from intercurrent infection on days 18-23, too early to be evaluated. Four had engraftment; however, one of the grafts was rejected, and that dog died by day 31. Three animals had sustained engraftment of littermate marrow, and two of these became long-term survivors. These experiments show the difficulties encountered when attempting to eradicate a once established unrelated marrow graft that has resulted in GVHD. Nevertheless, the idea of combining a conditioning program with subsequent deliberately-induced GVHD to exert a graft-versus-leukemia effect remains attractive, particularly if more uniformly successful methods were developed to ''rescue'' patients with either previously cryopreserved autologous marrow cells or marrow cells from histocompatible siblings.

Because of the generally accepted view that mature T cells contained in donor marrow inoculum are the primary initiators of acute GVHD, methods of removing T cells from transplanted marrow seem ideally suited to prevent acute GVHD. This way, the transplanted immune system would be returned to a prenatal state, and any new stem cell-derived T cells would accept the host antigenic environment as ''self'' and become tolerant to it. We have explored T-cell depletion with L-leucyl-L-leucine methylester (Leu-Leu-OME) which is a lysosomal tropic agent that selectively kills cytotoxic T cells and their precursors, natural killer cells, and monocytes, but not helper T cells or other hematopoietic cells. We first carried out *in vitro* studies which showed complete abrogation of cytotoxic T-lymphocyte responses in ^{51}Cr release assays at doses of Leu-Leu-OME of 500-1,000 μM (FIG. 6).[26] Similarly, natural killer cell activity was completely abrogated at 1,000 μM, although severe suppression was already seen at 250 and 500 μM (FIG. 7). We then investigated whether marrow incubation with Leu-Leu-OME would interfere with engraftment of autologous mar-

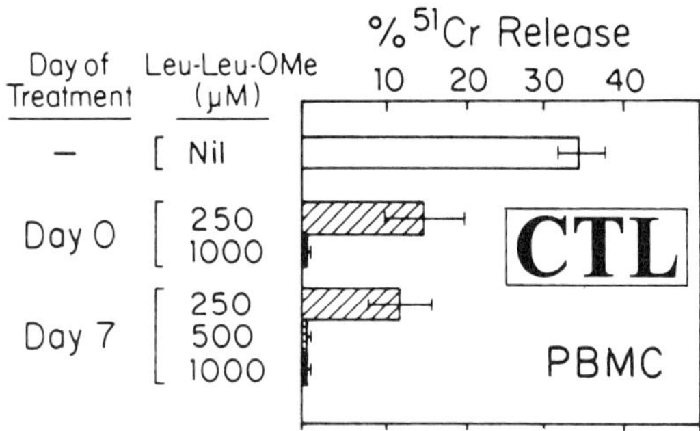

FIGURE 6. Effect of Leu-Leu-OME treatment suppresses cytotoxic lymphocyte activity. Cells were treated with Leu-Leu-OME on either day 0 or day 7 of the mixed leukocyte culture. The ordinate indicates mean percentage of ^{51}Cr release $\pm$ SEM using ^{51}Cr-labeled and concanavalin A-stimulated peripheral blood mononuclear cells as targets.

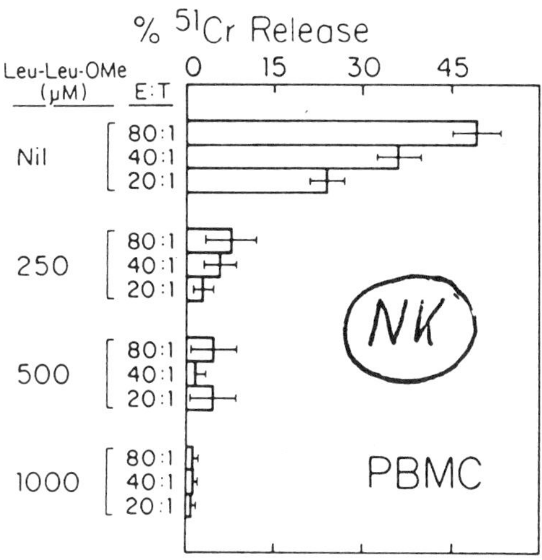

FIGURE 7. Leu-Leu-OME treatment of peripheral blood mononuclear cells eliminates natural killer (NK) cytolytic activity. The ordinate indicates mean percentage of ^{51}Cr release $\pm$ SEM from a CTAC target cell line at three different effector : target (E : T) ratios.

row. FIGURE 8 shows granulocyte recovery in seven dogs given Leu-Leu-OME-treated marrow autografts. Six of the seven showed engraftment patterns that could not be distinguished from those of 16 control dogs given untreated autologous marrow[26] (FIG. 8). The six received marrow cell doses of 0.7 to 1.7 × 10⁸ cells/kg. The seventh dog received a dose of only 0.05 × 10⁸ cells/kg which were treated with Leu-Leu-OME at a concentration of 2,000 µM; this dog did not have engraftment. Among the six dogs that had engraftment, three had marrow incubated with 1,000

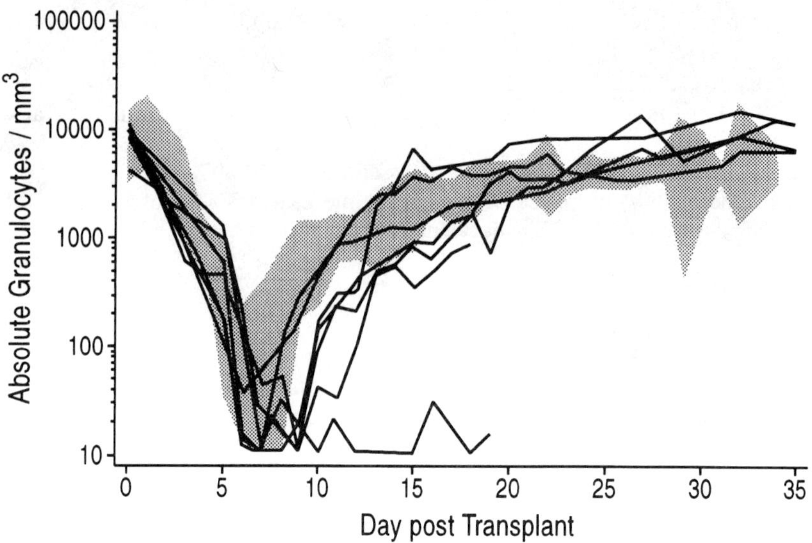

FIGURE 8. Hematologic recovery in recipients conditioned with 9.2 Gy total body irradiation (TBI) and infused with Leu-Leu-OME-treated autologous marrow. The ordinate indicates absolute granulocyte counts. The *shaded area* represents the range of granulocyte recovery (mean ± SD) in 16 dogs conditioned with 9.2 Gy of TBI and given untreated autologous marrow.

TABLE 6. Dogs Given 9.2 Gy Total Body Irradiation and Hematopoietic Grafts with or without Treatment of the Grafts by Leu-Leu-OME

Donor	Leu-Leu-OME 1,000 μM	No. of Dogs Studied	Graft Failure	Fatal GVHD	Surviving	Median Survival (days)
Unrelated	No	10	0	10	0	10
DLA-nonidentical	Yes	6	2	4	0	13
DLA-haploidentical	No	6	0	6	0	10.5
Littermate	Yes	5	3	3	0	17
DLA-identical	No	7	0	3	4	>80
Littermate	Yes	5	4	1	0	11

μM Leu-Leu-OME, one wiht 2,000 μM, and two with 4,000 μM. Next we investigated the effect of Leu-Leu-OME incubation of marrow in three allogeneic transplant settings, using as marrow donors either DLA-nonidentical unrelated dogs or DLA-haploidentical and DLA-identical littermates.[27] Results are summarized in TABLE 6 and are compared with those obtained in dogs transplanted with untreated marrow.

In all three donor-recipient settings studied, graft failure was a major problem, with two of six DLA-nonidentical unrelated dogs, three of five DLA-haploidentical littermates, and four of five DLA-identical littermates failing to engraft. Furthermore, all eight dogs that had engraftment developed fatal GVHD. Overall, survival was not improved over control in DLA-nonidentical recipients and was considerably worse than control among the DLA-identical littermates.

In other studies, we treated DLA-identical littermate recipients of Leu-Leu-OME-treated marrow with recombinant canine stem cell factor after transplant in an attempt to enhance engraftment (unpublished data). In those studies, 5 of 10 stem cell factor-treated dogs failed to have engraftment compared to 6 graft failures among 8 dogs not given stem cell factor; 4 of the 10 stem cell factor-treated dogs are surviving compared to only 1 of 8 control dogs. Although these data are not conclusive, they suggest that additional combinations of growth factors should be explored in studies of enhancing engraftment of T-cell-depleted marrow.

Finally, we studied GVHD after transplantation of allogeneic peripheral blood stem cells mobilized by either canine recombinant granulocyte colony-stimulating factor, stem cell factor, or a combination of the two (unpublished data). These studies were prompted by two findings. One was the observation of extremely rapid and sustained autologous engraftment of growth factor-mobilized peripheral blood stem cells. The other was changes in function of T lymphocytes from donors that had undergone mobilization with hematopoietic growth factors. Specifically, we found that T cells were no longer responsive to alloantigens in mixed leukocyte culture and also that mononuclear cells had lost their capacity to stimulate T lymphocytes from other dogs. Thus, we expected that allogeneic engraftment would be rapid and that GVHD might be absent or at least modified in a beneficial way. The expectation about rapid engraftment was fulfilled. However, the incidence and severity of acute GVHD after transplantation of mobilized peripheral blood stem cells were not different from those previously reported for nonmobilized peripheral blood mononuclear cell transplants. In fact, all nine dogs with DLA-haploidentical grafts died with acute GVHD, and eight of nine DLA-identical recipients developed GVHD which was fatal in three and transient in five.

In conclusion, the canine marrow graft model has been important in developing concepts and approaches for preventing and treating GVHD which have been effective in human marrow transplantation. Examples include the use of methotrexate, methotrexate/cyclosporine, methotrexate/tacrolimus, or trimetrexate/cyclosporine for GVHD prevention, and the treatment of acute GVHD by anti-T-cell reagents. Many of the drugs that looked promising in inbred murine models were found to be ineffective in dogs, presumably because of the random-bred nature of the species. Other drugs were not introduced clinically because they showed unacceptable associated toxicities in dogs. Despite the success achieved so far, the ideal approach to prevent GVHD and to induce stable graft-host tolerance has as yet not been found.

REFERENCES

1. STORB, R. & E. D. THOMAS. 1994. The scientific foundation of marrow transplantation based on animal studies. *In* Bone Marrow Transplantation. S. J. Forman, K. G. Blume, and E. D. Thomas, Eds.: 3-11. Blackwell Scientific Publications. Boston.

2. STORB, R. & E. D. THOMAS. 1985. Graft-versus-host disease in dog and man: The Seattle Experience. *In* Immunological Reviews. G. Möller, Ed. No. 88: 215–238. Munksgaard, Copenhagen.

3. STORB, R., T. C. GRAHAM, R. SHIURBA & E. D. THOMAS. 1970. Treatment of canine graft-versus-host disease with methotrexate and cyclophosphamide following bone marrow transplantation from histoincompatible donors. Transplantation **10:** 165–172.

4. STORB, R., H. J. KOLB, H. J. DEEG, P. L. WEIDEN, F. APPELBAUM, T. C. GRAHAM & E. D. THOMAS. 1986. Prevention of graft-versus-host disease by immunosuppressive agents after transplantation of DLA-nonidentical canine marrow. Bone Marrow Transpl. **1:** 167–177.

5. RAFF, R. F., R. STORB, T. GRAHAM, J. M. FIDLER, G. E. SALE, B. JOHNSTON, H. J. DEEG, M. PEPE, F. SCHUENING, F. R. APPELBAUM, R. J. BAUER, J. D. YOUNG, B. J. MARAFINO, D. G. ANDO & I. A. BRAUDE. 1992. Pharmacologic, toxicologic and marrow transplantation studies in dogs given succinyl acetone. Transplantation **54:** 813–820.

6. DEEG, H. J. & R. STORB. 1982. Experimental marrow transplantation, Chapter 10. *In* Cyclosporin A. Proceedings of an International Conference on Cyclosporin A. D. J. G. White, Ed.: 121–134. Elsevier Biomedical Press. Amsterdam.

7. STORB, R., R. F. RAFF, F. R. APPELBAUM, H. J. DEEG, W. FITZSIMMONS, T. C. GRAHAM, M. PEPE, M. PETTINGER, G. SALE, R. VAN DER JAGT & F. G. SCHUENING. 1993. FK506 and methotrexate prevent graft-versus-host disease in dogs given 9.2 Gy total body irradiation and marrow grafts from unrelated DLA-nonidentical donors. Transplantation **56:** 800–807.

8. RAFF, R. F., R. STORB, T. GRAHAM, H. J. DEEG, M. PEPE, R. SCHAFFER, G. E. SALE, F. SCHUENING & F. R. APPELBAUM. 1993. What role for 15-deoxyspergualin in enhancing engraftment of unrelated, histoincompatible canine marrow grafts and preventing graft-versus-host disease? Transplantation **55:** 684–688.

9. YU, C., R. STORB, I. BRAUDE, H. J. DEEG, F. G. SCHUENING, R. HUSS & T. C. GRAHAM. 1995. Corticotropin releasing factor (CRF) with or without methotrexate for prevention of graft-versus-host disease in DLA-nonidentical unrelated canine marrow grafts. Transplantation. In press.

10. STORB, R., R. B. EPSTEIN, T. C. GRAHAM & E. D. THOMAS. 1970. Methotrexate regimens for control of graft-versus-host disease in dogs with allogeneic marrow grafts. Transplantation **9:** 240–246.

11. SULLIVAN, K. M., R. STORB, C. D. BUCKNER, A. FEFER, L. FISHER, P. L. WEIDEN, R. P. WITHERSPOON, F. R. APPELBAUM, M. BANAJI, J. HANSEN, P. MARTIN, J. E. SANDERS, J. SINGER & E. D. THOMAS. 1989. Graft-versus-host disease as adoptive immunotherapy in patients with advanced hematologic neoplasms. N. Engl. J. Med. **320:** 828–834.

12. STORB, R., R. L. PRENTICE, C. D. BUCKNER, R. A. CLIFT, F. APPELBAUM, J. DEEG, K. DONEY, J. A. HANSEN, M. MASON, J. E. SANDERS, J. SINGER, K. M. SULLIVAN, R. P. WITHERSPOON & E. D. THOMAS. 1983. Graft-versus-host disease and survival in patients with aplastic anemia treated by marrow grafts from HLA-identical siblings. Beneficial effect of a protective environment. N. Engl. J. Med. **308:** 302–307.

13. STORB, R., H. J. KOLB, T. C. GRAHAM, H. KOLB, P. L. WEIDEN & E. D. THOMAS. 1973. Treatment of established graft-versus-host disease in dogs by antithymocyte serum or prednisone. Blood **42:** 601–609.

14. STORB, R., E. GLUCKMAN, E. D. THOMAS, C. D. BUCKNER, R. A. CLIFT, A. FEFER, H. GLUCKSBERG, T. C. GRAHAM, F. L. JOHNSON, K. G. LERNER, P. E. NEIMAN & H. OCHS. 1974. Treatment of established human graft-versus-host disease by antithymocyte globulin. Blood **44:** 57–75.

15. STORB, R., H. J. DEEG, M. PEPE, C. ANASETTI, F. R. APPELBAUM, W. BENSINGER, C. D. BUCKNER, R. A. CLIFT, K. DONEY, J. HANSEN, G. LONGTON, P. MARTIN, J. E. SANDERS,

J. SINGER, P. STEWART, K. M. SULLIVAN, E. D. THOMAS & R. P. WITHERSPOON. 1992. Long-term follow-up of three controlled trials comparing cyclosporine versus methotrexate for graft-versus-host disease prevention in patients given marrow grafts for leukemia (Letter). Blood **79:** 3091–3092.

16. DEEG, H. J., R. STORB, P. L. WEIDEN, R. F. RAFF, G. E. SALE, K. ATKINSON, T. C. GRAHAM & E. D. THOMAS. 1982. Cyclosporin A and methotrexate in canine marrow transplantation: Engraftment, graft-versus-host disease, and induction of tolerance. Transplantation **34:** 30–35.

17. DEEG, H. J., R. STORB, F. R. APPELBAUM, M. S. KENNEDY, T. C. GRAHAM & E. D. THOMAS. 1984. Combined immunosuppression with cyclosporine and methotrexate in dogs given bone marrow grafts from DLA-haploidentical littermates. Transplantation **37:** 62–65.

18. STORB, R., H. J. DEEG, V. FAREWELL, K. DONEY, F. APPELBAUM, P. BEATTY, W. BENSINGER, C. D. BUCKNER, R. CLIFT, J. HANSEN, R. HILL, G. LONGTON, L. LUM, P. MARTIN, R. McGUFFIN, J. SANDERS, J. SINGER, P. STEWART, K. SULLIVAN, R. WITHERSPOON & E. D. THOMAS. 1986. Marrow transplantation for severe aplastic anemia: Methotrexate alone compared with a combination of methotrexate and cyclosporine for prevention of acute graft-versus-host disease. Blood **68:** 119–125.

19. STORB, R., H. J. DEEG, J. WHITEHEAD, F. APPELBAUM, P. BEATTY, W. BENSINGER, C. D. BUCKNER, R. CLIFT, K. DONEY, V. FAREWELL, J. HANSEN, R. HILL, L. LUM, P. MARTIN, R. McGUFFIN, J. SANDERS, P. STEWART, K. SULLIVAN, R. WITHERSPOON, G. YEE & E. D. THOMAS. 1986. Methotrexate and cyclosporine compared with cyclosporine alone for prophylaxis of acute graft versus host disease after marrow transplantation for leukemia. N. Engl. J. Med. **314:** 729–735.

20. BEATTY, P. G., C. ANASETTI, J. A. HANSEN, G. M. LONGTON, J. E. SANDERS, P. J. MARTIN, E. M. MICKELSON, S. Y. CHOO, E. W. PETERSDORF, M. S. PEPE, F. R. APPELBAUM, S. I. BEARMAN, C. D. BUCKNER, R. A. CLIFT, F. B. PETERSEN, J. SINGER, P. S. STEWART, R. S. STORB, K. M. SULLIVAN, M. C. TESLER, R. P. WITHERSPOON & E. D. THOMAS. 1993. Marrow transplantation from unrelated donors for treatment of hematologic malignancies: effect of mismatching for one HLA locus. Blood **81:** 249–253.

21. ANASETTI, C., P. G. BEATTY, R. STORB, P. J. MARTIN, M. MORI, J. E. SANDERS, E. D. THOMAS & J. A. HANSEN. 1990. Effect of HLA incompatibility on graft-versus-host disease, relapse, and survival after marrow transplantation for patients with leukemia or lymphoma. Hum. Immunol. **29:** 79–91.

22. RAFF, R. F., R. STORB, T. GRAHAM, G. SALE, H. SHULMAN, M. PEPE, H. J. DEEG, F. SCHUENING, F. R. APPELBAUM, J. M. FIDLER & D. G. ANDO. 1992. succinyl acetone plus methotrexate as GVHD prophylaxis in DLA-haploidentical canine littermate marrow grafts (Letter). Transplantation **54:** 947–948.

23. APPELBAUM, F. R., R. F. RAFF, R. STORB, H. J. DEEG, T. C. GRAHAM, B. SANDMAIER & F. SCHUENING. 1989. Use of trimetrexate for the prevention of graft-versus-host disease. Bone Marrow Transplantation **4:** 421–424.

24. DONEY, K. C., R. STORB, K. BEACH, C. ANASETTI, H. J. DEEG, J. A. HANSEN, P. J. MARTIN, R. A. NASH, M. M. SCHUBERT, K. M. SULLIVAN, R. P. WITHERSPOON & F. R. APPELBAUM. 1995. A phase I study of trimetrexate used in combination with cyclosporine as acute graft-versus-host disease prophylaxis in HLA-mismatched, related donor bone marrow transplants. Transplantation **60:** 55–58.

25. STORB, R., R. B. EPSTEIN, T. C. GRAHAM, H. J. KOLB, H. KOLB & E. D. THOMAS. 1974. Rescue from canine graft-versus-host reaction by autologous or DL-A-compatible marrow. Transplantation **18:** 357–367.

26. RAFF, R. F., E. SEVERNS, R. STORB, P. MARTIN, T. GRAHAM, B. SANDMAIER, F. SCHUENING, G. SALE & F. R. APPELBAUM. 1988. L-Leucyl-L-Leucine methyl ester treatment of

canine marrow and peripheral blood cells: Inhibition of proliferative responses with maintenance of the capacity for autologous marrow engraftment. Transplantation **46:** 655-660.

27. RAFF, R. F., E. SEVERNS, R. STORB, T. C. GRAHAM, G. SALE, F. G. SCHUENING & F. R. APPELBAUM. 1993. Studies of the use of L-leucyl-L-leucine methyl ester in canine allogeneic marrow transplantation. Transplantation **55:** 1244-1249.

The Bidirectional Paradigm of Transplant Immunology[a]

THOMAS E. STARZL,[b] NORIKO MURASE,
ANGUS THOMSON, ANTHONY J. DEMETRIS,
SHIGUANG QIAN, ABDUL S. RAO, AND
JOHN J. FUNG

Pittsburgh Transplant Institute
University of Pittsburgh Medical Center
Pittsburgh, Pennsylvania 15213

Until 1992, the conventional view of transplantation immunology was what we have referred to as the one-way paradigm (FIG. 1A and B), a conceptual framework that had been extrapolated from the neonatal tolerance model of Billingham, Brent, and Medawar.[1,2] In Medawar's defenseless recipient experiments, and in the parent to offspring F_1 hybrid and recipient cytoablation models (FIG. 1A), it was learned in the 1950s that the risk of lethal graft-versus-host disease (GVHD) after splenocyte or bone marrow transplantation was directly proportional to the degree of MHC incompatibility.

As early as 1959, it was known that all the same rules applied when whole organs containing immunologically active cells, such as the intestine, were transplanted. Thus, any kind of hematolymphopoietic transplantation was conceived to be an essentially one-way cellular transaction, yielding either GVHD, rejection, or tolerance.

THE DEFECTIVE ONE-WAY PARADIGM

In this context, it was perfectly logical to view solid organ transplantation as a mirror image of the bone marrow experiments, the difference being that the graft was the defenseless victim instead of being the aggressor (FIG. 1B). This one-way paradigm in the opposite direction became the disorienting dogma upon which most clinically directed transplantation research was based for the next third of a century.

The One-Way In Vitro Tests

Ironically, the introduction of *in vitro* models beginning with the one-way mixed lymphocyte reaction (MLR) in 1963[3,4] further supported this dogma. These so-called

[a] This work was aided by Project Grant No. DK 29961 from the National Institutes of Health, Bethesda, Maryland.

[b] Address for correspondence: Thomas E. Starzl, MD, PhD, Department of Surgery, 3601 Fifth Avenue, 5C Falk Clinic, University of Pittsburgh, Pittsburgh, Pennsylvania 15213.

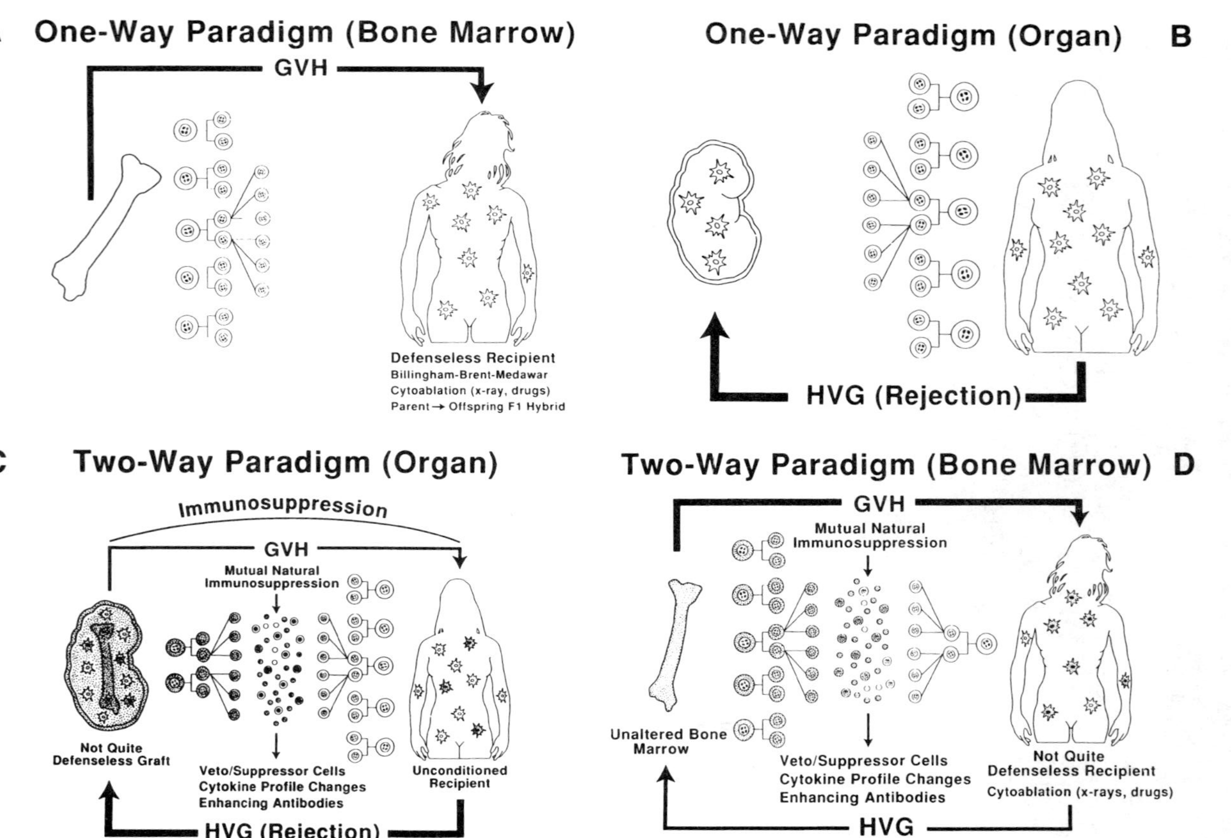

FIGURE 1. Transplantation immunology as seen with the conventional one-way paradigm (**A** for bone marrow and **B** for whole organ transplantation). The two-way paradigm is shown in **C** (whole organ) and **D** (bone marrow transplantation).

"minitransplant models" generated thousands of increasingly sophisticated cellular and ultimately molecular studies of immunologic interactions, the full understanding and clinical exploitation of which was hampered by the restrictive context of the one-way paradigm.

With Clinical Bone Marrow Transplantation

Aside from the overwhelming support provided by the unidirectional *in vitro* tests, the one-way paradigm was ostensibly strengthened in 1968 when the strategy of recipient cytoablation before bone marrow transplantation finally was extended from the mouse model to successful clinical application, emphasizing at every step the need for HLA compatibility if stable engraftment (called tolerance) was to be accomplished without the complication of GVHD.[5,6]

With Whole Organ Transplantation

However, the one-way paradigm never explained what was being observed and accomplished with organ transplantation without dependence on MHC matching, without host preconditioning, and with no GVHD. Because of these striking "violations of rules," organ transplantation was dissociated from the kind of rational scientific base enjoyed by those involved in bone marrow transplantation. In fact, the tumultuous development of the whole organ field can only be described as empirical. Treatment was based on the assumption that continuous immunosuppression would be required for life to maintain adequate graft function.

The avalanche of clinical whole organ cases began in 1962–1963 when kidney recipients were treated with the combination of azathioprine and prednisone at the University of Colorado.[7] A characteristic postoperative pattern was recognized in which rejection was found surprisingly to be easily reversed with augmented doses of prednisone. More importantly, maintenance immunosuppression could later be progressively reduced and even stopped in some cases. The same sequence of immunologic crisis and resolution has since been seen with all other organs successfully transplanted and with all of the clinical immunosuppressive regimens (FIG. 2). Something appeared to have changed in the host, the graft, or both. But what?

THE DISCOVERY OF CHIMERISM

A plausible answer was found in 1992, when a group of the original still surviving Colorado kidney recipients (then approaching 31 years posttransplantation) and more than 2 dozen liver recipients (10–23 years posttransplantation) were restudied.[8–13] A low level of donor leukocyte chimerism was ubiquitously found in biopsies obtained of the graft, of multiple host tissue sites, and in blood.

The chimerism was thought to be multilineage, but the dominant cell population had the morphologic characteristics of dendritic cells. Because the number of donor cells was small, skeptics claimed, and perhaps some still do, that these cells were

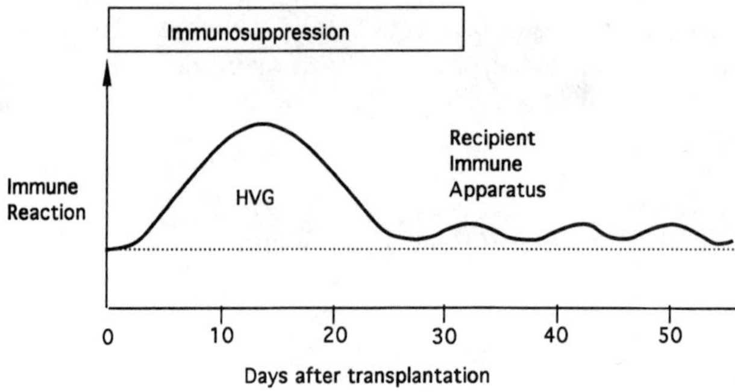

FIGURE 2. Postoperative events using the one-way paradigm to interpret events after successful whole organ transplantation.

merely an epiphenomenon of tolerance (or graft acceptance), not the cause of it. However, this position has become increasingly difficult to justify.

Confirmatory evidence of donor HLA alleles was obtained with polymerase chain reaction (PCR). Karyotyping in patients with opposite-sex donors, with either *in situ* hybridization or PCR, yielded similar results. All 30 of the chronically surviving kidney and liver recipients studied in 1992 were chimeras. The leukocytes of bone marrow origin, which are resident in all tissues, apparently had migrated and been assimilated by the overwhelmingly larger immunologic network of the host. In essence, a small fragment of disseminated extramedullary donor bone marrow, depicted in FIGURE 1C as a bone silhouette, had accidentally been engrafted. These observations provided the basis for the formulation of the two-way paradigm.

THE TWO-WAY PARADIGM

In the two-way paradigm, the immunologic confrontation following whole organ transplantation involved a graft-versus-host (GVH) as well as host-versus-graft (HVG) component in which the two cell populations were somehow reciprocally modulating, provided that both could survive (FIG. 3). Veto cells, suppressor cells, cytokine profile changes, and the development of enhancing antibodies seemingly had an accessory and ultimately crucial role in the development of reciprocal nonreactivity (FIG. 1C). However, these were derivative from the primary event of the David versus Goliath mutual cell engagement. The umbrella of immunosuppression that equally covered both in the empirically developed clinical protocols had permitted these changes.

It could be seen that the vast gap between the fields of bone marrow and whole organ transplantation merely reflected entrenched differences of treatment strategy, leaving intact the mutually censoring immunologic limbs with organ transplantation and deliberately trying to remove one of the limbs for bone marrow grafting procedures, following a recipient cytoablation.

However, one detail remained before the linkage was seamless. Although complete donor chimerism had long been assumed to be the objective of bone marrow trans-

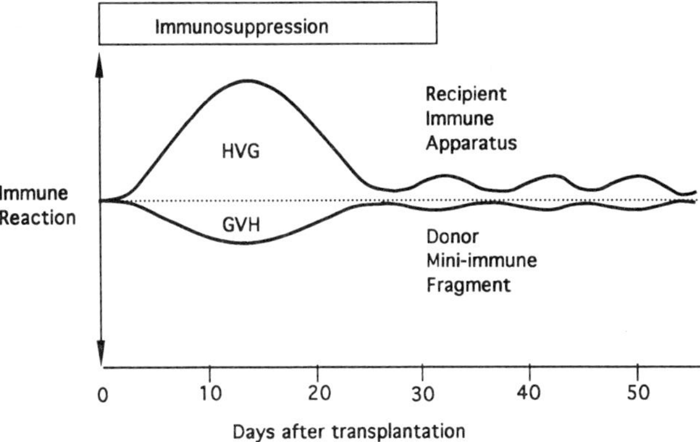

FIGURE 3. Postoperative events in the two-way paradigm after whole organ transplantation. The *small lower curve* is the graft-versus-host reaction which usually is silent.

plantation, Thomas and others[14,15] recently showed that in recipients of bone marrow from opposite sex donors, a trace population of recipient leukocytes can always be detected with sensitive molecular techniques. Thus, the veto and other accessory events at the cellular interface are the same in principle with bone marrow as with organ transplantation (FIG. 1D).

With either approach to treatment (that for whole organs versus that for bone marrow), the resulting reciprocal nonreactivity of the two populations is a natural event that apparently is only permitted, not caused, by the drugs we use. Chaperoned would be a better term, because it does not seem to matter where these agents interdict the allogeneic response: from the second signal transduction proximally (i.e., with CTLA4Ig fusion proteins) to the most distal inhibition of p70 S6 kinase activity by rapamycin or any site in between. By choosing an "easy" strain combination of rodents, these agents as well as dozens of less potent molecules sometimes have been made to look like Hercules, when a single dose or multiple doses were shown to induce permanent donor-specific tolerance, when in fact the model (not the drug) was the principal factor.

EXPERIMENTAL CLARIFICATION

A Rat Model

In an illustrative experiment of tolerance induction across a moderately difficult barrier,[16] Brown Norway rat recipients were transplanted with four different fully allogeneic Lewis organs (liver, heart, kidney, and intestine) or with a standard dose of Lewis cell suspensions from four different sources (bone marrow, thymus, spleen, and lymph node), with or without immunosuppression with tacrolimus.

No Treatment. As expected without immunosuppression, all Lewis cell suspensions were rejected by the Brown Norway recipients. There was no mortality, but after 100 days, there was no chimerism. The hearts, kidneys, and intestines were rejected after 7.5-12 days and the livers in 28 days.

Transient Tacrolimus (FK 506) Treatment. A 2-week course of treatment with tacrolimus with two supplementary single doses at days 20 and 27 dramatically changed the outcome.[16] All hearts, kidneys, and livers now survived to 100 days, drug free for the last three quarters of this time. Bone marrow engrafted silently with no overt evidence of GVHD. The intestines were not rejected. However, all of the bowel recipients died of GVHD at about 45 days. Spleen and lymph node cell suspensions behaved like intestine, always causing GVHD. Thymocytes failed to engraft.

The striking divergence of outcome with different allografts reflected their cellular composition.[16] The lack of some essential factor(s) may account for the failure of engraftment of T-cell-rich adult thymocytes. The infusion of T- and B-cell-rich splenocytes and lymph node cells led to GVHD, whereas engraftment of the clinically inocuous bone marrow correlated with a large component of immature cells of undetermined phenotype.

At 100 days, the animals successfully engrafted with bone marrow, heart, or liver underwent examination with *in vitro* mixed lymphocyte reaction and cytotoxic assays. These revealed consistent anti-donor reactivity (so-called split tolerance). Now drug free, the animals accepted challenge livers from donor, but not third-party animals. The hepatic allografts went through spontaneously resolving rejection in rats primed originally with either donor-strain hearts or bone marrow. After passing through these crises, all of the orthotopically transplanted challenge livers permanently supported life and thereafter were completely normal histopathologically.

Challenge heart grafts that normally are rejected in 8 days were also accepted by the drug-free animals primed with liver, bone marrow, or heart, with no clinical failures in any of these groups. However, when examined histologically, the challenge hearts appeared completely normal at 100 days posttransplantation only in rats primed originally with donor-strain liver. In rats that had been primed with bone marrow, challenge hearts had the subendothelial infiltration of recipient lymphoid cells (called Quilty lesions) that are generally considered as very early premonitors of chronic rejection.[16]

Animals primed originally with hearts were at the lowest end of the tolerance scale. Challenge hearts in these rats also escaped clinical rejection and continued to function along with the priming hearts, but at the 200-day milestone both first and second hearts showed the classic proliferative arterial lesions of chronic rejection as well as low grade cellular infiltration.

The Tolerance/Chimerism Relation. The spectrum of tolerogenicity defined by histopathologic outcome was liver best —> bone marrow next —> heart least. These results correlated with the chimerism produced by the priming transplant. The lineage composition of the chimerism caused by the tolerogenic priming allografts included T and B lymphocytes and was qualitatively similar to that caused by the transplantation of GVHD-inducing allografts such as intestine, lymph node cells, or splenocytes. However, there were fewer total number of donor leukocytes in the recipient tissues, a smaller proportion of T cells, and a more prominent population of cells of myeloid lineage, notably dendritic cells.[16]

Mouse Liver Transplantation

The use of drugs like tacrolimus in such models could obscure the search for fundamental mechanisms of natural tolerance. Consequently, the spontaneous tolerance induced by orthotopic liver transplantation in the mouse model has presented unique opportunities for investigation, particularly because so much about mammalian immunology is learned from this species. Qian *et al.*[17] have shown that in virtually all strain combinations, the majority of mouse liver recipients survive permanently without immunosuppression.

As in the rats, low levels of donor cell chimerism were typically observed in animals followed for more than 300 days posttransplantation. As expected, the liver recipients accepted subsequently transplanted donor heart and skin despite retention of donor specific MLR and CML reactivity (again split tolerance). It was noteworthy that the induction of donor-specific nonreactivity by primary heterotopic heart transplants in some strain combinations precluded completion of these experiments. This induced tolerance by the mouse heart as well as the observations made in rats showed that such tolerogenicity that is most readily induced with hepatic grafts is not organ-specific. Hepatic tolerogenicity is only an extreme illustration of a cardinal principle operational with all tissues and organs, based on donor leukocyte migration and chimerism.[17]

The Nature of Cell Migration

This trafficking of donor leukocytes after whole organ transplantation was described in the classic 1981 article by Nemlander and coworkers[18] of Helsinki. This was in the context of allosensitization as emphasized a decade later in the equally classic studies of dendritic leukocyte migration after heterotopic cardiac transplantation in mice by Larsen et al.[19] However, our investigations placed the phenomenon of donor cell migration squarely in the context of tolerance, both in transiently immunosuppressed rats[16,20] and in drug-free mice.[17] With both species, the migratory donor cells began to home to the central and secondary lymphoid organs within minutes after transplantation. After pausing there for 1 or 2 weeks,[17,20] they broke out and became generalized, including the skin where they can so easily be found in patients.

THE DONOR/RECIPIENT CELLULAR INTERFACE

The question of how the chimeric cells survive and induce donor-specific tolerance was examined by a team that included Angus Thomson, Anthony J. Demetris, and the husband and wife team of Drs. Lina Lu and Shiguang Qian. The hepatic leukocytes were the target of their investigation because of overwhelming evidence that the liver was more tolerogenic than any other organ. After discarding the hepatocytes and duct cells, approximately 10^7 nonparenchymal cells (NPCs) could be obtained from one mouse liver.[21]

The technology with which the suspect tolerogenic cells were studied was described in 1992 by Inaba and co-workers.[22,23] Following in their tracks, Thomson and

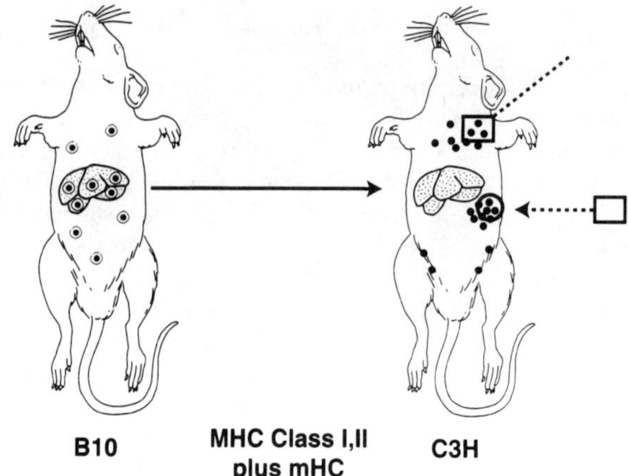

FIGURE 4. Experimental design in mice in which peripheralized donor leukocytes in whole organ allografts were shown to migrate and form self-perpetuating peripheral cellular oases. (See text for discussion.)

Lu cultured the NPCs in GM-CSF enriched medium. After 4 or 5 days of culture, approximately 2×10^6 cells with dendritic morphology and surface phenotype were identified.[21] A subpopulation of these cells formed clusters on the bottom of the culture wells. Loosely adherent cells were harvested and further cultured and studied according to the methods described by Inaba and co-workers.[22,23] Although they had the phenotype and function of precursor dendritic cells, it was difficult at first to prove their dendritic leukocyte origin because it was impossible to drive them to maturation, even with the addition of gamma-interferon and tumor necrosis factor. They had poor allostimulatory function, expressed low levels of MHC class II antigen, and were avidly phagocytic.[21]

This impasse was broken when the culture wells were coated with Type I collagen, thus stimulating the natural microenvironment of liver where mature dendritic cells are normally known to reside. Under these conditions, the precursor cells in the wells promptly assumed the properties of mature dendritic cells, now expressed high levels of MHC class II antigen, and acquired potent allostimulatory activity. The question of whether these unusual cells would mature and express class II antigen *in vivo* was investigated by injecting the purified precursor cells from B10.BR livers into the footpad of fully allogeneic B10 mouse recipients. The cells migrated promptly to the T-cell areas of the central lymphoid organs where they were easily phenotyped as donor and shown to express high levels of class II antigen.[21]

In the crucial next step, liver transplantation was carried out in the fully allogeneic but nonrejecting mouse stain combination (B10 to C3H).[24,25] The recipient animals were of course chimeric, and samples were collected from their bone marrow, spleen, thymus, and lymph nodes (FIG. 4). Donor as well as recipient precursor dendritic cells, at variable stages of maturation, were demonstrated in these samples, using the same culture techniques as had been used previously for study of liver-derived

NPCs. These observations suggest that these cells are derived from precursor dendritic cells and presumably pluripotent stem cells that have migrated from the graft and have widely distributed throughout the recipient tissues.[24,25] The profile and the ease with which these peripheralized cells (both donor and recipient) could be identified were much the same 4, 14, or 150 days after liver transplantation.

Although the same events occurred in heart recipients who rejected their allografts, the peripheralized donor cells were transient and could no longer be found 30 days after cardiac transplantation.[25] Although the cellular beachhead was the same, it was too feeble to be self-sustaining.

Thus, it appears that after transplantation, allografts export immature dendritic and probably stem cells, which establish residence in many preactive niduses within the recipient tissue, creating widespread and persistent cellular oases, presumably swimming in cytokines and other growth factors. Lu *et al.*[25] have obtained evidence that the dendritic precursor cells may be tolerogenic. These remarkable findings have suggested not only a mechanism for perpetuation of the migratory dendritic cells, but also a means by which the chimeric cells can exert a tolerogenic effect.

CLINICAL DONOR LEUKOCYTE AUGMENTATION

If our hypothesis of the mechanism of graft acceptance is correct, it should be possible to safely facilitate this process by adding unaltered donor bone marrow perioperatively to the minimal dose of the so-called passenger leukocytes contained in a whole organ allograft. Such a trial is well underway in Pittsburgh[26–28] and now includes 89 patients entered between December 1992 and February 1995. Donor bone marrow cells, obtained from cadaveric vertebral bodies, were not T-cell depleted or modified prior to infusion. Subsequent to organ placement, $3\text{-}5 \times 10^8$ cells/kg were infused into nonconditioned recipients who were then maintained on routine immunosuppression with tacrolimus and prednisone. No complication of bone marrow infusion was observed in any of the 89 primary whole organ transplant recipients, and their convalescence was rapid. The cumulative risk of rejection was similar in both bone marrow augmented and nonaugmented recipients and there was no incidence of serious GVHD. The results of this study are summarized in TABLE 1.

CONCLUSION

In FIGURE 1, the bottom panels (C, D) portray what transplantation immunology looks like after eliminating the blindfold of the one-way paradigm, which is depicted in the upper panels. A third of a century ago, Simonsen[29] and Michie, Woodruff, and Zeiss[30] challenged the one-way paradigm. While sound, their views were not accepted because the ideas could not be proved. In experiments prior to this, Martinez, Shapiro, and Good[31] described, without recipient cytoablation or immunosuppression, mutual immunologic tolerance in parabiotic mice, that could only be explained by the two-way paradigm. In retrospect, the resemblance its obvious of Good's mutually tolerogenic parabiotic partners, the allograft/host cellular relationship of our experiments, and for that matter the observations of chimerism in Freemartin cattle by Owen in 1945.[32]

TABLE 1. Function and Actuarial One-Year Graft Survival of Bone Marrow Augmented and Nonaugmented Whole Organ Transplant Recipients

			Function ($\bar{x} \pm$ SD)			
Organs Transplanted	n	Graft Survival[a]	Bilirubin (mg/dl)	Creatinine (mg/dl)	Cardiac Output (L/min)	FEV_1 (L)
Bone Marrow Augmented						
Liver	34[b]	31 (91%)	0.8 ± 0.6	—	—	—
Kidney	40[c]	39 (98%)	—	1.7 ± 0.6	—	—
Heart	10	08 (80%)	—	—	6.0 ± 1.7	—
Lungs	05	05 (100%)	—	—	—	2.0 ± 2.0
Controls						
Liver	33	26 (79%)	0.7 ± 0.3	—	—	—
Kidney	21[d]	18 (86%)	—	2.2 ± 1.5	—	—
Heart	04	06 (100%)	—	—	6.3 ± 3.2	—
Lung	01	0	—	—	—	—

[a] Actuarial 1-year graft survival.

[b] One type I diabetic also received pancreatic islets; not insulin-free.

[c] Nineteen type I diabetics also received either whole organ pancreas (n = 13) or isolated pancreatic islets (n = b); 11 patients (all recipients of pancreases) are insulin-free.

[d] Four type I diabetics also received whole organ pancreas transplants; two are currently off insulin.

The continuity of this theme was interrupted in the early 1960s and not restored until 1992, when our observation regarding the persistence of donor cells in long-term allograft recipients exposed the cellular events that transpire after organ transplantation. The therapeutic implications of the two-way paradigm, including the iatrogenic augmentation of spontaneous chimerism with perioperative unaltered donor bone marrow, are obvious. In our clinical trials, adjuvant bone marrow under conventional tacrolimus/prednisone immunosuppression has never caused clinically significant GVHD. Levels of chimerism 1,000 times greater than that occurring spontaneously have been regularly produced.

REFERENCES

1. BILLINGHAM, R. E., L. BRENT & P. B. MEDAWAR. 1953. "Actively acquired tolerance" of foreign cells. Nature **172:** 603–606.
2. BILLINGHAM, R., L. BRENT & P. MEDAWAR. 1956. Quantitative studies on tissue transplantation immunity. III. Actively acquired tolerance. Philos. Trans. R. Soc. Lond. (B.) **239:** 357–412.
3. BACH, F. & K. HIRSCHORN. 1954. Lymphocyte interaction: A potential histocompatibility test in vitro. Science **143:** 813–814.
4. BAIN, B., M. R. VAS & L. LOWENSTEIN. 1964. The development of large immature mononuclear cells in mixed leukocyte cultures. Blood **23:** 108–116.

5. GATTI, R. A., H. J. MEUWISSEN, H. D. ALLEN, R. HONG & R. A. GOOD. 1968. Immunological reconstruction of sex-linked lymphopenic immunological deficiency. Lancet **2:** 1366–1369.

6. BACH, F. H. 1968. Bone-marrow transplantation in a patient with the Wiskott-Aldrich syndrome. Lancet **2:** 1364–1366.

7. STARZL, T. E., T. L. MARCHIORO & W. R. WADDELL. 1963. The reversal of rejection in human renal homografts with subsequent development of homograft tolerance. Surg. Gynecol. Obstet. **117:** 385–395.

8. STARZL, T. E., A. J. DEMETRIS, N. MURASE, S. ILDSTAD, C. RICORDI & M. TRUCCO. 1992. Cell migration, chimerism, and graft acceptance. Lancet **339:** 1579–1582.

9. STARZL, T. E., A. J. DEMETRIS, M. TRUCCO, H. RAMOS, A. ZEEVI, W. A. RUDERT, M. KOCOUA, C. RICORDI, S. ILDSTAD & N. MURASE. 1992. Systemic chimerism in human female recipients of male livers. Lancet **340:** 876–877.

10. STARZL, T. E., A. J. DEMETRIS, M. TRUCCO, S. RICORDI, S. ILDSTAD, P. TERASAKI, N. MURASE, R. S. KENDALL, M. KOCOVA, W. A. RUDERT, A. ZEEVI & D. VAN THIEL. 1993. Chimerism after liver transplantation for type IV glycogen storage disease and Type I Gaucher's disease. N. Engl. J. Med. **328:** 745–749.

11. STARZL, T. E., A. J. DEMETRIS, M. TRUCCO, N. MURASE, C. RICORDI, S. ILDSTAD, H. RAMOS, S. TODO, A. TZAKIS, J. J. FUNG, M. NALESNIK, W. A. RUDERT & M. KOCOVA. 1993. Cell migration and chimerism after whole organ transplantation: The basis of graft acceptance. Hepatology **17:** 1127–1152.

12. STARZL, T. E., A. J. DEMETRIS, M. TRUCCO, A. ZEEVI, H. RAMOS, P. TERASAKI W. A. RUDERT, M. KOCOVA, C. RICORDI, S. ILDSTAD & N. MURASE. 1993. Chimerism and donor specific nonreactivity 27 to 29 years after kidney allotransplantation. Transplantation **55:** 1272–1277.

13. STARZL, T. E., A. J. DEMETRIS, N. MURASE, A. W. THOMSON, M. TRUCCO & C. RICORDI. 1993. Donor cell chimerism permitted by immunosuppressive drugs: A new view of organ transplantation. Immunol. Today **14:** 326–332.

14. PRZEPIORKA, D., E. D. THOMAS, D. M. DURHAM & L. FISHER. 1991. Use of a probe to repeat sequence of the Y chromosome for detection of host cells in peripheral blood of bone marrow transplant recipients. Am. J. Clin. Pathol. **95:** 201–206.

15. WESSMAN, M., S. POPP, T. RUUTU, L. VOLIN, T. CREMER & S. KNUUTILA. 1993. Detection of residual host cells after bone marrow transplantation using non-isotopic in situ hybridization and karyotype analysis. Bone Marrow Transplant. **11:** 279–284.

16. MURASE, N., M. TANABE, S. FUJISAKI, H. MIYAZAWA, Y. E. QING, C. P. DELANEY, A. J. DEMETRIS & T. E. STARZL. 1995. Variable chimerism, graft versus host disease, and tolerance after different kinds of cell and solid organ transplantation from Lewis to Brown-Norway rats. Transplantation **60:** 158–170.

17. QIAN, S., A. J. DEMETRIS, N. MURASE, A. S. RAO, J. J. FUNG & T. E. STARZL. 1994. Murine liver allograft transplantation: Tolerance and donor cell chimerism. Hepatology **19:** 916–924.

18. NEMLANDER, A., A. SOOTS, E. V. WILLEBRAND, B. HUSBERG & P. HAYRY. 1982. Redistribution of renal allograft responding leukocytes during rejection. II. Kinetics and specificity. J. Exp. Med. **156:** 1087–1100.

19. LARSEN, C. P., J. M. AUSTYN & P. J. MORRIS. 1990. The role of graft-derived dendritic leukocytes in the rejection of vascularized organ allografts. Ann. Surg. **212:** 308–317.

20. DEMETRIS, A. J., N. MURASE, S. FUJISAKI, J. J. FUNG, A. S. RAO & T. E. STARZL. 1993. Hematolymphoid cell trafficking, microchimerism, and GVHD reactions after liver, bone marrow, and heart transplantation. Transplant. Proc. **25:** 3337–3344.

21. LU, L., J. WOO, A. S. RAO, Y. LI, S. C. WATKINS, S. QIAN, T. E. STARZL, A. J. DEMETRIS & A. W. THOMSON. 1994. Propagation of dendritic cell progenitors from normal mouse liver using granulocyte/macrophage colony-stimulating factor and their maturational development in the presence of type-1 collagen. J. Exp. Med. **179:** 1823–1834.

22. INABA, K., R. M. STEINMAN, M. W. PACK, H. AYA, M. INABA, T. SUDO, S. WOLPE & G. SCHULER. 1992. Identification of proliferating dendritic cell precursors in mouse blood. J. Exp. Med. **175:** 1157.

23. INABA, K., M. INABA, N. ROMANI, H. AYA, M. DEGUCHI, S. IKEHARA, S. MURAMATSU & R. M. STEINMAN. 1992. Generation of large numbers of dendritic cells from mouse bone marrow cultures supplemented with granulocyte/macrophage colony-stimulating factor. J. Exp. Med. **176:** 1693.

24. THOMSON, A. W., L. LU, V. M. SUBBOTIN, Y. LI, S. QIAN, A. S. RAO, J. J. FUNG & T. E. STARZL. 1995. In vitro propagation and homing of liver-derived dendritic cell progenitors to lymphoid tissues of allogeneic recipients. Implications for the establishment and maintenance of donor cell chimerism following liver transplantation. Transplantation **59:** 544–551.

25. LU, L., W. A. RUDERT, S. QIAN, D. MCCASLIN, F. FU, A. S. RAO, M. TRUCCO, J. J. FUNG, T. E. STARZL & A. W. THOMSON. 1995. Growth of donor-derived dendritic cells from the bone marrow of liver allograft recipients in response to granulocyte/macrophage colony-stimulating factor. J. Exp. Med. **182:** August.

26. FONTES, P., A. RAO, A. J. DEMETRIS, A. ZEEVI, M. TRUCCO, P. CARROLL, W. RYBKA, C. RICORDI, F. DODSON, R. SHAPIRO, A. TZAKIS, S. TODO, K. ABU-ELMAGD, M. JORDAN, J. J. FUNG & T. E. STARZL. 1994. Augmentation with bone marrow of donor leukocyte migration for kidney, liver, heart, and pancreas islet transplantation. Lancet **344:** 151–155.

27. STARZL, T. E., A. J. DEMETRIS, A. S. RAO, A. W. THOMSON, M. TRUCCO, N. MURASE, A. ZEEVI & P. FONTES. 1994. Spontaneous and iatrogenically augmented leukocyte chimerism in organ transplant recipients. Transplant. Proc. **26:** 3071–3076.

28. RAO, A. S., P. FONTES, A. ZEEVI, M. TRUCCO, F. S. DODSON, W. B. RYBKA, R. SHAPIRO, M. JORDAN, S. M. PHAM, H. L. RILO, T. SESKEY, S. TODO, V. SCANTLEBURY, C. VIVAS, A. J. DEMETRIS, J. J. FUNG & T. E. STARZL. 1995. Augmentation of chimerism in whole organ recipients by simultaneous infusion of donor bone marrow cells. Transplant. Proc. **27:** 210–212.

29. SIMONSEN, M. 1962. Graft versus host reactions. Their natural history, and applicability as tools of research. Progr. Allergy **6:** 349–467.

30. MICHIE, D., M. F. A. WOODRUFF & I. M. ZEISS. 1961. An investigation of immunological tolerance based on chimera analysis. Immunology **4:** 413–424.

31. MARTINEZ, C., F. SHAPIRO & R. A. GOOD. 1960. Essential duration of parabiosis and development of tolerance to skin homografts in mice. Proc. Soc. Exp. Biol. Med. **104:** 256–259.

32. OWEN, R. D. 1945. Immunogenetic consequences of vascular anastomoses between bovine twins. Science **102:** 400–401.

Lymphocyte Migration Following Bone Marrow Transplantation

ROBERT SACKSTEIN

Division of Bone Marrow Transplantation
H. Lee Moffitt Cancer Center & Research Institute
University of South Florida
12902 Magnolia Drive
Tampa, Florida 33612

Bone marrow transplantation (BMT) results in immune deficits that can persist several years following hematologic engraftment. Immunologic recovery from either autologous or allogeneic BMT requires a quantitative and qualitative repopulation of lymphocyte effector cells. Lymphocytes are unique among leukocytes in that they are long-lived and can move (''migrate'' or ''home'') in a tissue-specific manner throughout the body. Increasing evidence indicates that lymphocyte migration to both lymphoid and nonlymphoid tissues is altered following BMT, raising the hypothesis that dysregulated migration compromises the kinetics of maturation and differentiation of immune effectors and the expression of immune responses at sites of inflammation. In addition, pathologic reactions such as graft-versus-host diseases (GVHD) are typified by lymphocytic infiltrates at selected target tissues (particularly the skin, but also the liver and gut), a consequence of directed migration to these sites. Enhanced understanding of the mechanisms regulating lymphocyte migration could yield therapeutic strategies to hasten immune recovery, improve localization of defense responses, and/or prevent pathologic inflammatory reactions following BMT. This article reviews our current understanding of the molecular basis of lymphocyte-endothelial interactions mediating lymphocyte migration into lymph nodes, the effects of BMT on these adhesion molecules, and the migration of lymphocytes to nonlymphoid tissues following BMT.

MEMBRANE ADHESION MOLECULES REGULATING LYMPHOCYTE MIGRATION TO LYMPH NODES

The first step in lymphocyte migration to both lymphoid and nonlymphoid tissues involves specific adhesive interactions between lymphocytes and the endothelial cells within the target tissue. These events occur under the shear forces of blood flow and require discrete receptor-ligand interactions between respective membrane structures on lymphocytes and endothelium. The expression of these adhesion molecules appears to be tightly regulated, consistent with their central role in the control of lymphocyte migration.

The physiology of lymphocyte migration has been most extensively characterized in the setting of cellular transit between the vasculature and lymph nodes. In this process, known collectively as ''lymphocyte recirculation,''[1] lymphocytes exit the blood at lymph nodes where they either reside for a variable period of time (depending on antigenic encounters and/or differentiation events) or exit via efferent lymphatics to the thoracic duct and thereon to the blood stream via the internal jugular vein (thus beginning again the recirculation cycle). This trafficking pattern is fundamental to the generation of the immune response in that it allows continuous reassortment of lymphocytes within nodal microenvironments architecturally specialized to promote cell-cell interactions and cytokine-mediated communication necessary for the differentiation and maturation of immune effector cells. In turn, the capacity of these "educated" immunologic effectors to reenter the vasculature and then to localize to target tissues is critical to the efficient delivery of the immune response(s), and, under both physiologic and pathophysiologic conditions, the tissue distribution of lymphocytes largely reflects these migration routes.

The trafficking ("homing") of lymphocytes from blood into lymph node is initiated by specific adherence of the cells to specialized nodal vascular structures known as high endothelial venules (HEV).[2] Several lymphocyte membrane glycoproteins mediate the attachment of lymphocytes to HEV, principal among which is the lymph node "homing receptor," now known as L-selectin or CD62L.[3] This glycoprotein is a member of the selectin class of adhesion molecules which includes E-selectin (CD62E or ELAM-1), an inducible endothelial protein, and P-selectin (also known as CD62P, GMP-140, or PADGEM), a protein found on activated platelets and endothelial cells. Selectins are characterized by an NH_2-terminal lectin domain, followed by an epidermal growth factor-like domain, and a variable number of repetitive units (two in L-selectin) showing homology to serum complement catalytic and regulatory proteins interacting with C3b or C4b.[3]

Human L-selectin is recognized by a variety of human monoclonal antibodies (TQ-1,[4] Leu 8,[5] DREG,[6] and LAM[7]) and has been characterized by monoclonal antibodies in mice (MEL-14[8]) and rats (A.11[9] and HRL-3[10]). Reduced SDS-PAGE analysis indicates that human lymphocyte L-selectin has a molecular weight of ~75,000, whereas the protein appears to be slightly larger (~90,000 mw) on murine and rat lymphocytes.[8,11] For each of these species, full-length cDNA clones encoding L-selectin have been characterized and sequenced,[11–18] revealing a predicted coding region of 372 amino acids containing a 38-residue leader sequence, a 23-residue COOH-terminal hydrophobic membrane insertion region, and a 17-residue cytoplasmic tail. Approximately 80% nucleotide and amino acid sequence homology exists between human and rodent L-selectin.[11] Biochemical studies reveal that the protein is heavily glycosylated, which accounts for the large discrepancy in molecular weight observed on SDS-PAGE compared to that predicted (~37,000 mw) for the core protein by cDNA sequencing.

Expression of L-selectin appears to be related to the activation state of the cells. For example, activation of lymphocytes with phorbol esters results in rapid shedding of L-selectin.[19] This process involves cleavage of the molecular off the membrane by a cell-associated protease that is activated by a protein kinase C-dependent phosphorylation pathway.[19] This shedding may be a physiologic event, allowing the lymphocyte to detach from HEV in order to enter the lymphoid parenchyma.

Transfection studies utilizing L-selectin cDNA demonstrated that expression of this protein is both necessary and sufficient to confer upon transfectants the capacity to bind HEV.[11,20] Studies of chimeric contructs of L-selectin have revealed that the lectin domain retains the property of HEV attachment, but that EGF and complement repeat domains are necessary for functional adherence to HEV.[21,22] However, in an accessory capacity, two other cell adhesion proteins that mediate non-organ-specific leukocyte-endothelial interactions, LFA-1 and CD44, cooperate with L-selectin to stabilize lymphocyte-HEV attachment. LFA-1, a member of the β_2 subfamily of the integrin class of adhesion molecules, is a heterodimer composed of two chains. CD11a (mw ~177,000) and CD18 (mw ~95,000). Its corresponding ligands include ICAM-1 (CD54) and ICAM-2, members of the immunoglobulin superfamily of proteins.[23] CD44 (also known as H-CAM or Hermes antigen) is a polymorphic glycoprotein of ~90,000 mw on lymphocytes.[24] By cDNA analysis, CD44 is composed of a core protein of ~37,000 mw which bears sequence homologies with cartilage link and proteoglycan core proteins.[25] Different molecular weight forms of CD44 are generated on various cells through alternative splicing of RNA and by variations in post-translational modifications (glycosylations or additions of chondroitin sulfate).[26,27] CD44 binds to extracellular matrix proteins, and CD44-dependent lymphocyte adherence to HEV appears to be mediated through binding to hyaluronate.[28] By contrast to L-selectin, both LFA-1 and CD44 function in a variety of cell-cell and cell-matrix interactions in addition to adhesive interactions between leukocytes and endothelium.

The adhesive interaction between L-selectin and its ligand(s) was first identified by an *in vitro* binding assay in which lymphocytes are overlaid onto frozen sections of lymph nodes.[29] This "lymphocyte-HEV adherence assay" is an *in vitro* approximation of physiologic adhesion mediated by L-selectin and has been the conventional approach for studying the adhesive function of L-selectin in its native state on the surface of leukocytes. Indeed, in early studies, antibodies directed against L-selectin were operationally identified by their ability to block lymphocyte-HEV adherence in the assay,[8,9] and these antibodies subsequently led to the identification of L-selectin at a molecular level. The adherence assay is performed under shear at 4°C, whereby binding mediated by L-selectin is maximized and effects of other adhesion molecules are minimized.[30,31] Under these conditions, lymphocytes will adhere specifically to lymph node HEV by interactions between L-selectin and its corresponding ligand(s). This event is calcium-dependent[32] and requires the presence of sialic acid[33,34] and sulfate[35] on the ligand(s). *In vitro* adherence of lymphocytes via L-selectin can be inhibited by carbohydrates such as mannose-6-phosphate (man-6-P), PPME (phosphomannan monoester core from *Hansenula hostii*, a phosphomannosyl-rich polysaccharide), and fucoidin (a sulfated, fucose-rich polysaccharide).[36,37]

To date, all endothelial ligands for L-selectin have been identified by an antibody known as MECA79.[38] Although this antibody was raised in rats against murine lymph nodes, it immunoprecipitates L-selectin ligands (known as addressins) from both murine and human lymph node endothelium, attaching to epitopes involved in functional adherence to L-selectin. In murine lymph nodes, this antibody precipitates two sulfated sialomucins of 50,000 and 90,000 molecular weight, initially designated Sgp50 and Sgp90, respectively.[39] In addition, a chimeric L-selectin-IgG molecule has been constructed consisting of the extracellular domain of murine L-selectin connected to the hinge-CH2-CH3 region of human IgG$_1$, and this reagent also immunoprecipitates these two proteins from lymph node lysates.[40] The 50,000 mw protein, now known as GlyCAM-1, has been cloned and its cDNA encodes a unique 132 amino acid protein with multiple potential O-linked glycosylation sites.[40] GlyCAM-

1 appears to be a secreted, soluble protein[41] that is most highly expressed among HEV of peripheral lymph nodes,[40] suggesting that this molecule may function to modulate L-selectin adhesive events at those sites.

The identity of the Sgp90 protein was revealed by utilizing the L-selectin-IgG chimera to immunoprecipitate Sgp90 followed by NH_2-terminal amino acid sequencing.[42] The NH_2-terminal sequence of Sgp90 matched the reported sequence of murine CD34. Furthermore, it was found that anti-murine CD34 antisera immunoprecipitated Sgp90 from detergent lysates of murine peripheral lymph nodes.[42] Thus, Sgp90 apparently is a vascular glycoform of murine CD34.

Although present on endothelial cells in most tissues,[43] CD34 is an integral membrane glycoprotein best known for its expression on the earliest multilineage colony-forming hematopoietic stem cells.[44] The observation that an L-selectin chimeric construct interacts with Sgp90 led us to examine whether L-selectin would interact with the CD34 present on human hematopoietic cells. To analyze this functional issue relative to the structure of native L-selectin (i.e., as expressed on cellular membranes), we used a modification of the *in vitro* lymphocyte-HEV binding assay.[45] Suspensions of human peripheral blood lymphocytes (PBL) or rat thoracic duct lymphocytes (TDL) were overlaid on cyto-spin preparations of KG1a cells, a primitive CD34-positive human hematopoietic cell line derived from acute myeloid leukemia,[44,46] as well as onto non-CD34-expressing myeloid, erythroid, and lymphocytic cell lines. Using identical assay conditions in which L-selectin mediates lymphocyte binding to HEV in lymph nodes, we observed lymphocyte binding to KG1a cells, whereas no binding was demonstrated with non-CD34-expressing hematopoietic cell lines.[45] Binding was completely inhibited by preincubation of PBL or TDL with the anti-L-selectin monoclonal antibodies LAM 1-3 (human) and A.11.5 (rat), respectively. Adherence of lymphocytes to KG1a was calcium-dependent, was strictly inhibited by coincubation with carbohydrate ligands of L-selectin such as PPME, mannose-6-phosphate, and fucoidin, and was abrogated by induction of L-selectin shedding from the lymphocyte membrane by treatment with phorbol esters. These data provided solid evidence that the lymphocytes attached via L-selectin; however, a variety of experimental approaches demonstrated that the ligand on KG1a is not CD34: (1) blocking studies using several anti-CD34 monoclonal antibodies singly and in combination did not decrease lymphocyte adherence to KG1a; (2) transfection of COS-7 cells with full-length CD34 cDNA did not confer capacity to support lymphocyte adherence despite high CD34 expression; (3) KG1a cells sorted into populations expressing high and low surface CD34 equally supported lymphocyte adherence; and (4) RPMI 8402 cells, another CD34[+] cell line, did not support lymphocyte adherence in the binding assay.[45] Treatment of KG1a with the enzymes neuraminidase, chymotrypsin, and bromelain abrogated lymphocyte binding to the cells, indicating that the ligand is a glycoprotein.[45] These experiments demonstrate that CD34 on human hematopoietic cells is not an L-selectin ligand and provide the first evidence of a ligand for L-selectin present on a nonendothelial cell.

The L-selectin ligand identified on KG1a is different from the L-selectin ligands previously described and likely represents a novel glycoprotein. In fact, although both mouse and rat lymphocytes bind to KG1a through an L-selectin-mediated interaction, the murine L-selectin chimera does not attach to KG1a cells.[47] We are currently investigating the structure of the KG1a L-selectin ligand. The relation between this structure and glycoproteins identified by the MECA 79 antibody currently remains to be determined. However, it must be emphasized that no information on the structure of human L-selectin ligands has been obtained to date; studies suggesting that endothelial CD34 is an L-selectin ligand were performed in mice, and there are major structural differences between human and murine CD34,[48,49] making problematic any extrapolation of data from mice to humans. Moreover, as CD34 is a constitutively expressed, ubiquitous, endothelial membrane protein, its role in mediating selective lymphocyte migration such as that into lymph nodes would require that it possess unique, tissue endothelium-specific, posttranslational modifications (e.g., glycosylations) for which no direct evidence currently exists.

MIGRATION OF LYMPHOCYTES TO LYMPH NODES FOLLOWING BONE MARROW TRANSPLANTATION

Considerable data from animal studies indicate that alterations in lymphocyte migration through lymph nodes occur after BMT. Studies in the mouse have shown that lymph nodes undergo structural changes, such as endothelial edema and microvascular occlusion, after transplantation which reduce the capacity of lymphocytes to migrate to these tissues[50]; similar changes are observed in human nodes.[50,51] These changes are accompanied by decreased expression of HEV-specific antigens such as those recognized by monoclonal antibody MECA-325, a reagent that identifies HEV in peripheral and mucosa-associated lymphoid tissues. Preparative regimens affect the integrity of HEV, causing diminished lymphocyte-HEV adherence and altering microcirculation of the lymph node.[50] These pathologic changes were shown to correlate with depression in the generation of immunologic functions such as contact hypersensitivity.[52] Other complications, such as opportunistic infections and the development of GVHD, also lead to alterations in lymph node structure,[51] which would be expected to affect trafficking of immune cells to and through lymph nodes.

In addition to changes in lymph node structure, alterations in lymphocyte migration can occur secondary to decreased expression of L-selectin on lymphocytes in the immediate posttransplant period. Even before it was known that L-selectin was identified by monoclonal antibody Leu8, there were reports that this marker was decreased among circulating lymphocytes after allogeneic transplants.[53] We observed that regardless of transplant type (autologous or allogeneic) or stem cell source (bone marrow or peripheral blood), both the percentage of lymphocytes bearing L-selectin and the level of L-selectin among the L-selectin-positive cells are markedly decreased posttransplantation compared with pretransplant values or levels in normal subjects. The decreased L-selectin expression is partly a reflection of the lymphocyte ontogeny program post-transplantation as high L-selectin expression is characteristic of mature recirculating cells, whereas immature lymphocytes are deficient in expression of the protein.[54-56]

Another major factor affecting the migration of lymphocytes to lymph nodes is the use of pharmacologic agents in the posttransplant period. In this regard, we extensively investigated methylprednisolone, a steroid commonly used in the prophylaxis of acute GVHD and in the treatment of both acute and chronic GVHD. It has been known for nearly two decades that steroids decrease lymphocyte migration to lymph nodes.[57,58] We tested whether this steroid effect in humans was mediated by alterations in expression of lymphocyte adhesion proteins directing lymphocyte attachment to HEV (L-selectin, LFA-1, and CD44) and/or was due to a decrease in the receptivity of HEV for lymphocytes.[59] The study protocol included flow cytometric measurements of adhesion protein levels on peripheral blood lymphocytes isolated at designated time points following methylprednisolone or placebo infusion in healthy volunteers as well as the use of fresh lymph nodes obtained from cadaveric, heart-beating organ donors before and after methylprednisolone infusion. Data revealed that the HEV of lymph nodes obtained after steroid administration were not deficient in the capacity to bind lymphocytes, but peripheral blood lymphocytes isolated following steroid infusion were unable to bind to HEV in the *in vitro* adherence assay. This alteration in lymphocyte adherence to HEV was accompanied by a marked reduction in the membrane levels of L-selectin principally, but also in CD44, indicating that the decreased migration of lymphocytes to lymph nodes after steroid administration is a result of changes in levels of lymphocyte adhesion proteins specific for entry into lymph node.[59] Further investigation of the effects on lymphocyte migration of other commonly used posttransplant medications, including other immunosuppressives, cytokines, and antibiotics, are indicated. These analyses must consider whether these agents may affect the lymphocyte, the HEV, or both, and whether the net physiologic effect is to promote or inhibit the capacity of lymphocytes to enter lymph nodes. Of note, recent data from *in vitro* studies of L-selectin expression in Jurkat cells indicate that cyclosporin A may attenuate the decrease in L-selectin levels seen after lymphocyte activation,[60] whereas GM-CSF has no effect on lymphocyte L-selectin levels.[61]

MIGRATION OF LYMPHOCYTES TO NONLYMPHOID TISSUES FOLLOWING BONE MARROW TRANSPLANTATION

Studies on the molecular basis of lymphocyte migration into nonlymphoid tissues have been hampered by the lack of histologically identifiable vascular structures, such as HEV, which are specialized to promote lymphocyte emigration from the blood stream into target tissues. Although HEV-like cuboidal endothelial cells are commonly observed in chronic inflammatory sites,[20] morphologic changes in endothelium are not themselves prerequisite for lymphocyte migration to the tissue. Instead, migration of lymphocytes appears to be dynamically associated with the development of the inflammatory response, during which specific phenotypic endothelial changes occur which yield an increased capacity to support lymphocyte adhesion. Concurrently, there is an apparent increased expression of lymphocyte membrane proteins specific for the altered endothelium of the target tissue, but, with few exceptions,[20,23] the nature of these adhesion proteins is unknown.

Despite the relative lack of information on the determinants of membrane interactions, there is no doubt that lymphocyte migration to nonlymphoid tissues is altered after BMT. For instance, quantitative analysis of leukocytes in bronchoalveolar lavage (BAL) fluid revealed a dramatic increase in the number of lymphocytes accumulating in the lung posttransplantation.[62] Compared to values obtained from healthy subjects, posttransplant peripheral blood lymphocyte counts were one third of normal, whereas lymphocyte counts in BAL fluid were sixfold greater than normal; thus, this tissue-blood stream ratio reflects a relative 18-fold enrichment of lymphocytes in the lung following BMT. The subset composition of BAL mirrored that of the peripheral blood in both normal subjects and posttransplant patients, in that normal subjects predominantly had a CD4$^+$ BAL population (~47%), whereas transplant patients had a low percentage of CD4$^+$ cells (~12%).[62] No variations in BAL lymphocyte composition were noted among patients undergoing different preparative regimens or receiving different stem cell sources. Most striking, however, was the absence of differences in cell characteristics in BAL in patients with and without posttransplant pneumonia, indicating that the usual physiologic mechanisms regulating local recruitment of lymphocytes to the lung in response to inflammation are compromised after BMT.

As reflected in the high incidence of pathologic reactions, the skin appears to be another major target tissue for lymphocytes traffic posttransplantation. Lymphocytic infiltrates are characteristic of a variety of cutaneous eruptions following BMT. As these eruptions most commonly arise in the setting of profound lymphopenia in the immediate posttransplant period, the adhesive system which is specialized to promote lymphocyte migration to skin must be highly efficient. In fact, the skin is an immunologic organ,[63] and increased migration of lymphocytes to the skin posttransplantation could represent an accentuation of normal immune physiology.

Several years ago, we demonstrated that dermal endothelium of normal skin did not support lymphocyte adherence in the *in vitro* adherence assay, but that vascular structures in inflamed skin, as in psoriatic plaques, did.[64,65] To determine if vascular endothelium of skin posttransplant promotes lymphocyte emigration, we used the adherence assay to investigate lymphocyte-endothelial interactions in punch biopsy specimens of cutaneous lesions in patients after both autologous and allogeneic transplantation. To date, biopsy specimens have been obtained from 31 patients (15 autologous, 16 allogeneic). Five of the allogeneic patients underwent biopsies at two different times: four patients before and after initiation of steroid therapy for GVHD, and one patient had two biopsies sequentially obtained as the skin changes progressed (total, 21 evaluable allogeneic biopsies). Eight micron frozen sections of skin were overlaid with suspensions of lymphocytes prepared from human peripheral blood or rat thoracic duct and were incubated under shear conditions at 4°C. After 30 minutes, sections were rinsed to remove nonadherent cells, fixed, and stained, and lymphocyte binding to sections was analyzed by light microscopy. Lymphocytes bound specifically to papillary dermal endothelium (identified by CD34 and factor VIII staining) in frozen sections of allogeneic BMT skin biopsies with histologically evident GVHD (9 biopsies), but not to that of posttransplant eruptions in the allogeneic BMT population without evident GVHD (10 biopsies). In the allogeneic BMT patient who had sequential biopsies, lymphocyte adherence to skin vessels was demonstrated in the first biopsy before the histologic or clinical diagnosis was made. The second biopsy clearly demonstrated GVHD. Another patient with GVHD whose skin initially demonstrated binding had resolution of binding 2 days after starting treatment for GVHD with high-dose steroids, although histologic evidence of GVHD remained; in the other three patients biopsied before and after initiation of steroid treatment, resolution of skin changes was accompanied by loss of lymphocyte binding capacity. Of the skin biopsies obtained from autologous BMT patients, only 2 of 15 specimens demonstrated lymphocyte binding to dermal vessels. These data provide evidence of changes in papillary dermal endothelial cells after BMT that mediate lymphocyte adhesion and that may promote migration of lymphocytes into skin. Expression of these adhesive structures appears to be highest in dermal endothelium of cutaneous GVHD. The molecular basis of the receptor-ligand interactions mediating the attachment of lymphocytes to endothelium in cutaneous GVHD is currently under investigation. Of note, the molecular determinant(s) mediating lymphocyte attachment is evidently conserved phylogenetically, as rat TDL adhere equally as well as human PBL to the dermal endothelium.

The pathologic diagnosis of cutaneous GVHD after allogeneic BMT is complicated by overlap with a number of histologic features seen in non-GVHD eruptions. To date, no specific and sensitive diagnostic test exists for establishing the diagnosis of cutaneous GVHD, and treatment at the onset of the earliest manifestations could alter the natural history of the disease. In this light, the lymphocyte-dermal endothelial adherence assay may be a useful adjunct in the diagnosis and clinical management of patients with GVHD. Moreover, these studies provide insights into the pathobiology of lymphocyte migration into the skin following BMT, and further information on the molecular basis of this interaction should be of benefit in designing therapeutic agents to treat cutaneous eruptions associated with BMT.

CONCLUSIONS

Transplantation of bone marrow requires the recipient to create a new immune system as stem cells divide and differentiate into lymphocyte effector cells. The establishment of host immune capabilities posttransplant is critically dependent on the migration of immature and mature lymphocytes to lymph nodes as these tissues function principally to promote a lymphocyte maturation and differentiation into immunologic effectors. Experimental evidence indicates that BMT results in perturbations in the migration of lymphocytes to lymph nodes by affecting lymphocyte-HEV adherence: pretransplant conditioning regimens have toxic effects on HEV which decrease their capacity to support lymphocyte adherence, circulating lymphocytes in the posttransplant period are deficient in membrane adhesion proteins which mediate attachment to HEV, and, furthermore, certain pharmacologic agents used posttransplantation may themselves alter the levels of relevant lymphocyte or endothelial adhesion proteins that direct migration to lymphoid tissues. A greater understanding of these issues may lead to the development of transplant regimens that preserve the physiologic trafficking of lymphocytes to lymph nodes, thereby accelerating the rate of immunologic recovery following transplant. Moreover, evidence indicates that lymphocyte migration to nonlymphoid tissues differs significantly from the trafficking patterns of normal physiology and that dysfunctional lymphocyte migration may contribute to the development of pathologic immune responses such as GVHD. The effects of BMT on the expression of lymphocyte adhesive molecules directing migration to nonlymphoid tissues and on their respective endothelial ligands is currently a subject of inquiry. Increasing knowledge of these molecular structures should prove useful in the development of therapies allowing selective preservation or modulation of tissue-specific lymphocyte migration patterns after BMT.

REFERENCES

1. GOWANS, J. L. & E. J. KNIGHT. 1964. The route of recirculation of lymphocytes in the rat. Proc. Roy. Soc. Lond. B. **159:** 257–282.
2. MARCHESI, V. T. & J. L. GOWANS. 1964. The migration of lymphocytes through the endothelium of venules in lymph nodes: An electron microscope study. Proc. Roy. Soc. Lond. B. **159:** 283–290.
3. BEVILACQUA, M. P. & R. M. NELSON. 1993. Selectins. J. Clin. Invest. **91:** 379–387.
4. REINHERZ, E. L., C. MORIMOTO, K. A. FITZGERALD et al. 1982. Heterogeneity of human T4 inducer T cells defined by a monoclonal antibody that delineates two functional subpopulations. J. Immunol. **128:** 463–468.
5. GATENBY, P. A., G. S. KANSAS, C. Y. XIAN et al. 1982. Dissection of immunoregulatory subpopulations of T lymphocytes within the helper and suppressor sublineages in man. J. Immunol. **129:** 1997–2000.
6. KISHIMOTO, T. K., M. A. JUTILA & E. C. BUTCHER. 1990. Identification of a human peripheral lymph node homing receptor: A rapidly down-regulated adhesion molecule. Proc. Natl. Acad. Sci. USA **87:** 2244–2248.
7. TEDDER, T. F., A. C. PENTA, H. B. LEVINE et al. 1990. Expression of the human leukocyte adhesion molecule, LAM-1. Identity with the TQI and Leu-8 differentiation antigens. J. Immunol. **144:** 532–540.
8. GALLATIN, W. M., I. L. WEISSMAN & E. C. BUTCHER. 1983. A cell-surface molecule involved in organ-specific homing of lymphocytes. Nature **304:** 30–34.
9. RASMUSSEN, R. A., Y. H. CHIN, J. J. WOODRUFF et al. 1985. Lymphocyte recognition of lymph node high endothelium. VII. Cell surface proteins involved in adhesion defined by monoclonal anti-HEBFLN (A.11) antibody. J. Immunol. **135:** 19–24.
10. TAMATANI, T., F. KITAMURA, K. KUIDA et al. 1993. Characterization of rat LECAM-1 (L-selectin) by the use of monoclonal antibodies and evidence for the presence of soluble LECAM-1 in rat sera. Eur. J. Immunol. **23:** 2181–2188.
11. SACKSTEIN, R., L. MENG, X. M. XU & Y. H. CHIN. 1995. Evidence of post-transcriptional regulation of L-selectin gene expression in rat lymphoid cells. Immunology **85:** 198–204.
12. LASKY, L. A., M. S. SINGER, T. A. YEDNOCK et al. 1989. Cloning of a lymphocyte homing receptor reveals a lectin domain. Cell **56:** 1045–1055.
13. BOWEN, B. R., T. NGUYEN & L. A. LASKY. 1989. Characterization of a human homologue of the murine peripheral lymph node homing receptor. J. Cell. Biol. **109:** 421–427.
14. SIEGELMAN, M. H. & I. L. WEISSMAN. 1989. Human homologue of mouse lymph node homing receptor: Evolutionary conservation at tandem cell interaction domains. Proc. Natl. Acad. Sci. USA **86:** 5562–5566.
15. TEDDER, T. F., C. M. ISAACS, T. J. ERNST et al. 1989. Isolation and chromosomal localization of cDNAs encoding a novel human lymphocyte cell surface molecule, LAM-1: Homology with the mouse lymphocyte homing receptor and other human adhesion proteins. J. Exp. Med. **170:** 123–133.
16. SIEGELMAN, M. H., M. VAN DE RIJN & I. L. WEISSMAN. 1989. Mouse lymph node homing receptor cDNA clone encodes a glycoprotein revealing tandem interaction domains. Science **243:** 1165–1172.
17. CAMERINI, D., S. P. JAMES, I. STAMENKOVIC & B. SEED. 1989. Leu-8/TQ-1 is the human equivalent of the lymph node homing receptor. Nature **342:** 78–82.
18. WATANABE, T., Y. SONG, Y. HIRCYAMA et al. 1992. Sequence and expression of a rat cDNA for LECAM-1. Biochim. Biophys. Acta **113:** 321–324.
19. JUNG, T. M. & M. O. DAILEY. 1990. Rapid modulation of homing receptors (gp90[MEL-14]) induced by activators of protein kinase C. J. Immunol. **144:** 3130–3136.
20. CHIN, Y. H., R. SACKSTEIN & J. P. CAI. 1991. Lymphocyte-homing receptors and preferential migration pathways. Proc. Soc. Exp. Biol. Med. **196:** 374–380.

21. BOWEN, B. R., C. FENNIE & L. A. LASKY. 1990. The MEL 14 antibody binds to the lectin domain of the murine peripheral lymph node homing receptor. J. Cell. Biol. **110:** 147–153.

22. WATSON, S. R., Y. IMAI, C. FENNIE *et al.* 1991. The complement binding-like domains of the murine homing receptor facilitate lectin activity. J. Cell. Biol. **115:** 235–243.

23. SPRINGER, T. A. 1994. Traffic signals for lymphocyte recirculation and leukocyte emigration: The multistep paradigm. Cell **76:** 301–314.

24. PICKER, L. J., M. NAKACHE & E. C. BUTCHER. 1989. Monoclonal antibodies to human lymphocyte homing receptors define a novel class of adhesion molecules on diverse cell types. J. Cell. Biol. **109:** 927–937.

25. GOLDSTEIN, L. A., D. F. ZHOU & L. J. PICKER. 1989. A human lymphocyte homing receptor, the hermes antigen, is related to cartilage proteoglycan core and link proteins. Cell **56:** 1063–1072.

26. JALKANEN, S., M. JALKANEN, R. BARGATZE *et al.* 1988. Biochemical properties of glycoproteins involved in lymphocyte recognition of high endothelial venules in man. J. Immunol. **141:** 1615–1623.

27. BROWN, T. A., T. BOUCHARD, T. St. JOHN *et al.* 1991. Human keratinocytes express a new CD44 core protein (CD44E) as a heparan-sulfate intrinsic membrane proteoglycan with additional exons. J. Cell. Biol. **113:** 207–220.

28. LESLEY, J., R. SCHULTE & R. HYMAN. 1990. Binding of hyaluronic acid to lymphoid cell lines is inhibited by monoclonal antibodies against Pgp-1. Exp. Cell. Res. **187:** 224–233.

29. STAMPER, H. B. & J. J. WOODRUFF. 1976. Lymphocyte homing into lymph nodes: *In vitro* demonstration of the selective affinity of recirculating lymphocytes for high-endothelial venules. J. Exp. Med. **144:** 828–833.

30. SHAW, S., G. E. G. LUCE, R. QUINONES *et al.* 1986. Two antigen-independent adhesion pathways used by human cytotoxic T-cell clones. Nature **323:** 262–264.

31. SPERTINI, O., F. W. LUSCINSKAS, G. S. KANSAS *et al.* 1991. Leukocyte adhesion molecule-1 (LAM-1, L-selectin) interacts with an inducible endothelial cell ligand to support leukocyte adhesion. J. Immunol. **147:** 2565–2573.

32. WOODRUFF, J. J., I. M. KATZ, L. E. LUCAS & H. B. STAMPER. 1977. An in vitro model of lymphocyte homing II. Membrane and cytoplasmic events involved in lymphocyte adherence to specialized high-endothelial venules of lymph nodes. J. Immunol. **119:** 1603–1610.

33. ROSEN, S. D., M. S. SINGER, T. A. YEDNOCK & L. M. STOOLMAN. 1985. Involvement of sialic acid on endothelial cells in organ-specific lymphocyte recirculation. Science **228:** 1005–1007.

34. TRUE, D. D., M. S. SINGER, L. A. LASKY & S. D. ROSEN. 1990. Requirement for sialic acid on the endothelial ligand of a lymphocyte homing receptor. J. Cell. Biol. **111:** 2757–2764.

35. IMAI, Y., L. A. LASKY & S. D. ROSEN. 1993. Sulphation requirement for GlyCAM-1, an endothelial ligand for L-selectin. Nature **361:** 555–557.

36. STOOLMAN, L. M. & S. D. ROSEN. 1983. Possible role for cell-surface carbohydrate-binding molecules in lymphocyte recirculation. J. Cell. Biol. **96:** 722–729.

37. STOOLMAN, L. M., T. S. TENFORDE & S. D. ROSEN. 1984. Phosphomannosyl receptors may participate in the adhesive interaction between lymphocytes and high endothelial venules. J. Cell. Biol. **99:** 1535–1540.

38. BERG, E., M. K. ROBINSON, A. WARNOCK *et al.* 1991. The human peripheral lymph node vascular addressin is a ligand for LECAM-1, the peripheral lymph node homing receptor. J. Cell. Biol. **114:** 343–349.

39. IMAI, Y., M. S. SINGER, C. FENNIE *et al.* 1991. Identification of a carbohydrate-based endothelial ligand for a lymphocyte homing receptor. J. Cell. Biol. **113:** 1213–1221.

40. LASKY, L. A., M. S. SINGER, D. DOWBENKO *et al.* 1992. An endothelial ligand for L-selectin is a novel mucin-like molecule. Cell **69:** 927–938.

41. KIKUTA, A. & S. D. ROSEN. 1994. Localization of ligands for L-selectin in mouse peripheral lymph node high endothelial cells by colloidal gold conjugates. Blood **84:** 3766-3775.

42. BAUMHUETER, S., M. S. SINGER, W. HENZEL *et al.* 1993. Binding of L-selectin to the vascular sialomucin CD34. Science **262:** 436-438.

43. BESCHORNER, W. E., C. I. CIVIN & L. C. STRAUSS. 1985. Localization of hematopoietic progenitor cells in tissue with the anti-My-10 monoclonal antibody. Am. J. Pathol. **119:** 1-4.

44. CIVIN, C. I., L. C. STRAUSS, C. BROVALL *et al.* 1984. Antigenic analysis of hematopoiesis III. A hematopoietic progenitor cell surface antigen defined by a monoclonal antibody raised against KG-1a cells. J. Immunol. **133:** 157-165.

45. OXLEY, S. M. & R. SACKSTEIN. 1994. Detection of an L-selectin ligand on a hematopoietic progenitor cell line. Blood **84:** 3299-3306.

46. KOEFFLER, H. P., R. BILLING, A. J. LUSIS *et al.* 1980. An undifferentiated variant derived from the human acute myelogenous leukemia cell line (KG-1). Blood **56:** 265-273.

47. MAJDIC, O., J. STÖCKL, W. F. PICKL *et al.* 1994. Signaling and induction of enhanced cytoadhesiveness via the hematopoietic progenitor cell surface molecule CD34. Blood **83:** 1226-1234.

48. SIMMONS, D. L., A. B. SATTERTHWAITE, D. G. TENEN & B. SEED. 1992. Molecular cloning of a cDNA encoding CD34, a sialomucin of human hematopoietic stem cells. J. Immunol. **148:** 267-271.

49. BROWN, J., M. F. GREAVES & H. V. MOLGAARD. 1991. The gene encoding the stem cell antigen, CD34, is conserved in mouse and expressed in haemopoietic progenitor cell lines, brain, and embryonic fibroblasts. Intern. Immunol. **3:** 175-184.

50. SAMLOWSKI, W. E., H. M. JOHNSON, E. H. HAMMOND *et al.* 1987. Marrow ablative doses of gamma-irradiation and protracted changes in peripheral lymph node microvasculature of murine and human bone marrow transplant recipients. Lab. Invest. **56:** 85-95.

51. SALE, G. E. 1984. Pathology of the lymphoreticular system. In Pathology of Bone Marrow Transplantation. G. E. Sale & H. M. Shulman, Eds.: 171-191. Yearbook Medical Publishers, Inc. Chicago.

52. SAMLOWSKI, W. E. & C. L. CRUMP. 1987. Recovery of contact hypersensitivity responses following murine bone marrow transplantation: Comparisons of gamma-irradiation and busulfan as preparative marrow-ablative agents. Blood **70:** 1910-1920.

53. KAGAN, J. M., R. E. CHAMPLIN & A. SAXON. 1989. B cell dysfunction following human bone marrow transplantation: Functional-phenotypic dissociation in the early posttransplant period. Blood **74:** 777-785.

54. KANSAS, G. S. & M. O. DAILEY. 1989. Expression of adhesion structures during B cell development in man. J. Immunol. **142:** 3058-3062.

55. PILARSKI, L. M., E. A. TURLEY, A. R. SHAW *et al.* 1991. FMC46 a cell protrusion associated leukocyte adhesion molecule-1 epitope on human lymphocytes and thymocytes. J. Immunol. **147:** 136-143.

56. TERSTAPPEN, L. W. M. M., S. HUANG & L. J. PICKER. 1992. Flow cytometric assessment of human T-cell differentiation in thymus and bone marrow. Blood **79:** 666-677.

57. FAUCI, A. S. & D. C. DALE. 1975. The effects of hydrocortisone on the kinetics of normal human lymphocytes. Blood **46:** 235-243.

58. FAUCI, A. S. & D. C. DALE. 1974. The effect of in-vivo hydrocortisone on subpopulations of human lymphocytes. J. Clin. Invest. **53:** 240-246.

59. SACKSTEIN, R. & M. BORENSTEIN. 1995. The effects of corticosteroids on lymphocyte recirculation in humans: Analysis of the mechanism of impaired lymphocyte migration to lymph node following methylprednisolone administration. J. Invest. Med. **43:** 68-77.

60. KALDJIAN, E. P. & L. STOOLMAN. 1995. Regulation of L-selectin mRNA in Jurkat cells. J. Immunol. **154:** 4351-4362.

61. GRIFFIN, J. D., O. SPERTINI, T. J. ERNST *et al.* 1990. Granulocyte-macrophage colony-stimulating factor and other cytokines regulate surface expression of the leukocyte

adhesion molecule-1 on human neutrophils, monocytes, and their precursors. J. Immunol. **145:** 576-584.
62. BOWDEN, R. A., M. MORI, S. DOBBS *et al.* 1993. Mononuclear cell reconstitution in the lung after marrow transplantation. Transplantation **55:** 557-561.
63. STREILEIN, J. W. 1983. Skin-associated lymphoid tissues (SALT): Origins and functions. J. Invest. Dermatol. **80:** 125-175.
64. SACKSTEIN, R., V. FALANGA, J. W. STREILEIN & Y. H. CHIN. 1988. Lymphocyte adhesion to psoriatic dermal endothelium is mediated by a tissue-specific receptor/ligand interaction. J. Invest. Dermatol. **91:** 423-428.
65. CHIN, Y. H., V. FALANGA, W. STREILEIN & R. SACKSTEIN. 1989. Lymphocyte recognition of psoriatic endothelium: Evidence for a tissue-specific receptor/ligand interaction. J. Invest. Dermatol. **93:** 82S-87S.

Antitumor Activity of Syngeneic/ Autologous Graft-versus-Host Disease[a]

ALLAN D. HESS,[b] M. JOHN KENNEDY,
PETER P. RUVOLO, GEORGIA B. VOGELSANG, AND
RICHARD J. JONES

Oncology Center
The Johns Hopkins University
Baltimore, Maryland 21287-8985

Cyclosporine (CsA) is an effective immunosuppressive drug that paradoxically disrupts the central and peripheral homeostatic mechanisms governing self-tolerance to self-MHC class II antigens during reconstitution of the immune system.[1] Administration of CsA after syngeneic or autologous bone marrow transplantation (BMT) in rodent models and in man results in the induction of a T-lymphocyte-dependent autoimmune syndrome with pathology identical to graft-versus-host disease (GVHD) occurring after allogeneic BMT.[2,3] The immunobiology of syngeneic/autologous GVHD is complex and requires both the induction of autoreactive $CD4^+$ and $CD8^+$ T cells and the elimination of a peripheral regulatory mechanism.[4,5] The autoreactive T cells recognize a "public" determinant on MHC class II molecules including self. Recognition of MHC class II molecules is, in fact, promiscuous.[6,7]

Despite many unresolved issues of this unique experimentally induced autoaggression syndrome, autologous/syngeneic GVHD appears to have significant antitumor activity that can be manipulated following autologous BMT. The present review summarizes the immunobiology of autologous/syngeneic GVHD with particular emphasis on the application of this syndrome as antitumor immunotherapy.

IMMUNOBIOLOGY OF SYNGENEIC GRAFT-VERSUS-HOST DISEASE

The experimental induction of syngeneic GVHD after autologous or syngeneic BMT was initially reported by Glazier *et al.*[2] Lethally irradiated Lewis rats that are reconstituted with syngeneic BMT and treated with CsA for 40 days develop a severe autoaggression syndrome 14–28 days after discontinuation of CsA treatment. Animals with this autoimmune disease exhibit erythroderma, dermatitis, and alopecia, classic

[a]This work was supported by grants AI24319, CA54203, CA58270, and CA15396 from the National Institutes of Health.

[b]Address for reprint requests: Dr. Allan D. Hess, Oncology Center 3-127, The Johns Hopkins University, 600 N. Wolfe Street, Baltimore, MD 21287-8985.

clinical signs of GVHD.[3] Histologic lesions in the tongue, skin, and liver are indistinguishable from the pathology observed in the same organs in acute GVHD following allogeneic BMT.[8,9] Recent studies indicate that after the initial onset of syngeneic GVHD there is rapid progression to a more chronic type of GVHD (complete alopecia, scleroderma, and fibrosis) along with its relevant histologic features.[9] The histologic damage in acute and chronic syngeneic GVHD also correlates with the activity of the autoreactive CD8[+] and CD4[+] T-lymphocyte subsets.[10] Adoptive transfer studies show that the acute phase is mediated by CD8[+] T cells. Progression of disease (amplification) and the development of chronic type syngeneic GVHD, although initially dependent on CD8[+]-mediated damage, requires the CD4[+] T-helper T-cell subset. Mechanisms accounting for the transition to chronic syngeneic GVHD and its dependence on distinct helper T-cell subsets are unknown, but they may be related to cytokine production.[11]

The autoreactive effector T cells in syngeneic GVHD have a unique specificity for MHC class II antigens. Initial studies by Hess *et al.*[6] demonstrated that the induction of syngeneic GVHD is associated with the development of autoreactive CD8[+] cytotoxic T cells that lyse blast cells from several different MHC disparate strains of rats. Lysis was effectively blocked by pretreating target cells with monoclonal antibodies (mAb), recognizing a public determinant on the MHC class II molecule. Of addition importance in the *in vitro* studies was the finding that in cold target inhibition studies, lysis mediated by the autoreactive T cells could be effectively blocked by blast cells from any MHC disparate strain of rat expressing MHC class II determinants. Similarly, Sorokin *et al.*[12] provided evidence that CD4[+] effector T cells in CsA-induced autoimmunity also were promiscuous in their recognition of MHC class II antigens. By contrast, anti-MHC class I-specific antibodies were ineffective. The recognition of class II MHC determinants in syngeneic GVHD is also supported by *in vivo* blocking studies.[7] Administration of mAb to the MHC class II determinant effectively delayed or prevented the onset of syngeneic GVHD after adoptive transfer of effector cells. These results suggest that a ''public determinant'' on MHC class II antigens is recognized by autoreactive CD8[+] T cells or that there is promiscuous recognition of these antigens.

The apparent recognition of a ''public'' epitope by the effector cells from animals with syngeneic GVHD as defined *in vitro* and *in vivo* is rather perplexing. Studies utilizing $F_1 \rightarrow$ parent (P) chimeras provide additional evidence that a ''public'' determinant on the MHC class II antigens is recognized in syngeneic GVHD.[7] Classically, GVHD does not develop in parental strain animals grafted with marrow from F_1 donors. Administration of CsA to $F_1 \rightarrow$P chimeras after BMT, however, induced syngeneic GVHD. Effector T cells from either $F_1 \rightarrow$P chimeric combination with syngeneic GVHD were able to transfer the disease into both parental strains. Thus, effector cells recognized the class II MHC antigens on both parental strains. Similarly, Babcock *et al.*[13] showed that the development of syngeneic GVHD in Lewis rats depends on the presence of a functioning thymus but is independent of its MHC haplotype. These data indicate that neither the thymic-dependent development nor the specificity of the autoreactive T cells is restricted by the MHC haplotype of the recipient thymus or target tissue. Rather, results suggest that autoreactive T cells recognize MHC class II determinants, but recognition of this antigen is not strain specific.

Molecular mechanisms accounting for the unique specificity of autoreactive T cells are not clear. Autoreactive T cells may directly recognize the molecule in a nonconventional manner (independent of the peptide presented by MHC class II determinants). Alternatively, we cannot exclude the recognition of a highly conserved common structural peptide bound to class II molecules that allows recognition independent of the MHC class II haplotype. It is also possible that promiscuous recognition of MHC class II antigens in syngeneic GVHD is driven by a superantigen-dependent process.[14] In this regard, the Vβ repertoire of both CD8[+] and CD4[+] autoreactive lymphocytes in the rat model is predominantly restricted to the Vβ 8.5 T-cell receptor (TcR) determinant.[15] T cells that express the Vβ 8.5 TcR determinant are responsive to the soluble superantigen staphylococcal enterotoxin B (SEB).[16,17] The hypothesis that promiscuous recognition of MHC class II antigens is driven by a superantigen may have some merit, because there are allelic variants of the Vβ 8 family of TcR genes that confer resistance to the induction of autoimmunity and the inability to respond to SEB.[16–20]

Mechanisms accounting for the production of autoreactive cells and the subsequent development of syngeneic GVHD are not fully understood. In addition to CsA treatment, two major factors have been identified that are critically important for the successful induction of this autoaggression syndrome. First, irradiation or other myeloablative therapy appears to be an important element in the induction of syngeneic GVHD.[21] Several studies clearly indicate that the principal effect of irradiation or other cytotoxic agents is the elimination of a peripheral T-lymphocyte-dependent regulatory system.[21–23] Elimination of this regulatory element provides a permissive environment for autoreactive T cells (see below). The second essential requirement is an intact thymus. Sorokin *et al.*[12] demonstrated that thymectomy prior to BMT and CsA therapy prevents the development of syngeneic GVHD, whereas thymectomy 2 weeks after BMT and the initiation of CsA therapy is ineffective in preventing the induction of this autoimmune response.

It is the effect of CsA thymic function, however, that is the critical element required for the induction of syngeneic GVHD. Recent studies show that CsA has remarkable effects on the thymus. Pharmacologic doses of CsA induce rapid ablation of the thymic medulla in both rats and mice.[24–26] There is a loss of medullary epithelium and a reduction of class II MHC antigen (Ia) expression. By contrast, Ia expression in cortical areas shows little change after CsA treatment. Recent data indicate that the thymic microenvironment including thymic epithelial cells and Ia antigen expression plays a critical role in triggering appropriate T-cell differentiation and the clonal deletion of autoreactive clones.[27–29] Jenkins, Gao, and co-workers[30–32] show in a murine system that in addition to inducing maturational arrest of thymocyte development and inhibition of positive selection, CsA also inhibits clonal deletion of anti-self I-E autoreactive T cells in the thymus. Moreover, these cells are exported to the peripheral lymphoid compartment. Clonal deletion of autoreactive thymocytes is thought to occur via apoptosis (programmed cell death) after engagement of cells having high affinity receptors for self-MHC antigens with epithelial and dendritic cells in the thymus.[27,28,33,34] In this regard, recent studies show that CsA inhibits anti-CD3-mediated thymocyte apoptosis.[35]

Despite the attractive hypothesis that the induction of syngeneic GVHD is primarily due to inhibition of clonal deletion by CsA, elimination of a T-lymphocyte-dependent regulatory mechanism is essential to allow development of active auto-aggression.[21,36] Direct support for an autoregulatory system was provided by the finding that normal splenic T lymphocytes, when cotransferred with autoimmune effector cells, prevent the development of syngeneic GVHD in secondary recipients.[22] This regulatory effect of normal splenic T lymphocytes was dose-dependent and sensitive to irradiation. Additional studies in our laboratory reveal that autoregulation of syngeneic GVHD is a dynamic process. Autoregulatory T cells specifically recognize and respond to autoreactive lymphocytes, resulting in activation, amplification, and maturation of the regulatory system.[37] This recognition requires a specific interaction between the α/β TcR on the regulatory cells and MHC class II determinants on the autoreactive T-cell compartment. Based on the finding that activated alloreactive T cells expressing MHC class II determinants fail to prime the autoregulatory component, it seems likely that the specificity of this system is conferred by other elements and may include a response to TcR idiotypic determinants.[38] The mechanism of regulation or suppression in this model has not been defined. It may include active suppression, induction of clonal anergy, or peripheral deletion of autoreactive T cells.

On the basis of these findings, a simplified working model of CsA-induced autoimmune disease can be constructed as shown in FIGURE 1. Treatment of animals with CsA leads to the production of autoreactive T cells with a novel specificity for MHC class II antigens. This occurs either by inhibiting clonal deletion in the thymus (through inhibition of the TcR signaling apoptotic process) or by altering normal selection mechanisms. These autoreactive T cells are then exported into the periphery. Upon discontinuation of CsA treatment and in the absence of regulatory compartment T cells (i.e., eliminated by irradiation), autoreactive T cells are activated and mediate autoaggression.

ANTITUMOR ACTIVITY OF SYNGENEIC/AUTOLOGOUS GRAFT-VERSUS-HOST DISEASE

Studies in our laboratory attempted to assess whether this experimentally induced autoimmune syndrome could be mobilized to mediate a significant antitumor effect against tumor cells expressing the target antigen (MHC class II determinants) of syngeneic GVHD. This is particularly important because one of the major limitations of autologous BMT as therapy for malignancy is the unacceptably high rate of tumor recurrence.[39,40] In comparison, the rate of tumor recurrence after allogeneic BMT is significantly lower than the rate observed after autologous BMT even though comparable preparative regimens are employed.[39,41] The enhanced antitumor effect of allogeneic BMT is thought to be due to the occurrence of GVHD and suggests that tumor cells can be recognized and eliminated by immune mechanisms.[41-43] Although autologous BMT avoids the morbidity and mortality associated with GVHD after allogeneic BMT, the graft-versus-tumor effect is absent. Certainly, the high rate of tumor recurrence in autologous BMT patients is in large part due to the lack of significant graft-versus-host disease. On the basis of significant antitumor activity of GVHD, it seems likely that immune modulation should enhance the efficacy of autologous BMT in the treatment of malignancy. Immunologic approaches for eradication of tumor in the autologous BMT setting should be particularly effective because

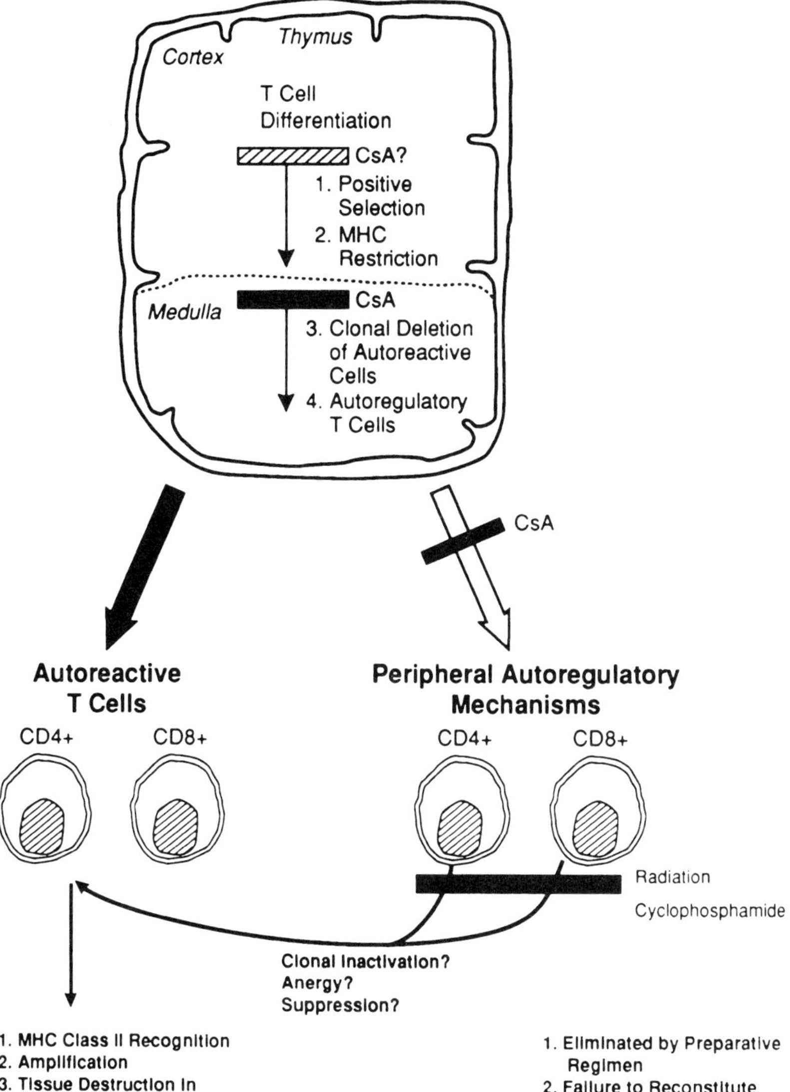

FIGURE 1. Autoreactive and autoregulatory immune mechanisms in autologous/syngeneic graft-versus-host disease.

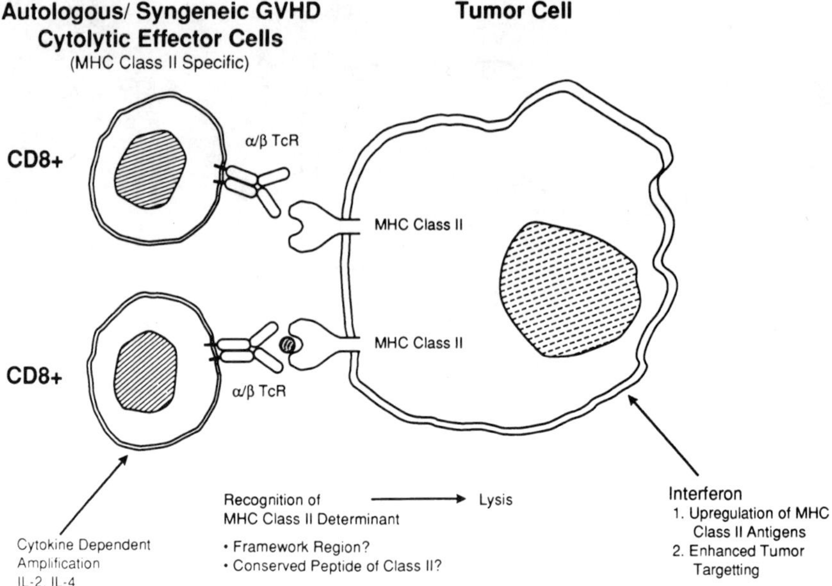

FIGURE 2. Tumor cell recognition by autoreactive T lymphocytes in autologous/syngeneic graft-versus-host disease.

they would be used at a time when residual disease is minimal, thus limiting the number of tumor cells needed to be eliminated by the immune system.

The induction of syngeneic/autologous GVHD as antitumor therapy after autologous BMT is particularly attractive for several reasons. First, immune recognition of tumor cells by autoreactive T lymphocytes appears to be dependent only on expression of MHC class II determinants because there is promiscuous recognition of these antigens as illustrated in FIGURE 2. Comparatively, recognition of tumor cells by lymphocytes mediating allogeneic GVHD (recognizing minor histocompatibility antigens restricted by class I MHC determinants in transplants performed between MHC matched siblings) requires that tumor cells express not only the MHC class I antigen but also the relevant minor antigen. Based on these differences in target cell recognition, it is conceivable that the antitumor effect of autologous/syngeneic GVHD may equal or exceed the antitumor activity observed with allogeneic GVHD. Second, expression of MHC class II antigens, the target antigen of autologous/syngeneic GVHD, can be upregulated by cytokines such as gamma-interferon (γ-INF), thereby potentiating tumor targeting (FIG. 2). Third, administration of interleukin-2 (IL-2) could amplify autoreactive T cells, providing maximum tumor kill. Together, several different strategies amplifying effector mechanisms and increased tumor cell targeting can be utilized singly or in concert to enhance the antitumor effect of autologous/syngeneic GVHD after autologous BMT.

TABLE 1. Antitumor Activity of Syngeneic GVHD and Potentiation by Cytokines following Adoptive Transfer of Effector T Cells[a]

Treatment	Estimated Log Tumor Cell Kill
Syngeneic GVHD effector cells + 0	1.5–2.0
Syngeneic GVHD effector cells + gamma-interferon	2.5–3.0
Syngeneic GVHD effector cells + IL-2	2.0–2.5
Syngeneic GVHD effector cells + gamma-interferon + IL-2	4.0–4.5

[a] Nylon wool nonadherent spleen cells (50×10^6) from Lou M animals with syngeneic GVHD were adoptively transferred into secondary Lou M recipients (irradiated, bone marrow reconstituted) challenged with 2.5×10^8 CRL 1662 myeloma cells. Animals were treated with gamma-interferon (50,000 U/d), IL-2 (10,000 U/d), or a combination for 10 days. Survival was assessed and log tumor cell kill was estimated from dose response studies.

ANIMAL STUDIES

Initial preclinical studies evaluated the antitumor effect of syngeneic GVHD in the rat model using the CRL 1662 myeloma derived from the Lou M strain rat. Not only does this tumor express MHC class II determinants, but also expression of these antigens can be significantly enhanced by treatment with γ-INF.[44] Studies by Geller *et al.*[44] demonstrated that CD8+ splenic T cells from Lou M rats that developed syngeneic GVHD were able to lyse myeloma cells *in vitro*. Lysis of tumor cells was blocked by pretreating tumor cells with antibodies to the MHC class II determinant but not antibodies to MHC class I antigens. Furthermore, incubation of tumor cells with γ-INF not only upregulated the expression of MHC class II antigen but also, and more importantly, increased their susceptibility to lysis by the effector lymphocytes from animals with syngeneic GVHD. These studies demonstrated that syngeneic GVHD could manifest significant antitumor activity *in vitro* and confirmed that the effector T cells recognized MHC class II antigens on the tumor cell.

Subsequent studies evaluated the antitumor activity of syngeneic GVHD *in vivo* and assessed if the administration of the recombinant lymphokines, γ-INF or IL-2, could potentiate this effect.[45,46] Results of these investigations, summarized in TABLE 1, indicate that syngeneic GVHD mediated a significant antitumor effect, achieving a 1-2 log tumor cell kill. Additionally, administration of γ-INF potentiated the antitumor effect of syngeneic GVHD, resulting in cure of 40% of the animals. These animals were resistant to rechallenge with the tumor cells, suggesting a concomitant development of specific antitumor immunity. Moreover, a two- to fivefold increase in MHC class II on the tumor cells *in vivo* was noted after treatment with γ-INF. Taken together with *in vitro* studies, it seems likely that the increased expression of MHC class II antigens on tumor cells resulted in enhanced recognition of tumor cells by autoreactive effector lymphocytes. On the other hand, the use of high dose (50–100,000 units/day) IL-2 treatment to amplify the effector mechanisms in syngeneic GVHD primarily exacerbated the autoaggression syndrome. Because of the potentiation of fatal autoaggression, the role of IL-2 in amplifying antitumor activity could not accurately be assessed. Lower doses (5-10,000 units/day) of IL-2 were more effective and appeared to have an additive effect with the administration of γ-INF as shown in TABLE 1. These data suggest that the antitumor activity of syngeneic GVHD can be enhanced by amplifying the autoreactive effector T cells and upregulating the target antigen on the tumor cells, thereby potentiating tumor cell recognition and destruction.

CLINICAL STUDIES

Encouraged by the results of animals studies, clinical studies were initiated to assess the feasibility of inducing an autoimmune GVHD in autologous BMT patients and to evaluate whether there was any antitumor activity. Initially, five consecutive patients with either aggressive non-Hodgkin's lymphoma or Hodgkin's disease in relapse who were not responsive to conventional salvage therapy underwent autologous BMT and CsA treatment.[47] Cyclosoporine was started on the day of BMT and was continued for 28 days at 1 mg/kg per day. Histologically proven grade II GVHD of the skin developed in all five patients at a median of 11 days (range 9-13 days) after BMT, at the time of initial evidence of hematologic recovery. The GVHD was confined to the skin (erythematous maculopapular rash affecting the face, ears, trunk, hands, and feet) with no evidence of extracutaneous involvement. The autologous GVHD resolved within 1-3 weeks either spontaneously or after a short course of corticosteroids. Moreover, cytolytic lymphocytes recognizing self- and MHC disparate lymphocytes could be detected during active disease, and lysis was blocked by pretreating target cells (self and unrelated) with monoclonal antibodies to class II MHC antigens. Autoreactive T cells could no longer be detected upon resolution of clinical autologous GVHD.

The findings in human autologous GVHD, for the most part, paralleled results in the animal model. The CsA-induced autoaggression syndrome in man is also associated with the development of autocytotoxic T cells that promiscuously recognize MHC class II determinants.[47,48] Clinical results with the induction of GVHD with CsA treatment after autologous BMT, including the detection of MHC class II restricted autoreactive T lymphocytes, now have been confirmed by several groups.[49-51] Additionally, recent studies by Ruvolo *et al.*[48] indicate that the appearance of MHC class II autocytolytic T cells coincides with the onset of clinical autologous GVHD. These lytic T cells were primarily CD8$^+$ CD4$^-$ α/β TcR$^+$; however, in a subgroup of patients the lytic T cells expressed both CD8 and CD4 cell surface accessory molecules. Also, it is of interest that the Vβ T-cell receptor repertoire expressed by the infiltrating lymphocytes was limited with a few common TcR elements including Vβ 15. The finding of Vβ 15$^+$ T cells infiltrating the skin in most patients tested (6 of 6 including 1 spontaneous case of autologous GVHD) is of interest because Vβ 15$^+$ T cells are responsive to the superantigen SEB.[52] These results, however, appear to parallel studies in the rat model (just described) and may explain the promiscuous recognition of MHC class II determinants. Although these findings were unexpected in an outbred species such as man, additional studies should define the importance of a restricted Vβ T-cell receptor repertoire in autologous GVHD.

TABLE 2. Characteristics of Clinical Autologous Graft-versus-Host Disease

Occurs in >70% of autologous bone marrow transplantation patients

Dose of cyclosporine 1-2 mg/kg/d iv

Confined primarily to skin; generally no involvement of internal organs

Onset occurs with initial phases of engraftment; can occur 1-2 weeks after cyclosporine withdrawal in a subset of patients

Lasts 1-3 weeks, resolves spontaneously, although a few patients require low dose steroid treatment

Gamma-interferon increases severity, has no effect on incidence

Associated with MHC class II autoreactive T cells; lysis of pretransplant lymphoblasts (phytohemagglutinin transformed) and tumor cell lines

Despite similar effector mechanisms and histologic lesions, a few differences exist between the induction of autologous/syngeneic GVHD in man and that in the rat model. One major difference is that autologous GVHD develops in patients while they are being treated with CsA. In the rat model, CsA must be discontinued, in most cases, prior to the onset of disease.[47,53,54] This difference may be related to the higher doses of CsA administered to animals, whereas the lower doses in man allow for activation of the autoreactive T cells. The second difference is that a chronic phase of the disease develops in most animals.[4,9] On the other hand, the development of a chronic phase in man is rare. Because the development of the chronic phase is principally due to autoreactive CD4[+] T cells, it seems likely that autoreactive helper T cells may develop infrequently in man or that they develop discordantly compared to CD8[+] autoreactive T cells.[4]

Encouraged by the fact that autologous GVHD could be induced in humans with similar effector mechanisms as defined in the animal model, several clinical trials were initiated to evaluate the antitumor activity of this experimentally induced auto-aggression syndrome especially because many lymphohematopoietic malignancies and solid tumors express MHC class II determinants. Included in these trials were a phase II study of high grade non-Hodgkin's lymphoma in sensitive relapse (still responsive to salvage chemotherapy), a phase I study in acute myelogenous leukemia, and a phase I/II study in metastatic breast cancer. An additional phase I/II study in metastatic breast cancer was also started with the induction of autologous GVHD and the adjuvant administration of recombinant human γ-INF. To date, over 200 patients have been on these clinical protocols. Although these clinical trials are ongoing, several important facts (as summarized in TABLE 2) have been established: (1) autologous GVHD can be induced in over 70% of patients; (2) this autoaggression syndrome in most cases is confined to the skin without any clinical evidence of internal organ disease (i.e., liver and gastrointestinal tract); (3) the appearance of autologous GVHD primarily occurs with the initial phases of engraftment while the patient is on CsA; (4) the autoimmune syndrome resolves spontaneously in most cases, although a small percentage of patients require a short course of corticosteroids; and (5) MHC class II restricted autoreactive T cells can be detected that not only lyse pretransplant lymphocytes but also lyse a number of tumor cell lines that express MHC class II determinants. Of further importance is the finding that the administration of γ-INF significantly increases the severity (greater incidence of grade II disease as defined by an erythematous rash covering >50% of the body) of autologous GVHD. Subsequent studies revealed that γ-INF administration results in the upregulation of class II MHC antigens in the skin and probably accounts for the increased severity of skin lesions.

More recently, a series of phase I pilot trials was initiated to maximize the induction of autologous GVHD in patients with metastatic breast cancer.[55] Administration of G-CSF mobilized progenitor cells to the bone marrow graft plus CsA and γ-INF treatment resulted in a significant increase in grade II autologous GVHD with a third of the patients requiring some corticosteroid therapy. This increase in the intensity of autologous GVHD was associated with an increase in the number of autoreactive cytolytic T cells and a rapid repopulation of CD4⁺ T helper cell compartment.[55] The increased frequency of autocytolytic T cells appears to be due to cytokine amplification provided by the proportional increase in helper T lymphocytes.

Ongoing analyses suggest that autologous GVHD does have significant antitumor activity.[56,57] The increase in the event-free survival (62%) and the decrease in the relapse rate (29%) of high grade non-Hodgkin's lymphoma with autologous GVHD were significant compared to recent historical controls (event-free survival, 40%; relapse rate, 50%). Similarly, breast cancer patients who develop autologous GVHD have a marked early survival advantage over those who do not develop this autoaggression syndrome. Moreover, the antitumor effect is apparently enhanced by the administration of recombinant γ-INF.[58,59] From these encouraging results several randomized trials with adjuvant administration of γ-INF in a variety of lymphohematopoietic malignancies are now underway to confirm the antitumor effect of autologous GVHD in man.

CONCLUSIONS

The disruption of immunologic homeostasis and self-tolerance during reconstitution of the immune system after syngeneic/autologous BMT by the administration of CsA results in induction of the autoaggression syndrome called syngeneic/autologous GVHD. Two components are essential for the induction of syngeneic/autologous GVHD. They include: (1) inhibition of clonal deletion in the thymus by CsA treatment, and (2) elimination of a peripheral T-lymphocyte-dependent autoregulatory mechanism. These two elements alter the balance of autoreactive and autoregulatory cells in the periphery, leading to the onset of autoaggression.

This experimentally induced autoaggression syndrome, however, can be mobilized to mediate a significant antitumor effect after autologous BMT that is similar in magnitude to the antitumor activity of allogeneic GVHD without its posttransplant mortality. Current studies also suggest that the antitumor activity of syngeneic/autologous GVHD can be modulated by the administration of cytokines such as IL-2 and γ-INF which amplify the effector mechanisms and upregulate the target antigen on the tumor cell, respectively. Certainly, the use of other cytokines such as GM-CsF to enhance the repopulation of antigen-presenting cells, IL-6 to stimulate the differentiation of cytolytic T cells and IL-15 to amplify effector mechanisms, may even further potentiate the antitumor activity of autologous/syngeneic GVHD. Taken together, the induction of autologous/syngeneic GVHD in combination with specific cytokine therapy after autologous BMT provides a unique and exciting approach for immunotherapy of neoplastic disease.

REFERENCES

1. SANTOS, G. W. 1988. Problems and strategies for BMT in acute leukemia and chronic myelogenous leukemia. Cancer Detect. Prev. **12:** 589–596.
2. GLAZIER, A., P. J. TUTSCHKA, E. R. FARMER & G. W. SANTOS. 1983. GVHD in CsA treated rats after syngeneic and autologous bone marrow reconstitution. J. Exp. Med. **158:** 1–8.
3. GLAZIER, A., P. J. TUTSCHKA & E. R. FARMER. 1983. Studies on immunobiology of syngeneic and autologous GVHD in cyclosporine treated rats. Transpl. Proc. **15:** 3035–3041.
4. HESS, A. D., A. C. FISCHER & W. E. BESCHORNER. 1990. Effector mechanisms in cyclosporine A-induced syngeneic graft-versus-host disease. Role of CD4⁺ and CD8⁺ T lymphocyte subsets. J. Immunol. **145:** 526–533.
5. FISCHER, A. C., W. E. BESCHORNER & A. D. HESS. 1989. Requirements for the induction and adoptive transfer of cyclosporine-induced syngeneic graft-versus-host disease. J. Exp. Med. **169:** 1031–1041.
6. HESS, A. D., L. R. HORWITZ, W. E. BESCHORNER & G. W. SANTOS. 1985. Development of GVHD-like syndrome in CsA-treated rats after syngeneic BMT. J. Exp. Med. **161:** 718–730.
7. HESS, A. D., L. R. HORWITZ, M. K. LAULIS & E. J. FUCHS. 1994. Cyclosporine-Induced syngeneic GVHD: Prevention of autoaggression by treatment with monoclonal antibodies to T lymphocyte cell surface determinants and to MHC Class II antigens. Clin. Immunol. Immunopathol. **69:** 341.
8. BESCHORNER, W. E., A. D. HESS, C. A. SHINN & G. W. SANTOS. 1988. Transfer of cyclosporine-associated syngeneic GVHD by thymocytes: Resemblance to chronic GVHD. Transplantation **45:** 209–215.
9. BESCHORNER, W. E., C. A. SHINN, A. C. FISCHER, G. W. SANTOS & A. D. HESS. 1988. Cyclosporine-induced pseudo GVHD in the early post-cyclosporine period. Transplantation **46**(Suppl): 112s–117s.
10. HESS, A. D., A. C. FISCHER & W. E. BESCHORNER. 1990. Effector mechanisms in cyclosporine A induced syngeneic graft-versus-host disease: Role of CD4⁺ and CD8⁺ T lymphocyte subsets. J. Immunol. **145:** 526–533.
11. PARKMAN, R. 1990. Clonal Analysis of Graft-versus-Host Disease. IV. Graft-versus-Host Disease. : 51–60. Marcel Dekker. New York.
12. SOROKIN, R., H. KIMURA, K. SCHRODER & D. B. WILSON. 1986. Cyclosporine-induced autoimmunity: Conditions for expressing disease, requirement for intact thymus, and potency estimates of autoimmune lymphocytes in drug-treated rats. J. Exp. Med. **164:** 1615–1625.
13. BABCOCK, S., K. NISWENDER, D. B. WILSON & D. BELLGRAU. 1990. Cyclosporine-induced autoimmunity in rats carrying thymus allografts. Transplantation **50:** 1278–1281.
14. WOODLAND, D. L. & M. A. BLACKMAN. 1993. How do T-cell receptors, MHC molecules and superantigens get together? Immunol. Today **14:** 208–212.
15. FISCHER, A. C., P. P. RUVOLO, R. BURT, L. R. HORWITZ, E. C. BRIGHT, J. M. HESS, W. E. BESCHORNER & A. D. HESS. 1995. Characterization of the autoreactive T cell repertoire in cyclosporine-induced syngeneic graft-versus-host disease: A highly conserved repertoire mediates autoaggression. J. Immunol. **154:** 3713–3725.
16. GOLD, D. P., C. D. SURH, K. S. SELLINS, K. SCHRODER, J. SPRENT & D. B. WILSON. 1994. Rat T cell responses to superantigens. II. Allelic differences in Vβ8.2 and Vβ8.5 β

chains determine responsiveness to staphylococcal enterotoxin B and mouse mammary tumor virus-encoded proteins. J. Exp. Med. **179:** 63–69.

17. SURH, C. D., D. P. GOLD, S. WILEY, D. B. WILSON & J. SPRENT. 1994. Rat T cell response to superantigens. I. Vβ-restricted clonal deletion of rat T cells differentiating in rat mouse chimeras. J. Exp. Med. **179:** 57–62.

18. BLANKENHORN, E. P., P. D. SMITH, C. B. WILLIAMS & G. A. GUTMAN. 1992. Alleles of the rat T-cell receptor β chain gene complex. Immunogenetics **35:** 324–331.

19. FU, Y., P. A. VILLAS & E. P. BLANKENHORN. 1991. Genetic control of rat T-cell response to Staphylococcus aureus entertoxins. Immunology **75:** 484–489.

20. BLANKENHORN, E. P., S. A. STRANFORD, P. D. SMITH & W. F. HICKEY. 1991. Genetic differences in the T cell receptor alleles of LEW rats and their encephalomyelitis-resistant derivative, LER, and their impact on the inheritance of EAE resistance. Eur. J. Immunol. **21:** 2033–2041.

21. FISCHER, A. C., W. E. BESCHORNER & A. D. HESS. 1989. Requirements for the induction and adoptive transfer of syngeneic GVHD. J. Exp. Med. **169:** 1031.

22. FISCHER, A. C., M. K. LAULIS, L. R. HORWITZ, W. E. BESCHORNER & A. D. HESS. 1989. Host resistance to cyclosporine induced syngeneic graft-versus-host disease. Requirement for two distinct lymphocyte subsets. J. Immunol. **143:** 827–832.

23. URDAHL, K. B., D. M. PARDOLL & M. K. JENKINS. 1992. Self-reactive T cells are present in the peripheral lymphoid tissues of CsA-treated mice. Int. Immunol. **4:** 1341–1349.

24. RYFFEL, B., R. DEYSSEROTH & J. F. BOREL. 1981. Cyclosporin A: Effects on the mouse thymus. Agents Actions **11:** 373–381.

25. BESCHORNER, W. E., J. D. NAMMORIM, A. D. HESS, C. A. SHIN & G. W. SANTOS. 1987. Cyclosporin A and the thymus. Amer. J. Pathol. **126:** 487–496.

26. FABIEN, N. H., C. AUGER & A. MOREIRA. 1992. Effects of CsA on mouse thymus: Immunochemical and ultrastructural studies. Thymus **2092:** 153–162.

27. GOSS, J. A., Y. NAKAFUSA & M. W. FLYE. 1993. MHC class II presenting cells are necessary for the induction of intrathymic tolerance. Ann. Surg. **217:** 492–501.

28. AGUILAR, L. K., E. AGUILAR-CORDOVA, Jr., J. CARTWRIGHT & J. W. BELMONT. 1994. Thymic nurse cells are sites of thymocyte apoptosis. J. Immunol. **152:** 2645–2651.

29. VON BOEHMER, H., W. SWAT & P. KISIELOW. 1993. Positive selection of immature αβ T cells. Immunol. Rev. **135:** 67–79.

30. JENKINS, M.K., R. H. SCHWARTZ & D. M. PARDOLL. 1988. Effects of CsA on T cell development and clonal deletion. Science **241:** 1655–1658.

31. GAO, E. K., D. LO, R. T. CHENEY, O. KANAGAWA & J. SPRENT. 1989. Abnormal differentiation of thymocytes in mice treated with cyclosporine. Nature **336:** 176–179.

32. URDAHL, K. B., D. M. PARDOLL & M. K. JENKINS. 1994. Cyclosporin A inhibits positive selection and delays negative selection in αβ TCR transgenic mice. J. Immunol. **152:** 2853–2859.

33. KAPPLER, J., U. STAERZ & J. WHITE. 1988. Self-tolerance eliminates T cells specific for MLS-modified products of the MHC complex. Nature **332:** 35–38.

34. KAPPLER, J. W., U. STAERZ & J. WHITE. 1987. T cell tolerance by clonal elimination in the thymus. Cell **49:** 273–280.

35. SHI, Y., B. M. SAHAI & D. R. GREEN. 1989. Cyclosporine A inhibits activation induced cell death in the T cell hybridomas and thymocytes. Nature **339:** 625–626.

36. HESS, A. D. & A. C. FISCHER. 1989. Immune mechanisms in cyclosporine-induced syngeneic graft-versus-host disease. Transplantation **48:** 895–900.

37. HESS, A. D., A. C. FISCHER, L. R. HORWITZ, E. C. BRIGHT & M. K. LAULIS. 1994. Characterization of peripheral autoregulatory mechanisms that prevent the development of cyclosporin-induced syngeneic graft-versus-host disease. J. Immunol. **153:** 400–411.

38. OFFNER, H., M. K. H. MALOTKY, L. POPE, M. VAINIENE, B. CELNIK, S. D. MILLER & A. A. VANDERBARK. 1995. Increased severity of experimental autoimmune encephalomy-elitis in rats tolerized as adults but not neonatally to a protective TcR Vβ8 CDR2 idiotype. J. Immunol. **154:** 928.

39. KERSEY, J. H., D. WEISDORF, N. E. NESBIT, T. W. LEBIEN, W. G. WOODS, P. B. MCGLAVE, T. KIM, D. A. VALLERA, A. I. GOLDMAN, B. BOSTROM, D. HURD & N. K. C. RAMSEY. 1987. Comparison of autologous and allogeneic bone marrow transplantation for treatment of high-risk refractory acute lymphoblastic leukemia. N. Engl. J. Med. **317:** 461.

40. SANTOS, G. W., A. M. YEAGER & R. J. JONES. 1989. Autologous bone marrow transplantation. Ann. Rev. Med. **40:** 99–112.

41. WEIDEN, P. L., N. FLOURNOY, E. D. THOMAS, R. PRENTICE, A. FEFER, C. D. BUCKNER & R. STORB. 1979. Antileukemic effect of GVHD in human recipients of allogeneic-marrow grafts. N. Engl. J. Med. **300:** 1068–1073.

42. WEIDEN, P. L., K. M. SULLIVAN, N. FLOURNOY, R. STORB & E. D. THOMAS. 1981. Antileukemic effect of chronic GVHD. N. Engl. J. Med. **304:** 1529–1533.

43. BUTTURINI, A., M. M. BORTIN & R. P. GALE. 1987. Graft-vs-leukemia following BMT. Bone Marrow Transplant. **2:** 233–242.

44. GELLER, R. B., A. H. ESA, W. E. BESCHORNER, C. G. FRONDOZA, G. W. SANTOS & A. D. HESS. 1989. Successful in vitro graft-versus-tumor effect against an Ia-bearing tumor using cyclosporine-induced syngeneic graft-versus-host disease in the rat. Blood **74:** 1165–1171.

45. NOGA, S. J., L. R. HORWITZ, H. KIM, M. K. LAULIS & A. D. HESS. 1992. Interferon-τ potentiates the antitumor effect of cyclosporine-induced autoimmunity. J. Hematother. **1:** 75–84.

46. HESS, A. D. & S. J. NOGA. 1992. Cyclosporine-induced syngeneic graft-versus-host disease: An immunotherapeutic approach after autologous bone marrow transplantation. Int. J. Cell. Cloning **10** (Suppl. 1): 179.

47. JONES, R. J., G. B. VOGELSANG, A. D. HESS, E. R. FARMER, R. B. MANN, R. B. GELLER, S. PIANTADOSI & G. W. SANTOS. 1989. Induction of graft-versus-host disease after autologous bone marrow transplantation. Lancet **1:** 754–757.

48. RUVOLO, P. P., E. C. BRIGHT, M. J. KENNEDY, L. E. MORRIS, A. C. FISCHER, G. B. VOGELSANG, R. J. JONES & A. D. HESS. 1995. Cyclosporine-induced autologous graft-versus-host disease: Assessment of cytolytic effector mechanisms and the Vβ T cell receptor repertoire. Transplant. Proc. **27:** 1363–1365.

49. DALE, B. M., K. ATKINSON, D. KOTASEK, J. C. BIGGS & R. E. SAGE. 1989. Cyclosporine-induced graft-versus-host disease in two patients receiving syngeneic bone marrow transplants. Transplant. Proc. **21:** 3816.

50. CARELLA, A. M., E. GAOZZA & G. PIATTI. 1990. Induction of graft-versus-host disease (GVHD) after ABMT for high risk ALL in first CR and second chronic phase of chronic myeloid leukemia (Abstr.). Exp. Hematol. **18:** 684.

51. CARELLA, A. M., E. GAOZZA, A. CONGIU *et al.* 1991. Cyclosporine-induced graft-versus-host disease after autologous bone marrow transplantation in hematological malignancies. Ann. Hematol. **62:** 156–159.

52. LUNDIN, K. E. A., J. E. BRINCHMANN & T. HANSEN. 1994. Interactions between Staphylococcal superantigens and human T-cell clones are predominantly but not exclusively governed by their T-cell receptor Vβ usage. Scand. J. Immunol. **39:** 387–394.

53. YEAGER, A. M., G. B. VOGELSANG, R. J. JONES, E. R. FARMER, V. ALTOMONTE, A. D. HESS & G. W. SANTOS. 1992. Induction of cutaneous graft-versus-host disease by administration of cyclosporine to patients undergoing autologous bone marrow transplantation for acute myeloid leukemia. Blood **79:** 3031–3035.

54. KENNEDY, M. J., G. B. VOGELSANG, R. A. BEVERIDGE, E. R. FARMER, V. ALTOMONTE, A. M. HUELSKAMP & N. E. DAVIDSON. 1993. Phase I trial of intravenous cyclosporine to induce GVHD in women undergoing autologous BMT for breast cancer. J. Clin. Oncol. **11:** 478–484.

55. HESS, A. D., M. J. KENNEDY, E. C. BRIGHT, G. B. VOGELSANG & R. J. JONES. 1994. Induction of autoimmune graft-versus-host disease after autologous bone marrow transplantation augmented with peripheral blood stem cells: Analysis of immune function (Abstr). Blood **83** (Suppl. 1): 33.

56. JONES, R. J., G. B. VOGELSANG, R. F. AMBINDER, G. W. SANTOS & A. D. HESS. 1991. Autologous marrow transplantation (ABMT) with cyclosporine (CsA)-induced autologous graft-versus-host disease (GVHD) for relapsed aggressive non-Hodgkin's lymphoma (NHL) (Abstr.). Blood **78:** 287a.

57. JONES, R. J. & A. D. HESS. 1995. Autologous graft-versus-host disease. *In* Immunotherapy and Bone Marrow Transplantation. T. Spitzer & A. Mazumder, Eds.: 59–70. Futura Publishing Co., Inc. Armonk, NY.

58. KENNEDY, M. J., R. A. BEVERIDGE, G. B. VOGELSANG, E. R. FARMER, S. D. ROWLEY, R. J. JONES & N. E. DAVIDSON. 1991. Phase I study of cyclosporine (CsA) to induce graft-versus-host disease (GVHD) following high dose chemotherapy (HDC) with autologous marrow infusion (AMR) for metastatic breast cancer (MBC) (Abstr.). Am. Soc. Clin. Oncol. **10:** 43.

59. KENNEDY, M. J., G. B. VOGELSANG, R. J. JONES, E. R. FARMER, A. D. HESS, V. ALTOMONTE, A. M. HUELSKAMP & N. E. DAVIDSON. 1994. Phase I trial of interferon-gamma to potentiate cyclosporine A-induced graft-versus-host disease in women undergoing autologous bone marrow transplantation for breast cancer. J. Clin. Oncol. **12:** 249.

Strategies to Enhance the Graft-versus-Malignancy Effect in Allogeneic Transplants

JOHN A. BARRETT

Bone Marrow Transplant Unit
Hematology Branch
National Heart Lung and Blood Institute
National Institutes of Health
Bethesda, Maryland 20892

The curative effect of bone marrow transplantation (BMT) in hematologic malignancies derives in part from pretransplant myeloablation and in part from a donor immune response to the leukemia, termed graft-versus-leukemia (GVL).[1,2] Overall, 55-70% disease-free survival can be expected for standard risk leukemias transplanted from a human leukocyte antigen (HLA)-matched sibling, whereas results are generally below 40% for poor risk patients.[3,4] Improved results in BMT for leukemia, especially from mismatched donors, depend on devising strategies to conserve GVL while preventing graft-versus-host disease (GVHD). New understanding of the alloresponse, the responder cells in GVL, the antigens on leukemia cells, and the mechanism involved in leukemia killing, should contribute to the goal of improving the BMT outcome.

GRAFT-VERSUS-LEUKEMIA IN CLINICAL BONE MARROW TRANSPLANTATION

Evidence for GVL following BMT for leukemia comes from observations that relapse rates for identical twin BMT (when there is no allo-effect) are higher than those for allogeneic BMT.[5] The GVL effect is closely linked to GVHD; patients who develop clinically significant acute or chronic GVHD have a lower relapse rate than do those who do not.[6,7] The GVL effect is linked to the presence of donor lymphocytes in the transplant; for example, T-cell depletion of donor marrow increases the 10% relapse rate in chronic myelogenous leukemia transplants to about 60%.[8] Evidence for a powerful antileukemic effect of alloreacting lymphocytes comes from recent observations that prolonged remission and probable cures of leukemia relapsing after BMT have been achieved with transfusions of donor lymphocytes.[9-12] Although evidence of a GVL effect is uncontested, its distinction from GVHD remains debated. Certain circumstances, however, suggest that the processes are not inevitably linked; patients with chronic myelogenous leukemia not developing GVHD but given non-T-cell depleted BMT have a sevenfold lower risk of relapse than do recipients of T-cell depleted marrow.[6] Donor lymphocyte transfusion can induce remission without causing GVHD.[12] In a comparative analysis of BMT from Japan and the United

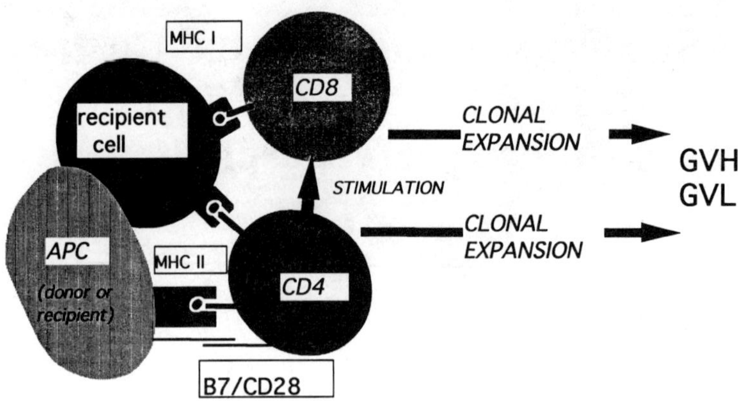

FIGURE 1. T-cell alloresponse to recipient.

Kingdom, we reported identical low relapse rates (<10%) in Japanese patients despite a GVHD incidence less than half that of transplant recipients from the UK.[13] These results suggest that GVL may be mediated by both GVHD-dependent and GVHD-independent mechanisms.

THE ALLORESPONSE

The process of allorecognition of the host involves T lymphocytes. In HLA-matched sibling BMT, minor histocompatibility antigens (mHA) are the targets presented to the donor either via host or recipient antigen-presenting cells (APC) (FIG. 1). Lymphocytes responding to host antigens undergo clonal expansion under the influence of interleukin-2 (IL-2). T cells, natural killer (NK) cells, tumor necrosis factor, IL-1, and interferons have all been implicated in the effector component of the alloresponse producing the clinical syndrome of GVHD.[14,15] Target tissues for GVHD (bone marrow cells, mucosal cells of the gastrointestinal tract, biliary endothelium, and epithelial cells) include cells with rapid turnover, capable of expressing major histocompatibility complex class I and II. The susceptibility of bone marrow to immune attack is further illustrated by the ease with which the recipient can reject the allograft. Host T cells target mHA on hematopoietic progenitor cells and, in conjunction with NK cells, mediate graft rejection.[16,17] Although T cells mediate both GVL and GVHD, the mechanisms may differ because of either antigenic differences between GVHD and leukemia targets or different susceptibilities of leukemic and normal cells to effector cells and cytokines.

T-CELL RESPONSES TO LEUKEMIA

The molecular structures involved in tumor recognition by T cells are well defined. Antigen receptors on the T-cell surface bind to peptides positioned in the groove of

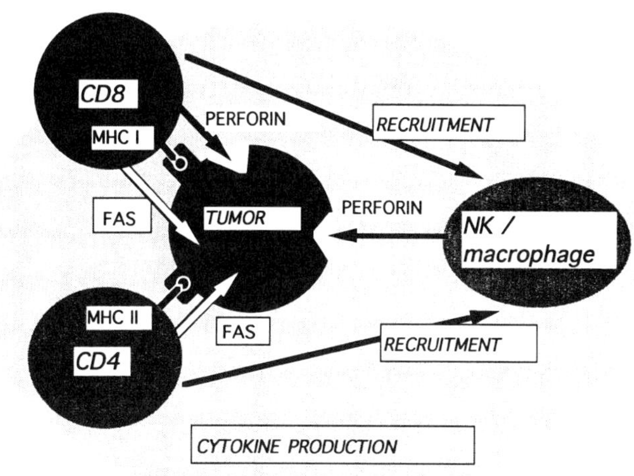

FIGURE 2. T-cell killing of malignant cells.

MHC molecules. Initial studies suggested that cellular proteins processed internally are presented by MHC class I molecules to cytotoxic CD8 cells. MHC class II molecules bind peptides derived from exogenous proteins that are picked up by antigen-presenting cells. These are recognized by CD4 cells. According to this paradigm, tumor-derived proteins are either processed by the tumor cell itself and presented to CD8 cells via MHC class I or taken up by various antigen-presenting cells and bound to class II molecules.[18] However, there are exceptions to these rules. MHC class I molecules can present exogenous antigens and MHC class II molecules can present endogenously derived proteins.[19] As some CD4 cells are cytotoxic, both CD4 and CD8 cells are capable of recognizing and killing leukemia cells.[20,21] The mechanism whereby alloreactive T cells kill leukemia cells is complex. CD8 cells kill their target by perforin-induced lysis. T cells also use the fas ligand to activate fas on the target cell surface, causing apoptosis.[22] Cytotoxic CD4 cells exclusively use this mechanism, and therefore only target cells expressing fas are susceptible to CD4-mediated killing.[23] CD4 cells also inhibit leukemia cell growth by producing gamma-interferon and tumor necrosis factor.[24] *In vivo*, GVL may involve several effector cell types employing different cytotoxic and cytostatic mechanisms[25] (FIG. 2).

NATURAL KILLER CELL RESPONSES TO LEUKEMIA

Although NK cells and IL-2 activated NK cells are cytotoxic to leukemia cell lines and fresh leukemia cells,[26,27] the role of NK cells in GVL is not known with certainty. Evidence that NK cells mediate GVL in man comes from observations that T-cell depletion techniques that spare NK cells are associated with a lower relapse rate than are those that deplete both T cells and NK cells.[28] The remissions achieved in patients with chronic myelogenous leukemia given donor leukocyte transfusions may partly be attributable to the effect of NK cells: Both cytotoxic T-cell precursors and NK-cell activity increases following donor lymphocyte transfusions.[29]

LEUKEMIA ANTIGENS

Leukemia antigens have been categorized under three overlapping systems: minor histocompatibility antigens, tissue-restricted antigen, and leukemia-specific antigens.

Minor Histocompatibility Antigens. This antigen system was first identified using T cells recognizing MHC-restricted alloantigens on HLA-matched targets. The system is extensive and poorly characterized. Minor histocompatibility antigens (mHA) are encoded by possibly hundreds of genes scattered throughout the genome.[30] It is now known that mHA are allelic self-peptides presented by MHC molecules. Minor histocompatibility antigen disparity is largely responsible for GVHD, GVL, and graft rejection following HLA-matched sibling BMT and contributes to these alloresponses in BMT from unrelated and less than fully HLA-matched donors.[31] Many mHA are ubiquitous, but some are tissue-restricted.[32] T-cell-mediated immune responses against mHA expressed on normal hematopoietic progenitors are responsible for marrow graft rejection.[16] Some mHA may be restricted to myeloid tissue. Distinct T-cell responses to lymphoid and myeloid cells can be detected in HLA-matched donor-recipient pairs, suggesting that lymphoid and myeloid cells express different mHA.[33] The molecular separation of GVL from GVHD may therefore reside in the recognition by donor T cells of mHA exclusively expressed on leukemic myeloid or lymphoid cells.

Tissue-Restricted Antigens. Recent studies of autologous T-cell responses to melanoma suggest that several proteins that are products of nonmutated genes serve as T-cell targets.[34,35] These antigens are tissue-specific, but not tumor-specific. It is equally possible that lymphoid and myeloid leukemia cells may present tissue-restricted antigens as targets for both alloreacting and autologous T cells. Several well characterized proteins that could function as T-cell targets are known to be exclusively expressed in bone marrow-derived cells. They include myeloid differentiation surface antigens CD33 and CD13 and primary and secondary granule enzymes.

Leukemia-Specific Antigens. The presence of the Ph chromosome in chronic myelogenous leukemia has raised the possibility that the p210 fusion protein derived from the t9;22 translocation could generate a leukemia-specific antigen. p210 contains a unique junctional peptide sequence in both splicing variants b2a2 and b3a2, which could serve as a T-cell target. It is hypothesized that p210 undergoes cytoplasmic degradation to peptides which then enter the class I antigen-processing pathway, eventually reaching the cell surface as 8-9mer peptides in the peptide-binding groove of the HLA molecule.[36] To function as T-cell targets, the fusion protein would have to be cytoplasmically processed and presented by HLA molecules in sufficient quantities for subsequent recognition by T cells. The T cells would have to contain HLA/p210 peptide complex within their repertoire.

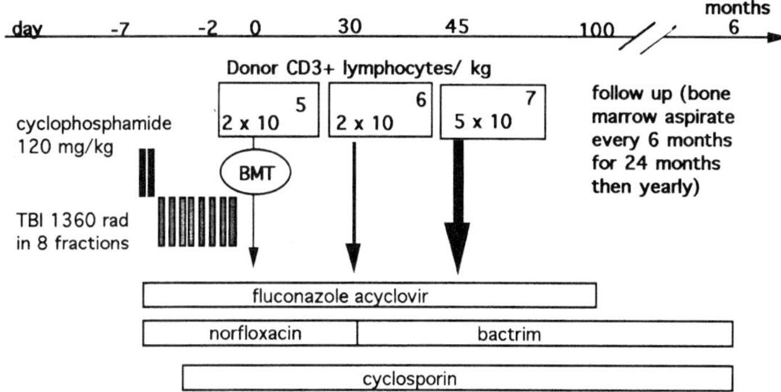

FIGURE 3. T-cell–depleted BMT with delayed T-cell add-back for hematologic malignancies.

NEW WAYS TO MANIPULATE GRAFT-VERSUS-LEUKEMIA AND GRAFT-VERSUS-HOST REACTIONS

While in current practice GVL cannot reliably be separated from GVHD, new approaches exploiting differences in the two reactions are being evaluated clinically.

Delayed Add-Back of Donor T Cells. T cells transplanted together with bone marrow cells into a recently irradiated recipient are prone to provoke GVHD, because they become activated by cytokines released during pregraft radiation. The hypothesis that the delayed addition of T cells, after the "cytokine storm,"[15] might cause less GVHD was tested in a murine GVHD model by Johnson *et al.*[37] They showed that add-back of large numbers of allogeneic donor spleen cells 21 days after BMT did not cause GVHD. Furthermore, the mice were able to mount a GVL response to AKR murine leukemia. A similar protective effect of delayed transfusion of lymphocytes is observed in man. In a previous study using donor lymphocytes to treat relapse after BMT, we noted that the frequency and severity of GVHD were often less after lymphocyte transfusions than they were at the time of transplantation.[12] We therefore tested the hypothesis that T-cell depletion followed by delayed lymphocyte add-back would cause minimal GVHD but preserve GVL in a clinical leukemia BMT protocol. The features of this ongoing study are shown in FIGURE 3. Patients received cyclophosphamide and total body irradiation as immunosuppressive and myeloablative preparation. The countercurrent elutriation procedure was used to achieve a greater than 3 log T-cell depletion of bone marrow. To improve marrow engraftment a low dose of CD3 cells (2×10^5/kg) was given. (This T-cell dose has a low probability of inducing GVHD.) As additional GVHD prophylaxis, cyclosporine was given from day 4 to day 180. Patients received increasing doses of donor lymphocytes on day 30 and day 45 posttransplant. Those developing GVHD of grade II or greater before or after the day 30 add-back did not receive lymphocytes. Marrow aspirates to detect the presence of residual leukemia were examined at regular intervals. The end points are relapse, GVHD, and survival. Between September 1993 and February 1995, 19 patients received an HLA-matched sibling BMT for chronic myelogenous leukemia (13), acute myeloblastic leukemia or myelodysplasia (4), or multiple myeloma (2).

Fourteen patients received T-cell add-back. The reasons for not adding back T cells in the remaining five were: grade II GVHD associated with incomplete T-cell depletion (3), and early death (2). Three of the 14 patients receiving T-cell add-back developed GVHD. This was transient, grade I-II, in two patients but severe in one who developed grade IV skin and gastrointestinal GVHD 83 days after the last T-cell transfusion. Chronic GVHD occurred in 4 of 11 evaluable patients given T-cell add-back, a rate similar to that observed in non-T-cell depleted BMT. One patient with high risk leukemia had a relapse. Overall, 13 of 19 patients survive (11 of 14 receiving T-cell add-back). The main causes of death were cytomegalovirus or other viruses (5) and aspergillosis (1). Our preliminary conclusions are that delayed add-back of T cells confers a low risk of acute GVHD and may protect against relapse.

Selective Depletion of CD8 Cells. In mHA mismatched murine marrow transplants, both CD8 and CD4 T cells contribute to GVHD. However, CD4 cells alone do not cause GVHD.[38] On this basis, Champlin *et al.*[39] explored CD8 depletion of donor marrow for patients with chronic myelogenous leukemia undergoing BMT. Patients had a low relapse rate, comparable to that seen with unmanipulated BMT, but a low GVHD incidence, comparable to that seen with T-cell depleted marrow. These results indicate that CD8 depletion may conserve GVL while reducing GVHD in HLA-matched donor-recipient pairs.

Functional T-Cell Depletion. In a murine mismatched BMT model, Cavazzana-Calvo *et al.*[40] showed that GVHD could be significantly reduced in severity if donor cells with antihost activity were first eliminated *in vitro*. Donor lymphocytes were cultured with recipient cells and a toxin-conjugated antibody to the IL-2 receptor to eliminate activated T cells. There was abrogation of the proliferative response to the stimulator but conservation of the third party response. In man, similar experiments demonstrated that in HLA-matched donor-recipient pairs, distinct donor T-cell populations recognized nonleukemic cells and leukemic cells in the recipient.[33] We are now developing a method to eliminate GVHD-reactive donor cells and conserve GVL by depleting donor cells reacting to host lymphocytes with toxin-conjugated antibodies to T-cell activation markers. Elimination of the donor anti-host response and conservation of third party cells and host leukemia response are measured by comparing proliferation of donor to recipient cells with and without antibody treatment. Haplo-identical (parent-child) stimulator-responder pairs were studied. Responder mononuclear cells were incubated with equal numbers of stimulator lymphocytes for 1-4 days and exposed to antibody for 2-24 hours. Cells were washed and rechallenged with the original stimulator or third party mononuclear cells. Five-day tritiated thymidine uptakes were compared with those of non-antibody-treated responders. Irrelevant antibody, unconjugated anti-CD25 antibodies, and toxin-conjugated interleukin-4 (IL-4) receptor antibodies did not reduce donor anti-recipient reactivity. A pseudomonas exotoxin antibody conjugated to the high affinity IL-2 receptor, expressed only on activated lymphocytes (kindly provided by Dr. I. Pastan) showed consistent, dose-dependent, and selective cytotoxicity to activated lymphocytes. In six experiments there was a mean of $7 \pm 3.5\%$ residual reactivity to the original stimulator and $66 \pm 7\%$ preservation of the third party response on rechallenge. Measurement of donor-versus-recipient cytotoxic lymphocyte precursor frequency has been shown to correlate with the risk of GVHD in matched but unrelated donor BMT.[41] To be effective, antibody treatment should reduce cytotoxic lymphocyte precursor frequency to levels associated with no or minimal GVHD. This functional T-cell depletion technique could then be evaluated in mismatched BMT for leukemia.

Generating Leukemia-Reacting Clones. While HLA-matched donor T-cell lines with antileukemia specificity can readily be generated *in vitro*,[42,43] many obstacles must be overcome before T-cell lines can be used for adoptive immunotherapy after BMT. In particular, since antigens recognized by T-cell lines are not known, there is a risk of inducing GVHD. Molecular characterization of the antigens would help to improve techniques for leukemia-specific T-cell clone expansion. We therefore investigated the possibility of generating leukemia-reactive T-cell clones with peptides derived from leukemia-specific fusion proteins or myeloid differentiation proteins. We used HLA-A2.1 as the restriction element in our studies because it is frequently expressed in the population. The ability of various peptides to bind to HLA-A2.1 was tested in the MHC class I deficient, antigen-processing defective, T2 lymphoid cell line. Peptide binding causes increased surface expression of HLA class I molecules in T2 cells. This is measured as increased anti-class I fluorescence by flow cytometry.[44] We were unable to demonstrate binding of a series of 9-mer peptides from the junction region of the b2a2 and b3a2 splicing variants of the Ph chromosome-derived protein P210. Because CD33 on myeloid leukemia cells could serve as a target for antileukemic T-cell responses, we screened CD33 for peptide sequences conforming to the known anchor motifs described for the HLA A2.1 molecule.[45] Two peptides from the myeloid-specific antigen CD33, predicted by their amino acid sequence to bind, increased HLA-A2.1 expression in T2 cells. We plan to generate CD33 peptide-specific T-cell clones to investigate their cytotoxicity and specificity for leukemia. This approach could ultimately be used to generate highly specific leukemia immuno-therapy using adoptively transferred T cells or peptide vaccines.

CONCLUSIONS

New understanding of the mechanisms of alloreactivity after BMT has opened up new possibilities of rendering the GVL response both more specific and more powerful. Several clinical studies suggest that immune manipulation of donor lympho-cytes could lead to safer and more strongly antileukemic BMT. In the future these approaches may improve the outlook for mismatched donor-recipient pairs and extend the use of alloreacting T cells to other malignancies.

REFERENCES

1. THOMAS, E. D. 1982. The role of marrow transplantation in the eradication of malignant disease. Cancer **49:** 1963-1969.
2. MATHE, G., J. L. AMIEL, L. SCHWARTZENBERG et al. 1963. Haematopoietic chimeras after allogeneic (homologous) bone marrow transplant. Br. Med. J. **11:** 1633.
3. HOROWITZ, M. M. & M. M. BORTIN. 1992. The role of registries in evaluating the results of bone marrow transplantation. *In* Bone Marrow Transplantation in Practice. J. G. Treleaven & A. J. Barrett, Eds. : 367-375. Churchill Livingstone, Edinburgh, UK.
4. ANASETTI, C., P. G. BEATTY, R. STORB et al. 1990. Effect of HLA incompatibility on graft-vs-host disease, relapse, and survival after marrow transplantation for patients with leukemia and lymphoma. Hum. Immunol. **29:** 79-84.

5. GALE, R. P., M. M. HOROWITZ *et al.* 1994. Identical twin bone marrow transplants for leukemia. Ann. Intern. Med. **120:** 646–652.

6. HOROWITZ, M. M., R. P. GALE, P. M. SONDEL *et al.* 1990. Graft-versus-leukemia reactions after bone marrow transplantation. Blood **75:** 555–562.

7. SULLIVAN, K. M., P. L. WEIDEN, R. STORB *et al.* 1989. Influence of acute and chronic graft-vs-host disease on relapse and survival after bone marrow transplantation from HLA-identical siblings as treatment of acute and chronic leukemia. Blood **73:** 1720–1726.

8. GOLDMAN, J. M., R. P. GALE, M. M. HOROWITZ *et al.* 1988. Bone marrow transplantation for chronic myelogenous leukemia in chronic phase: Increased risk of relapse associated with T cell depletion. Ann. Intern. Med. **108:** 806–814.

9. KOLB, H. J., J. MITMULLER, C. H. CLEMM *et al.* 1990. Donor leukocyte transfusions for treatment of recurrent chronic myelogenous leukemia in marrow transplant patients. Blood **76:** 2462–2465.

10. DROBYSKI, W. R., C. A. KEEVER, M. S. ROTH *et al.* 1993. Salvage immunotherapy using donor leukocyte infusions as treatment for relapsed chronic myelogenous leukemia after allogeneic bone marrow transplantation. Blood **82:** 2310–2318.

11. KOLB, H. J., T. de WITTE, B. MITMULLER *et al.* 1994. Graft-versus-leukemia effect of donor buffy coat transfusions on recurrent leukemia after marrow transplantation. Bone Marrow Transplantation, 20th Annual Meeting of the European Group for Bone Marrow Transplantation. Abstract, p. 96.

12. VAN RHEE, F., L. FENG, J. O. CULLIS *et al.* 1994. Relapse of chronic myeloid leukemia after allogeneic bone marrow transplantation: The case for giving donor leucocyte transfusions before the onset of hematological relapse. Blood **83:** 3377–3383.

13. MIAMURA, K., A. J. BARRETT, Y. KODERA & H. SAITO. 1994. Minimal residual disease after bone marrow transplantation for chronic myelogenous leukemia and implications for graft-versus-leukemia effect: A review of recent results. Bone Marrow Transplant. **14:** 201–210.

14. BARRETT, A. J. 1992. Graft-vs-host disease. *In* Bone Marrow Transplantation in Practice. J. G. Treleaven & A. J. Barrett, Eds. : 257–272. Churchill Livingstone. Edinburgh.

15. ANTIN, J. & J. L. M. FERRARA. 1992. Cytokine dysregulation and acute graft versus host disease. Blood **80:** 2964–2968.

16. MARTIN, P. J. 1992. Determinants of engraftment after allogeneic marrow transplantation. Blood **79:** 1647–1650.

17. MARIJT, W. A. F., W. F. J. VEENHOF, E. GOULMY *et al.* 1993. Minor histocompatibility antigen HA-1, –2, –4, and H-Y specific cytotoxic T cell clones inhibit human hematopoietic progenitor cell growth by a mechanism that is dependent on direct cell-cell contact. Blood **82:** 3778–3785.

18. MOUDGIL, K. D., A. AMETANIS, I. S. GREWAL *et al.* 1993. Processing of self-protein and its impact on shaping T cell repertoire. Rev. Immunol. **10:** 365–377.

19. STAERZ, U. D., H. KARASUGAMA & A. M. GARNER. 1987. Cytotoxic T lymphocytes against a soluble protein. Nature **327:** 449–451.

20. WOODS, G., K. KITAGAMI & A. OCHI. 1989. Evidence for an involvement of T4 cytotoxic T cells in tumor immunity. Cell. Immunol. **118:** 126–135.

21. SOSMAN, J. A., K. R. OETTEL, S. D. SMITH *et al.* 1990. Specific recognition of human leukemic cells by allogeneic T cells. II. Evidence for HLA-D restricted determinants on leukemic cells that are crossreactive with determinants present on unrelated leukemic cells. Blood **75:** 2005–2016.

22. KAGI, D., F. VIGNAUX, G. LEDERMANN *et al.* 1994. Fas and perforin pathways as major mechanisms of T-cell mediated cytotoxicity. Science **265:** 528–530.

23. STADLER, T. 1994. Fas antigen is the major target molecule for CD4$^+$ mediated cytotoxicity. J. Immunol. **152:** 1127–1134.

24. JIANG, Y. Z. & A. J. BARRETT. 1995. Cellular and cytokine-mediated effects of CD4-positive lymphocyte lines generated in vitro against chronic myelogenous leukemia. Exp. Hematol. *In press.*

25. SLAVIN, S., A. ACKERSTEIN & E. NAPARSTEK. 1990. The graft-versus-leukemia (GVL) phenomenon: Is GVL separable from GVHD? Bone Marrow Transplant. **6:** 155-158.

26. LOTZOVA, E., C. A. SAVARY & R. B. HERBERMAN. 1987. Induction of NK activity against fresh human leukemia in culture with the interleukin-2. J. Immunol. **138:** 2718-2723.

27. HAUCH, M., M. V. GAZZOLA, T. SMALL *et al.* 1990. Anti-leukemia potential of interleukin-2 activated natural killer cells after bone marrow transplantation for chronic myelogenous leukemia. Blood **75:** 2250-2262.

28. MARMONT, A. M., M. M. HOROWITZ, R. P. GALE *et al.* 1991. T-cell depletion of HLA-identical transplants in leukemia. Blood **78:** 2120-2130.

29. JIANG, Y. Z., J. O. CULLIS, E. J. KANFER, J. M. GOLDMAN & A. J. BARRETT. 1990. T-cell and NK cell mediated graft-versus-leukaemia reactivity following donor buffy coat transfusion to treat relapse after bone marrow transplantation for chronic myeloid leukaemia. Bone Marrow Transplant. **11:** 133-138.

30. PERRAULT, C., F. DECARY, S. BROCHU *et al.* 1990. Minor histocompatibility antigens: A review. Blood **76:** 1269-1280.

31. GOULMY, E. 1988. Minor histocompatibility antigens in man and their role in transplantation. Transplant. Rev. **2:** 29-53.

32. DE BUEGER, M., A. BAKKER, J. J. VAN ROOD *et al.* 1992. Tissue distribution of human minor histocompatibility antigens: Ubiquitous versus restricted tissue distribution indicated heterogeneity among human cytotoxic lymphocyte defined non-MHC antigens. J. Immunol. **149:** 1788-1794.

33. DATTA, A. R., A. J. BARRETT, Y. Z. JIANG *et al.* 1994. Distinct T-cell populations distinguish chronic myeloid leukemia cells from lymphocytes in the same individual: A model for separating GVHD from GVL reactions. Bone Marrow Transplant. **14:** 517-524.

34. COX, A. L., J. SKIPPER, Y. CHEN, R. A. HENDERSON *et al.* 1994. Identification of a peptide recognized by five melanoma-specific human cytotoxic T cell lines. Science **264:** 716-719.

35. STORKUS, W. J., H. J. ZEH, M. J. MAEURER *et al.* 1993. Identification of human melanoma peptides recognized by class I restricted tumor infiltrating lymphocytes. J. Immunol. **37:** 19-27.

36. BARRETT, A. J. & Y. Z. JIANG. 1991. Immune responses to chronic myeloid leukaemia. Bone Marrow Transplant. **9:** 305-311.

37. JOHNSON, B. D., W. R. DROBYSKI & R. L. TRUITT. 1993. Delayed infusion of normal donor cells after MHC mismatched bone marrow transplantation provides an antileukemia reaction without graft-versus-host disease. Bone Marrow Transplant. **11:** 329-337.

38. KORNGOLD, R. & J. SPRENT. 1987. T cell subsets and graft versus host disease. Transplantation **44:** 335-339.

39. CHAMPLIN, R., W. HO, J. GAJEWSKI *et al.* 1990. Selective depletion of CD8[+] lymphocytes for prevention of graft-versus-host disease after allogeneic bone marrow transplantation. Blood **76:** 418-423.

40. CAVAZZANA-CALVO, M., J. L. STEPHAN, S. SARNAKI *et al.* 1994. Attenuation of graft-versus-host disease and graft rejection by ex-vivo immunotoxin elimination of alloreactive T cells in an H-2 haplotype disparate mouse combination. Blood **83:** 288-298.

41. KAMINSKI, E., J. HOWS, S. MAN *et al.* 1989. Prediction of graft versus host disease by frequency analysis of cytotoxic T cells after unrelated donor bone marrow transplantation. Transplantation **48:** 608-613.

42. VAN LOCHEM, E., B. DE GAST & E. GOULMY. 1992. In vitro separation of host specific GVH and GVL cytotoxic T cell activities. Bone Marrow Transplant. **10:** 181-183.

43. FALKENBERG, J. H., L. M. FABER, M. VAN DEN ELSHOUT, F. VAN LUXEMBERG-HEIJS, A. HOOFTMAN VAN DEN OTTER, W. M. SMIT, P. J. VOOGT & R. WILLEMZ. 1993.

Generation of donor-derived antileukemic cytotoxic T-lymphocyte responses for treatment of relapsed leukemia after allogeneic HLA-identical bone marrow transplantation. J. Immunother. **14:** 305–309.

44. CULLIS, J., A. J. BARRETT, R. LECHLER & J. M. GOLDMAN. 1994. Binding of bcr/abl junctional peptides to MHC class I molecules: Studies in antigen processing defective cell lines. Leukemia **8:** 165–170.

45. RAMMENSEE, H. G., F. FALK & O. ROETSCHKE. 1993. Peptides naturally presented by MHC class I molecules. Ann. Rev. Immunol. **11:** 213–244.

Lymphopoiesis, Apoptosis, and Immune Amnesia[a]

ALBERT D. DONNENBERG,[b,c]
JOSEPH B. MARGOLICK,[d] AND
VERA S. DONNENBERG[b]

[b]University of Pittsburgh School of Medicine
Department of Medicine
Division of Hematology/Bone Marrow Transplantation
Pittsburgh, Pennsylvania 15213

[d]Johns Hopkins University
School of Hygiene and Public Health
Baltimore, Maryland

Mechanisms of immune deficiency appear to be relatively straightforward. Patients are immunodeficient after bone marrow transplantation (BMT) because their entire immune system is ablated and with it the repertoire of immune memory cells nurtured over a lifetime of successful encounters with potential pathogens. Similarly, patients infected with the human immune deficiency virus HIV-1 have a loss of CD4$^+$ T cells, the cornerstone of the immune system. Formulating the problem in this way fails to address a fundamental issue: Why, when other hematopoietic functions return with relative speed, does it take so long to regenerate immune competence after BMT? In HIV-1 infection, the mirror image of this question remains problematic: Why does it take, on average, almost a decade to develop AIDS when the greatest decline in the CD4$^+$ T-cell count occurs in the first year after HIV-1 infection?[1]

LYMPHOPOIESIS, IMMUNE MEMORY, AND IMMUNE AMNESIA

Much of what we know about the development and maintenance of the immune system we have learned from small animal models. Such studies have elucidated the central role of the thymus in T-cell poiesis, development of self-tolerance, and selection of clonal specificities capable of recognizing foreign peptides in the context of self major histocompatibility determinants. As much as these studies have helped us understand the generation and regulation of the immune system in man, they have also erected a conceptual roadblock of sorts; the rodents on which these studies were

[a]This work was supported by grants RO1 CA44887 and RO1 AI32376 from the Department of Health and Human Services. Dr. Donnenberg is the recipient of a Carter-Wallace fellowship for AIDS research.

[c]Address for correspondence: 3459 5th Avenue, Pittsburgh, PA 15213.

performed have short life spans relative to humans and remain euthymic for much of their lives. How then do we meet our need for T-lymphocyte replacement through our adult lives after thymic involution has occurred in late childhood/early adolescence? One can argue that in man, the thymus plays a once-in-a-lifetime role of "bootstrapping" the immune system, populating it for the first time with a cohort of diverse, nonautoreactive naive T cells which, through a process of antigen-driven clonal selection, evolve to form a dynamic but stable memory compartment. Once this has been accomplished, T-cell generation becomes decentralized to the peripheral lymphoid tissues, and the thymus becomes irrelevant. The adult immune system specializes in the maintenance of useful clonal specificities (immune memory) while retaining the capacity for primary response to newly encountered antigens through expansion of *de novo* generated naive T cells. Accordingly, T cells can be generated from two very different progenitor compartments. They may arise from antigen-mediated selection and clonal expansion of existing mature T cells, or they may be generated from lymphohematopoietic progenitors by a process equivalent to that which occurred in the thymus on a much broader scale earlier in life. In the former case, progeny T cells express the clonal idiotype of their "memory cell" progenitor. In the latter case, first generation progeny T cells display the T-cell receptor diversity characteristic of naive cells, pose the same clonal censorship problems encountered during immune ontogeny, but are generated in an environment that differs from that of early development in at least two important respects: the absence of robust thymic function and the presence of a cohort of functional, self-tolerant, clonally diverse memory T cells. In this report we will argue that memory cells play a central, albeit mysterious, role in the selection of *de novo* generated T cells, perhaps by providing signals that rescue a proportion of them from a pre-programmed apoptotic death. We hypothesize that in the adult, ablation of memory T cells (by therapy or disease) not only destroys the ability to mount specific anamnestic responses mediated by the individual memory clones, but also undermines the ability of newly generated T cells to make the transition from naive to memory cells. It is this pathologic state, the loss of anamnestic response combined with the inability to generate memory T cells upon encountering antigen, that we have termed *immune amnesia*. As will be described, it is characterized by increased T-cell turnover and the substitution of short-lived hypofunctional replacement cells for longer lived, biologically selected memory cells.

REBUILDING THE IMMUNE SYSTEM AFTER BONE MARROW TRANSPLANTATION

Origin of Newly Generated T Cells

In bone marrow transplantation the immune system is completely ablated by the preparative regimen and is explosively reconstituted by progenitor cells present in the graft. Unmanipulated bone marrow grafts contain a substantial number of T cells ($2.6 \pm 0.3 \times 10^9$, mean $\pm$ standard error in a recent series of 30 allografts prepared by the Pittsburgh Cancer Institute Bone Marrow Processing Laboratory). Peripheral stem cell grafts contain even more mature T cells. Despite the large scale infusion of mature donor T cells in the graft, adoptive transfer of donor immune memory cells can be demonstrated only rarely. Immunization studies in man[2,3] and animal models[4] highlight the requirement for exposure to antigen immediately after graft infusion. In our own studies of transfer of T-cell immunity to tetanus toxoid, we found that booster immunization on the day of transplant ensured adoptive transfer of specific immunity,[2] but delaying immunization until 28 days after transplant did not elicit a detectable lymphoproliferative response (unpublished data). Thus, allogeneic BMT recipients remain anergic to most recall antigens until a year or more after transplant, after which time they regain the ability to respond to immunization.[5] The exceptions are microbial antigens such as herpesviruses[6,7] and polyomaviruses,[8] both of which are endogenous viruses present at the time of graft infusion. It is of interest that the hypofunctional state, the characteristic immunophenotypic profile, and the increased rate of spontaneous T-cell apoptosis are indistinguishable between recipients of allografts, autografts, T-cell depleted grafts, and purified CD34+ progenitor grafts (see below). This finding weighs against the interpretation that regenerating T cells are predominantly the progeny of mature graft T cells that have been disproportionately expanded in the new host. On the contrary, data suggest that following BMT most newly generated T cells are generated from prelymphoid progenitor cells and therefore are prototypically naive.

Role of the Thymus

Recent data on the recovery of CD4+ T cells in leukemic children undergoing intensive chemotherapy shed some light on the role of the thymus in T-cell replacement after catastrophic T-cell loss.[9] Although these patients did not receive a fully myeloablative regimen, they became severely lymphopenic. Both thymic rebound (enlargement of the thymus as measured by CT scan) and the speed of CD4+ T-cell recovery were correlated with patient age. Although older patients (>14 years of age) did not evidence thymic enlargement, their CD4+ T-cell counts normalized with time after therapy, albeit at a slower pace than that in younger children. This conclusively demonstrates that large scale T-cell replacement occurs in older individuals without demonstrable participation of the thymus and agrees with anecdotal observations in adult BMT recipients who died early after transplant without evidence of thymic enlargement. Interestingly, in both young and older children, the earliest CD4+ T cells to return after chemotherapy were uniformly CD45RO+. In young, euthymic children, CD45RA+ CD4+ T cells were recovered more rapidly than in older children. The authors resisted the conventional interpretation which would identify the early reconstituting CD45RO+ cells as memory cells, but noted that naive T cells exported from the thymus are CD45RA+.[10] The significance of CD45 isoform expression in reconstituting BMT recipients will be addressed subsequently herein.

Kinetics of T-Cell Replacement

As just noted, CD4+ T cells were replaced faster in euthymic children than in their slightly older counterparts. Although this may reflect faster T-cell generation time, it should be emphasized that recovery of peripheral T-cell counts after therapy requires a net increase in birth rate related to death rate. It is equally plausible that in older children lacking thymic mechanisms for clonal censoring,[11] replacement T cells generated in an extrathymic environment lack central mechanisms of tolerance and therefore have a far higher turnover rate in the periphery. Beyond thymus-mediated central tolerance, newly generated T cells can be tolerized (reviewed in ref. 12) or deleted[13] in peripheral lymphoid organs. The latter mechanism is mediated by apoptosis as shown in several experimental systems (reviewed in ref. 14). Thus, we reasoned that generation of replacement T cells in adult BMT recipients might also result in the deletion of a large proportion of newly produced T cells. To test this hypothesis, we examined apoptosis of peripheral blood T cells from BMT recipients. We chose an assay of spontaneous apoptosis occurring in short-term culture in the hope that it mirrors as closely as possible the *in vivo* behavior of T cells. FIGURE 1 shows spontaneous apoptosis of CD3$^+$, CD4$^+$, and CD8$^+$ T cells cultured for 18 hours, as a function of time after BMT. These data indicate that early after BMT most CD4$^+$ (65.6 ± 4.2% [mean ± standard error]) and CD8$^+$ (70.2 ± 0.1%) T cells apoptose in short-term unstimulated culture. These findings graphically explain why cells obtained in the first weeks after BMT are largely unresponsive in *in vitro* assays. Although peripheral T-cell counts approach the lower limits of normal at 3 months after BMT,[15] in many patients T-cell apoptosis did not begin to approach levels observed in healthy control subjects (10–20%) until much later. Assuming that our *in vitro* apoptosis assay provides a valid indication of the *in vivo* fate of these cells, it can be inferred that T-cell turnover remains elevated long after peripheral counts have normalized. The predominance of T cells of extremely short life span presents an obvious impediment to the development of immune memory.

Considerable heterogeneity was present in our patient population with respect to both disease and transplant type. T-cell apoptosis was indistinguishable in all transplant types except autologous peripheral stem cell (PSC) grafts (FIG. 2). Recipients of PSC grafts, which contain several-fold more mature T cells than does autologous marrow, and several orders of magnitude more T cells than do purified progenitor grafts or T-cell-depeleted grafts, had significantly lower T-cell apoptosis. These data suggest that the introduction of large numbers of autologous T cells in the graft can reduce T-cell apoptosis rates weeks to months after graft infusion. This observation can be understood in the context of the hypothesis just discussed, in which preexisting memory cells provide signals that rescue newly generated T cells from an apoptotic death. If correct, this strategy could be exploited to decrease T-cell turnover and thus hasten stabilization of the immune system after autologous and possibly allogeneic BMT.

Identity of Replacement Cells

From the studies just described we demonstrated that most T cells present in the circulation early after BMT apoptose in short-term unstimulated culture; from this, we infer that a major factor limiting immune reconstitution is the short life span of the newly generated T cells. Numerous immunophenotypic studies have been performed to understand the functional T-cell deficit that occurs in the posttransplant period. The findings are remarkably concordant across transplant types. Virtually all

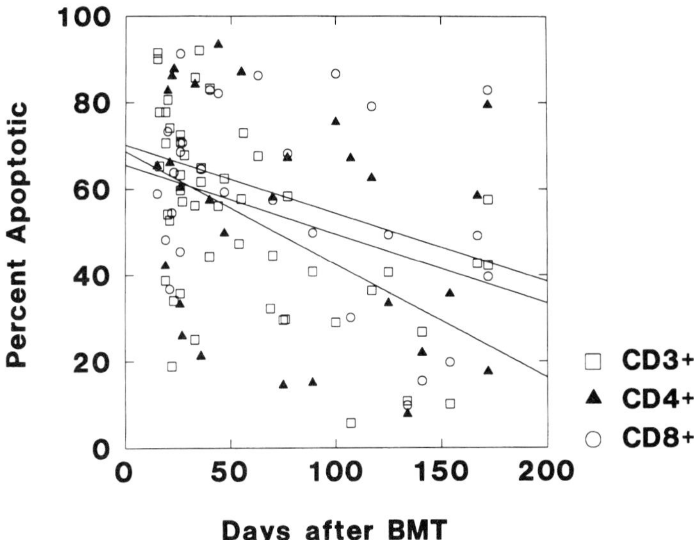

FIGURE 1. Apoptosis of CD3[+], CD4[+], and CD8[+] lymphocytes decreases with time after bone marrow transplantation. Percentage of CD3 apoptosis is plotted as a function of days after transplantation. The least squares lines of best fit are shown (slope coefficients and standard errors for CD3[+], CD4[+], and CD8[+] lymphocytes are –0.26 ± 0.06, –0.16 ± 0.09, and –0.16 ± 0.07, respectively. Slopes did not differ significantly from each other). A total of 50 observations were made in 43 patients studied between 14 and 175 days after transplantation. Informed consent was obtained from all study participants. The patients are listed by transplant type in the legend to FIGURE 2. The percentage of apoptotic cells (cells with <2N DNA) was measured by flow cytometry after staining with the DNA-binding dye PI (modified from Nicoletti *et al.*[33]). Following removal of erythrocytes from peripheral blood by ammonium chloride lysis, leukocytes were resuspended at 10^6 cells/ml in RPMI + 10% human AB serum and incubated in 24-well plates (2.5 ml/well) for 18 hours at 37°C, 5% CO_2 in air. Cells were then washed in Dulbecco's phosphate-buffered saline solution (PBS) without CA^{+2} or Mg^{+2} (PBS) + 0.1% NaN_3 + 4% newborn calf serum + 2% human AB serum + 1% mouse serum, resuspended in 0.5 ml of washing solution, and 100 μl of cells/sample were transferred into 4 wells of a round-bottomed 96-well plate. Cells were pelleted and the following were added to 4 replicate wells, respectively: (1) FITC-conjugated anti-mouse IgG1 (Becton-Dickinson, San Jose, California) as a negative control, (2) anti-CD3-FITC mAb (IOT3b, Immunotech, Westbrook, California), (3) anti-CD4-FITC (IOT4a, Immunotech), and (4) anti-CD8 (IOT8a, Immunotech). After incubating 30 minutes at 4°C, cells were pelleted, washed twice, and fixed and permeablized with 200 μl cold 70% ethanol for 1 hour. After washing twice, cells were pelleted and resuspended in 50 μl PBS with 50 μl ribonuclease A (1 mg/ml) and 100 μl PI (100 μg/ml) in PBS. Cells were incubated for 15 minutes at room temperature and stored at 4°C overnight. Fresh noncultured peripheral blood leukocytes were permeablized and incubated with PI to determine the fluorescence intensity of 2N DNA. Data were acquired using an FACScan flow cytometer (Becton-Dickinson). The Becton-Dickinson LYSIS analysis program was used to determine the percentage of CD3[+], CD4[+], and CD8[+] cells with <2N DNA.

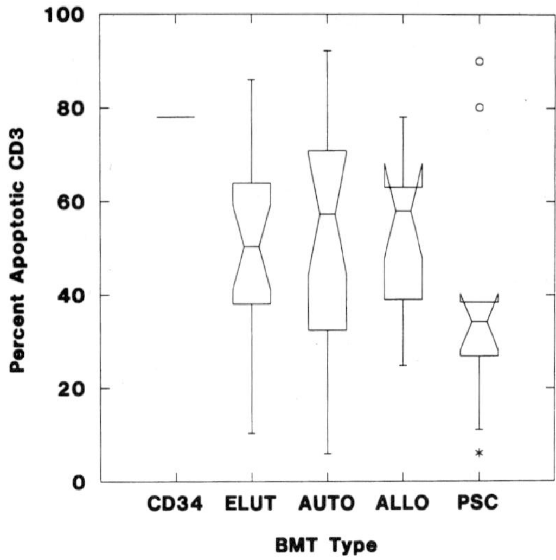

FIGURE 2. Proportion of apoptotic CD3[+] T cells by transplant type. Bone marrow transplant recipients were inpatients and outpatients of the Pittsburgh Cancer Institute Bone Marrow Transplantation Program. In order of approximate graft T-cell content they included recipients of the following grafts: 1 autologous purified CD34[+] stem cell graft, 8 elutriated (lymphocyte-depleted) allografts, 12 autologous bone marrow grafts, 11 unmanipulated HLA-matched sibling allografts, and 10 autologous peripheral stem cell grafts. The data are expressed as notched box plots which provide nonparametric tests of significance. The waist indicates the group median; the hinges (upper and lower boundaries of the box) indicate interquartile distances. The notches show 95% confidence intervals about the median (boxes with nonoverlapping notches are significantly different at a confidence level of at least 95%). The whiskers (*bars*) give the ranges, exclusive of outliers. Outliers (more than 1.5 times the hinge spread from the median) are shown by stars and far outliers (more than 3 times the hinge spread from the median) are shown by circles.

point to the abundance of CD45RO[+], CD29[high], CD38[+], HLA-DR[+] T cells during reconstitution.[16–18] As just discussed, CD45RO[+] cells also predominate in patients recovering from high dose chemotherapy[9] in the absence of transplantation. The conventional interpretation of these results poses a conundrum: Expression of the low molecular weight RO isoform of CD45 and high expression of CD29 have both been associated with memory T cells.[19] Abundant evidence exists that CD45RA[+] cells stimulated in culture switch isoforms and express CD45RO,[20] that CD45RO[+] but not CD45RA[+] T cells respond to recall antigens in culture,[19] and that CD45RO[+] cells predominate *in vivo* at sites of inflammation.[21] Equally puzzling, CD38 and HLA-DR have been described as activation markers, low or absent on resting T cells and upregulated during antigen- or mitogen-mediated activation. Why then should activated memory cells comprise the dominant population in the early phases of immune reconstitution? One possible answer is that graft memory T cells have undergone aberrant selection and expansion to fill the *T-cell niche* opened up during ablative therapy. Driven by host minor histocompatibility antigens or infectious

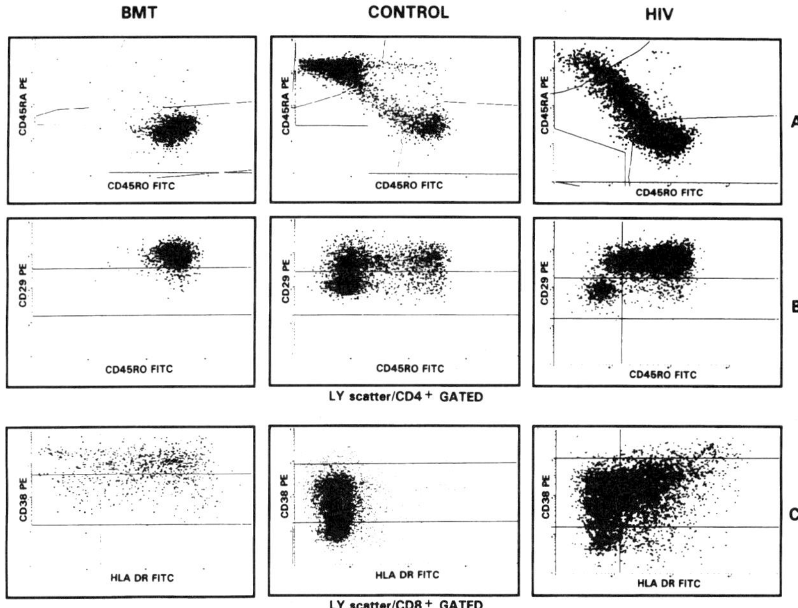

FIGURE 3. Expression of activation and differentiation markers on T cells from a BMT recipient, a healthy control subject, and an HIV-1⁺ individual. Three-color flow cytometry was performed on whole blood specimens after lysis of erythrocytes. Events were gated on a "lymphocyte forward and side light scatter gate" and CD4 (*rows A and B*) or CD8 (*row C*). For analysis, CD45RO versus CD45RA was divided into three populations (CD45RA⁺, CD45RO⁺, and transitional). CD45RO versus CD29 and HLA-DR versus CD38 were divided into six populations (negative, low and high for CD29 and CD38).

agents, they have expanded far beyond the physiologic norm. This interpretation is unattractive from several standpoints. First, BMT recipients, even those with immunologic abnormalities such as graft-versus-host disease or low response to mitogens, have T-cell receptor spectrotypes of high complexity,[22] indicating a high level of T-cell clonal diversity. Second, in the early posttransplant period, T cells are refractory to mitogen-driven stimulation, a state uncharacteristic of memory cells. Third, unlike memory T cells obtained from healthy subjects, most cells obtained early after transplant apoptose in unstimulated short-term culture. And finally, highly apoptotic T cells bearing *activated memory* markers predominate in recipients of autologous purified stem cell grafts and T-cell depleted allogeneic grafts, both of which contain few mature T cells. FIGURE 3 shows representative phenotypic profiles of peripheral blood T cells from a recipient of a lymphocyte-depleted matched unrelated donor allograft (40 days after BMT), a concurrently analyzed healthy control subject, and an HIV-1⁺ subject (peripheral CD4⁺ T-cell count 220/μl). These data illustrate the virtual absence of CD45RA⁺ cells among CD4⁺ T cells examined early after BMT and the predominance of the CD45RO⁺/CD29ʰⁱᵍʰ phenotype. CD8⁺ T cells were largely CD38ʰⁱᵍʰ (and uniformly CD38⁺), with a high proportion of CD8⁺ T cells expressing HLA-DR. By contrast, CD45RO[+] cells represent about half the CD4[+] T cells from healthy subjects, and CD38[high], HLA-DR[+] cells are rare. Interestingly, the phenotype of T cells from the HIV-1[+] subject, although not as skewed as that of the BMT recipient, also displays a predominance of CD45RO[+]/CD29[high] cells among CD4[+] T cells and an abundance of HLA-DR[+], CD8[+] T cells. The extent to which the immunopathology occurring after BMT and that in HIV-1[+] disease parallel each other will be explored.

PARALLELS BETWEEN BONE MARROW TRANSPLANTATION AND HIV-1 DISEASE

The kinetics of T-cell turnover in HIV-1 disease is a matter of recent excitement.[23] Studies from two laboratories[24,25] revealed an unexpectedly high rate of CD4[+] T-cell turnover in HIV-1 infected subjects. The CD4[+] T-cell turnover rate was estimated from the slope of CD4[+] T-cell recovery after administration of the antiviral drug ABT-538. It was assumed that CD4[+] T-cell birth rate was constant before and after drug administration, thereby allowing estimation of the CD4[+] turnover during steady state conditions (i.e., before drug administration). Both studies concluded that CD4[+] T-cell replacement occurs at a remarkably high rate (0.2 to 5.4 × 10[9] cells/day). This interpretation strongly supports the notion that compensatory lymphopoiesis is prominent in HIV-1 infection, but probably greatly underestimates the CD4[+] T-cell death rate and fails entirely to take into account the CD8[+] T-cell death rate. The earlier studies of Gougeon *et al.*[26] and Gougeon and Montagnier[27] clearly demonstrated elevated apoptosis in peripheral blood T cells from HIV-1 infected subjects. In their studies and ours as well,[28,29] elevated apoptosis was observed in both CD4[+] and CD8[+] T-cell subsets. Furthermore, the magnitude of T-cell apoptosis was inversely correlated with the absolute CD4 count, a surrogate for disease status.[29] FIGURE 4 compares CD4[+] and CD8[+] T-cell apoptosis rates in short-term cultured cells from BMT recipients, healthy control subjects, and HIV-1 infected subjects. The concordance between T-cell subsets and between patient groups is remarkable. The observation of elevated apoptosis in both CD4[+] and CD8[+] T cells weighs against the interpretation that increased lymphocyte turnover is due solely (or even chiefly) to direct virus-mediated effects. The remarkable immunophenotypic similarities between HIV-1[+] subjects and reconstituting BMT recipients (FIG. 3) cast doubt on the conventional interpretation that most of these cells are activated memory cells responding to HIV-1 or other pathogens, especially in the later stages of disease when T cells obtained from HIV-1[+] subjects are as hyporesponsive as those of reconstituting BMT recipients.

CONCLUSIONS

Bone marrow transplant recipients and HIV-1 infected individuals both suffer massive T-cell losses. In BMT recipients, the loss is catastrophic and acute; rescue is effected by infusion of a marrow graft which contains the hematopoietic progenitors necessary to reconstitute the system. In HIV-1 infected individuals the depletion of CD4[+] T cells, although initially less dramatic than marrow ablative therapy, is chronic and relentless. In BMT, the immune system gradually recovers. In HIV-1 disease,

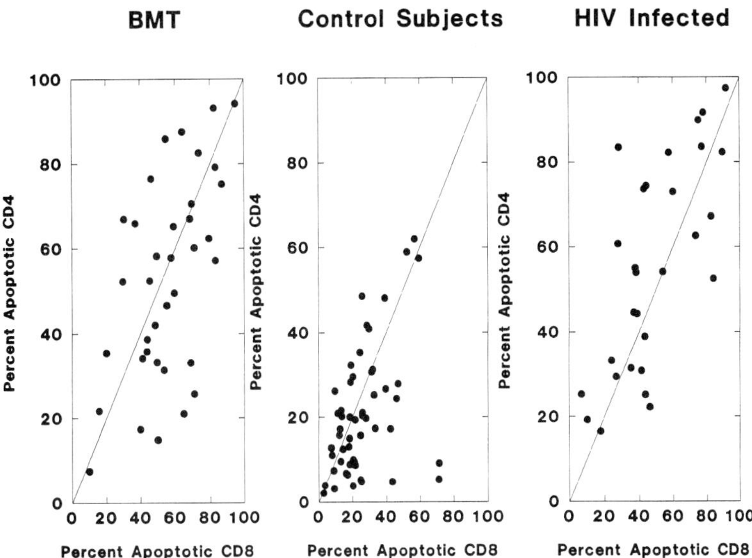

FIGURE 4. Comparison of CD8 apoptosis (x-axis) and CD4 apoptosis (y-axis) in BMT recipients, HIV-1 infected subjects, and healthy control subjects. The number of points above and below the diagonal lines are indicated and represent subjects in whom apoptosis of CD4 T cells was greater (above the line) or less than (below the line) that of CD8 T cells. Peripheral blood cells were held in short-term culture as described (FIG. 1, legend). Twenty-eight HIV-1[+] patients were studied, representing the entire disease spectrum. Their peripheral CD4[+] T-cell counts ranged from 10-968/μl (mean 315).

it inexorably declines. We presented the available evidence to support the hypothesis that in both states, hyporesponsiveness occurs not because of an inability to replace lost T cells, but because ablation of immune memory cells, as a diverse population of selected clonotypes, prevents the maturation and selection of newly generated naive T-cells, resulting in their untimely death. FIGURE 5 shows this hypothesis in schematic. The left side of the diagram is speculative, whereas the right side is supported by a wealth of experimental evidence. Beginning on the left side, the steady state T-cell concentration (T-cell count) is governed by an antigen-independent feedback mechanism that can be likened to a thermostat (*T-cell stat*) which senses T-cell number but does not distinguish between CD4[+] and CD8[+] subsets. T-cell loss triggers lymphopoiesis from a pre-T lymphohematopoietic progenitor cell. The progeny, shown as *pre-naive*, are TCR positive, CD4 or CD8 single positive, and, although not actively cycling, express phenotypic markers typical of T cells that have recently undergone activation. Many will undergo apoptosis unless actively rescued by memory cells. This process is rendered in FIGURE 5 as a *black box* but could conceivably occur in lymphoid tissues when pre-naive cells contact, as bystanders, mature memory lymphocyte cells engaged in antigen-specific responses. Memory cells can be envisioned to interact with naive cells in many ways, especially in a context where complex antigens are processed and presented as diverse arrays of

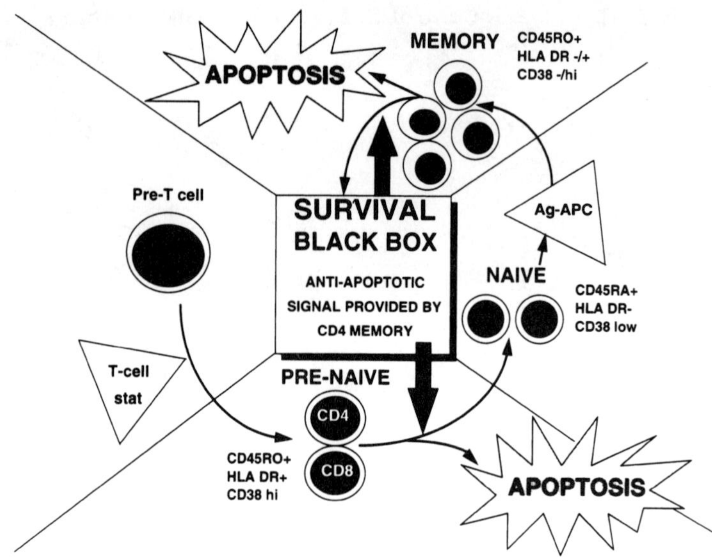

FIGURE 5. The role of memory T cells in T-cell replacement.

peptides. The present hypothesis requires only that signals provided by functioning memory cells rescue a proportion of naive cells that are otherwise programmed to die. Such a mechanism may also play a role in the peripheral enforcement of self-tolerance.[14] Once rescued, newly generated T cells become *stabilized* and assume the phenotype commonly attributed to naive cells. From this point (the right of the figure), naive cells encountering cognate antigen on appropriate antigen-presenting cells (again in the proximity of memory cells) are activated and clonally expanded, recapitulating the array of phenotypic markers expressed in the *pre-naive* stage. The majority of such cells apoptose when activation signals or antigen is removed, but a fraction survive, downregulating activation markers but retaining *memory markers* including the low molecular weight isoform of CD45 (RO) and high expression of the integrinβ chain, CD29. In FIGURE 5, memory cells are depicted as being involved in this selection process as well. Thus, memory cells are envisioned as arbiters of their own replacement. Without a cohort of memory cells engaged in the baseline responses that constitute immune surveillance, the probability that a newly generated T cell will receive the required signals for survival and proliferation is greatly diminished. The neonate has the advantage of several months of protection *in utero,* maternal antibodies, and a robust thymus, which supplies a steady stream of self-tolerant naive CD45RA⁺ T cells until this task is accomplished. The adult reconstituting BMT recipient must rely solely on peripheral mechanisms of tolerance and gradually accumulate a cohort of memory cells. In the interim, short-lived hypofunctional naive T cells masquerading as activated memory cells populate the immune system. In HIV-1 disease, the opposite scenario ensues. The immune system responds to infection with its characteristic efficacy. Virus reactivation and mutation are countered by anamnestic responses to conserved determinants and *de novo* responses to novel epitopes. As was so elegantly demonstrated,[24,25] CD4[+] T-cell losses are severe, far greater than those evidenced by the decline in circulating CD4[+] T cells. The immune system responds to such losses by generating replacement T cells (FIG. 5, left side). Because the *T-cell stat* does not recognize CD4/CD8 subset distinctions,[1,30] total T-cell number is maintained but the proportion of CD8[+] cells increases relative to CD4[+] T cells. This process is well tolerated for years, because replacement T cells, aided by existing memory cells, can make the naive to memory transition. This capacity, resilient as it is, is eroded after years of virus-mediated CD4[+] T-cell destruction. As HIV-1 disease progresses, the proportion of *pre-naive* T cells (CD4[+] and CD8[+]) increases and the probability that these cells will survive to maturity decreases. Finally, 12–24 months preceding the onset of clinical AIDS, T-cell homeostasis fails and absolute CD3 count declines,[31,32] signaling the point at which the rate of T-cell loss outstrips the capacity for T-cell replacement. If correct, this interpretation predicts that even a completely effective antiviral agent would not normalize T-cell turnover in the short term. Depending on the extent to which the memory compartment has been ablated, reconstitution would take place over the course of months as it does after BMT. From a practical perspective, the viewpoint that immune memory governs selection of naive replacement T cells suggests ways in which the immune system could be *jump started* following BMT. It may also help identify ways in which the war of attrition between HIV-1 and the immune system can be fought to a draw in the time frame of the human life span.

ACKNOWLEDGMENTS

The authors wish to thank Lisa Beltz, PhD, Deborah Griffin, E. Michael Meyer, and Timothy Patton for their participation in the apoptosis and immunophenotype studies, Charles Rinaldo, PhD, Robert Thackery, and the Pittsburgh Men's study for providing specimens from HIV-1 positive subjects, and Denise Thomas, RN, and Erin Weston, RN, for coordinating samples from BMT recipients.

SUMMARY

Bone marrow transplant recipients have a functional T-cell deficit long after T-cell counts have returned to normal levels. Early after BMT, T-cell phenotype is predominantly CD45RO[+]/CD29[high]/HLA-DR[+]/CD38[high]. This profile is associated with activated memory cells in healthy subjects, but also appears on the earliest mature naive T-cells in times of lymphopoietic stress. Most of these cells apoptose in short-term unstimulated culture, suggesting that they would have had a similar fate *in vivo*. Twelve to 24 months after BMT, CD45RA[+]/CD29[low]/HLA-DR[−]/CD38[low] T cells increase, apoptosis decreases, and T-cell function normalizes. We hypothesize that in the adult, mature memory T cells regulate their own replacement by rescuing a proportion of newly generated naive cells from apoptosis. Ablation of memory cells consequent to high dose therapy disrupts this process, resulting in a protracted period of high lymphocyte turnover with few cells surviving to make the antigen-driven transition to memory cells. Infection with HIV-1 also eventuates in immune deficiency associated with a loss in CD4$^+$ T cells and dominance of the phenotypic/apoptotic profile which we have associated with lymphopoietic stress. Recent data independently confirm that T-cell turnover is greatly elevated in HIV infection. Catastrophic or chronic depletion of memory T cells due to marrow ablative therapy or HIV-1 infection interferes with memory replacement, substituting short-lived hypofunctional naive T cells which characterize the state of immune amnesia.

REFERENCES

1. MARGOLICK, J. B., A. D. DONNENBERG, A. MUÑOZ, L. P. PARK, K. D. BAUER, J. V. GIORGI, J. FERBAS, A. J. SAAH & the Multicenter AIDS Cohort Study. 1993. Changes in T and non-T lymphocyte subsets following seroconversion to HIV-1: Stable CD3$^+$ and declining CD3$^-$ populations suggest regulatory responses linked to loss of CD4 lymphocytes. J. AIDS **6:** 153-161.

2. DONNENBERG, A. D., A. D. HESS, S. C. DUFF, E. BRIGHT, S. J. NOGA, R. SARAL & G. W. SANTOS. 1987. Regeneration of genetically restricted immune functions following human marrow transplantation: Influence of four different strategies for graft-versus-host disease (GVHD) prophylaxis. Transplant Proc. **19** (Suppl. 7): 144-152.

3. WIMPERIS, J. Z., M. K. BRENNER, H. G. PRENTICE, J. E. REITTIE, P. KARAYIANNIS, P. D. GRIFFITHS & A. V. HOFFBRAND. 1986. Transfer of a functioning humoral immune system in transplantation of T-lymphocyte-depleted bone marrow. Lancet **1**(8477): 339-343.

4. MARKHAM, R. B. & A. D. DONNENBERG. 1992. Effect of donor and recipient immunization protocols on primary and secondary human antibody responses in SCID mice reconstituted with human peripheral blood mononuclear cells. Infect. Immunity **60:** 2305-2308.

5. LJUNGMAN, P., M. WIKLUND-HAMMARSTEN, V. DURAJ, L. HAMMARSTROM, B. LONNQVIST, T. PAULIN, O. RINGDEN, M. S. PEPE & G. GAHRTON. Response to tetanus toxoid immunization after allogeneic bone marrow. J. Infect. Dis. **162:** 496-500.

6. QUINNAN, G. V., JR., N. KIRMANI, A. H. ROOK, J. F. MANISCHEWITZ, L. JACKSON, G. MORESCHI, G. W. SANTOS, R. SARAL & W. H. BURNS. 1982. Cytotoxic T cells in cytomegalovirus infection: HLA-restricted T-lymphocyte and non-T-lymphocyte cytotoxic responses correlate with recovery from cytomegalovirus infection in bone-marrow-transplant recipients. N. Engl. J. Med. **307:** 7-13.

7. WIMPERIS, J. Z., N. J. BERRY, H. G. PRENTICE, A. LEVER, P. D. GRIFFITHS & M. K. BRENNER. 1987. Regeneration of humoral immunity to herpes simplex virus following T-cell-depleted allogeneic bone marrow transplantation. J. Med. Virol. **23:** 93-99.

8. DRUMMOND, J. E., K. V. SHAH, R. SARAL, G. W. SANTOS & A. D. DONNENBERG. 1987. BK virus specific humoral and cell mediated immunity in allogeneic bone marrow transplant (BMT) recipients. J. Med. Virol. **23:** 331-344.

9. MACKALL, C. L., T. A. FLEISHER, M. R. BROWN, M. P. ANDRICH, C. C. CHEN, I. M. FEUERSTEIN, M. E. HOROWITZ, I. T. MAGRATH, A. T. SHAD, S. M. STEINBERG, L. H. WEXLER & R. E. GRESS. Age, thymopoiesis and CD4 T lymphocyte regeneration after intensive chemotherapy. N. Engl. J. Med. **332:** 143-149.

10. PILARSKI, L. M., R. GILLITZER, H. ZOLA, K. SHORTMAN & R. SCOLLAY. 1989. Definition of the thymic generative lineage by selective expression of high molecular weight isoforms of CD45 (T200). Eur. J. Immunol. **19:** 589-597.

11. KAPPLER, J. W., N. ROEHM & P. MARRACK. 1987. T cell tolerance by clonal elimination in the thymus. Cell **49:** 273-280.

12. SCHWARTZ, R. H. 1989. Acquisition of immunologic self-tolerance. Cell **57:** 1073-1081.

13. WEBB, S., C. MORRIS & J. SPRENT. 1990. Extrathymic tolerance of mature T-cells: Clonal elimination as a consequence of immunity. Cell **63:** 1249-1256.

14. DONNENBERG, A. D. & V. S. DONNENBERG. 1994. Apoptosis, autoimmunity and lymphopoiesis in the adult. Clin. Immunol. Newsletter **14:** 140-144.

15. STOREK, J., S. FERRARA, C. RODRIGUEZ & A. SAXON. 1992. Recovery of mononuclear cell subsets after bone marrow transplantation: Overabundance of CD4$^+$CD8$^+$ dual-positive T cells reminiscent of ontogeny. J. Hematother. **1:** 303-316.

16. DONNENBERG, A. D., B. M. A. M. BÄR, J. P. BARBER & G. W. SANTOS. 1990. Lymphocyte phenotype early after BMT: Expression of "memory" markers on naive T cells. Exp. Hematol. **18:** 584.

17. MOLLER, J., E. DICKMEISS, L. P. RYDER, N. JACOBSEN & A. SVEJGAARD. 1991. Increased frequencies of the CD29 and CD57 markers and decreased frequency of CD45RA within CD4$^+$ and CD8$^+$ subsets after allogeneic bone marrow transplantation in man. Scand. J. Immunol. **33:** 499-504.

18. VAN DER HARST, D., A. BRAND, S. A. VAN LUXEMBURG-HEIJS, Y. M. KOOIJ-WINKELAAR, E. ZWAAN & F. KONING. 1991. Selective outgrowth of CD45RO$^+$ V gamma 9$^+$/V delta 2$^+$ T-cell receptor gamma/delta T cells early after bone marrow transplantation. Blood **78:** 1875-1881.

19. PLEBANSKI, M., M. SAUDERS, S. S. BURTLES, S. CROWE & D. C. HOPPER. 1992. Primary and secondary human in vitro T cell responses to soluble antigens are mediated by subsets bearing different CD45 isoforms. Immunology **75:** 86-91.

20. AKBAR, A. N., L. TERRY, A. TIMMS, P. C. L. BEVERELY & G. JANOSSY. 1988. Loss of CD45R and gain of UCHL1 reactivity is a feature of primed T cells. J. Immunol. **140:** 2171-2178.

21. JANOSSY, G., M. BOFILL, D. ROWE, J. MUIR & P. C. BEVERLEY. 1989. The tissue distribution of T lymphocytes expressing different CD45 polypeptides. Immunology. **66:** 517-525.

22. GORSKI, J., M. YASSAI, X. ZHU, B. KISSELLA, C. KEEVER & N. FLOMENBERG. 1994. Circulating T cell repertoire complexity in normal individuals and bone marrow recipients analyzed by CDR3 size spectratyping. Correlation with immune status. J. Immunol. **152:** 5109-5119.

23. WAIN-HOBSON, S. 1995. Virological mayhem. Nature **373:** 102.

24. HO, D. D., A. U. NEUMANN, A. S. PERELSON, W. CHEN, J. M. LEONARD & M. MARKOWITZ. 1995. Rapid turnover of plasma virions and CD4 lymphocytes in HIV-1 infection. Nature **373:** 123-126.

25. WEI, X., S. K. GHOSH, M. E. TAYLOR, V. A. JOHNSON, E. A. EMINI, P. DEUTSCH, J. D. LIFSON, S. BONHOEFFER, M. A. NOWAK, B. H. HAHN, M. S. SAAG & G. M. SHAW. 1995. Viral dynamics in human immunodeficiency virus type 1 infection. Nature **373:** 117-122.

26. GOUGEON, M. L., S. GARCIA, J. HEENEY, R. TSCHOPP, H. LECOEUR, D. GUETARD, V. RAME, C. DAUGUET & L. MONTAGNIER. 1993. Programmed cell death in AIDS-related HIV and SIV infections. AIDS Res. Human Retroviruses 9(6): 553-563.

27. GOUGEON, M. L. & L. MONTAGNIER. 1993. Apoptosis in AIDS. Science **260:** 1269-1270.

28. DONNENBERG, A. D., J. B. MARGOLICK, L. A. BELTZ, V. X. SVOBODOVA & C. R. RINALDO. 1993. Apoptosis and lymphopoiesis: Positive correlation with progression in HIV disease, inverse in reconstitution of bone marrow transplant (BMT) patients. Abstracts of the Paris Conference on Apoptosis in AIDS and Cancer. p. 138.

29. DONNENBERG, A. D., J. B. MARGOLICK, L. A. BELTZ, V. S. DONNENBERG & C. R. RINALDO. 1995. Apoptosis and lymphopoiesis in bone marrow transplantation (BMT) and HIV disease. Res. Immunol. In press.

30. ADLEMAN, L. M. & D. WOOFSY. 1993. T cell homeostasis: Implications in HIV infection. J. AIDS **6:** 144-152.

31. MARGOLICK, J. B., A. D. DONNENBERG & A. MUÑOZ. 1994. T lymphocyte homeostasis after HIV seroconversion. J. AIDS **7:** 415-416.

32. Margolick, J. B., A. Muñoz, A. D. Donnenberg, L. P. Park, N. Galai, J. V. Giorgi, M. O'Gorman & J. Ferbas for the multicenter AIDS cohort study. 1995. Failure of T-cell homeostasis and the onset of AIDS in HIV-1 infection. Nature Med. **1:** 674–681.

33. Nicoletti, I., G. Migliorati, M. C. Pagliacci, F. Grignani & C. Riccardi. 1991. A rapid and simple method for measuring thymocyte apoptosis by propidiumiodide staining and flow cytometry. J. Immunol. Methods **139**(2): 271–279.

Cytokine Inhibitors and Graft-versus-Host Disease

JAMES L. M. FERRARA

Division of Pediatric Hematology/Oncology
Dana-Farber Cancer Institute
Childrens Hospital
Boston, Massachusetts 02115

Although bone marrow transplantation (BMT) is the therapy of choice for a number of diseases, the toxicities associated with allogeneic transplantation are pronounced. Graft-versus-host disease (GVHD) is the leading transplant-related complication, and during the 1980s multiple clinical trials attempted to eliminate the problem through T-cell depletion. Unfortunately, T-cell depletion presents its own risks, including graft rejection, leukemic relapse, and impaired immunologic reconstitution. Therefore, improved understanding of GVHD pathophysiology is an important objective in transplantation biology, and new approaches to this difficult problem are still needed.

We recently proposed that the pathophysiology of acute GVHD can be considered a "cytokine storm."[1] We envisage this storm as having three parts. First, the conditioning regimen damages host tissues (intestinal mucosa, liver, etc.) which release inflammatory cytokines tumor necrosis factor-alpha (TNF-α) and interleukin-1 (IL-1). These cytokines increase the expression of human leukocyte antigen (HLA) and other critical adhesion molecules. During autologous transplantation this generation of cytokines is self-limited and resolves in 7–10 days. However, in allogeneic transplantation, mature donor T cells recognize alloantigens in the host and become activated. This recognition is facilitated by consequences of the first step, that is, cytokine-induced increases in host cell surface receptors. Activated donor T cells then proliferate and secrete IL-2. When the principal T-cell response is a "Th1" or inflammatory response (mainly IL-2 and gamma-interferon [IFN-γ]), these cytokines activate additional donor (and residual host) mononuclear cells and macrophages to secrete IL-1 and TNF-α. The resulting inflammatory response causes additional release of cytokines that amplifies local tissue injury, at least in part through active nitrogen intermediates such as the nitric oxide. The overall result is the acute "suppressive" form of GVHD. When the principal T-cell response is a Th2 or "helper" response in which IL-4 and IL-10 predominate, the overall result is the chronic or "stimulatory" form of GVHD with increased IgE synthesis and exaggerated lymphoproliferation.

This conceptual framework explains a number of unique and seemingly unrelated aspects of GVHD. For example, analyses of clinical transplants have noted an increased risk of GVHD associated with advanced leukemia, certain intensive conditioning regimens, and a history of viral infections.[2-4] The epithelial and endothelial injury associated with these processes stimulates the release of inflammatory cytokines and increases the expression of cell-surface adhesion molecules. Similarly, the importance of bowel decontamination in the prevention of GVHD is explained by the ability of endotoxin to leak through damaged intestinal mucosa and stimulate gut-associated lymphocytes and macrophages to produce cytokines such as IL-1, TNF-α, and IFN-γ. The growth of certain virulent *Escherichia coli* strains is enhanced by IL-1, suggesting that local production of IL-1 in the gut mucosa can amplify the effects of endotoxin.[5] Endotoxin from gram-negative rods on the skin may stimulate keratinocytes, dermal fibroblasts, and macrophages to produce similar cytokines in the dermis and epidermis. The effect of gamma globulin in reducing GVHD is also probably related to the cytokine hypothesis.[6] When IgG is bound to macrophages, IL-1 receptor antagonist (IL-1ra) production is preferentially increased over that of IL-1-α.[7] Exogenously administered IgG *in vivo* may thus directly modulate the cytokine storm.

An excellent review of the involvement of cytokines in GVHD appeared in 1992.[8] This article provides a sweeping review of the field as it developed throughout the 1980s, and it also suggests a very similar model of the progression of GVHD through a cytokine cascade. One point of difference is the lack of initial cytokine release in their model, probably because of its reliance on animal models in which GVHD is induced in unirradiated hosts. Many of the studies reviewed are essentially correlative, because most antagonists had not been identified at the time of the initial publications. There is, however, a fine appreciation of the interactive nature of many cytokine circuits and constant stress on the multistep pathway in the generation of target organ damage during GVHD.

With this cytokine hypothesis as background, the rest of this article reviews individual cytokines as they relate to GVHD. References to some experimental systems that are particularly relevant to cytokine dysregulation are also made even though there is as yet no direct connection with GVHD.

INTERLEUKIN-2

Interleukin-2 has long been considered by many to be the primary cytokine involved in GVHD both because of its centrality as a T-cell growth factor and because cyclosporine, a powerful prophylactic agent against GVHD, inhibits IL-2 secretion. Several reports demonstrate the importance of IL-2 in the development of GVHD. Two separate European groups have shown that the precursor frequency of host-specific IL-2-producing T cells (pHTL) predicts the occurrence of GVHD in the recipients of HLA-identical, mixed lymphocyte culture nonreactive bone marrow. Theobald and colleagues[9] in Ulm used a limiting dilution analysis technique for pHTL in 16 donor/recipient pairs. They found that the critical precursor frequency of host-specific IL-2-secreting cells (pHTL) was 1/100,000. Eight patients whose donor bone marrow contained fewer host-specific pHTL later developed only grade 0-1 GVHD, whereas eight patients whose donor bone marrow contained greater frequencies all developed significant grade II or III GVHD. Schwarer *et al.*[10] in London reported similar results, although their method of performing LDA was considerably simpler than the German technique and therefore more likely to be widely applied. The important frequency of IL-2-secreting cells again was approximately 1/100,000. The Ulm group published a follow-up study of the pHTL frequencies in the peripheral blood of patients after allogeneic transplantation.[11] In accordance with their earlier study, eight patients with grade 0-1 GVHD never developed detectable frequencies of host specific pHTL, whereas six patients with grade II-III had pHTL frequencies ranging between 1/13,000 and 1/174,000. These cells were detectable as early as day 20 after transplantation, often preceding the onset of acute GVHD by a couple of weeks and persisting until the GVHD resolved. These data are consistent with experimental data showing that IL-2 secreted by T cells is an early event in the pathology of GVHD and can be seen as early as 2 days after GVHD induction.[12]

The relationship of IL-2 to early events of GVHD is actively being investigated. The observation that the administration of exogenous IL-2 decreases GVHD in a murine model[13] is the subject of intense exploration, and the potential mechanisms involved form another chapter in this volume. In terms of clinical treatment or prophylaxis against GVHD, not all antagonism of IL-2 is equally effective. For example, the addition of an anti-IL-2 receptor to a prophylactic regimen of cyclosporine and methotrexate did not change the incidence of severe GVHD in a clinical trial in 64 patients.[14] There are always many possible reasons for negative results, particularly in clinical research where concomitant variables are difficult to control; this trial employed a murine monoclonal antibody, and whether a humanized version will be more efficacious is still open to question.

INTERFERON-γ

Gamma interferon (IFN-γ) has been implicated in the pathophysiology of experimental GVHD for several years. The characteristic immunosuppression of GVHD lymphocytes could be partially reversed *in vitro* by an anti-IFN-γ monoclonal antibody;[15] the intestinal pathology of GVHD could also be reduced by the administration of anti-IFN-γ antibody.[16]

An important earlier observation was that both IFN-γ and TNF-α, were directly involved in producing the cytopathic effects of GVHD in a skin explant model.[17] High levels of both of these cytokines correlated with intense cellular damage. These two cytokines alone are not likely to mediate GVHD, because one third of the supernatants from activated mixed lymphocyte reactions contained large amounts of both cytokines, but they did not cause GVHD pathology. (See a later section on nitric oxide.)

Gamma interferon serum levels are also increased during clinical GVHD, but the increase is not dramatic, and small numbers of patient studies did not permit statistically meaningful differences to be achieved.[18] The importance of IFN-γ in the pathology was recently demonstrated unexpectedly.[19] Twice weekly injections of IFN-γ could prevent GVHD elicited by MHC antigens in a murine model; survival of mice was significantly increased and intestinal lesions were significantly reduced. The mechanism by which these injections prevented GVHD was the reduction in the number of IFN-γ-secreting T cells in mice undergoing the reaction. Administration of exogenous IFN-γ thus appeared to reduce GVHD by acting in a negative feedback loop. It is interesting that maximum IFN-γ production in animals with untreated GVHD peaked at day 7, before the clinical manifestations of GVHD were apparent, suggesting that the release of this cytokine is an early event in the process. This notion is consistent with the schema of the cytokine storm that we proposed.

Gamma interferon secretion was greatly increased during GVHD using an interesting method to enumerate lymphokine mRNA-containing cells that combined limiting dilution analysis and polymerase chain reaction (PCR) amplification of cDNA.[20] Mice with acute GVHD had 2.6% unstimulated cells that contained IFN-γ mRNA compared to 0.07% in controls, a nearly 40-fold increase. When cells were stimulated with anti-CD3 antibody, the number containing IFN-γ mRNA rose dramatically to 67.0%, which was 70 times greater than that in the controls (0.92%). Increased frequencies were also noted for IL-4, GM-CSF, and IL-3. A much less quantitative approach also determined that IFN-γ was increased 14 days after induction of acute GVHD in an unirradiated GVHD model.[21] Polymerase chain reaction (PCR) amplification of multiple cytokines showed that IL-1-α, IFN-γ, IL-10, and MIP 1-α were all increased in acute GVHD, whereas only IL-4 was significantly elevated in chronic GVHD. A second group found similar results using a semiquantitative PCR technique in the same murine model of chronic GVHD.[22] Interleukin-2 increased dramatically 2 days after GVHD induction, but then decreased to normal levels. By contrast, IL-4 continued to rise until day 7, and IL-10 showed the largest increases at that time. This group demonstrated the importance of IL-4 in chronic GVHD by injecting anti-IL-4 antibodies in mice with chronic GVHD.[23] The kidney damage and death that are characteristic of this chronic GVHD model were delayed by anti-IL-4, and IgE serum levels were decreased. Injections of IFN-γ, an IL-4 antagonist, decreased IgE levels but had no effect on kidney damage or mortality. Analysis of cytokine secretion *in vitro* by lymphocytes from animals with chronic GVHD showed elevated IL-4 production but diminished IL-2 and IFN-γ secretion.[24] Data from several laboratories thus consistently showed a difference in the patterns of cytokine expression during acute and chronic GVHD, with Th1 cytokines predominating in acute GVHD and Th2 cytokines more prominent in chronic GVHD.

TUMOR NECROSIS FACTOR-ALPHA

Piguet *et al.*[25] first demonstrated that TNF-α was an important mediator of GVHD in an experimental murine model system. The role of TNF-α in GVHD was further elucidated in a study by Nestel and colleagues.[26] Using an experimental GVHD model in unirradiated recipients, they showed that macrophages in animals with GVHD were activated and primed to release TNF-α after stimulation with small amounts of lipopolysaccharide, a cell wall component of gram-negative bacteria. Small, normally nonlethal amounts of lipopolysaccharide caused elevated TNF-α serum levels in animals with GVHD that led to shock and death. This sequence could be prevented with rabbit anti-TNF-α antiserum, demonstrating the importance of TNF-α to the systemic pathology of GVHD. These experiments strongly support the role of mononuclear cells, or macrophages, as sources of inflammatory cytokines during the effector arm of acute GVHD.

An important role for TNF-α in clinical acute GVHD was suggested by a retrospective study of Holler *et al.*[27] describing elevated TNF-α levels in patients with acute GVHD and endothelial complications such as veno-occlusive disease.[27] Measurement of TNF-α in serum has been particularly difficult to standardize because of the large amounts of soluble, circulating TNF-α receptors.[28] Such soluble receptors interfere with the detection of cytokines depending on the specific epitopes recognized by monoclonal antibodies in any given assay system. Holler and colleagues[27] have now performed a prospective evaluation of serum TNF-α levels in over 100 patients. Increased serum TNF-α levels correlated with more severe GVHD and with veno-occlusive disease. More importantly, timing of the elevated levels was predictive of severe complications and overall survival. Patients with elevated serum TNF-α levels during the conditioning regimen (prior to transplantation) had a greater than 90% incidence of acute GVHD and less than 30% overall survival. In addition, a phase I/II trial of a monoclonal anti-TNF-α receptor during the conditioning regimen was initiated in high risk patients, with 7 of 10 patients requiring additional immunosuppression for acute GVHD compared to 15 of 16 historical controls. These preliminary data as well as animal and laboratory studies suggest that this approach to TNF-α inhibition will be a very exciting avenue of investigation.

A second phase I/II study used an anti-TNF-α monoclonal antibody in patients with severe acute GVHD.[29] In this study of 19 patients (15 of whom had grade IV GVHD), there were no complete responses but approximately 75% partial responses. In responding patients, there was 100% response in intestinal lesions, 85% in skin lesions, and 37% in liver lesions. In most patients, GVHD flared after discontinuation of treatment (median time to flare, 3 days). It is not surprising that a single agent used in this setting did not induce complete responses, particularly in light of the synergistic actions of the proinflammatory cytokines TNF-α and IL-1. The significant partial response rate deserves notice, however, and future trials will presumably use this antibody in a more prophylactic mode. Finally, it should be noted that not all studies agree on the relation of elevated TNF-α in the serum and increased GVHD. Robinet *et al.*[30] could not find a correlation in a small series from France. The assay for TNF-α was different from that used in Germany, and this point is clearly a critical component of the accuracy of quantitation. The eventual usefulness of this assay awaits further standardization of these laboratory techniques.

INTERLEUKIN-1

Investigations of the role of IL-1 in GVHD intensified after the discovery of a naturally occurring IL-1 receptor antagonist, a third member of the IL-1 protein family.[31] Using a mouse model of acute GVHD to minor histocompatibility antigens, Ferrara *et al.*[32] examined cytokine dysregulation in two major GVHD target organs, the spleen and the skin. At 4 weeks after transplantation when most animals have died of GVHD and surviving animals clearly have active disease, IL-2 transcripts were not elevated in either the skin or the spleen. By contrast, TNF-α transcripts were significantly increased about sixfold in both organs. Most strikingly, IL-1α mRNA was induced at least 200 times above controls in both organs. Intraperitoneal administration of IL-1ra starting on day 10 after transplantation when animals were already showing clinical signs of disease reversed the disease in most animals, providing a significant survival advantage in treated animals (75 vs 28%). These animal data thus emphasize the role of IL-1 in the effector phase of the cytokine storm and support further examination of IL-1ra in the treatment of clinical GVHD. In phase I/II trial of IL-1ra for steroid-resistant GVHD,[32] IL-1ra in a dose ranging from 400–3,200 mg/day was administered in a continuous infusion over 7 days in 17 patients. Stage-specific improvement of acute GVHD occurred in the skin (8 of

14, 57%), gut (9 of 11, 82%), and liver (2 of 11, 18%). Overall, acute GVHD improved by at least one grade in 10 of 16 (63%) patients. Response to therapy was associated with a reduction in TNF-α mRNA levels in blood mononuclear cells ($p =$ 0.001) The only toxicity observed was reversible elevation in liver enzymes in two patients.

INTERLEUKIN-6

Interleukin-6 might be expected to play a role in the pathophysiology of GVHD, particularly because it is known to have inflammatory properties among its pleiotropic effects and it is induced in monocytes after stimulation by IFN-γ and TNF-α. Little experimental work has been done in animal models, but there is one report of elevated serum IL-6 levels in patients with acute GVHD and hepatorenal syndrome.[33] Several patterns of elevated IL-6 levels were observed which did not always correlate with active disease among the 22 patients studied. The strongest conclusion that can be drawn from this study is that there may be a correlation between elevated IL-6 and acute GVHD and hepatorenal syndrome, but what specific role IL-6 plays in this complex process is yet to be defined.

NITRIC OXIDE

Nitric oxide (NO) is a short-lived biologic mediator that has recently received much attention as a messenger molecule with pleiotropic effects in several tissue types. The molecule certainly plays an important role in host defense and the antimicrobial and tumoricidal functions of macrophages. Inhibitors of NO synthesis, particularly L-NG monomethyl arginine (L-NMMA), permit analysis of the role of NO in different physiologic processes. An important contribution to understanding the role of NO in GVHD was published by Garside and colleagues[34] from Glasgow who examined nitric oxide as it relates to intestinal GVHD. L-NMMA treatment of mice with GVHD reduced the pathology of the intestinal mucosa and diminished lymphocytic infiltration of the epithelium. L-NMMA treatment in these animals did not affect splenomegaly, which is an early sign of T-cell proliferation in GVHD. Nitric oxide is therefore more likely to be involved in the effector arm of the process, and indeed in another study serum NO levels were increasingly elevated as GVHD progressed or after the immunosuppressive agent FK506 was discontinued.[35] The observation that NO mediates important aspects of GVHD pathology is particularly relevant to the notion of a cytokine storm: inflammatory cytokines in combination with endotoxin are the principal stimulators of NO in a variety of systems. Nussler and colleagues[36] showed that an inducible form of NO synthase (NOS) is present in human hepatocytes after stimulation with IL-1, TNF-α, IFN-γ, and endotoxin. Individually, none of these cytokines induced NOS, and in pairwise combinations, less than 5% elevation in NO synthesis was observed. Three cytokines together were more effective in inducing NO than was the combination of lipopolysaccharide and any two, and the addition of lipopolysaccharide to the trio of TNF-α, IL-1, and IFN-γ increased NO production by 33%. This system appears to model the pathologic mechanisms of GVHD in the liver, where lymphokines, monokines, and endotoxin act synergistically to produce the damage that none of them causes alone. Inflammatory cytokines and lipopolysaccharide also synergize to produce NO in another system that utilizes articular chondrocytes.[37] In this system, IL-1 and lipopolysaccharide alone were able to induce significant NO levels, whereas TNF-α and INF-γ were unable to generate NO alone, although they increased the maximal production when added to IL-1 and lipopolysaccharide. This observation supports the notion described earlier that IL-1 may dominate the hierarchy of cytokines causing GVHD. In addition, the unusual tissue distribution of GVHD pathology may reflect not only differences in the combination of cytokines and endotoxin present in a particular tissue but also the reaction of different cell types to local cytokine dysregulation. Investigations in this area are likely to lead to important mechanistic insights into the pathophysiology of GVHD in the near future.

SUMMARY

Graft-versus-host disease (GVHD) remains the major complication of allogeneic bone marrow transplantation. T cells in donor bone marrow recognize and react to host alloantigens and thereby initiate GVHD, but the precise mechanisms by which host tissues are damaged remain unclear. Recently, several convergent lines of evidence suggested that inflammatory cytokines act as mediators of acute GVHD. Most of the clinical manifestations of GVHD may, in fact, be due to the dysregulated production of cytokines by T cells and other inflammatory cells. The complex interactions among cytokines and their cellular targets suggest that individual cytokines may play an important and distinctive role in the pathophysiology of GVHD. Perturbation of the cytokine network may function as a final common pathway of target organ damage, and the rapid onset of severe, acute GVHD can be considered a ''cytokine storm.''

REFERENCES

1. ANTIN, J. H. & J. L. M. FERRARA. 1992. Cytokine dysregulation and acute graft-versus-host disease. Blood **80:** 2964–2968.
2. GALE, R. P., M. M. BORTIN, D. W. VAN BEKKUM, J. C. BIGGS, K. A. DICKEL, E. GLUCKMAN, R. A. GOOD, R. G. HOFFMAN, H. E. M. KAY, J. H. KERSEY, A. MARMONT, T. MASAOKA, A. A. RIMM, J. J. VAN ROOD & F. E. ZWAAN. 1987. Risk factors for acute graft-versus-host disease. Br. J. Haematol. **67:** 397.
3. RINGDEN, O. 1990. Viral infections and graft-vs.-host disease. In Graft-vs.-Host Disease. S. J. Burakoff, H. J. Deeg, J. Ferrara & K. Atkinson, : 467. New York. Marcel Dekker.
4. CLIFT, R. A., C. D. BUCKNER, F. R. APPELBAUM, S. I. BEARMAN, F. B. PETERSON, L. B. FISHER, C. ANASETTI, P. BEATTY, W. I. BENSINGER, K. DONEY, R. S. HILL, G. B. MCDONALD, P. MARTIN, J. SANDERS, J. SINGER, P. STEWART, K. M. SULLIVAN, R. WITHERSPOON, R. STORB, J. A. HANSEN & E. D. THOMAS. 1990. Allogeneic marrow transplantation in patients with acute myeloid leukemia in first remission. A randomized trial of two irradiation regimens. Blood **76:** 1867.
5. PORAT, R., B. D. CLARK, A. M. WOLFE, C. A. DINARELLO. 1991. Enhancement of growth of virulent *Escherichia coli* by interleukin-1. Science **254:** 431.
6. SULLIVAN, K. M., K. J. KOPECKY, J. JOCOM, L. FISHER, C. D. BUCKNER, J. D. MEYERS, G. W. COUNTS, R. A. BOWDEN, F. B. PETERSON, R. P. WITHERSPOON, M. D. BUDINGER,

R. S. SCHWARTZ, F. R. APPELBAUM, R. A. CLIFT, J. A. HANSEN, J. E. SANDERS, E. D. THOMAS & R. STORB. 1990. Immunomodulatory and antibmicrobial efficacy of intravenous immunoglobulin in bone marrow transplantation. N. Engl. J. Med. **323:** 705.

7. AREND, W. P., M. F. SMITH, Jr., R. W. JANSON & F. G. JOSLIN. 1991. IL-1 receptor antagonist and IL-1-beta production in human monocytes are regulated differently. J. Immunol. **147:** 1530-1536.

8. JADUS, M. R. & H. T. WEPSIC. 1992. The role of cytokines in graft-versus-host reactions and disease. Bone Marrow Transplant. **10:**1-14.

9. THEOBALD, M., T. NIERLE, D. BUNJES, R. ARNOLD & H. HEIMPEL. 1992. Host-specific interleukin-2-secreting donor T-cell precursors as predictors of acute graft-versus-host disease in bone marrow transplantation between HLA-identical siblings. N. Engl. J. Med. **327:** 1613-1617.

10. SCHWARER, A. P., Y. Z. JIANG, P. A. BROOKES, A. J. BARRETT, J. R. BATCHELOR, J. M. GOLDMAN & R. I. LECHLER. 1993. Frequency of anti-recipient alloreactive helper T-cell precursors in donor blood and graft-versus-host disease after HLA-identical sibling bone-marrow transplantation. Lancet **341:** 203-205.

11. NIERLE, T., D. BUNJES, R. ARNOLD, H. HEIMPEL & M. THEOBALD. 1993. Quantitative assessment of posttransplant host-specific interleukin-2-secreting T-helper cell precursors in patients with and without acute graft-versus-host disease after allogeneic HLA-identical sibling bone marrow transplantation. Blood **81:** 841-848.

12. VIA, C. S. 1991. Kinetics of T cell activation in acute and chronic forms of graft versus host disease. J. Immunol. **146:** 2603-2609.

13. SYKES, M., M. L. ROMICK, K. A. HOYLES & D. H. SACHS. 1990. In vivo administration of interleukin 2 plus T cell-depleted syngeneic marrow prevents graft-versus-host disease mortality and permits alloengraftment. J. Exp. Med. **171:** 645-658.

14. BELANGER, C., H. ESPEROU-BOURDEAU, P. BORDIGONI, J. P. JOUET, G. SOUILLET, N. MILPIED, X. TROUSSARD, M. KUENTZ, P. HERVE, J. REIFFERS, F. DEMEOCQ, C. DAURIAC, D. BLAISE, M. MICHALLET, D. FRIERE, F. FREYCON, N. GRATECOS, B. RIO, V. LEBLOND, N. IFRAH, M. ATTAL, J. P. BERGERAT, E. VILMER, J. PICO, C. RAFFOUX, P. CAUDRELIER & E. GLUCKMAN. 1993. Use of an anti-interleukin-2 receptor monoclonal antibody for GVHD prophylaxis in unrelated donor BMT. Bone Marrow Transplant. **11:** 293-297.

15. WALL, D. A., S. D. HAMBERG, D. S. REYNOLDS, S. J. BURAKOFF, A. K. ABBAS & J. L. M. FERRARA. 1988. Immunodeficiency in graft-versus-host disease. I. Mechanism of immune suppression. J. Immunol. **140:** 2970-2976.

16. MOWAT, A. 1989. Antibodies to IFN-gamma prevent immunological mediated intestinal damage in murine graft-versus-host reactions. Immunology **68:** 18-24.

17. DICKINSON, A. M., L. SVILAND, J. DUNN, P. CAREY & S. J. PROCTOR. 1991. Demonstration of direct involvement of cytokines in graft-versus-host reactions using an *in vitro* skin explant model. Bone Marrow Transplant. **7:** 209-216.

18. NIEDERWIESER, D., M. HEROLD, W. WOLOSZCZUK, W. AULITSKY, B. MEISTER, H. TILG, G. GASTL, R. BOWDEN & C. HUBER. 1990. Endogenous IFN-gamma during human bone marrow transplantation. Transplantation **50:** 620-625.

19. BROK, H. P. M., P. J. HEIDT, P. H. VAN DER MEIDE, C. ZURCHER & J. M. VOSSEN. 1993. Interferon-gamma prevents graft-versus-host disease after allogeneic bone marrow transplantation in mice. J. Immunol. **151:** 6451-6459.

20. TROUTT, A. B. & A. KELSO. 1992. Enumeration of lymphokine mRNA-containing cells *in vivo* in a murine graft-versus-host reaction using the PCR. Proc. Natl. Acad. Sci. USA **89:** 5276.

21. ALLEN, R. D., T. A. STALEY & C. L. SIDMAN. 1993. Differential cytokine expression acute and chronic murine graft-versus-host disease. Eur. J. Immunol. **23:** 333-337.

22. GARLISI, C. G., K. J. PENNLINE, S. R. SMITH, M. I. SIEGEL & S. P. UMLAND. 1993. Cytokine gene expression in mice undergoing chronic graft-versus-host disease. Molec. Immunol. **30:** 669-677.

23. UMLAND, S. P., S. RAZAC, D. K. NAHREBNE & B. W. SEYMOUR. 1992. Effects of in vivo administration of interferon (IFN)-gamma, anti-IFN-gamma, or anti-interleukin-4 monoclonal antibodies in chronic autoimmune graft-versus-host disease. Clin. Immunol. Immunopathol. 63: 66–73.

24. DE WIT, D., M. VAN MECHELEN, C. ZANIN, J.-M. DOUTRELEPONT, T. VELU, C. GERARD, D. ABRAMOWICZ, J.-P. SCHEERLINCK, P. DE BAETSELIER, J. URBAIN, O. LEO, M. GOLDMAN & M. MOSER. 1993. Preferential activation of Th2 cells in chronic graft-versus-host disease. J. Immunol. 150: 361–366.

25. PIGUET, P. F., G. E. GRAU, B. ALLET & P. J. VASSALLI. 1987. Tumor necrosis factor/cachectin is an effector of skin and gut lesions of the acute phase of graft-versus-host disease. J. Exp. Med. 166: 1280–1289.

26. NESTEL, F. P., K. S. PRICE, T. A. SEEMAYER & W. S. LAPP. 1992. Macrophage priming and lipopolysaccharide-triggered release of tumor necrosis factor alpha during graft-versus-host disease. J. Exp. Med. 175: 405–413.

27. HOLLER, E., H. J. KOLB, R. HUNTERMEIER-KNABE, J. MITTERMULLER, S. THIERFELDER, M. KAUL & W. WILMANNS. 1993. Role of tumor necrosis factor alpha in acute graft-versus-host disease and complications following allogeneic bone marrow transplantation. Transplantation 25: 1234–1236.

28. HINTERMEIER-KNABE, R., M. BROCKHAUS, E. HOLLER, W. LESSLAUER, J. KEMPENI, H. J. KOLB & W. WILMANNS. 1992. Sequential release of tumor necrosis factor alpha and tumor necrosis factor receptors in complications of human bone marrow transplantation. In Cytokines in Hemopoiesis, Oncology, and AIDS II. Freund, Link, Schmidt & Welte, Eds. Berlin. Springer-Verlag.

29. HERVE, P., M. FLESCH, P. TIBERGHIEN, J. WIJDENES, E. RACADOT, P. BORDIGONI, E. PLOUVIER, J. L. STEPHAN, H. BOURDEAU, E. HOLLER, B. LIOURE, C. ROCHE, E. VILMER, F. DEMEOCQ, M. KUENTZ & Y. J. CAHN. 1992. Phase I-II trial of a monoclonal anti-tumor necrosis factor alpha antibody for the treatment of refractory severe acute graft-versus-host disease. Blood 79: 3362–3368.

30. ROBINET, E., A. IBRAHIM, A. TRUNEH, M. OSTRONOFF, Z. MISHAL, E. ZAMBON, F. GAY, M. HAYAT, J.-L. PICO & S. CHOUAIB. 1992. Serum levels and receptor expression of tumor necrosis factor-alpha following human allogeneic and autologous bone marrow transplantation. Transplantation 53: 574–579.

31. MCCARTHY, P. L., S. ABHYANKAR, S. NEBEN, G. NEWMAN, C. SIEFF, R. C. THOMPSON, S. J. BURAKOFF & J. L. M. FERRARA. 1991. Inhibition of interleukin-1 by an interleukin-1 receptor antagonist prevents graft-versus-host disease. Blood 78: 1915–1918.

32. FERRARA, J. L. M., S. ABHYANKAR & D. G. GILLILAND. 1993. Cytokine storm of graft-versus-host disease: A critical effector role for interleukin-1. Transplant. Proc. 25: 1216–1217.

33. SYMINGTON, F. W., B. E. SYMINGTON, P. Y. LIU, H. VIGUET, U. SANTHANAM & P. B. SEHGAL. 1992. The relationship of serum IL-6 levels to acute graft-versus-host disease and hepatorenal disease after human bone marrow transplantation. Transplantation 54: 457–462.

34. GARSIDE, P., A. K. HUTTON, A. SEVERN, F. Y. LIEW & A. M. MOWAT. 1992. Nitric oxide mediates intestinal pathology in graft-vs-host disease. Eur. J. Immunol. 22: 2141–2145.

35. LANGREHR, J. M., N. MURASE, P. M. MARKUS, X. CAI, P. NEUHAUS, W. SCHRAUT, R. L. SIMMONS & R. A. HOFFMAN. 1992. Nitric oxide production in host-versus-graft and graft-versus-host reactions in the rat. J. Clin. Invest. 90: 679–683.

36. NUSSLER, A. K., M. DI SILVIO, T. R. BILLIAR, R. A. HOFFMAN, D. A. GELLER, R. SELBY, J. MADARIAGA & R. L. SIMMONS. 1992. Stimulation of the nitric oxide synthase pathway in human hepotocytes by cytokines and endotoxin. J. Exp. Med. 176: 261–264.

37. STADLER, J., M. STEFANOVIC-RACIC, T. R. BILLIAR, R. D. CURRAN, L. A. MCINTYRE, H. I. GEORGESCU, R. L. SIMMONS & C. H. EVANS. 1991. Articular chondrocytes synthe-

size nitric oxide in response to cytokines and lipopolysaccharide. J. Immunol. **147:** 3915–3920.

38. ANTIN, J. H., H. J. WEINSTEIN, E. C. GUINAN, P. McCARTHY, B. E. BIERER, D. G. GILLILAND, S. K. PARSONS, K. K. BALLEN, I. J. RIMM, G. FALZARANO, D. C. BLOEDOW, L. ABATE, M. LEBSACK, S. J. BURAKOFF & J. L. M. FERRARA. 1994. Recombinant human interleukin 1 receptor antagonist in the treatment of steroid-resistant graft-versus-host disease. Blood **84:** 1342–1348.

Pharmacology of Bone Marrow Transplantation Conditioning Regimens[a]

RICHARD J. JONES[b] AND LOUISE B. GROCHOW

Johns Hopkins Oncology Center
Johns Hopkins Medical Institutions
Baltimore, Maryland 21287

Therapeutic monitoring is widely used in clinical practice for a variety of drugs including theophylline, cardiovascular agents, and antibiotics. However, it has played a relatively small role in the treatment of cancer, even though anticancer agents have narrow therapeutic ratios. Bone marrow transplantation (BMT) conditioning regimens, in particular, are at or near nonhematologic dose-limiting toxicity. To provide the greatest antitumor effect, BMT conditioning regimens have been escalated beyond doses that produce the usual toxicity associated with anticancer agents, bone marrow failure. The doses employed in BMT conditioning regimens produce a substantial incidence in severe end-organ damage, particularly that involving lungs, liver, or heart. Therefore, small interpatient differences in the handling of drugs used at very high doses as conditioning therapy for BMT could produce major differences in toxicity. Substantial evidence now exists that the pharmacokinetics of high-dose BMT conditioning regimens predict regimen-related toxicity.[1-3] Moreover, recent data demonstrate that individualized dosing of drugs used in BMT conditioning regimens can significantly decrease toxicity and hopefully improve tumor control.

BUSULFAN PHARMACOKINETICS

Busulfan, a bifunctional alkylating agent, has been widely used in conditioning regimens for BMT for many years, usually in combination with cyclophosphamide. The dose-limiting nonhematopoietic toxicity of busulfan is venoocclusive disease of the liver.[4] However, the incidence of VOD (about 20%) with the usual doses of busulfan employed in BMT is not different from that with most other BMT conditioning regimens.[5,6] Venocclusive disease is a serious complication of BMT conditioning regimens, with death occurring in 40-50% of affected patients.[5,6] Approximately half the cases of VOD occur in patients with mild to moderate underlying liver damage

[a] This work was supported in part by National Institutes of Health grant CA15396. R.J.J. is a Leukemia Society of America Scholar.

[b] Address for correspondence and reprint requests: Richard J. Jones, MD, Johns Hopkins Oncology Center, Room 2-127, 600 North Wolfe Street, Baltimore, Maryland 21287-8967.

at the time of BMT.[5,6] It has been difficult to establish causal associations in most other patients in whom VOD develops after BMT.

Only an oral formulation of busulfan is currently available for clinical use; it can produce major differences in busulfan exposure among patients given the same dose. We investigated whether interpatient differences in busulfan exposure could explain the development of VOD in some patients. We found nearly a 10-fold variance in busulfan exposure in a study of 30 BMT patients receiving the same dose of drug (1 mg/kg orally every 6 hours for 16 doses).[1] The area under the curve (AUC) contributed by this dose of busulfan ranged from 606 to 5,144 μmol/min/L (mean 2,012 ± 1,223). Moreover, there was a strong association between busulfan levels and the risk of VOD. All six patients who developed VOD on this study had an AUC that was above the mean, and five of the six had an AUC that was greater than 1 standard deviation above the mean. By contrast, only one patient with a busulfan AUC less than 1 standard deviation above the mean developed VOD. Hence, the variability in busulfan levels among patients was substantial and appeared to contribute to differences in outcome among patients receiving high-dose busulfan as conditioning for BMT.

Age clearly is one feature that influences the interpatient variability in busulfan pharmacokinetics. The incidence of busulfan-related toxicities after allogeneic BMT apparently was less[5] and the rate of engraftment failure higher[7] in young children than in adults, suggesting that busulfan levels may be lower in young children dosed as adults. In fact, this has now been shown in multiple groups.[7–9] Children under 6 demonstrated both a higher clearance and a higher volume of distribution, resulting in an AUC that was less than half that in adults. Children above 6 handled busulfan similarly to adults.

For several drugs, children require higher doses than adults when dosing is by milligrams per kilogram.[10] We investigated pediatric busulfan dosing by body surface area,[11] because it may more closely approximate adult drug levels.[10,12] However, normalizing pediatric busulfan doses to body surface area was still associated with twice the clearance rate in adults.[7] Therefore, to provide young children with busulfan levels similar to adults levels, pediatric dosing was also increased by about 60% (40 mg/m^2 per dose for a total dose of 640 mg/m^2) over the normal body surface area dosing equivalent to 16 mg/kg. We initially studied seven patients under the age of 6. Expressed as a function of body weight, their median busulfan total dose was 26.4 mg/kg (range 24.3-28.2). Using this body surface area-derived dosing, young children had busulfan levels similar to those in adults. Nonfatal VOD developed in one patient, but with no life-threatening regimen-related toxicity. Although this approach in young children provided busulfan levels that were closer to adult levels, substantial variation in busulfan levels was still seen.

PHARMACOKINETICS OF OTHER DRUGS USED IN BONE MARROW TRANSPLANTATION CONDITIONING REGIMENS

Although less information is available about other drugs used in BMT conditioning regimens, pharmacokinetic monitoring may now have important implications for all drugs used in BMT conditioning regimens. Cyclophosphamide is the most commonly used drug in BMT conditioning regimens. Not only is it a potent antineoplastic agent that can be safely and significantly dose escalated, but also its powerful immunosuppressive effects make it indispensable for inducing allogeneic graft tolerance. Studying cyclophosphamide pharmacokinetics has been complicated by the fact that its cytotoxicity is caused not directly by the parent compound, but by an unstable derivative, 4-hydroxycyclophosphamide. Nevertheless, the pharmacokinetics of high-dose cyclophosphamide appear to provide useful clinical information.

Acute cardiomyopathy is the dose-limiting nonhematologic toxicity of high-dose cyclophosphamide.[13] However, it has been difficult to directly relate this complication to any specific administered dose of cyclophosphamide.[14] To determine if an association exists between cyclophosphamide pharmacokinetics and cardiac dysfunction, 19 women undergoing autologous BMT for metastatic breast cancer after high-dose cyclophosphamide, thiotepa, and carboplatin were studied.[3] As with high-dose busulfan, wide interpatient variation in cyclophosphamide levels was noted even though cyclophosphamide was administered intravenously; cyclophosphamide levels varied fourfold among patients. Pharmacokinetics revealed an association between the levels of total cyclophosphamide (the inactive parent compound) and cardiac toxicity.[3] Congestive heart failure occurred in six patients; these patients had a significantly lower AUC for cyclophosphamide (median 2,888 μmol/L/hour) than did the 13 patients who did not develop heart failure (median 6,121 μmol/L/hour). The six patients who developed heart failure also exhibited a more durable tumor response (median duration 22 months) than did the other 13 patients (median duration 5.25 months). These data suggested that lower levels of the inactive parent compound resulted from enhanced activation, with both greater toxicity and tumor cytotoxicity. Furthermore, like busulfan, cyclophosphamide levels displayed substantial interpatient variability and predicted outcome.

A retrospective analysis of 38 patients undergoing autologous BMT after high-dose cyclophosphamide, cisplatin, and BCNU also showed a strong correlation between BCNU pharmacokinetics and toxicity.[2] The AUC of BCNU varied more than 10-fold among patients, again despite the fact that BCNU was administered intravenously. Acute lung injury, the dose-limiting nonhematologic toxicity of BCNU, developed in 20 of 38 patients. Of these 20 patients, 12 had a BCNU AUC over 600 μg/ml/min, whereas only 2 of 18 patients without lung injury had an AUC above this value. Thus, 12 of 14 patients with a BCNU AUC over 600 μg/ml/min developed lung injury.

THERAPEUTIC MONITORING OF HIGH-DOSE BUSULFAN

Multiple studies (summarized above) demonstrate that the pharmacokinetics of high-dose chemotherapy used in BMT conditioning regimens correlate with toxicity.[1-3,8,9] Not surprisingly, evidence also indicates that antitumor effect also correlates with BMT conditioning regimen pharmacokinetics.[3] Moreover, wide interpatient variability in exposure to these agents exists even when administered intravenously. This interpatient variability is of particular concern because of the narrow therapeutic ratio and hence the high incidence of life-threatening toxicity associated with BMT conditioning regimens. Strategies aimed at more uniform drug exposure should reduce the incidence of toxicity associated with high-dose chemotherapy and BMT. However, the basis for the variability in drug levels among patients is unknown. Therefore, individualization of drug dosing offers the only real prospect for providing uniform drug exposure in patients receiving BMT conditioning regimens.

To establish the use of therapeutic monitoring in patients receiving BMT conditioning regimens, we began a prospective trial of individualized busulfan dose adjustment in patients undergoing BMT after conditioning with busulfan and cyclophosphamide.[15] Pharmacokinetic studies were performed after the first dose of busulfan. Patients with a busulfan AUC more than 1 standard deviation either above or below the median received dose-adjusted busulfan for the fifth through sixteenth doses. Repeat pharmacokinetic studies were performed after the fifth dose of busulfan to document the success of dose adjustment. Individualized dosing of busulfan was successful in that the AUC for busulfan was normalized to within 1 standard deviation of the median in virtually every patient who was dose modified. The overall incidence of VOD was markedly reduced especially in patients whose busulfan dose was decreased because of initially high levels. Moreover, dose escalation in those patients whose initial levels were low could be performed safely, as none of these patients developed life-threatening VOD.

CONCLUSIONS

Bone marrow transplantation is effective in patients with high-risk hematologic malignancies and is probably the treatment of choice in patients with these diseases at relapse. Autologous BMT has also shown promising preliminary results in drug-responsive solid tumors such as breast, ovarian, and testicular cancer. However, the toxicity resulting from high-dose BMT conditioning regimens is substantial and has restricted more universal application of this approach.

Knowledge of the pharmacokinetics of drugs used in very high-dose BMT conditioning regimens holds great promise for improving the outcome of BMT. Wide interpatient variations in handling these drugs make drug dosing on the basis of either weight or body surface area an inadequate means of establishing uniform drug exposure among patients. Therapeutic monitoring of drugs used in BMT conditioning regimens appears to decrease the incidence and mortality of nonhematologic regimen-related toxicities such as venocclusive disease. Perhaps as importantly, this approach has allowed safe increases in drug doses for previously "undertreated" patients. Thus, therapeutic monitoring should produce improved results in patients undergoing BMT by both decreasing treatment-related toxicity and improving antitumor activity. Busulfan therapeutic monitoring has become the standard of care at our institution. Ongoing studies should allow a similar statement to be made for cyclophosphamide in the near future.

REFERENCES

1. GROCHOW, L. B., R. J. JONES, R. B. BRUNDRETT, H. G. BRAINE, T-L. CHEN, R. SARAL, G. W. SANTOS & O. M. COLVIN. 1989. Pharmacokinetics of busulfan: Correlation with veno-occlusive disease in patients undergoing bone marrow transplantation. Cancer Chemother. Pharmacol. **25:** 55–61.

2. JONES, R. B., S. MATTHES, E. J. SHPALL, J. H. FISHER, S. M. STEMMER, C. DUFTON, J. K. STEPHENS & S. I. BEARMAN. 1993. Acute lung injury following treatment with high-dose cyclophosphamide, cisplatin, and carmustine: Pharmacodynamic evaluation of carmustine. J. Natl. Cancer Inst. **85:** 640-647.

3. AYASH, L. J., J. E. WRIGHT, O. TRETYAKOV, R. GONIN, A. ELIAS, C. WHEELER, J. P. EDER, A. ROSOWSKY, K. ANTMAN & E. FREI, III. 1992. Cyclophosphamide pharmacokinetics: Correlation with cardiac toxicity and tumor response. J. Clin. Oncol. **10:** 995-1000.

4. PETERS, W. P., W. D. HENNER, L. B. GROCHOW, G. OLSEN, S. EDWARDS, H. STANBUCK, A. STUART, J. GOCKERMAN, J. MOORE, R. C. BAST, JR., H. F. SEIGLER & O. M. COLVIN. 1987. Clinical and pharmacologic effects of high dose single agent busulfan with autologous bone marrow support in the treatment of solid tumors. Cancer Res. **47:** 6402-6406.

5. JONES, R. J., K. S. K. LEE, W. E. BESCHORNER, V. G. VOGEL, L. B. GROCHOW, H. G. BRAINE, G. B. VOGELSANG, L. L. SENSENBRENNER, G. W. SANTOS & R. SARAL. 1987. Venoocclusive disease of the liver following bone marrow transplantation. Transplantation **44:** 778-783.

6. MCDONALD, G. B., P. SHARMA, D. E. MATTHEWS, H. M. SHULMAN & E. D. THOMAS. 1964. Venocclusive disease of the liver after bone marrow transplantation: Diagnosis, incidence, and predisposing factors. Hepatology **4:** 116-122.

7. GROCHOW, L. B., W. KRIVIT, C. B. WHITLEY & B. BLAZAR. 1990. Busulfan disposition in children. Blood **75:** 1723-1727.

8. HASSAN, M., P. LJUNGMAN, P. BOLME, O. RINGDEN, Z. SYRUCKOVA, A. BEKASSY, J. STARY, I. WALLIN & N. KALLBERG. 1994. Busulfan bioavailability. Blood **84:** 2144-2150.

9. VASSAL, G., A. FISCHER, D. CHALLINE, I. BOLAND, F. LEDHEIST, S. LEMERLE, E. VILMER, C. RAHIMY, G. SOUILLET, E. GLUCKMAN, G. MICHEL, A. DEROUSSENT & A. GOUYETTE. 1993. Busulfan disposition below the age of three: Alteration in children with lysosomal storage disease. Blood **82:** 1030-1034.

10. EVANS, W. E., M. V. RELLING, S. DE GRAAF, J. H. RODMAN, J. A. PIEPER, M. L. CHRISTENSEN & W. R. CROM. 1989. Hepatic drug clearance in children: Studies with indocyanine green as a model substrate. J. Pharm. Sci. **78:** 452-456.

11. YEAGER, A. M., J. E. WAGNER, M. L. GRAHAM, R. J. JONES, G. W. SANTOS & L. B. GROCHOW. 1992. Optimization of busulfan dosage in children undergoing bone marrow transplantation: A pharmacokinetic study of dose escalation. Blood **80:** 2425-2428.

12. MORSELLI, P. L., R. FRANCO-MORSELLI & L. BOSSI. 1980. Clinical pharmacokinetics in newborns and infants. Age related differences and therapeutic implications [Review]. Clin. Pharmacokinet. **5:** 485-527.

13. GOLDBERG, M. A., J. H. ANTIN, E. C. GUINAN & J. M. RAPPEPORT. 1986. Cyclophosphamide cardiotoxicity: An analysis of dosing as a risk factor. Blood **68:** 1114-1118.

14. HERTENSTEIN, B., M. STEFANIC, T. SCHMEISER, M. SCHOLZ, V. GOLLER, M. CLAUSEN, D. BUNJES, M. WIESNETH, J. NOVOTNY, M. KOCHS, W.-E. ADAM, H. HEIMPEL & R. ARNOLD. 1994. Cardiac toxicity of bone marrow transplantation: Predictive value of cardiologic evaluation before transplant. J. Clin. Oncol. **12:** 998-1004.

15. GROCHOW, L. B. 1993. Busulfan disposition: The role of therapeutic monitoring in bone marrow transplantation induction regimens. Semin. Oncol. **20:** (Suppl. 4): 18-25.

Detection of Minimal Residual Disease in Hematopoietic Tissues[a]

J. G. SHARP,[b] M. BISHOP,[c] W. C. CHAN,[d]
T. GREINER,[d] S. S. JOSHI,[b] A. KESSINGER,[c] E. REED,[c]
W. SANGER,[e] S. TARANTOLO,[c] M. TRAYSTMAN,[d]
AND J. VOSE [c]

[b]Departments of Cell Biology and Anatomy,
[c]Internal Medicine,
[d]Pathology/Microbiology,
and
[e]Pediatrics
University of Nebraska Medical Center
Omaha, Nebraska 68198-6395

The concept of minimal disease or minimal residual disease (MRD) was originally developed to explain treatment failure in leukemia,[1] particularly in the context of high dose therapy and allogeneic transplantation. The few remaining leukemic cells in the normal-appearing bone marrow of patients in clinical complete remission that were undetectable by techniques available at the time were believed to be the source of subsequent relapses.[1] In subsequent studies, occult tumor cells in hematopoietic tissues, detected by techniques such as molecular and immunologic methods in acute leukemia,[2] molecular and culture methods in lymphoma,[3–6] or culture and/or immunocytochemistry in breast cancer[7–9] and lung cancer,[10] were statistically associated with a poorer clinical outcome. This was demonstrated in patients in whom bone marrow or blood autografts containing occult tumor cells were transplanted after high dose therapy for cancer[5,6,11] and in nontransplanted patients in whom occult tumor in blood or bone marrow predicted subsequent relapse.[9,12–14]

The application of molecular techniques such as Southern analysis to detect clonality of lymphoid populations in leukemia and lymphoma and polymerase chain reaction (PCR) to identify translocations[2,15] such as *bcl-2* in follicular lymphomas[5] and *bcr-abl* in chronic myelogenous leukemia[16] has increased the sensitivity of occult tumor detection, but clinical correlations establishing the significance of positivity at such sensitive levels are limited.[2] Often, chronic myelogenous leukemia cells positive for the *bcr-abl* translocation detected by the PCR can be found in the marrow of patients who are in a state of clinical and cytogenetic remission in the first few months following allogeneic transplantation. However, persistence of such cells beyond 6 months has indicated a higher likelihood of relapse.[17,18] An increasing

[a]These studies were supported by the National Institutes of Health (grants CA61453 and NCI P30 CA36727), the Nebraska Department of Health (LB 506 and LB 595 funds), and the American Cancer Society.

proportion of *bcr-abl* positive cells over time has presaged relapse, but PCR-negative patients occasionally have had a relapse. Conversely, patients in clinical complete remission long-term may continue to have PCR-positive cells in marrow.[19,20] Studies of changes in the frequency of detectable MRD in such patients hint at the mechanisms of maintenance of posttransplantation complete remissions and suggest that precursor or "stem" cells of the malignant clone may be present without actively producing progeny. Such quiescence might be maintained by microenvironmental or growth factor influences or by immunologic mechanisms, because immunosuppression can lead to expansion of the malignant clone and cessation of immunosuppression can produce its death.[21] Infusion of donor leukocytes into allogeneic recipients has eliminated PCR-positive cells. Similar phenomena appeared to occur in myeloma[22] and virus-associated lymphomas,[23] but these diseases are less well studied than is chronic myelogenous leukemia. Recently, Brenner and colleagues,[24,25] using retroviral mediated transfer of marker genes to hematopoietic harvests destined for autologous transplantation, provided formal proof that tumor cells inadvertently reinfused with hematopoietic cells can be a source of disease relapse.

For this review, two forms of minimal disease are considered: (1) minimal disease in the patient that survived high dose therapy, and (2) minimal disease in hematopoietic harvests transplanted to restore hematopoiesis following high dose therapy which may cause tumor relapse. Both forms of minimal disease can be detected by the techniques to be described; both can lead to relapse and both may predict outcome after high dose therapy and transplantation. Following allogeneic transplantation, inasmuch as the stem cells are from a normal donor, the only source of relapse is tumor cells surviving therapy. In autologous transplantation the source of relapse may be either tumor that survives high dose therapy or tumor cells in the infused harvest. A current problem is to determine the relative contribution to relapse of minimal disease in the patient versus minimal disease in the harvest. The optimal approaches to the solution of this dilemma depend on whether the problem lies with the harvest, for which *ex vivo* manipulation might provide a solution, or with the patient, for whom additional therapeutic interventions such as immunotherapy or cytokine therapy should be considered in the posttransplant period. Early intervention when the extent of residual disease is minimal seems most likely to be effective, emphasizing the need for rapid, sensitive, and relevant methods of MRD detection.

This review centers around the application of state-of-the-art molecular techniques to detect minimal lymphoma and leukemia. This is illustrated by a comparison of the extent of MRD in bone marrow versus blood stem cells for transplantation in non-Hodgkin's lymphoma and the use of an oligonucleotide for purging chronic myelogenous leukemia cells from hematopoietic harvests. A comparison of immuno-cytochemical versus PCR methods of detecting cytokeratins in breast cancer cells is also presented, followed by a discussion of the future challenges in MRD detection and treatment of malignancies.

DETECTION OF MINIMAL LYMPHOMAS, MYELOMAS, AND LEUKEMIAS WITH KNOWN TRANSLOCATIONS

General approaches to the detection of these tumor cell types are similar. They fall into two categories, and both use PCR analysis with primer pairs that amplify across translocated sequences unique to the disease in question, such as *myc*-immuno-globulin genes in Burkitt's lymphoma, *bcl*-2 immunoglobulin genes in follicular lymphoma, or *bcr-abl* translocation in chronic myelogenous leukemia. Potential applications of this technique continue to increase as more of the translocations that underlie the development of acute myelogenous and acute lymphocytic leukemias are defined. The second approach to tumors of T- or B-cell lineage is the detection of neoplastic clones based on the specific immunoglobulin heavy chain gene (J_H) or T-cell receptor (TCR-β, -γ, or -δ) of the malignant clone. T-cell receptor gamma gene rearrangements are most frequently used to identify tumor-specific primers and probes for detecting MRD.[26–28] T-cell receptor rearrangements with TCR-δ and TCR-β are also used. In our laboratory, TCR-γ gene rearrangements have been identified by denaturing gradient gel electrophoresis. In denaturing gradient gel electrophoresis, the PCR products have incorporated a 40-basepair GC-clamp at the 5′ end of one primer. Incorporation of the GC-clamp enables high-resolution separation of each specific T-cell gene rearrangement present in the samples. Because denaturing gradient gel electrophoresis separates DNA strands primarily on the basis of sequence rather than length, it facilitates recovery of the clonal fragment for direct sequencing of the PCR product. This allows for two approaches to MRD detection. A sensitivity of 0.1% or 1 in 1,000 cells can be attained by analyzing the sample in question in a lane adjacent to a diagnostic tumor amplification with a known TCR-γ gene rearrangement.[29] Additional sensitivity approaching one tumor cell in 10^5-10^6 nucleated cells can be attained by sequencing the initial TCR-γ gene rearrangement to produce a tumor-specific primer from the unique junctional sequence.[29] Additionally, B-cell neoplasms can be detected using PCR to detect cells with a specific complementarity determinant region (CDRIII).[30] The CDRIII where the V_H, D, and J_H segments of the IgH gene are joined during gene rearrangement is unique for each individual B cell.[31] This region has therefore been widely used as a tumor-specific marker for the detection of residual B-lineage neoplasia. The general approach involves amplification of the CDRIII of the original tumor using primers flanking the region. This set of primers is not specific for the tumor clone, but because tumor cells are the dominant population, most products are tumor derived. The tumor-specific CDRIII product can be purified and its unique sequence determined. From this unique sequence, tumor-specific primers and probes that will only hybridize with tumor CDRIII can be designed and used to detect residual tumor cells at high sensitivity levels.[32]

When applying IgH CDRIII PCR amplification to DNA extracted from either fresh tumor or paraffin block, it is advisable to examine the sample morphologically to ensure that tumor is indeed being amplified. In our experience, fresh tumor is the best starting material because it has only been possible to obtain CDRIII sequences in about 60-70% of patients when paraffin blocks are employed as the starting material. Additionally, unfixed material is amenable to amplification by primer sets for IgH amplification of additional conserved regions in the J_H gene.

Serial dilution studies have established that lymphoma cells can be detected at a frequency of 1 in 10^4-10^5 nucleated cells by this approach.[32] The PCR technique apparently is more sensitive than previously described Southern analysis or culture techniques (FIG. 1).

Polymerase chain reaction amplification of *bcl*-2 translocations on the IgH CDRIII is being employed to compare levels of tumor contamination in granulocyte colony-stimulating factor (G-CSF) mobilized blood stem cell harvests versus bone marrow harvests in a prospective randomized study of these modalities for restoration of hematopoiesis in patients with intermediate or high grade non-Hodgkin's lymphoma[33] and to determine if the existence of MRD is predictive of outcome. In addition, by comparing blood obtained before chemotherapy and/or cytokine mobilization to the mobilized apheresis harvest and to blood obtained subsequently, the question of whether cytokine mobilizes breast tumor cells into the blood[34] along with hematopoietic stem and progenitor cells and other normal cells, as suggested by the study of Brugger *et al.*,[35] may be answerable. This issue may be difficult to unravel, because we detected tumor cells in the blood before cytokine administration, but the leukapheresis harvest subsequently was negative on direct examination. When this apheresis harvest was cultured, tumor again became evident. Tumor becomes more apparent because culture leads to loss of normal cells by apoptosis and differentiation. Normal hematopoietic cells mobilized by the cytokine may have diluted out tumor cells in the apheresis harvest to levels below the limit of detection. In other instances, the leukapheresis harvest was positive in situations in which blood obtained before cytokine administration was negative, suggesting that mobilization of tumor cells had occurred. Similar observations have been made with myeloma.[36] No prospective studies are currently available on the clinical risks of infusing cytokine-mobilized tumor cells. However, a retrospective analysis was performed in two groups of patients with low grade lymphoma who received either nonmobilized or mobilized blood stem cells after similar high dose therapy regimens. No differences in progression-free survival between the two groups were found, suggesting that if low grade lymphoma cells had been mobilized by cytokine, their infusion was not clinically significant.[37] Clearly the issue of the clinical relevance of mobilized tumor cells will require time to resolve.

To determine if MRD in the patient or MRD in the harvest is most important, insight can be gained by comparing samples from patients after infusion of tumor-positive or tumor-negative harvests.[5,38] In patients with lymphoma undergoing high dose therapy and receiving immunologically purged marrow, the inability to purge residual lymphoma cells was the most important prognostic indicator of relapse. The inability to purge residual lymphoma was not associated with the degree of bone marrow involvement or the previous response to therapy. In our own studies of the outcome of patients with non-Hodgkin's lymphoma undergoing high dosage therapy and autologous transplantation, we compared recipients with histologically positive bone marrow who received tumor-negative blood stem cell transplantation with recipients with histologically negative bone marrow, some of whom in retrospect received minimally contaminated marrow transplants and some of whom received tumor-negative transplants. Extrapolated to 5 years with a median follow-up of 3 years, the proportion of patients who achieved complete remission at 100 days and who were still disease-free was respectively 58%, 50%, and 17%.[39] Thus, regardless of whether the marrow was histologically positive, recipients of tumor-negative harvests had disease-free survival of 55-60% at 5 years, but survival of the recipients of minimally contaminated marrow was only 20%. This suggests that about 40% of relapses arose from disease surviving high dose therapy and about 40% from reinfused tumor and that in the autologous setting, the contributions of minimal disease (in both patient and harvest) may be equivalent. These results also predict that the maximum benefit that might be derived from *ex vivo* manipulation of the harvest (purging) is a 40% improvement in disease-free survival and 40% of patients would still have a relapse. Consequently, improvement in the methods of delivering high dose therapy in the autologous setting and the development of additional therapies targeting MRD posttransplantation are still important objectives.

APPLICATIONS OF TECHNIQUES TO DETECT MINIMAL LEUKEMIC CELLS

In chronic myelogenous leukemia, acute lymphoblastic leukemia, and myeloma, studies of outcome suggest that the absence of PCR-detectable tumor cells in marrow after transplantation is a good prognostic sign. In allotransplantation, if this status is not achieved by the transplant, infusion of donor leukocytes,[23] and for chronic myelogenous leukemia treatment with immunotherapy,[40] interferon,[41] or G-CSF,[42] has brought about this state. Although about 50-60% long-term disease-free survival can be achieved in acute myelogenous leukemia treated with high dose therapy and infusion of unpurged autologous marrow, especially from patients who have under- gone consolidation therapy, purging of the hematopoietic stem cell source may be of benefit. Currently, favorable clinical results are still limited to small subgroups of patients,[43] but trends towards a broader benefit are becoming evident.[44]

PURGING OF MINIMAL RESIDUAL DISEASE AND POSITIVE SELECTION OF STEM CELLS

A variety of purging approaches have been attempted, many of which use cytotoxic agents (chemopurging).[43] The major disadvantage to effective chemopurging is that normal progenitor cells as well as tumor cells are killed in the harvest. This may be significant, because we believe rapid restoration of hematopoiesis and immune recov- ery are important to the outcome. As an alternative, the use of oligonucleotides complementary to the mRNA of chimeric genes transcribed from translocated genes of the tumor cells[45] or upregulated cell cycle genes of the tumor has been proposed.[46,47] Theoretically, cytotoxicity using such oligonucleotides is limited to tumor cells that are killed by induction of apoptosis.[48] Normal hematopoietic progenitor cells that are not transcribing the targeted mRNA sequences are spared. An example of the use of *in situ* hybridization to detect chronic myelogenous leukemia cells[49] in hematopoietic harvests is shown in FIGURE 2 and RT-PCR for *bcr-abl* positive cellular DNA to monitor the purging of chronic myelogenous leukemia cells by an oligonucleotide complementary to *brc-abl* is shown in FIGURE 3. In the *in situ* hybridization approach (FIG. 2) *bcr-abl* translocation was detected using a probe mixture from Oncor ac- cording to the procedure supplied by the manufacturer, with slight modifications. The *bcr* gene was detected using FITC/Avidin (green-G) and the *abl* gene by rhoda- mine-labeled anti-digoxigenin (red-R). Because these genes are paired and on different chromosomes in normal metaphases, the visible paired dots of the same color of fluorescence are separated. In chronic myelogenous leukemia cells with the *bcr-abl* translocation a pair of closely juxtaposed fusion signals (F) is evident and appears as a mixture of the two colors (FIG. 2). The technique can be applied to both metaphase

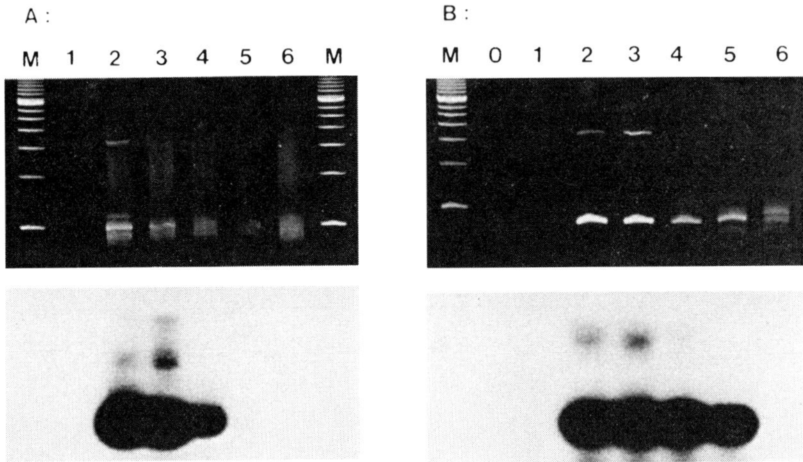

FIGURE 1. A B-cell line, Namalwa, has been used to establish the sensitivity and specificity of tumor detection. The CDRIII sequence of the rearranged IgH gene of this cell line was determined and a tumor-specific primer as well as a tumor-specific probe was designed. Namalwa cells were serially diluted in normal peripheral blood mononuclear cells and extracted DNA was amplified using consensus primers (**A**) and the tumor-specific primer together with primers to the J_H segment (**B**). The amplified product was electrophoresed and transferred to a nylon membrane which was hybridized with the tumor-specific probe labeled with ^{32}P (lane M-100 bp molecular weight marker; (1) placental DNA; (2-6) 10-fold dilutions of Namalwa cell line DNA starting at 1 : 10 on lane 2). Tumor cells were detectable to a dilution of 10^{-4} when the tumor-specific primer was used and 10^{-3} when consensus primers were employed, while the negative controls show no detectable signal.

and interphase cells, and the frequency of positive cells can be quantitated by counting. The PCR approach uses the method of Margello *et al.*[50] In these experiments, a known number of chronic myelogenous leukemia cells was mixed with normal human peripheral blood cells, and then the mixture was treated with antisense oligonucleotides to the *bcr-abl* fusion gene-specific region for 36 hours. Treated cells were analyzed for the presence of *bcr-abl*-positive cellular DNA using DNA PCR techniques as we described recently.[48] FIGURE 3 shows the results of these experiments. The mixture of chronic myelogenous leukemia and normal cells treated with *bcr-abl* antisense oligonucleotides showed significantly decreased PCR-amplified bands, particularly the lower molecular weight band (lane B), when compared to the untreated control cell mixture (lane A) or the mixture of cells treated with sense oligonucleotides of the same length (lane C). It is much more difficult to perform quantitative PCR. Because of the effort and intrinsic uncertainty involved in quantitating minimal numbers of chronic myelogenous leukemia cells among many normal cells by *in situ* hybridization, the PCR technique is probably more sensitive and practical for detection purposes. However, the two techniques complement each other.

An alternative approach to purging tumor cells employs positive stem cell selection based on the CD34 marker.[51-53] The potential concerns with this approach are that it

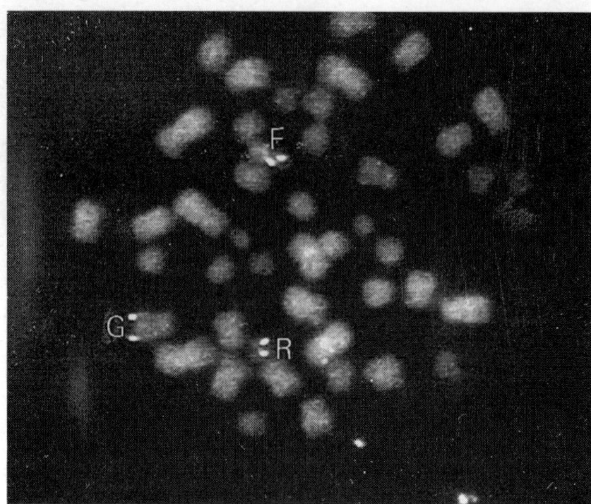

FIGURE 2. Detection of a chronic myelogenous leukemia cell using *in situ* hybridization probes for the *bcr* and *abl* genes. In the original color preparation the *bcr* probe fluoresces green (G) and the *abl* probe red (R). In addition to the pairs of green and red dots, a closely juxtaposed pair of fusion signals (F) appear as a mixture of the two colors, indicating the *bcr-abl* gene created by translocation. Although this illustration depicts a metaphase nucleus, the technique is also applicable to interphase nuclei.

cannot be employed for leukemia cells that express the CD34 antigen, although the use of other markers (Thyl) might circumvent this problem.[54] Additionally, it might also deplete antitumor cytotoxic cells or their precursors or other cells involved in immune reconstitution of the recipient.[55] If these cells are involved in the control of MRD in the early posttransplantation period, as they might be in chronic myelogenous leukemia, the advantage of reducing the burden of reinfused tumor cells by positive stem cell selection may be compromised or lost.

DETECTION OF BREAST CANCER CELLS

Over the last several years immunocytochemistry has become the standard method for detection of breast cancer cells in hematopoietic tissues.[9] The immunocytochemistry approach, which we prefer, employs CAM 5.2, a murine monoclonal antibody specific for human cytokeratin proteins 8 and 18, and the MAK 6 antibody cocktail which detects cytokeratin proteins 8, 14, 15, 16, 18, and 19. This assay is used routinely by our pathology department to evaluate bone marrow biopsies from patients with breast cancer. The mononuclear cell fraction is separated on lymphocyte separation medium and enumerated as previously described,[56] an aliquot is removed for PCR analysis, and remaining cells are deposited on slides using a Shandon cytospin centrifuge. The slides are fixed in cold acetone for 10 minutes, air dried, and stored at –20°C for batch processing with appropriate controls (known positive and negative

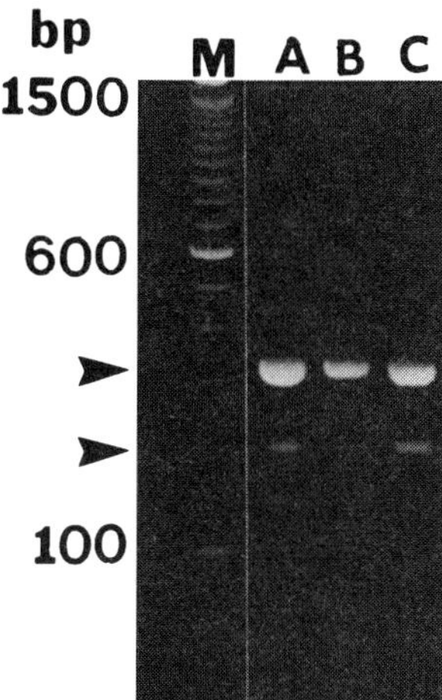

FIGURE 3. The successful purging of chronic myelogenous leukemia cells from a hematopoietic harvest employing an oligonucleotide complementary (antisense) to [*bcr-abl*]. There is a significant decrease of the *bcr-abl* product in the antisense oligonucleotide-treated sample (*lane B*). *Arrows* indicate the two different-sized PCR products obtained using the *bcr-abl*-specific primers.

cells as well as antibody isotype controls). The slides are stained by standard immunocytochemical procedures employing the glucose oxidase method.[57] The detection of breast tumor cells in bone marrow by immunocytochemistry in several studies of nontransplanted patients was associated with a poorer outcome.[14] In the transplant situation, only limited studies of patients have been reported, largely all patients with metastatic disease. None of the recipients of stem cell grafts that we determined retrospectively to be contaminated with immunocytochemistry-detected tumor cells were long-term survivors. Unfortunately, progression in autotransplanted patients with metastatic breast cancer is rapid, and with current treatment regimens only approximately 20% experience long-term (3 years) disease-free survival.[11] This suggests that current preparative regimens for patients with extensive and/or resistant disease are inadequate, and most relapses occur from tumor cells that survive high dose therapy. The outcome of patients with earlier stages of disease currently undergoing high dose therapy and transplantation will likely be more informative as to the role of MRD detection in breast cancer.

The immunocytochemistry approach can be supplemented if the cells in question are cultured before assay. A short-term clonal culture method was employed by Ross *et al.*[8] and the colonies obtained were then stained by immunocytochemistry. A long-term culture method was used by Sharp *et al.*[7,58] In the latter situation, the period of culture amplifies both the relative and the absolute numbers of tumor cells present, probably because normal hematopoietic cells differentiate and are lost from the cultures and tumor cells replicate in the cultures. In a preliminary study, the frequency of immunocytochemistry-detected breast tumor cells in four hematopoietic harvests examined directly was 0.5 ± 1 tumor cell/10^5 nucleated cells. After 8-10 weeks of culture the frequency of immunocytochemistry-positive cells had risen to 43 ± 22 tumor cells/10^5 nucleated cells, an average 86-fold increase which is compatible with the 2 log increase predicted from calibration studies.[57]

Recently a PCR technique to detect breast cancer cells was introduced based on their expression of cytokeratin 19 (CK 19) mRNA.[59,60] Using the RT-PCR technique, Datta *et al.*[59] were the first to analyze blood or bone marrow from 34 patients with stages I-IV breast cancer and 39 control patients without breast cancer. Results showed that 4 of 19 patients (21%) with stage IV breast cancer and 5 of 6 (83%) with histologically negative bone marrow biopsies after adjuvant chemotherapy and before autologous bone marrow transplantation were positive for the CK 19 transcript by the RT-PCR technique. Briefly, RNA is extracted from the sample suspected to contain breast tumor cells. A nested primer set is employed in RT-PCR to detect CK 19 transcripts. The initial product is 1069 bp and the ultimate product 745 bp. This PCR method can detect 1 tumor cell in 10^6 hematopoietic cells, but it does not always do so. Statistical variations inherent in low frequency event analysis or whether or not all tumor cells are transcribing CK 19 mRNA may both have an impact on the reproducibility of the assay.

Immunocytochemistry and PCR techniques are currently being compared on harvests from consecutive breast cancer patients and in a multicenter study of breast cancer cell detection sponsored by the International Society for Hematotherapy and Graft Engineering (ISHAGE). When the frequency of tumor cells is greater than 1 in 10^5 nucleated cells, the results of immunocytochemistry and PCR techniques applied directly to the harvests correspond (FIG. 4a and b). However, direct immunocytochemistry studies of 10 PCR-positive patients indicated that only one was positive at a level of 2 breast tumor cells/10^5 nucleated cells. When harvests were cultured, most cultures were then immunocytochemistry-positive, although not all harvests grew in culture. This illustrates a limitation of the immunocytochemistry technique, because even when 100,000 cells are screened, tumor contamination can be missed. This suggests that the PCR technique to detect breast cancer cells is more sensitive than the immunocytochemistry technique when applied directly to hematopoietic harvests and at least as sensitive as culture combined with immunocytochemistry. However, as the RT-PCR approach currently only detects cytokeratin 19 which is not detected by the CAM 5.2 antibody often employed in immunocytochemistry, then the correspondence of RT-PCR and immunocytochemistry depends on the coexpression of cytokeratin 19. Additional methodologic development is clearly required. The correlation of the presence of tumor cells detected by the PCR technique with clinical outcome is currently being evaluated; however, emphasis has been on early stage patients undergoing high dose therapy and autotransplantation, and fortunately to date, none of the patients evaluated has relapsed.

MINIMAL RESIDUAL DISEASE IN BLOOD VERSUS BONE MARROW

Debate has been increasing as to the relative merits of employing cytokine-mobilized blood versus bone marrow for autologous hematopoietic reconstitution

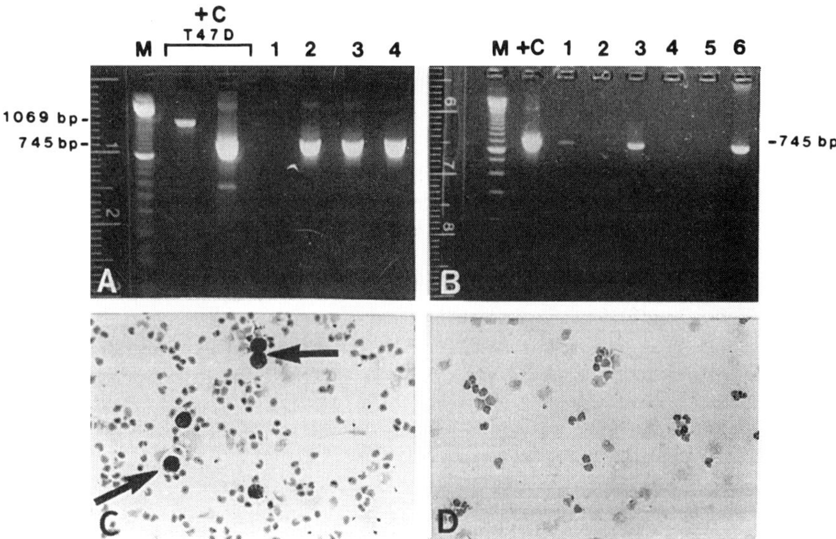

FIGURE 4. The application of RT-PCR to detect cytokeratin 19 transcript and immunocyto-chemistry employing the CAM 5.2 antibody to detect cytokeratins 8 and 18 in breast cancer cells. (**A**) This ethidium bromide–stained minigel shows the amplification products from the outer primer (1,069-bp product) and the nested primers (745-bp product). *Lane M* shows a 100-bp molecular weight marker. *Lanes +C* show the two different-sized CK 19 PCR products obtained from the positive control sample, T47D, a human mammary breast carcinoma cell line. *Lanes 1-4* represent the results on test samples. *Lanes 1-3* represent apheresis samples and *lane 4* is a blood sample. Sample 1 is negative; samples 2-4 show the 745-bp amplification product. (**B**) This ethidium bromide–stained minigel shows nested PCR results on six test samples from five patients. *Lane M* is a 100-bp molecular weight marker. *Lane +C* is the T47D-positive control. *Lanes 1 and 3* are blood stem cell harvests, both of which are positive. *Lanes 2 and 4* are bone marrow aspirates for which *lane 2* is negative and *lane 4* faintly positive. *Lanes 5 and 6* from the same patient are bone marrow harvests obtained at different times, the first of which was negative (*lane 5*) and the second positive (*lane 6*). **Immunocyto-chemistry Analysis:** (**C**) Low power (100X) view of a field containing positively stained breast carcinoma cells (*arrows*) obtained from an apheresis sample that was positive by RT-PCR for the CK 19 transcript (see sample 3 in **A**). This immunocytochemistry result was obtained by staining the preparation using a complex including monoclonal antibody CAM 5.2 with avidin-biotin-glucose-oxidase in the presence of nitroblue tetrazolium. (**D**) Low power (100X) view from a cytospin slide prepared from an apheresis sample which was negative by RT-PCR for CK 19 transcript (see sample 1 in **A**).

after high dose therapy.[61] Consequently, the relative MRD status of these two tissues has become an issue.[62] The approach of immunocytochemistry and culture has been used to compare blood stem cell harvests versus bone marrow harvests of breast cancer patients.[8,12] The studies suggested that blood stem cell harvests may be less contaminated and/or less frequently contaminated than bone marrow harvests.[63] Similar findings were noted in non-Hodgkin's lymphoma.[64] These observations were controversial, because other studies noted that if marrow was contaminated, so was blood.[66] More recently, several studies support the notion that blood may have lower levels of MRD in non-Hodgkin's lymphoma or leukemia.[38,67] Similar observations were made in myeloma[68] and neuroblastoma.[69,70] Resolution of this issue would clearly influence future choices of stem cell product for hematopoietic reconstitution. With the culture technique, factors other than frequency could be important, including the ability of the tumor cells to grow in the culture system and the potential for immune cells to "kill" tumor cells during the culture period. Apheresis products apparently have greater intrinsic cytotoxic properties than do bone marrow harvests.[71] Cytokine-mobilized apheresis products can have a significant content of activated large granular lymphocytes after several weeks of culture. Consequently, tumor cells in the original harvest may be eliminated by a period of culture, and this has been observed in leukemia[72,73] although the mechanism is unclear. This topic merits more thorough evaluation.

FUTURE CHALLENGES IN DETECTION OF MINIMAL RESIDUAL DISEASE

A significant challenge in MRD detection is to extend the application of modern cellular and molecular techniques to other tumor types including leukemias for which the molecular defects are known. Immunocytochemistry has been developed and applied in lung,[10,74] colon,[75] and gastric cancers.[76] Other candidate tumors for study are melanoma and carcinomas of the ovary, cervix, and prostate. Detection of MRD in hematopoietic tissues may also be a useful indicator of prognosis in diseases for which high dose therapy is not currently advocated. For patients with early stage disease this information might motivate a better selection of patients for adjuvant therapy or further treatment.

Minimal residual disease detection techniques currently emphasize detection of tumor cells based on clonal markers (lymphoma/leukemia) or markers of cellular function unanticipated in the tissue being evaluated (cytokeratin expression of breast cancer cells in blood and bone marrow). Additional characteristics of clinically predictive tumor cells could possibly be evaluated by molecular analysis (PCR) even on small numbers of tumor cells. The potential of this approach may be illustrated by considering an alternative explanation of the observation that 30–40% of histologically normal appearing bone marrow harvests from patients with non-Hodgkin's lymphoma contain lymphoma cells that can be grown in culture.[6] These observations have led to the conclusion that 30–40% of such harvests are minimally contaminated with lymphoma and 60–70% are uncontaminated. However, in an analysis of bone marrow cultures in a small series of patients with low grade lymphoma, over half (57%) were contaminated with lymphoma, which was not unexpected because a significant proportion of such bone marrow harvests are contaminated with cells with clonal translocations of the *bcl-2* gene.[65] However, in a more recent study of patients with an original diagnosis of low grade lymphoma, no cultures of tumor cells from patients with a diagnosis of primary follicular lymphoma could be established. Rather, culture growth was obtained from patients whose lymphoma displayed areas of aggressive histology. Reevaluation of the original series of patients with low grade lymphoma[65] showed that positive cultures were obtained only in patients whose lymphoma contained similar aggressive areas. Therefore, primary follicular lymphomas apparently do not grow in culture, but *in vitro* growth can be obtained once lymphomas show evidence of aggressive histology. Mutations of the p53 gene are associated with progression of low grade lymphoma to higher grade tumors.[77] Other genetic changes may also occur. The wild-type p53 gene detects DNA damage and may induce apoptosis of lymphoma cells with such damage.[78] The mutant p53 gene is associated with failure of lymphomas with DNA damage to undergo apoptosis[79] and also with resistance of tumor cells to chemotherapy.[80] The transfer of cells from physiologic levels of oxygen to higher levels in culture may lead to oxygen radical damage.[81] Conceivably, this could explain why follicular lymphoma cells with wild-type p53 might undergo apoptosis in culture. By contrast, lymphoma cells with mutant p53 might survive and grow. If this were the case, a much greater proportion than 30-40% of non-Hodgkin's lymphoma patient bone marrows might be contaminated with lymphoma cells and be detectable by molecular techniques. However, only 30-40% would grow in culture because this potentially would be the proportion with p53 mutations. The association of p53 mutations with resistance of tumor cells to chemotherapy could explain the ability of lymphoma cell growth in culture to predict the patient's clinical outcome and may be independent of infused tumor cells.[82] In the future, it may be necessary to move studies of MRD beyond simple detection of tumor cells and to define their clinically relevant characteristics.

Currently, MRD detection techniques focus solely on tumor cell detection with little attention to the environment in which such tumor cells grow and metastasize. However, lung tumor cells have an affinity for bone marrow stromal cells.[83,84] Similarly, breast cancer cells appear to interact symbiotically with hematopoietic cells. Multipotential hematopoietic progenitor cells (colony-forming units-granulocyte, erythroid, monocyte, megkarocyte: CFU-GEMM) are more frequent in bone marrow cultures that are minimally contaminated with breast tumor cells than in uncontaminated cultures.[85] In addition, hematopoietic cells cluster around such cells, forming small colonies in the CFU-GEMM assay. Such interactions are potential therapeutic targets in the treatment of MRD. The normal cells from which lymphomas derive, B and T lymphocytes, have very specific ligand-controlled patterns of migration and distribution in the body.[86] The nature of the molecules involved in the interaction of tumor cells with stromal cells of bone marrow and other tissues is only beginning to be defined. Some are adhesion molecules and their ligands. In lymphoma and myeloma, some of the relevant ligands bind to members of the tumor necrosis factor receptor molecule family (CD30 and CD40).[87,88] When lymphoma cells grow in long-term bone marrow cultures, their distribution is not random. Rather, tumor cells associate preferentially with stromal cells. Such cultures generally cannot be passaged by supernatant cells alone. However, if tumor cells and associated stroma are scraped and the aggregate reseeded, the culture usually can be successfully passaged. Even when the most aggressive lymphomas, which grow and passage from supernatant cells, are placed in cultures with appropriate stroma, the lymphoma cells adhere to the stroma and are largely lost from the supernatant.[85] This is also observed when circulating lymphoma cells are placed in culture with stroma and raises the question as to whether stromal abnormalities or competition for "niches" exists in some patients which promotes the dissemination of tumor cells. Lymphoma cells may also alter the stromal cells with which they interact in a symbiotic relationship which facilitates lymphoma growth.

When MRD is inadvertently reinfused at transplantation, these tumor cells may reassociate with stroma at sites of previous tumor growth in the patient. This explains why the sites of relapse in patients suspected of receiving tumor-containing harvests mirror those of prior disease rather than exhibiting a systemic distribution which might be expected of intravenously infused tumor cells.[6] This notion is also compatible with the anecdotal observation that relapses are less common at sites that have been subjected to high doses of local radiation therapy for control of bulk tumor. Potentially, these radiation doses sterilize the stroma and disrupt its ability to attract/interact with reinfused tumor cells. Local radiation therapy could be expanded as an approach to minimizing relapses due to reinfused MRD. The environments in which minimal tumor survives and with which reinfused tumor associates deserve more attention in the evaluation of MRD.

Other unresolved questions more directly related to high dose therapy requiring rescue include the choice of blood or bone marrow as the source of stem cells,[61] whether chemotherapy and/or cytokines employed to mobilize stem/progenitor cells into the circulation increase the risk of relapse,[34] and the circumstances under which tumor cells detected by highly sensitive molecular techniques are clinically relevant.[19] The mobilization of tumor cells into the circulation by chemotherapy and/or cytokines is not a simple problem to quantify especially if the tumor detection technique employs PCR methods that require meticulous technique for accurate quantitation. Both the white blood cell count and the mononuclear cell count in these patients are changing rapidly at the time of cytokine administration. Consequently, any circulating tumor cells present before cytokine administration are diluted by mobilized normal cells, and any mobilized tumor cells are poured into this mixture of everchanging proportions. Conclusions that tumor cells are not mobilized if their relative level stays constant in previously positive harvests should be drawn carefully, because without additional mobilized tumor cells, the addition of normal cells would otherwise diminish the proportion of tumor cells. Quantification of the amount of MRD in an individual patient may need more attention to establish the clinical relevance of MRD. Rather, most studies on MRD have reported the sensitivity levels of their assays, because quantitative PCR is difficult to calibrate. Hetu *et al.*[89] reported a quantitative method that helps mitigate the problems of low frequency, rare event Poisson statistics that impact on MRD. Their calibration curves are based on double-round PCR in which dilutions of the positive first round result can be quantitated in the second round. Variations of this model may become useful in assessing MRD. As noted earlier, even with immunocytochemical approaches, quantitation of low levels of tumor contamination is fraught with difficulties, and therefore only gross mobilization of tumor cells by cytokines may be readily detectable. Because of these inadequacies in our current knowledge and technologies and, in particular, because of our lack of information on the clinical implications of MRD, imposition of regulatory standards based on MRD detection is probably inappropriate at this time, even though the ethical dilemma posed by the possible reinfusion of tumor cells in patients is very real.

ACKNOWLEDGMENTS

We thank our fellows, Drs. G. Q. Wu, G. Wu, and A. G. Wu, and students C. Weekes and B. Murphy for their efforts in support of these studies. It is a pleasure to thank S. Mann, P. Reilly, S. Clausen, R. Wickert, D. Lytle, and E. Zuvanich for excellent technical assistance. The Hem/Onc clinical coordinators provided outstanding support in the collection and distribution of clinical samples. We thank J. Huey who typed the manuscript. A debt of gratitude is acknowledged to all patients who gave freely of their time and tissues and who made these studies possible. We thank the Nebraska Lymphoma Study Group and Leukemia Network for obtaining tissues as well as collecting and maintaining data bases.

REFERENCES

1. HAGENBEEK, A., Y. LU, G. ARKESTEIJN, Y. YING & A. C. M. MARTENS. 1991. Minimal residual disease in acute leukemia: Preclinical studies. *In* New Strategies in Bone Marrow Transplantation. R. Champlin & R. Gale, Eds.: 193-199. Wiley-Liss, Inc. New York.

2. CAMPANA, D. & C. PU. 1995. Detection of minimal residual disease in acute leukemia: Methodologic advances and clinical significance. Blood **85:** 1416-1434.

3. BENJAMIN, D., I. T. MAGRATH, E. C. DOUGLASS & L. M. CORASH. 1983. Derivation of lymphoma cell lines from microscopically normal bone marrow in patients with undifferentiated lymphomas: Evidence of occult bone marrow involvement. Blood **61:** 1017-1019.

4. SMITH, S. D., S. KISKER, L. BUSH & R. C. TRUEWORTHY. 1983. Utilization of a human tumor cloning system to monitor for bone marrow involvement in children with non-Hodgkin's lymphoma. Cancer **53:** 1724-1729.

5. GRIBBEN, J. G., A. S. FREEDMAN, D. NEUBERG, D.C. ROY, K. W. BLAKE, S. D. WOO, M. L. GROSSBARD, S. N. RABINOWE, F. CORAL & G. J. FREEMAN. 1991. Immunologic purging of marrow assessed by PCR before autologous bone marrow transplantation for B-cell lymphoma. N. Engl. J. Med. **325:** 1525-1533.

6. SHARP, J. G., S. S. JOSHI, J. O. ARMITAGE, P. F. COCCIA, D. S. HARRINGTON, A. KESSINGER, D. A. CROUSE, S. L. MANN & D. D. WEISENBURGER. 1992. Significance of detection of occult non-Hodgkin's lymphoma in histologically uninvolved bone marrow by a culture technique. Blood **79:** 1074-1080.

7. SHARP, J. G., S. L. MANN & A. KESSINGER. 1987. Detection of occult breast cancer cells in cultured pretransplantation bone marrow. *In* Autologous Bone Marrow Transplantation, III. K. Dicke, G. Spitzer & S. Jagannath, Eds.: 497-502. The University of Texas, MD Anderson Cancer Center. Houston.

8. ROSS, A. A., B. W. COOPER, H. M. LAZARUS, W. MACKAY, T. J. MOSS, N. CIOBANU, M. S. TALLMAN, M. J. KENNEDY, N. E. DAVIDSON & D. SWEET. 1993. Detection and viability of tumor cells in peripheral blood stem cell collections from breast cancer patients using immunocytochemical and clonogenic assay techniques. Blood **82:** 2605-2610.

9. OSBORNE, M. P. & P. P. ROSEN. 1994. Detection and management of bone marrow micrometastases in breast cancer. Oncology **8:** 25-31.

10. HAY, F. G., A. FORD & R. C. F. LEONARD. 1988. Clinical applications of immunocytochemistry in the monitoring of the bone marrow in small cell lung cancer (SCLC). Int. J. Cancer Suppl. 2: 8-10.

11. SHARP, J. G., A. KESSINGER, J. O. ARMITAGE, P. J. BIERMAN, S. L. MANN, E. C. REED & D. D. WEISENBURGER. 1993. Influence of minimal tumor contamination of hematopoietic harvests on clinical outcome of patients undergoing high-dose therapy and transplanta-

tion. *In* ABMT VI. K. Dicke, A. Keating, N. Gorin, C. Nichols & A. Yeager, Eds.: 223-226. Cancer Treatment Research Education Fund. Arlington, TX.

12. SHARP, J. G., W. P. VAUGHAN, A. KESSINGER, S. L. MANN, J. M. DEBOER, W. G. SANGER & D. D. WEISENBURGER. 1991. Significance of detection of tumor cells in hematopoietic stem cell harvest of patients with breast cancer. *In* Autologous Bone Marrow Transplantation V. K. Dicke, J. Armitage & M. Dicke-Evinger, Eds.: 385-391. University of Nebraska Medical Center. Omaha.

13. KNAUF, W. U., A. D. HO, G. HEGER, D. HOELZER, W. HUNSTEIN & E. THIEL. 1991. Detection of minimal residual disease in adult acute lymphoblastic leukemia by analysis of gene rearrangements and correlation with early relapses. Leukemia Lymphoma **5:** 57-63.

14. DIEL, I. J., M. KAUFMANN, R. GOERNER, S. D. COSTA, S. KAUL & G. BASTERT. 1992. Detection of tumor cells in bone marrow patients with primary breast cancer: A prognostic factor for distant metastasis. J. Clin. Oncol. **10:** 1534-1539.

15. BIONDI, A. & A. RAMBALDI. 1994. Polymerase chain reaction (PCR) approach for the evaluation of minimal residual disease in acute leukemia. Stem Cells **12:** 394-401.

16. CROSS, N. C., L. FENG, J. BUNGEY & J. M. GOLDMAN. 1993. Minimal residual disease after bone marrow transplant for chronic myeloid leukemia detected by the polymerase chain reaction. Leukemia Lymphoma. **11**(Suppl. 1): 39-43.

17. DELAGE, R., R. J. STOIFFER, K. DEAR & J. RITZ. 1991. Clinical significance of *bcr-abl* gene rearrangement detected by polymerase chain reaction after allogeneic bone marrow transplantation in chronic myelogenous leukemia. Blood **78:** 2759-2767.

18. PREUDHOMME, C., E. WATTEL, J. L. LAI, L. MEYER, N. HENIC, M. P. NOEL-WALTER, T. FACON, P. FENAUX, A. COSSON & J. P. JOUET. 1994. High correlation between detection of minimal residual disease (MRD) by polymerase chain reaction (PCR) and relapse in chronic myelogenous leukemia (CML) after allogeneic bone marrow transplantation (BMT). Bone Marrow Transplant. EBMT, p 225.

19. HUGHES, T. P. & J. M. GOLDMAN. 1990. Review: Biological importance of residual leukaemic cells after BMT for CML: Does the polymerase chain reaction help? Bone Marrow Transplant. **5:** 3-6.

20. HUGHES, T. P., G. J. MORGAN, P. MARTIAT & J. M. GOLDMAN. 1991. Detection of residual leukemia after bone marrow transplant for chronic myeloid leukemia: Role of polymerase chain reaction in predicting relapse. Blood **77:** 874-878.

21. KUMAR, L. 1993. Chronic myeloid leukemia: Management of relapse after allogeneic bone marrow transplantation. Leukemia Lymphoma **10:** 165-171.

22. BIRD, J. M., N. H. RUSSELL & D. SAMSON. 1993. Minimal residual disease after bone marrow transplantation for multiple myeloma: Evidence for cure in long-term survivors. Bone Marrow Transplant. **12:** 651-654.

23. PAPADOPOULOS, E. B., M. LADANYI, D. EMANUEL, S. MACKINNON, F. BOULAD, M. H. CARABASI, H. CASTRO-MALASPINA, B. H. CHILDS, A. P. GILLIO, T. N. SMALL, J. W. YOUNG, N. A. KERNAN & J. O'REILY. 1994. Infusions of donor leukocytes to treat Epstein-Barr virus-associated lymphoproliferative disorders after allogeneic bone marrow transplantation. N. Engl. J. Med. **330:** 1185-1191.

24. BRENNER, M. K., D. R. RILL, R. C. MOEN, R. A. KRANCE, J. MIRRO, JR., W. F. ANDERSON & J. N. IHLE. 1993. Gene-marking to trace origin of relapse after autologous bone marrow transplantation. Lancet **341**(8837): 85-86.

25. RILL, D. R., V. M. SANTANA, W. M. ROBERTS, T. NILSON, L. C. BOWMAN, R. A. KRANCE, H. E. HESLOP, R. C. MOEN, J. N. IHLE & M. K. BRENNER. 1994. Direct demonstration that autologous bone marrow transplantation for solid tumors can return a multiplicity of tumorigenic cells. Blood **84:** 380-383.

26. HANSEN-HAGGE, T. E., S. YOKOTA & C. R. BARTRAM. 1989. Detection of minimal residual disease in acute lymphoblastic leukemia by *in vitro* amplification of rearranged T-cell receptor δ sequences. Blood **74:** 1762-1767.

27. TYCO, B., J. D. PALMER, M. P. LINK, S. D. SMITH & J. SKLAR. 1989. Polymerase chain reaction amplification of rearranged antigen receptor genes using junction-specific oligonucleotides: Possible application for detection of minimal residual disease in acute lymphoblastic leukemia. *In* Cancer Cells 7: Molecular Diagnostics of Human Cancer.: 47-52. Cold Spring Harbor Laboratory Press. Cold Spring Harbor, NY.

28. D'AURIOL, L., E. MACINTYRE, F. GALIBERT & F. SIGAUX. 1989. *In vitro* amplification of T cell γ gene rearrangements: A new tool for the assessment of minimal residual disease in acute lymphoblastic leukemias. Leukemia **3:** 155-158.

29. GREINER, T. C., M. R. RAFFELD, C. LUTZ, F. DICK & E. S. JAFFE. 1995. Analysis of T cell receptor-γ gene rearrangements by denaturing gradient gel electrophoresis of GC-clamped PCR products: Correlation with tumor specific sequences. Am. J. Pathol. **136:** 46-55.

30. YAMADA, M., S. HUDSON, O. TOURNAY, S. BITTENBENDER, S. S. SHANE, B. LANGE, Y. TSUJIMOTO, A. J. CATON & G. ROVERA. 1989. Detection of minimal disease in hematopoietic malignancies of the B-cell lineage by using third-complementarity-determining region (CDRIII) specific probes. Proc. Natl. Acad. Sci. USA **86:** 5123-5127.

31. STEWART, A. K. & R. S. SCHWARTZ. 1994. Review Article: Immunoglobulin V regions and the B cell. Blood **83:** 1717-1730.

32. CHAN, W. C., G. WU, T. GREINER, J. VOSE & J. G. SHARP. 1994. Detection of tumor contamination in peripheral stem cells in patients with lymphoma using cell culture and PCR technology. J. Hematother. **3:** 175-184.

33. SHARP, J. G., J. CHAN, G. WU, T. GREINER, S. S. JOSHI, P. IVERSEN, J. JACKSON, S. PIRRUCCELLO, E. BAYEVER & J. VOSE. 1994. Progress in the detection of minimal lymphoma and new approaches to the treatment of minimal disease. *In* Autologous Bone Marrow Transplantation VII. K. Dicke & A. Keating, Eds.: 633-640. Cancer Treatment Research Education Fund. Arlington, TX.

34. SHPALL, E. J. & R. B. JONES. 1994. Release of tumor cells from bone marrow. Blood **83:** 623-625.

35. BRUGGER, W., K. J. BROSS, M. GLATT, F. WEBER, R. MERTELSMANN & L. KANZ. 1994. Mobilization of tumor cells and hematopoietic progenitor cells into peripheral blood of patients with solid tumors. Blood **83:** 636-640.

36. VORA, A. J., C. H. THO, J. PEEL & M. GREAVES. 1994. Use of granulocyte colony-stimulating factor (G-CSF) for mobilizing peripheral blood stem cells: Risk of mobilizing clonal myeloma cells in patients with bone marrow infiltration. Br. J. Hematol. **86:** 180-182.

37. KESSINGER, A., J. ANDERSON, P. BIERMAN, J. VOSE, M. BISHOP & J. ARMITAGE. 1994. Mobilized versus non-mobilized peripheral stem cell transplantation after high-dose therapy for low grade non-Hodgkin's lymphoma: Effect on progression free survival. Blood **84**(Suppl 1): 394a.

38. GRIBBEN, J. G., D. NEUBERG, M. BARBER, J. MOORE, K. W. PESEK, A. S. FREEDMAN & L. M. NODLER. 1994. Detection of residual lymphoma cells by polymerase chain reaction in peripheral blood is significantly less predictive for relapse than detection in bone marrow. Blood **83:** 3800-3807.

39. SHARP, J. G., A. KESSINGER, S. MANN, D. A. CROUSE, J. O. ARMITAGE, P. BIERMAN & D. D. WEISENBURGER. 1995. Outcome of high-dose therapy and autologous transplantation in non-Hodgkin's lymphoma based on the presence of tumor in the marrow or infused hematopoietic harvest. J. Clin. Oncol. (Accepted)

40. PORTER, D. L., M. S. ROTH, C. MCGARIGLE, J. L. M. FERRARA & J. H. ANTIN. 1994. Induction of graft-versus-host disease as immunotherapy for relapsed chronic myeloid leukemia. N. Engl. J. Med. **330:** 100-106.

41. HIGANO, C. S., W. H. RASKIND & J. W. SINGER. 1992. Use of α interferon for the treatment of relapse of chronic myelogenous leukemia in chronic phase after allogeneic bone marrow transplantation. Blood **80:** 1437-1442.

42. GIRALT, S., S. ESCUDIER, H. KANTARJIAN, A. DEISSEROTH, E. J. FREIREICH, B. S. ANDERS-
SON, S. O'BRIEN, M. ANDREEFF, H. FISHER, A. CORK, C. HIRSCH-GINSBERG, J. TRUJILLO,
S. STASS & R. E. CHAMPLIN. 1993. Preliminary results of treatment with filgrastim for
relapse of leukemia and myelodysplasia after allogeneic bone marrow transplantation.
N. Engl. J. Med. **329:** 757–761.

43. GORIN, N. C., M. LABOPIN & G. MELONI. 1991. Autologous bone marrow transplantation
for acute myeloblastic leukemia in Europe: Further evidence of the role of marrow
purging by mafosfamide. Leukemia **5:** 896–904.

44. GORIN, N. C. 1995. Stem cell transplantation in acute leukemia. N.Y. Acad. Sci. This
volume.

45. SZCZYLIK, C., T. SKORSKI, N. C. NICOLAIDES, L. MANZELLA, L. MALAGUARNERA,
D. VENTURELLI, A. M. GEWIRTZ & B. CALABRETTA. 1991. Selective inhibition of
leukemia cell proliferation by *bcr/abl* antisense oligodeoxynucleotides. Science **253:**
562–565.

46. REED, J. C., C. STEIN, C. SUBASINGHE, S. HALDAR, C. M. CROCE, S. YUM & J. COHEN.
1990. Antisense mediated inhibition of *bcl-2* protoncogene expression and leukemic
phosphorothioate oligodeoxynucleotides. Cancer Res. **50:** 6565–6570.

47. GEWIRTZ, A. M. 1993. Potential therapeutic application of antisense oligonucleotides in
the treatment of chronic myelogenous leukemia. Leukemia Lymphoma. **11**(Suppl. 1):
131–137.

48. WU, A. G., S. S. JOSHI, W. C. CHAN, P. L. IVERSEN, J. D. JACKSON, A. KESSINGER, S. J.
PIRRUCCELLO, W. G. SANGER, J. G. SHARP, D. J. VERBIK, V. L. WHALEN & M. R.
BISHOP. 1995. Effects of *bcr-abl* antisense oligonucleotides (as-odn) on human chronic
myeloid leukemic cells: As-odn as effective purging agents. Leukemia Lymphoma.
In press.

49. BENTZ, M., G. CABOT, M. MOOS, M. R. SPEICHER, A. GANSER, P. LICHTER & H. DOHNER.
1994. Detection of chimeric *bcr-abl* genes on bone marrow samples and blood smears
in chronic myeloid and acute lymphoblastic leukemia by in situ hybridization. Blood
83: 1922–1928.

50. MARGELLO, B., L. C. KENYON & R. DALLA-FAVERA. 1986. Human c-myb proto-oncogene:
Nucleotide sequences of cDNA organization of the genomic locus. Proc. Natl. Acad.
Sci. USA **83:** 9636–9640.

51. COLLINS, R. H. 1993. CD34+ selected cells in clinical transplantation. Stem Cells **12:**
577–585.

52. BENSINGER, W. 1994. Isolating stem and progenitor cells. *In* Blood Stem Cell Transplants.
R. Gale, C. Juttner & P. Henon, Eds.: 32–42. Cambridge University. New York.

53. GORIN, N., M. LOPEZ, J. LAPORTE, P. QUITTET, S. LESAGE, F. LEMOINE, R. J. BERENSON,
F. ISNARD, M. GRANDE, J. STACHOWIAK, M. LABOPIN, L. FOUILLARD, P. MOREL, J. JOUET,
M. NOEL-WALTER, L. DETOURMIGNIES, M. AOUDJHANE, F. BAUTERS, A. NAJMAN &
L. DOUAY. 1995. Preparation and successful engraftment of purified CD34+ bone marrow
progenitor cells in patients with non-Hodgkin's lymphoma. Blood **85:** 1647–1654.

54. VANDEN BERG, D., A. CARELLA, R. NEGRIN, D. SNYDER, N. C. GORIN, A. DEISSEROTH,
C. READING, D. CLAXTON, J. LIANG, M. WESSMAN, D. SIMONETTI, S. CHEN, L. MURRAY &
R. HOFFMAN. 1994. Potential use of normal stem cells isolated from mobilized peripheral
blood of CML patients as an autograft. Blood **84**(Suppl. 1): 400a.

55. KESSINGER, A. 1993. High dose therapy and peripheral blood stem cell transplants. *In*
Peripheral Blood Stem Cells. D. Smith & R. Sacher, Eds.: 33–44. American Association
of Blood Banks. Bethesda.

56. JOSHI, S. S., A. KESSINGER, S. L. MANN, M. STEVENSON, D. D. WEISENBURGER, W. P.
VAUGHAN, J. O. ARMITAGE & J. G. SHARP. 1987. Detection of tumor cells in histologically normal bone marrow using culture techniques. Bone Marrow Transplant. **1:**
303–310.

57. JOSHI, S. S., D. L. NOVAK, L. MESSBARGER, V. MAITREYAN, D. D. WEISENBURGER & J. G. SHARP. 1990. Levels of detection of tumor cells in human bone marrow with or without prior culture. Bone Marrow Transplant. **6:** 179-183.

58. SHARP, J. G., J. ARMITAGE, D. CROUSE, S. JOSHI, A. KESSINGER, S. MANN, W. VAUGHAN & D. WEISENBURGER. 1989. Recent progress in the detection of metastatic tumor in bone marrow by culture techniques. *In* Autologous Bone Marrow Transplantation IV. K. Dicke, G. Spitzer, S. Jagannath & M. J. Evinger-Hodges, Eds.: 421-425. M. D. Anderson Press. Houston.

59. DATTA, Y. H., P. T. ADAMS, W. R. DROBYSKI, S. P. ETHIER, V. H. TERRY & M. S. ROTH. 1994. Sensitive detection of occult breast cancer by the reserve transcriptase polymerase chain reaction. J. Clin. Oncol. **12:** 475-482.

60. SCHOENFELD, A., Y. LUQMANI, D. SMITH, S. O'REILLY, S. SHOUSHA, H. D. SINNETT & R. C. COOMBES. 1994. Detection of breast cancer micrometastases in axillary lymph nodes by using polymerase chain reaction. Cancer Res. **54:** 2986-2990.

61. KORBLING, M., C. JUTTNER, P. HENON & A. KESSINGER. 1994. Blood versus bone marrow transplants. *In* Blood Stem Cell Transplants. R. Gale, C. Juttner & P. Henon, Eds.: 87-98. Cambridge University. New York.

62. SHARP, J. G. & A. KESSINGER. 1994. Minimal residual disease and blood stem cell transplants. *In* Blood Stem Cell Transplants. R. Gale, C. Juttner & P. Henon, Eds.: 75-86. Cambridge University. New York.

63. SHARP, J. G., J. O. ARMITAGE, D. A. CROUSE, J. DEBOER, S. S. JOSHI, S. L. MANN, D. D. WEISENBURGER & A. KESSINGER. 1989. Are occult tumor cells present in peripheral stem cell harvests of candidates for autologous transplantation? *In* Autologous Bone Marrow Transplantation IV. K. Dicke, G. Spitzer, S. Jagannath & M. Evinger-Hodges, Eds.: 693-702. University of Texas. Houston.

64. SHARP, J. G., A. KESSINGER, W. P. VAUGHAN, S. MANN, D. A. CROUSE, K. DICKE, A. MASIH & D. D. WEISENBURGER. 1992. Detection and clinical significance of minimal tumor cell contamination of peripheral stem cell harvests. Int. J. Cell Cloning **10:** 92-94.

65. SHARP, J. G., A. KESSINGER, J. O. ARMITAGE, P. J. BIERMAN, D. A. CROUSE, S. L. MANN, S. PIRRUCCELLO, J. VOSE & D. D. WEISENBURGER. 1992. Clinical significance of occult tumor cell contamination of hematopoietic harvests in non-Hodgkin's lymphoma and Hodgkin's disease. *In* Autologous Bone Marrow Transplantation in Lymphoma, Hodgkin's Disease and Multiple Myeloma. A. Zander, Ed.: 123-132. Springer-Verlag. Berlin.

66. NAGAFUJI, K., M. HARADA, Y. TAKAMATSU, T. ETO, T. TESHIMA, T. KAMURA, T. OKAMURA, S. HAYASHI, K. AKASHI & M. MURAKAWA. 1993. Evaluation of leukaemic contamination in peripheral blood stem cell harvest by reverse transcriptase polymerase chain reaction. Br. J. Hematol. **85:** 578-583.

67. CRAIG, J. I., K. LANGLANDS, A. C. PARKER & R. S. ANTHONY. 1994. Molecular detection of tumor contamination in peripheral blood stem cell harvests. Exper. Hematol. **22:** 898-902.

68. MARIETTE, X., J. P. FERMAND & J. C. BROUET. 1994. Myeloma cell contamination of peripheral blood stem cell grafts in patients with multiple myeloma treated by high-dose therapy. Bone Marrow Transplant. **14:** 47-50.

69. DOMINICI, C., G. DEB, A. ANGIONI, A. LANDALFO, F. PARISI, L. HELSON & A. DONFRANCESCO. 1993. Peripheral blood stem cells in children with solid tumors. Part II. Immunocytologic detection of tumor cells in bone marrow and peripheral blood stem cell harvests. Anticancer Res. **13:** 2573-2575.

70. DI-CARO, A., B. BOSTROM, T. J. MOSS, J. NEGLIA, N. K. RAMSAY, J. SMITH & L. C. SASKY. 1994. Autologous peripheral blood cell transplantation in the treatment of advanced neuroblastoma. Am. J. Pediat. Hematol. Oncol. **16:** 200-206.

71. VERBIK, D. J., J. D. JACKSON, S. J. PIRRUCCELLO, K. D. PATIL, A. KESSINGER & S. S. JOSHI. 1995. Functional and phenotypic characterization of human peripheral blood stem cell harvests: A comparative analysis of cells from consecutive collections. Blood **85:** 1964-1970.

72. CHANG, J., T. D. ALLEN & T. M. DEXTER. 1989. Long-term bone marrow cultures: Their use in autologous marrow transplantation. Cancer Cells **1:** 17-24.

73. BARNETT, M. J., C. J. EAVES, G. L. PHILLIPS, R. D. GASCOYNE, D. E. HOGGE, D. E. HORSMAN, R. K. HUMPHRIES, H. G. KLINGEMAN, P. M. LANSDORP, S. H. NANTEL, D. E. REECE, J. D. SHEPHERD, J. J. SPINELLI, H. J. SUTHERLAND & A. C. EAVES. 1994. Autografting with cultured marrow in chronic myeloid leukemia: Results of a pilot study. Blood **84:** 724-732.

74. PANTEL, K., J. R. IZBICKI, M. ANGSTWURM, S. BRAUN, B. PASSLICK, O. KARG, O. THETTER & G. RIETHMULLER. 1993. Immunocytological detection of bone marrow micrometastasis in operable non-small cell lung cancer. Cancer Res. **53:** 1027-1031.

75. LINDEMANN, F., G. SCHLIMOK, P. DIRSCHEDL, J. WITTE & G. RIETHMULLER. 1991. Prognostic significance of micrometastatic tumor cells in bone marrow of colorectal cancer patients. Lancet **340**(8821): 685-689.

76. SCHLIMOK, G., I. FUNKE, K. PANTEL, F. STROBEL, F. LINDEMANN, J. WITTE & G. RIETHMULLER. 1991. Micrometastatic tumor cells in bone marrow of patients with gastric cancer: Methodological aspects of detection and prognostic significance. Eur. J. Cancer **27:** 1461-1465.

77. SANDER, C. A., T. YANO, H. M. CLARK, C. HARRIS, D. L. LONGO, E. S. JAFFE & M. RAFFELD. 1993. p53 mutation is associated with progression in follicular lymphomas. Blood **82:** 1994-2004.

78. KOHN, K. W., J. JACKMAN & P. M. O'CONNOR. 1994. Cell cycle control and cancer chemotherapy. J. Cell Biochem. **54:** 440-452.

79. O'CONNOR, P. M., J. JACKMAN, D. JONDLE, K. BHATIA, I. MAGRATH & K. W. KOHN. 1993. Role of the p53 tumor suppressor gene in cell cycle arrest and radiosensitivity of Burkitt's lymphoma cell lines. Cancer Res. **53:** 4776-4780.

80. LOWE, S. W., S. BODIS, A. MCCLATCHEY, L. REMINGTON, H. E. RULEY, D. E. FISHER, D. E. HOUSMAN & T. JACKS. 1994. p53 status and the efficacy of cancer therapy in vivo. Science **266:** 807-810.

81. COPPLE, B., E. BAYEVER & P. L. IVERSEN. 1994. Oligonucleotides directed to p53 mRNA cause increased sensitivity to radical oxygen induced cytotoxicity. Proc. Am. Assoc. Cancer Res. **35:** 307.

82. DOHNER, H., K. FISHCHER, M. BENTZ, K. HANSEN, A. BENNER, G. CABOT, D. DIEHL, R. SCHLENK, J. COY, S. STILGENBAUER, M. VOLKMANN, P. R. GALLE, A. POUSTKA, W. HUNSTEIN & P. LICHTER. 1995. p53 gene detection predicts for poor survival and non-response to therapy with purine analogs in chronic B cell leukemias. Blood **85:** 1580-1589.

83. ZIPORI, D., M. KRUPSKY & P. RESNITZKY. 1987. Stromal cell effects on clonal growth tumors. Cancer **60:** 1757-1762.

84. STROBEL, E. S., H. G. STROBEL, K. J. BROSS, B. WINTERHALTER, H. H. FIEBIG, J. V. SCHILDGE & G. W. LOHR. 1989. Effects of human bone marrow stroma on the growth of human tumor cells. Cancer Res. **49:** 1001-1007.

85. SHARP, J. G., S. L. MANN, B. MURPHY & C. WEEKES. 1995. Culture methods for the detection of minimal tumor contamination of hematopoietic harvests: A review. J. Hematother. **4:** 141-148.

86. SACHSTEIN, R. 1995. The physiology of lymphocyte migration following bone marrow transplantation. N.Y. Acad. Sci. This volume.

87. GRUSS, H., N. BOIANI, D. E. WILLIAMS, R. J. ARMITAGE, C. A. SMITH & R. G. GOODWIN. 1994. Pleiotropic effects of the CD30 ligand on CD30 expressing cells and lymphoma cell lines. Blood **83:** 2045-2056.

88. JOHNSON, P. W. M., S. M. WATT, D. R. BETTS, D. DAVIES, S. JORDAN, A. J. NORTON & T. A. LISTER. 1993. Isolated follicular lymphoma cells are resistant to apoptosis and can be grown in vitro in the CD40/stromal cell system. Blood **82:** 1848–1857.
89. HETU, F., F. COUTLEE & D. C. ROY. 1994. A non-isotopic nested polymerase chain reaction method to quantitate minimal residual disease in patients with non-Hodgkin's lymphoma. Mol. Cell. Probes **8:** 449–457.

Stem Cell Transplantation in Acute Leukemia

NORBERT-CLAUDE GORIN[a]

Bone Marrow Transplant Unit
Hôpital Saint-Antoine
Paris, France
and
European Cooperative Group for Blood and Marrow
Transplantation (EBMT)
Paris, France

In the last 30 years, treatment of acute myelocytic (AML) and lymphocytic (ALL) leukemias has evolved considerably.[1] From the first historical treatments with steroids, monochemotherapy, and exsanguino-transfusion to the more complex strategies of today, the general evolution has invariably been in the direction of more aggressive therapy, culminating in total body irradiation or high dose, ''ablative'' polychemotherapy regimens in conjunction with bone marrow transplantation (BMT).

Allogeneic BMT was first employed in the 1970s in patients with end-stage overt acute leukemias,[2,3] with the initial, perhaps naive, idea of destroying the leukemic marrow and replacing it with normal, HLA-identical, family-related marrow. Results were poor because of toxicity, including graft-versus-host disease (GVHD),[4-6] and a very high rate of persisting leukemia, recurring leukemia, or both. Performing allogeneic BMT earlier in remission[7] to deliver the same high dose therapy on a much lower residual tumor (that is in complete remission) has considerably improved the outcome. An important finding, at least on theoretical grounds, was that GVHD is associated with antileukemic activity, the graft-versus-leukemia effect (GVL).[8,9] However, although GVHD-GVL is associated with a lower incidence of recurrent leukemia, it is not yet of clear benefit to patients because of the increased mortality resulting from GVHD per se.

Autologous bone marrow transplantation, which developed later,[3,10-14] has been applied by the same principles previously used for allogeneic BMT: marrow collected in remission was first reinfused after high dose therapy in patients in relapse,[12,15] producing high remission rates but no cure. Subsequently, autologous BMT was performed earlier in the disease to enable high dose consolidation, again in complete remission. First considered essentially for patients with no available HLA-identical donor for an allograft, autologous BMT was recently applied more widely in view of its reduced toxicity, in part linked to the absence of GVHD. However, a major theoretical impediment to autologous BMT has been the potential contamination of

---

[a] Address for correspondence: Service des maladies du sang, Hôpital Saint-Antoine, 184, rue du Fg St-Antoine, 75012 Paris, France.

collected marrow by residual leukemic cells and the risk of reinfusing them into the patient.

The introduction of techniques to purge the marrow of leukemic residual cells, using cyclophosphamide derivatives (4-hydroperoxycyclophosphamide and mafosfamide) essentially for AML[16-19] or monoclonal antibodies (mAb) essentially for ALL,[20-22] has led several teams, including ours, to systematically purge the marrow.[20-31] In contrast, other teams relying on high dose conventional chemotherapy consolidation courses given to the patient in remission before marrow collection and referring to this as "*in vivo* purging" have advocated against unnecessary and potentially harmful additional *in vitro* purging and obtained good results, raising controversy over whether purging is indeed necessary.[32-35] However, in 1988-1991, for the first time, retrospective analyses of the registry of the European cooperative group for blood and marrow transplantation (EBMT) demonstrated that marrow purging with mafosfamide was associated with a lower relapse rate in patients with AML autografted in first complete remission (CR1).[36,37] In 1993, by gene-marking experiments using the transduction of the neomycin resistance gene in unpurged AML autografts, Brenner *et al.*[38] showed that at least in some instances, leukemic cells infused with the graft do contribute to relapse. Although much clinical evidence in favor of purging concerns AML rather than ALL, purging is still more widely applied to ALL, and most teams in Europe but not in the United States still use unpurged marrow in AML. However, even with purged marrow, autologous BMT, especially if done in second or third remission (CR2 or CR3) is associated with higher relapse rates than is allogeneic BMT. This as well as the finding in the last 5 years that T-cell depletion of donor marrow for allografting, in an effort to reduce the incidence and severity of GVHD, is associated with an increased incidence of relapse[39] further outlined the specific GVL potential of allografting, absent with autologous BMT. Peripheral blood stem cell autografting was introduced in the last 10 years after the first observation that a sufficient amount of stem cells could be collected by leukapheresis at the time of recovery from aplasia after induction or consolidation courses and produce sustained engraftment.[40,41] Although it indeed produced more rapid engraftment than did autologous marrow, with a clear benefit to the patient, the risk of reinfusing circulating leukemic cells with this unpurged material, supported by the observation of a possibly increased relapse rate greater than that observed with purged marrow, has at least for the moment reduced its use.[42,43] More recent approaches, however, in which leukaphereses are not done immediately after induction, as in the past, but after several courses of consolidation chemotherapy to take advantage of *in vivo* purging produce better results.[44,45]

While both allogeneic and autologous BMT were being developed, important progress was also being made in the field of conventional chemotherapy, for example, in the promulgation of the concept of double induction (tandem chemotherapy), the demonstration that more than one consolidation course is needed, the development of the principles for early or late intensification, the introduction of new schedules for administration of existing drugs such as high dose cytosine arabinoside (ARAC), and the introduction of new drugs such as idarubicin, mitoxantrone, and etoposide. Therefore, the current situation is complex, and controversy exists over which strategy should be applied in the treatment of AML and ALL. This situation is further clouded by the development of new research areas such as the administration of GM-CSF or

G-CSF with chemotherapy[46] or after transplantation, the use interleukin-2,[47] and attempts to separate GVHD and GVL[9,48] in allografting and to induce GVHD/GVL[49] in autografting. The amount of information in the field of stem cell transplantation for acute leukemias is considerable, and results of recent analyses comparing allogeneic to autologous BMT and chemotherapy are now available.

We present the results of ABMT in our institution and review the worldwide experience. We then present the preliminary results of two EBMT retrospective studies, the first comparing ABMT to allogeneic transplantation from an HLA-identical related donor and the second comparing ABMT to allogeneic BMT from an HLA-identical unrelated donor (MUD). Finally, we summarize the results of the EORTC-GIMEMA AML-8 study comparing allogeneic and autologous BMT to conventional chemotherapy in AML. One must keep in mind that comparison of autologous to allogeneic BMT, however, is always biased because only younger patients with a matched sibling can get an allogeneic transplant, whereas ABMT primarily concerns all patients who lack a suitable related donor and those who are too old for an allogeneic transplant; MUD transplants, when possible, concern younger patients with refractory or evolving leukemia. Although comparisons are of scientific interest, they presently compare complementary rather than competing transplantation modalities. There are cases, however, when in the presence of a suitable donor (related or unrelated) for an allograft, the question of whether an autograft is preferred is raised, and this situation may well become increasingly more frequent in the near future.

AUTOLOGOUS BONE MARROW TRANSPLANTATION FOR ACUTE LEUKEMIA: 10-year Experience at Hôpital Saint-Antoine/ Paris Using Marrow Purged by Mafosfamide

In the late 1970s, our team designed a program of high dose consolidation therapy containing total body irradiation followed by ABMT with bone marrow purged by mafosfamide, a directly active congener of cyclophosphamide, in an effort to reduce or eliminate residual leukemic cells that might contaminate the graft and later contribute to relapse. To purge the bone marrow by mafosfamide, we used two techniques. First, from January 1982 to January 1990, we adjusted the doses of mafosfamide to the individual sensitivity of the normal GM-CFU in each patient to reach the highest tolerable dose that would achieve maximum antileukemic activity without jeopardizing bone marrow engraftment. This dose was defined as the GM-CFU LD95 on buffy-coat bone marrow cells, sparing 5% ± 5% GM-CFU. A total of 95 patients had bone marrow treatment according to this technique.[17,26,27,50] Second, in the period from January 1990 to January 1993, 30 patients had a Ficoll-Hypaque separation of their bone marrow; the mononuclear cell fraction was adjusted to a final concentration of 10^7/ml and treated with a constant dose of 50 μg/ml of mafosfamide. Whatever the dose, the bone marrow suspension was incubated with mafosfamide for 30 minutes in a water bath at 37°C and then immediately cooled and centrifuged at 4°C to block the action of the drug abruptly. After two washes, bone marrow cells were then resuspended in irradiated autologous plasma (40 Gy) and TC 199 medium and finally frozen with 10% dimethylsulfoxide in Teflon-Kapton DF 1000 Gambro bags (Gambro

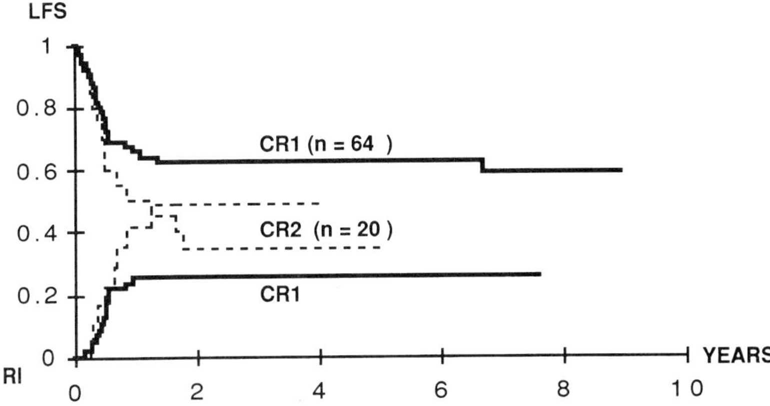

FIGURE 1. Leukemia-free survival (LFS) and relapse incidence (RI) in patients with acute myelocytic leukemia (AML) autografted in first (CR1) or second (CR2) remission with marrow purged by mafosfamide at Hôpital Saint-Antoine, Paris, France. Reproduced, with permission, from Laporte *et al.*[27]

Dialysatoren, GmbH, Germany) in a Nicool 316 programmed biologic freezer (CFPO, Sassenage, France), using our previously reported freezing techniques.[26,51-56] The purged bone marrow was then stored in the gas phase of liquid nitrogen at a temperature constantly below −190°C. Cell counts and GM-CFU evaluations were performed at each step in the procedure. The number of residual progenitor cells after incubation with mafosfamide in each patient were known before ABMT. A total of 125 adult patients with acute leukemia were autografted with bone marrow purged by mafosfamide from January 1983 to January 1993. The median follow-up period was 64 months (range 3-126) There were 84 acute myeloblastic leukemias (AMLs) and 41 acute lymphoblastic leukemias (ALLs). At the time of autologous BMT, 64 AMLs were in first complete remission (CR1) and 20 were in CR2. Thirty-five ALL were in CR1 and six in CR2. The median age of the patients was 33 years (range 16-55). The median interval between complete remission and autografting was 5 months (range 1.3-23). The pretransplant regimen consisted of cyclophosphamide (120 mg/kg) and total body irradiation. The initial richness in granulomacrophagic progenitors GM-CFU of the harvested bone marrows was 5.16×10^4 GM-CFU/kg (range 0.55-33). After mafosfamide purging, the residual number of GM-CFU was 0.021×10^4/kg (range 0-1.78). The probability of successful engraftment was significantly higher and the time to engraftment was significantly shorter in ALL. Of 33 patients grafted with bone marrow containing no residual CFU-GM, those with AML ($n = 22$) had platelet recoveries that were significantly longer than those for AML patients receiving bone marrow with residual GM-CFU. At 8 years, patients autografted in CR1 for AML and ALL had a leukemia-free survival (LFS) of 58% and 56%, respectively, with a relapse incidence of 25% and 37%, respectively (FIGS. 1 and 2). Patients autografted in CR2 for AML had an LFS of 34% and a relapse incidents of 48% at 5 years. The incidence of late relapses was significantly higher in ALLs. By multivariate

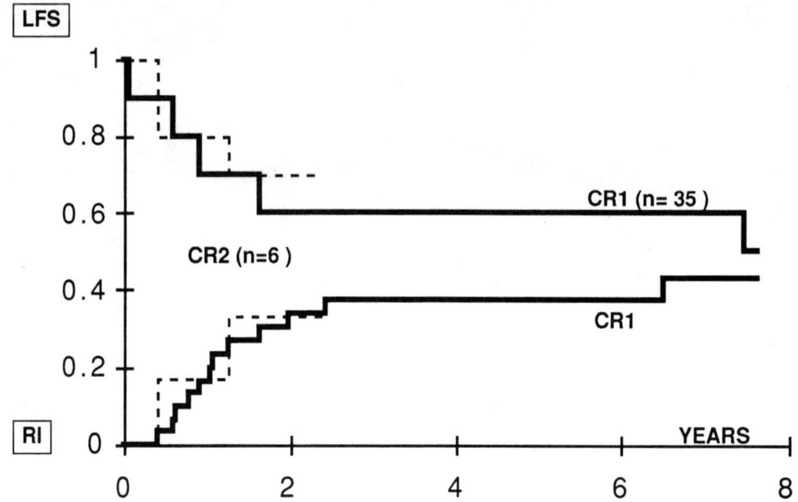

FIGURE 2. Leukemia-free survival (LFS) and relapse incidence (RI) in patients with acute lymphocytic leukemia (AML) autografted in first (CR1) or second (CR2) remission with marrow purged by mafosfamide at Hôpital Saint-Antoine, Paris, France. Reproduced, with permission, from Laporte *et al.*[27]

TABLE 1. 125 Adult Patients with Primary Acute Leukemia Autografted with Marrow Purged by Mafosfamide at Hôpital St-Antoine, Paris; Factors Influencing Engraftment: Multivariate Analyses[a]

Factor	Neutrophils		Platelets	
	RR[b]	*p*	RR[b]	*p*
Patient age >33 years	0.4	0.0001	0.38	0.003
Purging with mafosfamide at adjusted levels	2.16	0.002	2.23	0.012
Transplant in CR2	0.53	0.02	0.44	0.014
Interval from CR to ABMT <5 mo	0.65	0.048	0.61	0.044

[a] Stratified on diagnosis.

[b] Relative risk for probability of engraftment. Higher doses of marrow in GM-CFU/kg prepurging tended to be associated with faster neutrophil engraftment ($p = 0.06$).

analysis, four factors in addition to a diagnosis of ALL were found to favorably influence engraftment: younger age, ABMT performed in CR1, the adjusted dose technique of purging (TABLE 1, FIGS. 3 and 4), and a shorter interval from complete remission to ABMT. Two factors were correlated with a better outcome: (1) Leukemia-free survival was significantly higher and transplant-related mortality significantly

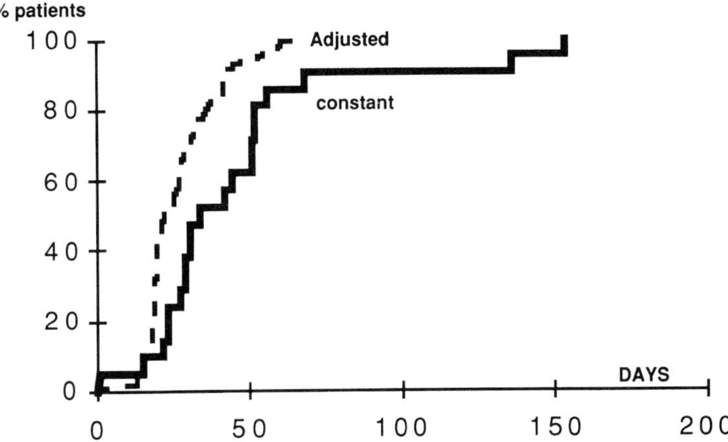

FIGURE 3. Percentage of patients engrafted on neutrophils with time, in relation to whether they received marrow purged by mafosfamide at an adjusted level or at a constant dose at Hôpital Saint-Antoine, Paris, France.

lower in patients who received richer bone marrow (FIG. 5); and (2) The relapse incidence was significantly lower in patients autografted within 150 days from complete remission.

We drew the following conclusions from this experience: (1) For patients autografted in CR1, an LFS of 58% for AML and 56% for ALL is very similar to the best results reported with allogeneic BMT using related donors. (2) The dose of

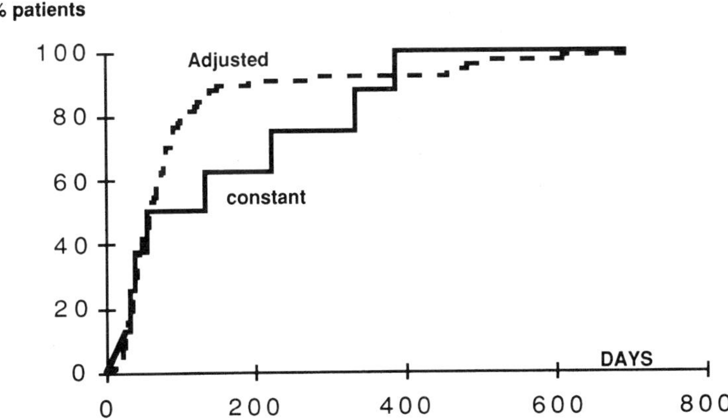

FIGURE 4. Percentage of patients engrafted on platelets with time, in relation to whether they received marrow purged by mafosfamide at an adjusted level or at a constant dose at Hôpital Saint-Antoine, Paris, France.

marrow to be infused is important; the more the better. The opposite observation was made in AML with unpurged marrow[57] and in high risk ALL with purged marrow,[21] where the LFS was lower and the relapse rate higher in patients receiving more marrow. A possible explanation for these apparently conflicting observations is the persisting contamination and therefore the infusion of tumor cells with the grafts if unpurged in AML and also despite purging because of its insufficient effectiveness in high risk ALL. By contrast, in AML CR1 where supposedly clean marrow can be obtained through purging, the infusion of richer marrows would induce an outcome advantage not clouded by a parallel deleterious infusion of a contaminating high tumor load. The reason that patients receiving higher doses of clean marrow do better, however, is unclear; patients receiving the richer bone marrow tended to engraft faster on neutrophils, but this had no impact on outcome. The ability to collect rich bone marrow may reflect a high-quality complete remission and is therefore a good prognostic indicator. Alternatively, one may hypothesize the intervention of a stem cell competition effect whereby an expanded normal stem cell pool would express a growth advantage and/or higher resistance (e.g., to inhibitors of leukemic origin) when faced with a minimal residual tumor population. This mechanism was recently suggested to explain the complete remission in patients with relapse of leukemia after allogeneic BMT, by the administration of granulocyte colony-stimulating factor.[58] Our finding supports the collection and infusion of the highest possible dose of bone marrow and might even question the routine putting aside of back-up bone marrow. The second factor influencing outcome, namely, the timing of ABMT, had an impact on relapse with a lower incidence in patients autografted earlier. The explanation is uncertain; however, it may be that patients reaching ABMT earlier were in a better clinical and hematologic condition and, in a way, selected for good prognostic criteria pertaining to the leukemia itself. This hypothesis may be supported by the finding that bone marrow before ($p = 0.07$) and after ($p = 0.07$) purging in this group of patients tended to be richer.

We presently continue to autograft our adult patients with both AML and ALL as early as possible in CR1, collecting as much marrow as possible and purging it with mafosfamide. Our current research program focuses on improving marrow purging through the use of protective agents such as amifostine (ethiofos) to spare immature normal hematopoietic progenitors and hopefully to further increase leukemic progenitor killing with higher doses of mafosfamide. Preliminary *in vitro* studies with amifostine at our institution indicate that this compound, by both protecting normal and sensitizing leukemic progenitors, induces up to 6 log differential resistance to mafosfamide in favor of the normal stem cells.[59]

WORLDWIDE AUTOLOGOUS STEM CELL TRANSPLANTATION IN ACUTE LEUKEMIA

Overall Review of Marrow Autografting. We reviewed existing published information on ABMT in acute leukemias. TABLES 2, 3, 4, and 5 summarize the LFS reported in AML-CR1 with purged marrow (TABLE 2), with unpurged marrow for adults (TABLE 3) and children (TABLE 4), and the LFS reported in AML CR2 (TABLE 5). TABLE 6 summarizes the data for ALL autografted in CR1, all with purged marrow.

TABLE 2. Results of ABMT with Purged Marrow in AML CR1[a]

Group	Patients (n)	Pretransplant Regimen	LFS (%)
St-Antoine, Paris	64	CY-TBI	58
Heidelberg	35	CY-TBI	58
Parma	20	CY-TBI	69
Manchester	30	CY-TBI	78
Atlanta	27	Various	63
Baltimore	48	BU-CY	38
ECOG	39	BU-CY	54
Stanford	34	BU-E	57
San Francisco	35	BU-E	79
Total/median	332		~58

Abbreviations: LFS = leukemia-free survival; CY-TBI = cyclophosphamide + total body irradiation; BU-CY = busulfan + cyclophosphamide; BU-E = busulfan + etoposide.

[a] No late relapse.

TABLE 3. Results of ABMT with Unpurged Marrow in Adult AML CR1[a]

Group	Patients (n)	Pretransplant Regimen	LFS (%)
UCH-London	82	CT	48
Glasgow	73	CY-TBI	44
Barcelona	24	CY-TBI	48
Genoa	55	CY-TBI	49
Belgium	33	+ ARA-C	31
Roma	101	CY-TBI/BAVC	41
Stanford	34	BU-E	32
Total/median	402		~45
EBMT	598	Various	42

Abbreviations: BAVC = BCNU, AMSA, VP16, ARAC. For other abbreviations, see footnote to TABLE 2.

TABLE 7 is a compendium of the results in both AML and ALL, as estimated from individual centers and from EBMT.

Evidence in Favor of Purging. Growing evidence indicates that purging the autograft indeed diminishes the relapse rate in AML; however, evidence is still lacking in ALL. In AML, in addition to animal preclinical modes.[16,60] clinical data have also been progressively accumulated in favor of purging with cyclophosphamide derivatives. The Baltimore team has provided indirect evidence in favor of purging by reporting that more *in vitro* treatment of bone marrow as assessed by the elimination of GM-CFU colonies was associated with a significant decrease in relapses.[61] Later,

TABLE 4. Results of ABMT with Unpurged Marrow in Childhood AML CR1

Group	Patients (n)	Pretransplant Regimen	LFS (%)
Parkville-Australia	25	HDM	68
EBMT	49	CY-TBI	63
Total/median	74		~65

Abbreviations: HDM = high dose melphalan; CY-TBI = cyclophosphamide + total body irradiation.

TABLE 5. Results of ABMT in AML CR2

Group	Patients (n)	Pretransplant Regimen	LFS (%)
		Purged Marrow	
St-Antoine, Paris	20	CY-TBI	34
Heidelberg	30	CY-TBI	34
Atlanta	28	Various	39
Baltimore	82	BU-CY	38
Pittsburgh	27	BU-CY	48
San Francisco	21	BU-E	52
Total/median	208		~35
		Unpurged Marrow	
Roma	31	BAVC	56
Barcelona	18	CY-TBI	28
EBMT	190 adults	Various	30
	35 children	Various	40

For abbreviations, see TABLES 2 and 3.

the same team correlated the sensitivity to 4-hydroperoxycyclophosphamide (4-HC) of clonogenic leukemia cells grown in remission with the posttransplant outcome.[62] Analyses from EBMT[36,37] showed a lower relapse rate with purged bone marrow that is more pronounced in patients transplanted early and in slow remitters, two situations that were interpreted as corresponding to a higher probability for persistence of a higher residual tumor load. Recent analyses have indicated a possibly higher probability of cure with purged rather than unpurged bone marrow (91 vs 80%) for patients autografted in CR1 after total body irradiation who did not have a relapse at 1 year.[37] Different relapse patterns were observed in the two populations, with late relapses at 32 months occurring only in the group receiving unpurged bone marrow (FIGS. 6 and 7). Recently, Brenner *et al.*[38] were able to mark the unpurged autograft by

TABLE 6. Results of ABMT in ALL CR1

Group	Patients (n)	Purging	LFS (%)
St-Antoine, Paris	35	Mafosfamide	56
Barcelona	20	mAb	49
London	27	mAb	32
Seattle	10	mAb	50
Newcastle	13	None	48
Royal Marsden	38	mAb ±	50 (maintenance)
Total/median	143		~50
EBMT	265	±	40

Abbreviations: mAb = monoclonal antibodies.

TABLE 7. ABMT for Acute Leukemia: Compendium of Results from Individual Teams and EBMT

Disease/Status	LFS (%)	RI (%)
AML CR1		
Purged	58	25
Unpurged	45	45
AML CR2	35	55
ALL CR1 (adults)	40	55
ALL CR2		
Children	40	60
Adults	30	65

transferring the neomycin-resistance gene in 12 ABMTs for AML. In the two cases in which relapse occurred, the presence of the marker was subsequently shown in leukemic cells and in leukemic colonies grown in culture. This observation suggests that at least in certain cases, the graft itself contributes to relapse. In contrast to AML, despite anecdotal reports in ALL,[63] evidence in favor of *in vitro* treatment with cyclophosphamide derivatives has only come from *in vitro* studies on cell lines, and there has been no demonstration of benefit in terms of lower relapse rate or higher leukemia-free survival in human clinical situations. TABLE 8 lists the arguments for marrow purging in AML, and TABLE 9 details the multifactorial role of mafosfamide used *in vitro*. This role goes far beyond a mere tumor cytotoxic effect. TABLE 10 lists data that may suggest that purging may be effective, but this has not been established in ALL. Our own interpretation of these contrasting observations in AML and ALL relies on the basic principle that leukemia can be cured in an autograft setting only if both the recipient and the autograft are made tumor free. Only in a tumor-free recipient can the possible impact of purging of the autograft be evaluated. We believe that this corresponds to AML CR1, a chemosensitive disease in which

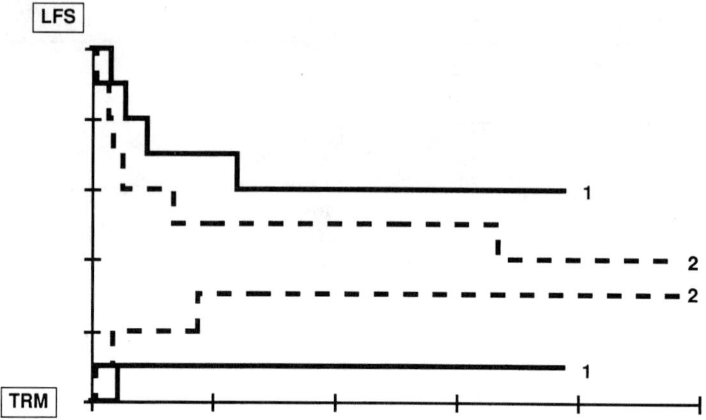

FIGURE 5. Leukemia-free survival (LFS) and transplant related mortality (TRM) in relation to the dose of marrow infused (evaluated before purging): (1) CFU-GM/kg > 5.15 × 10^4 (n = 62), and (2) CFU-GM/kg ≤ 5.15 × 10^4 (n = 63) multivariate analysis, p = 0.045 for LFS, p = 0.003 for TRM. Reproduced, with permission, from Laporte *et al.*[27]

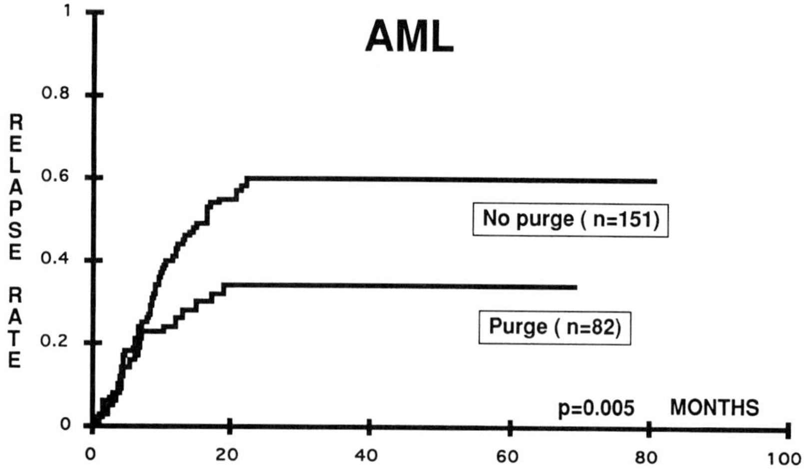

FIGURE 6. Relapse rates in patients with AML in CR1 autografted after TBI with purged or unpurged marrow, within 6 months of obtention of remission. (EBMT survey). Reproduced, with permission, from Gorin *et al.*[37]

in vitro purging is effective, in contrast to ALL even in CR1 which is more resistant to both *in vivo* and *in vitro* therapies.

Peripheral Blood Autografting. After early concern about the possibility of obtaining sustained engraftment with peripheral blood stem cells, this technique has been routinely used since 1985.[64-73] Currently, peripheral blood stem cells are usually

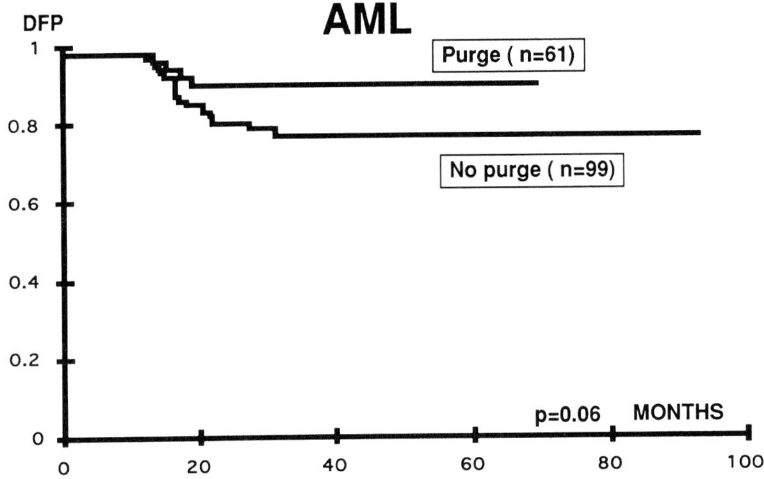

FIGURE 7. Probability of persisting remission (cure) in patients with AML in CR1 autografted after TBI, who did not relapse 1 year posttransplant. Patients receiving purged marrow are compared with those receiving unpurged marrow (EBMT survey). Reproduced, with permission, from Gorin *et al.*[37]

TABLE 8. Evidence in Favor of Purging in ABMT for AML

BNML rat model (Sharkis, 1980; Wiley, 1991)

Characteristics of the purged graft predict outcome:
    Better leukemia-free survival for:
        residual GM-CFU <1% (Rowley, 1989)
        CR LPC sensitive to 4 HC (Miller, 1991)

EBMT surveys (Gorin, 1990, 1991)
    Better leukemia-free survival with purged marrow
        Slow remitters
        Early transplants

Gene marking
    In AML (Brenner, 1993)
    In CML (Deisseroth, 1994)

Abbreviations: BNML = Brown Norway myelocytic leukemia rat model; LPC = leukemic progenitor cells.

collected after chemotherapy followed by the administration of hematopoietic growth factors, and they are used for autografting of solid tumors and lymphomas. In the field of acute leukemia, most of the existing experience concerns AML. In the context of AML the initial rationale was appealing for two reasons. First, contamination of peripheral blood by leukemic clones at the time of complete remission was thought

TABLE 9. Role of Mafosfamide in Marrow Treatment

Direct cytotoxic effect on committed progenitor cells

Induction of apoptosis in human AML, enhancement by IL-3, IL-6 (Bullock, 1993)

Increase of natural killer cell population and activity in mice after mafosfamide
    ABMT (Skorski, 1988)
    In lymphocytes of normal volunteers cultured *in vitro* with 4HC (Sharma, 1984)

In patients autografted for
    AML
    NHL
    but not ALL (Carlo Stella, 1994)

likely to be less important than the estimated contamination of marrow or even nil; therefore, the risk of reinfusing tumor would be lower or nonexistent, and purging would no longer be necessary. The second reason was related to the long duration of aplasia observed with autologous BMT, which has a median duration of thrombocytopenia of around 90 days, sometimes necessitating platelet support longer than 1 year; preliminary results of peripheral blood stem cells autografting had indicated very rapid kinetics of recovery of hematopoiesis. Therefore, several teams started collecting peripheral blood stem cells at the time of recovery from aplasia, after either induction or consolidation courses. Yields of collected GM-CFU were better after induction and decreased after each additional consolidation course. As the minimum dose for safe engraftment was considered to be greater than 10^5 GM-CFU per kilogram, three to six leukaphereses were usually needed, requiring considerable effort in terms of harvesting, freezing, storage facilities, and hence finances. The initial experience of our own team was disastrous, with a very high early relapse rate.[72]

We postulated that in contrast to the initial hypothesis of the absence of or reduction in contamination of peripheral blood by leukemic cells, leukemic clonogenic cells might in fact circulate in peripheral blood precisely at the time of marrow

TABLE 10. Data Suggesting an Efficacy of Purging in ABMT for ALL

BCL 1 mouse model

Correlation of the number of leukemic progenitor cells infused to the outcome
    Simonsson, 1989
    Uckun, Kersey 1990, 1992

EBMT survey
    Possible efficacy in early remitters, i.e., chemosensitive disease
    (Unpublished, 1992)

Occasional observations
    Grande, Gorin, 1994

Effective marrow purging in NHL (BCL2-PCR) predicts favorable outcome
    Gribben, Nadler, 1991

regeneration, especially after induction. We considered that the large volume of blood processed (15 liters or so per patient) may have increased the probability of collecting tumor cells. Finally, we suggested that leukapheresis be done after additional courses of consolidation, to take advantage of *in vivo* purging.

Recently, Reiffers *et al.*[67] for EBMT retrospectively reviewed the data of patients who underwent either autologous blood stem cell transplantation ($n = 63$) or autologous bone marrow transplantation ($n = 886$) in first remission. They also compared the data of 57 peripheral blood stem cell transplanted patients with the data of 114 patients who underwent unpurged autologous BMT matched for age, interval between diagnosis and transplantation, and conditioning regimen. The 4-year leukemia-free survival was 35% ± 7% for peripheral blood stem cell and 44% ± 5% for autologous BMT with unpurged marrow, with a higher relapse risk in peripheral blood stem cell transplanted patients (63% ± 7% versus 44% ± 6%, $p = 0.04$). The transplant-related mortality, on the other hand, was higher after unpurged autologous BMT (21% ± 5% versus 9% ± 5%, $p = 0.06$). The patients undergoing purged autologous BMT had a longer leukemia-free survival (51% ± 4%) and a lower risk of relapse (43% ± 4%) than did peripheral blood stem cell transplanted patients (36% ± 6% and 63% ± 7%; $p < 0.002$ and $p < 0.0004$). After peripheral blood stem cell autograft, the median time to recover 500 PMN/mm^3 was 15.5 days (9-60), which was shorter than that observed after autologous BMT (27 days). Platelet engraftment was similar after either a peripheral blood stem cell autograft or an autologous BMT. The benefit and inconvenience of peripheral blood stem cell autografts were clear in a comparative study conducted by Körbling in which patients with AML in CR1 received either infusion of peripheral blood stem cells ($n = 20$) or autologous BMT with marrow purged with mafosfamide ($n = 23$).[66] In both cases the pretransplant regimen combined cyclophosphamide and fractionated total body irradiation (FTBI) at a higher dosage than usual (14.4 Gy). The major differences in the two approaches were as follows: (1) The blood stem cell autograft contained 17-fold more mononuclear cells. (2) White blood cell reconstitution was initiated earlier with peripheral blood stem cells. The median time to reach 10^9 leukocytes/l was 10 days with peripheral blood stem cells versus 28 days with purged autologous BMT. (3) Platelet reconstitution occurred faster after peripheral blood stem cell infusion than after purged autologous BMT, although the significance was borderline. (4) The patient's hospital stay was significantly shorter following peripheral blood stem cell autografting, 45 versus 73 days for purged autologous BMT. (5) However, more relapses occurred after peripheral blood stem cell autografting, and leukemia-free survival at 2 years was higher in the group receiving purged marrow, 51% compared to 35%.

Thus, the only advantage of peripheral blood stem cell infusion over autologous BMT was to shorten the duration of granulocytopenia, certainly not to decrease the risk of relapse. This suggests that the leukemic contamination of peripheral blood stem cells is not different from that of bone marrow or even that it may be greater, as recently observed for ALL.[74] At the present time, peripheral blood stem cell autografting plays a minor role in the general management of acute leukemias. This, however, may change.

In more recent trials in both Spain and Japan, peripheral blood stem cells have been collected later after one or several consolidation courses at supposedly a better time to take advantage of *in vivo* purging. Preliminary results with a short follow-

TABLE 11. Allogeneic versus Autologous BMT in Adults with AML CR1: 4-Year Results[a]

	LFS	RI	TRM
Autologous BMT ($n = 598$)	42 ± 3%	52 ± 3%	13 ± 2%
Allogeneic BMT ($n = 516$)	55 ± 3%	25 ± 3%	27 ± 2%
p. Univariate	0.006	$<10^{-4}$	$<10^{-4}$
p. Multivariate	0.003	$<10^{-4}$	$<10^{-4}$

[a] EBMT 1994

up suggest considerable improvement in leukemia-free survival, now comparable to the one achieved with marrow.[44,45]

EUROPEAN COOPERATIVE GROUP FOR BLOOD AND MARROW TRANSPLANTATION COMPARATIVE STUDIES

The European Cooperative Group for Blood and Marrow Transplantation (EBMT) recently conducted two retrospective studies to compare autologous BMT to allogeneic BMT in patients with acute leukemia. The first one concerned allogeneic BMT with HLA-identical siblings and the second one allogeneic BMT with unrelated donors.

ABMT versus Allogeneic Transplantation Using HLA-Identical Siblings. We retrospectively analyzed data from 1,696 patients with AML transplanted in Europe between 1987 and 1992.[75] Of 1,114 adult patients transplanted in CR1, 598 received an autograft and 516 an allograft. The TRM was significantly higher following allogeneic bone marrow transplantation (BMT) (27% vs 13%, $p <10^{-4}$), the relapse incidence (RI) was higher following autologous BMT (52% vs 25%, $p < 10^{-4}$), and in the end the leukemia-free survival was higher following allogeneic BMT (55% vs 42%, $p = 0.003$). 288 adult patients were transplanted in CR2. In these patients, the leukemia-free survival (LFS) was 39 and 30%, respectively, for allogeneic BMT and ABMT, but this difference was not statistically significant. Finally, when comparing 113 children autografted to 129 allografted in CR1, the LFS was better following allogeneic BMT: 68% vs 47% ($p = 0.007$). Results are detailed on TABLES 11 (adult AML CR1), 12 (adult AML CR2), and 13 (childhood AML CR1).

TABLE 12. Allogeneic versus Autologous BMT in Adults with AML CR2: 4-Year Results[a]

	LFS	RI	TRM
Autologous BMT ($n = 190$)	30 ± 4%	63 ± 5%	20 ± 3%
Allogeneic BMT ($n = 98$)	39 ± 7%	42 ± 8%	32 ± 5%
p. Univariate	0.22	0.001	0.02
p. Multivariate	NS	0.0002	0.004

[a] EBMT 1994.

TABLE 13. Allogeneic versus Autologous BMT in Childhood AML CR1: 4-Year Results[a]

	LFS	RI	TRM
Autologous BMT	47 ± 6%	48 ± 6%	8 ± 4%
Allogeneic BMT	68 ± 5%	25 ± 5%	9 ± 3%
p. Univariate	0.0014	10^{-4}	0.56
p. Multivariate	0.007	0.002	NS

[a] EBMT 1994

TABLE 14. Allogeneic versus Autologous BMT after TBI in Adults with ALL CR1: 4-Year Results[a]

	LFS	RI	TRM
Autologous BMT	40 ± 4%	55 ± 4%	11 ± 3%
Allogeneic BMT	47 ± 3%	35 ± 4%	27 ± 3%
p. Univariate	0.19	$<10^{-4}$	$<10^{-4}$
p. Multivariate	NS (0.06)	$<10^{-4}$	$<10^{-4}$

[a] EBMT 1994.

TABLE 15. Allogeneic versus Autologous BMT after TBI in Adult Patients with ALL CR2: 4-Year Results[a]

	LFS	RI	TRM
Autologous BMT	30 ± 6%	64 ± 7%	16 ± 7%
Allogeneic BMT	25 ± 6%	52 ± 8%	48 ± 8%
p. Univariate	0.30	0.17	0.0002
p. Multivariate	NS	NS	0.0002

[a] EBMT 1994.

The EBMT database for the same analyses in ALL consisted of 1,336 patients,[76] 850 adults and 486 children. The adults had 326 allografts in CR1 vs 300 ABMT, 108 allografts in CR2 vs 116 ABMT. Of the children 79 were allografted and 52 autografted in CR1, and 174 were allografted and 181 autografted in CR2. Analyses focused on those who received total body irradiation (TBI) as the pretransplant regimen because TBI in all was consistently associated with a better outcome. Results are shown on TABLES 14 (adult ALL CR1), 15 (adult ALL CR2), and 16 (childhood ALL CR2). In adults, the TRM was significantly lower after ABMT in CR1 and CR2 and the incidence of relapse significantly higher after ABMT in CR1. The LFS was not significantly different after ABMT or allogeneic BMT, but the trend favored

TABLE 16. Allogeneic versus Autologous BMT after TBI in Childhood ALL CR2: 4-Year Results[a]

	LFS	RI	TRM
Autologous BMT	36 ± 4%	60 ± 5%	11 ± 3%
Allogeneic BMT	54 ± 4%	32 ± 5%	21 ± 4%
p. Univariate	0.003	$<10^{-4}$	0.09
p. Multivariate	0.003	$=10^{-4}$	NS

[a] EBMT 1994.

allogeneic BMT in CR1 (47 ± 3% vs 40 ± 4%, $p = 0.06$). In children in CR2, the TRM was small after either ABMT or allogeneic BMT; the incidence of relapse was significantly higher after ABMT (60 ± 5% vs 32 ± 5%, $p < 10^{-4}$), and consequently the LFS was significantly higher after allogeneic BMT (54 ± 4% vs 36 ± 4%, $p = 0.003$).

Finally, we investigated the occurrence of late events (beyond 2 years) in patients with acute leukemia who received an allogeneic BMT ($n = 1,059$) or an ABMT ($n = 656$) in Europe from January 1979 to December 1990.[77] Patients with no recurrence of leukemia at 2 years had an 82% overall chance of being alive in complete remission at 9 years after transplantation regardless of the nature of the leukemia, the status at transplant, and the type of transplant. The incidence of late relapses continuously decreased with time. The latest relapses in AML were observed following BMT at 6.6 years in a patient transplanted in CR1 and at 3.7 years in a patient transplanted in CR2 and after ABMT at 6 years and 5.1 years, respectively. The latest relapses in ALL were observed after BMT at 4 years in a patient transplanted in CR1 and at 6.8 years in a patient transplanted in CR2, and after ABMT at 5.3 years and 4.5 years, respectively. Several factors predictive of late relapse or death were identified. Allografted patients had a lower frequency of late relapse than did autografted patients. Consequently, LFS and survival were better after allogeneic BMT for ALL, but not for AML because of a parallel increase in procedure-related mortality. Of the numerous prognostic factors studied, female sex in AML, TBI for ALL, and status in CR1 rather than CR2-3 for both ALL and AML allografts were correlated with a lower incidence of relapse. The use of TBI in ALL was also associated with better LFS and survival. This study indicates that patients alive and well 2 years posttransplant have a high probability of cure, but the possibility of late relapse remains. FIGURE 8 (AML) and FIGURE 9 (ALL) indicate the LFS and incidence of relapse in autografted patients who are alive and well 2 years posttransplant.

ABMT versus Allogeneic Transplantation Using Matched Unrelated Donors. In a pair-match analysis, 123 patients with acute leukemia receiving a bone marrow transplant from an HLA, A, B, and DR identical unrelated donor were compared with 246 recipients of an (unpurged) autograft.[78] Patients were pair matched for diagnosis (AML and ALL), age (less than 20 years, 20-40 years, and above 40 years of age), disease status (CR1, intermediate, and more advanced disease), and finally the year the transplant took place.

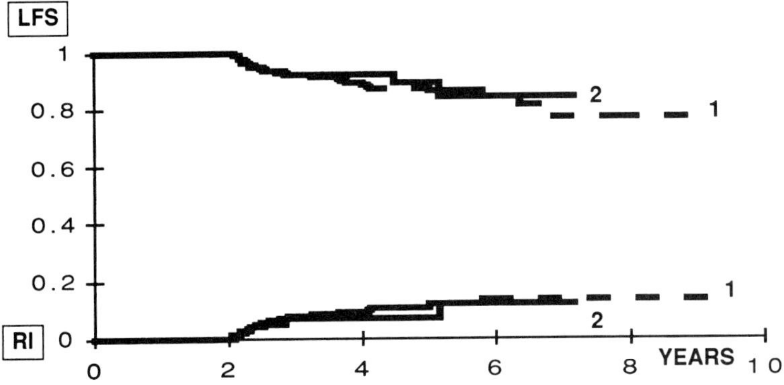

FIGURE 8. Leukemia-free survival (LFS) and relapse incidence (RI) in patients autografted for acute myelocytic leukemia who are alive and well 2 years posttransplant (EBMT analysis). (1) patients transplanted in CR1, and (2) patients transplanted CR2 and CR3. Reproduced, with permission, from Frassoni *et al.*[77]

In AML, 55 matched unrelated donor (MUD) transplants (16 in CR1, 37 in intermediate, and 2 in more advanced disease), were compared to 110 ABMT (32 in CR1, 74 in intermediate, 4 and in advanced). At 2 years, LFS for ABMT and MUD transplants was $35 \pm 5\%$ vs $31 \pm 7\%$ (p = NS), the incidence of relapse was $58 \pm 6\%$ vs $37 \pm 10\%$ (p = 0.06), and the TRM $17 \pm 4\%$ vs $51 \pm 8\%$ (p = 0.0001) (TABLE 17).

In ALL, 68 MUD transplants (12 in CR1, 55 in intermediate, and 1 in more advanced disease) were compared to 136 ABMT (24 in CR1, 110 in intermediate, and 2 in advanced). At 2 years, the LFS for ABMT and MUD transplants was 36

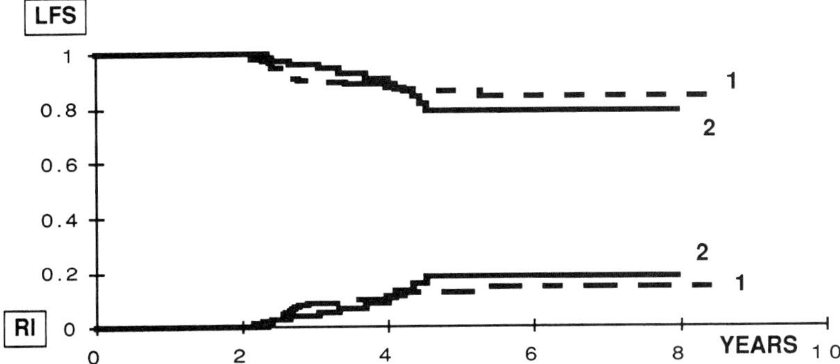

FIGURE 9. Leukemia-free survival (LFS) and relapse incidence (RI) in patients autografted for acute lymphocytic leukemia who are alive and well 2 years posttransplant (EBMT analysis). (1) patients transplanted in CR1, and (2) patients transplanted in CR2 and CR3. Reproduced, with permission, from Frassoni *et al.*[77]

TABLE 17. Comparison between BMT Using Unrelated Donors and Autologous BMT in Patients with Acute Leukemia: AML Patients, 2-Year Results[a]

	LFS	RI	TRM	Survival
MUD	31 ± 7	37 ± 10	51 ± 8	36 ± 7
ABMT	35 ± 5	58 ± 6	17 ± 4	45 ± 5
p Value	0.30	0.056	0.0001	0.07

[a] EBMT 1995

± 5% vs 40 ± 7% (p = NS), the relapse incidence was 59 ± 5% vs 25 ± 7% (p = 0.0001), and the TRM was 12 ± 3% vs 47 ± 7% (p <0.0001) (TABLE 18).

These results indicate that currently ABMT is just as good as MUD transplantation in this population of patients for the majority beyond CR1. This observation, however, is retrospective and justifies a randomized study between the two modalities. Considering the numerous difficulties and the low likelihood to reach a MUD transplant in a patient with acute leukemia, the answer to such a study would be of considerable practical importance.

COMPARISON OF ALLOGENEIC OR AUTOLOGOUS BONE MARROW TRANSPLANTATION WITH INTENSIVE CHEMOTHERAPY

Prospective randomized comparisons of allogeneic, autologous BMT, and conventional chemotherapy (CT) have essentially been done in AML. The most important study currently available is the EORTC-GIMEMA-AML8A trial, which from November 1986 to April 1993 included 992 adult AML patients.[79] In this randomized study, patients achieving CR after one or two induction courses with daunorubicin (DNR) and cytosine-arabinoside (conventional doses) then received an intensive consolidation course combining intermediate dose ARA-C and M-AMSA. They then were eligible for an allogeneic BMT if an HLA-identical sibling was available or were randomized for either an ABMT with unpurged marrow or a second intensive consolidation (IC2) chemotherapy course with high dose ARA-C and daunorubicin. As of

TABLE 18. Comparison between BMT Using Unrelated Donors and Autologous BMT in Patients with Acute Leukemia: ALL Patients, 2-Year Results[a]

	LFS	RI	TRM	Survival
MUD	40 ± 7	25 ± 7	47 ± 7	40 ± 6
ABMT	36 ± 5	59 ± 5	12 ± 3	45 ± 5
p Value	0.85	0.0001	<0.0001	0.13

[a] EBMT 1995.

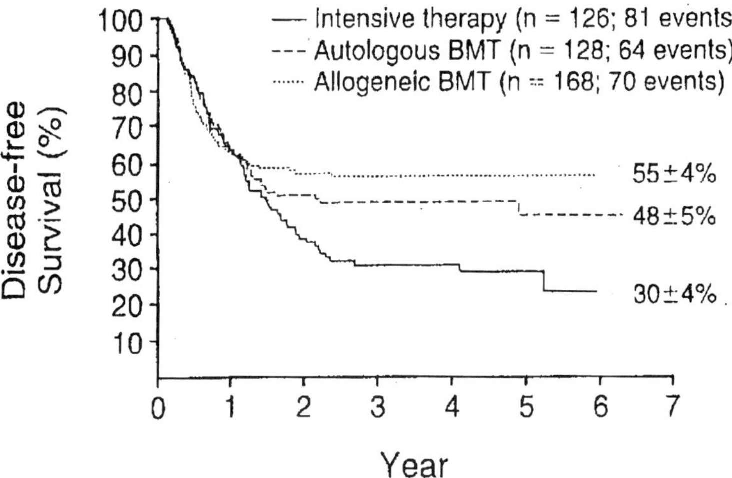

FIGURE 10. EORTC-GIMEMA AML-8 trial: Comparison of disease-free survival in patients maintained with intensive therapy or transplanted with autologous or allogeneic marrow. Reproduced, with permission, from Zittoun *et al.*[79]

December 1993, 623 patients had entered into CR; 168 patients were eligible for allogeneic BMT, 128 were randomized for ABMT, and 126 for IC2. With a median follow-up of 3 years, LFS at 4 years was globally 40%. By intention to treat, LFS at 4 years was significantly different in favor of allo-BMT (55%) and ABMT (48%) as compared to IC2 (30%), with a *p* value between ABMT and IC2 of 0.026 (FIG. 10). The overall survival of the remitters in the three arms was not significantly different (59%, 56%, and 46% respectively) as more patients who had relapses after IC2 entered into a CR2 and were then salvaged by ABMT. Globally, these results were interpreted as strongly in favor of ABMT over conventional chemotherapy. As a consequence, the EORTC-GIMEMA AML10 trial, in combination with EBMT, now proposes ABMT to all patients with no available HLA-identical related donor. Another important multicenter trial in progress in the United Kingdom (MRC 10 study), designed along the same lines, has currently gathered more than 500 patients. The overall LFS at 4 years is impressingly good, but results of the three arms are not currently available. An Eastern Cooperative Oncology Group (ECOG) trial is currently evaluating ABMT with marrow purged with 4HC; in this trial, patients with de novo AML 15-55 years old receive one or two induction courses with daunorubicin, ARA-C, and thioguanine. One to 3 months after CR, they then either receive ABMT or undergo allogeneic BMT if they are less than 41 years of age and have a histocompatible sibling. In an interim analysis recently presented, the CR rate was 74%. Thirty-five patients underwent ABMT and 16 allogeneic BMT. The Kaplan-Meier estimate of event-free survival at 2 years was 52 ± 29% versus 46 ± 26% for ABMT and allogeneic BMT, respectively.

In ALL, very few randomized studies exist. Recently, a French prospective study[80] in adults in CR1, following a high dose induction regimen (similar to the one used

TABLE 19. Variables to Consider and Selection of Postinduction Treatment(s) in AML CR1 According to the Patient

Variables	Maintenance CT	Possible Strategy(ies) alloBMT	autoBMT	Comments
Age ≥55–60 yr and/or major organ dysfunction	+	–	–	
Age between 45 and 60	+	–	+	
Age below 45	–	+	+	Allo BMT with the highest early toxicity but the lowest risk of relapse

by the German BFM group), compared the use of allogeneic BMT and autologous unpurged BMT. After autologous BMT, patients were further randomized to receive Interleukin-2 or not. By intention to treat at 3 years, the allografted arm ($n = 43$) had a DFS of 68%, while the autografted arm ($n = 77$) had a DFS of only 26%. There was no difference whether IL-2 was then given or not. This study conveys the generally accepted message that results of allogeneic BMT in ALL are superior to those of ABMT. However, results of ABMT in this trial are far below those of the EBMT registry, and the use of unpurged marrow in ALL can be criticized.

CONCLUSION

It is difficult to draw a valuable conclusion because the field is evolving quickly. However, we propose our own possible strategy in the management of AML (TABLES 19 and 20): we consolidate in CR1 all adult patients with AML and all children with poor-risk features by cyclophosphamide 60 mg/kg/day × 2 and single dose TBI at 10 Gy with lung shielding at 8 Gy, followed by ABMT with marrow purged by mafosfamide. We believe that marrow should be collected after a minimum of two consolidation courses to take advantage of *in vivo* purging. We even recommend this procedure in CR1 for a patient having an HLA-identical related sibling, because transplant-related mortality is lower with ABMT. We use exactly the same approach in CR2. We would recommend allografting for patients with an available HLA-identical sibling only in CR3 or in early relapse after CR2. We never consider allografting with an HLA-identical unrelated donor for AML. TABLES 19 and 20 summarize the treatment strategy in AML CR1.

In ALL, for adult patients in CR1 and CR2, for children in CR1 with high risk features [t (4;11) or t (9;22)], and children in CR2, we consider allogeneic transplantation first when there is a sibling donor. In the absence of a donor, we consider autografting with marrow purged by mafosfamide. However, we would consider a MUD allograft favorably in adult ALL CR2 in a case of full-matched donor availability in view of the poor results of ABMT in this situation.

TABLE 20. Variables to Consider and Selection of Postinduction Treatment(s) in AML CR1 According to the Disease

Variables	Maintenance CT	Possible Strategy(ies)		Comments
		alloBMT	autoBMT	
Standard risk	–	±	+	Less toxicity ABMT purging suggested for slow remitters and/or early transplant
High risk of relapse: Related donor available	–	+	±	Allo BMT associated with the lowest risk of relapse
No related donor	–	–	+	
Refractory AML: related or unrelated donor	–	+	–	

REFERENCES

1. CLARKSON, B. D., T. GEE, K. MERTELSMANN *et al.* 1986. Current status of treatment of acute leukemia in adults: An overview of the Memorial experience and review of literature. CRC. Crit. Rev. Oncol. Hematol. **4:** 221.
2. THOMAS, E. D., R. STORB, R. A. CLIFT, *et al.* 1975. Bone marrow transplantation. N. Engl. J. Med. **292:** 832-843, 895-902.
3. SANTOS, G. 1983. History of bone marrow transplantation. Clin. Haematol. **12:** 611-663.
4. MATHE, G., J. BERNARD & M. J. DE VRIES. 1960. Nouveaux essais de greffe de moëlle osseuse homologués après irradiation totale chez des enfants atteints de leucémie aiguè en rémission. Le problème du syndrome secondaire chez l'homme. Rev. Fr. Clin. Biol. **15:** 115.
5. ATKINSON, K., M. M. HOROWITZ, J. C. BIGGS *et al.* 1988. The clinical diagnosis of acute graft versus host disease: A diversity of views amongst marrow transplant centers. Bone Marrow Transplant **3:** 5-10.
6. ATKINSON, K., M. M. HOROWITZ, R. P. GALE *et al.* 1989. Consensus among bone marrow transplanters for diagnosis grading and treatment of chronic graft versus host disease. Bone Marrow Transpl. **4:** 247-254.
7. THOMAS, E. D., C. D. BÜCHNER, R. A. CLIFT *et al.* 1979. Marrow transplantation for acute non lymphoblastic leukemia in first remission. N. Engl. J. Med. **301:** 597-599.
8. WEIDEN, P. L., N. FLOURNOY, E. D. THOMAS *et al.* 1979. Antileukemia effect of graft versus host disease in human recipients of allogeneic marrow grafts. N. Engl. J. Med. **300:** 1068.
9. HOROWITZ, N. M., R. P. GALE & P. M. SONDEL. 1990. Graft versus leukemia reactions after bone marrow transplantation. Blood **75:** 555-562.
10. GORIN, N. C., A. NAJMAN & G. DUHAMEL. 1977. Autologous bone marrow transplantation in acute myelocytic leukemia. Lancet **14:** 1050.
11. GORIN, N. C., G. HERZIG, M. I. BULL *et al.* 1978. Long term preservation of bone marrow and stem cell pool in dogs. Blood **51:** 257-265.

12. DICKE, K. A., A. ZANDER, G. SPITZER *et al.* 1979. Autologous bone marrow transplantation in relapsed adult acute leukemia. Lancet **1:** 514–517.
13. GORIN, N. C. & G. DUHAMEL. 1987. L'autogreffe de Moëlle Osseuse. New York. Masson.
14. GOLDSTONE, A. H. (Ed). 1986. Autologous bone marrow transplantation. Clin. Haematol. **1:** 150.
15. GORIN, N. C., R. DAVID, J. STACHOWIAK *et al.* 1981. High dose chemotherapy and autologous bone marrow transplantation in acute leukemias, malignant lymphomas and solid tumors: Study of 23 patients. Eur. J. Cancer **17:** 557–568.
16. SHARKIS, S. J., G. W. SANTOS & O. M. COLVIN. 1980. Elimination of acute myelogenous leukemia cells from marrow and tumor suspensions in the rat with 4 hydroperoxy-cyclophosphamide. Blood **55:** 521–523.
17. DOUAY, L., J. Y. MARY, M. C. GIARRATANA *et al.* 1989. Establishment of a reliable experimental procedure for bone marrow purging with mafosfamide (Asta Z 7557). Exp. Hematol. **17:** 429–432.
18. JONES, R. J., M. ZUEHLDORF, S. D. ROWLEY *et al.* 1987. Variability in 4 hydroperoxycyclo-phosphamide activity during clinical purging for autologous bone marrow transplanta-tion. Blood **70:** 1490–1494.
19. CARLO-STELLA, C., L. MANGONI, C. ALMICI *et al.* 1992. Differential sensitivity of adherent CFU-blast, CFU-mix, BFUE and CFUGM to mafosfamide: implications for adjusted dose purging in autologous bone marrow transplantation. Exp. Hematol. **20:** 328–333.
20. UCKUN, F. M., J. KERSEY, R. HAAKE *et al.* 1992. Autologous bone marrow transplantation in high-risk remission-B lineage acute lymphoblastic leukemia using a cocktail of three monoclonal antibodies (BA-1/CD24, BA-2/CD9 and BA-3/CD10) plus complement and 4-hydroperoxycyclophomamide for ex vivo bone marrow purging. Blood **79:** 1094–1104.
21. BILLETT, A., E. KORNMEHL, N. J. TARBELL *et al.* 1993. Autologous bone marrow trans-plantation after a long first remission for children with recurrent acute lymphoblastic leukemia. Blood **81:** 1651–1657.
22. SELVAGGI, K. J., J. W. WILSON, L. E. MILLS *et al.* 1994. Improved outcome for high-risk acute myeloid leukemia patients using autologous bone marrow transplantation and monoclonal antibody-purged bone marrow. Blood **83:** 1698–1705.
23. YEAGER, A. M., H. KAIZER, G. W. SANTOS *et al.* 1986. Autologous bone marrow trans-plantation in patients with acute non lymphoblastic leukemia using ex vivo marrow treatment with 4 hydroperocyclophosphamide. N. Engl. J. Med. **315:** 141–147.
24. KÖRBLING, M., W. HUNSTEIN, J. M. FLIEDNER *et al.* 1989. Disease free survival after autologous bone marrow transplantation in patients with acute myelocytic leukemia. Blood **74:** 1898–1904.
25. RIZZOLI, V., L. MANGONI & C. CARLO-STELLA. 1992. Autologous bone marrow transplanta-tion in acute myelogenous leukemias. Leukemia **6:** 1101–1106.
26. GORIN, N. C., L. DOUAY, J. P. LAPORTE *et al.* 1986. Autologous bone marrow transplanta-tion using marrow incubated with Asta Z 7557 in adult acute leukemia. Blood **67:** 1367–1376.
27. LAPORTE, J. P., L. DOUAY, M. LOPEZ. *et al.* 1994. One hundred twenty-five adult patients with primary acute leukemia autografted with marrow purged by mafosfamide: A 10 year single institution experience. Blood **84:** 3810–3818.
28. DEXTER, M. & H. SCARFFE. Personal communication.
29. VOGLER, W. R., W. E. BERDEL, W. S. DALTON *et al.* 1994. Autologous bone marrow transplant (ABMT) in acute leukemia using marrow purged with Edelfosine (ET-18-OCH). Exp. Hematol. **22:** 778a.
30. CHAO, N. J., A. S. STEIN, G. D. LONG *et al.* 1993. Busulfan/Etoposide initial experience with a new preparatory regimen for autologous bone marrow transplantation in patients with acute non lymphoblastic leukemia. Blood **81:** 319–323.

31. SIERRA, J., A. GRANENA, J. GARCIA *et al.* 1993. Autologous bone marrow transplantation for acute leukemia: Results and prognostic factors in 90 consecutive patients. Bone Marrow Transplant. **12:** 517-523.

32. BURNETT, A. K., P. TANSEY, R. WATKINS *et al.* 1984. Transplantation of unpurged autologous bone marrow in acute myeloid leukemia in first remission. Lancet **2:** 1068-1070.

33. McMILLAN, A. K., A. H. GOLDSTONE, D. C. LINCH *et al.* 1990. High dose chemotherapy and autologous bone marrow transplantation in acute myeloid leukemia. Blood **76:** 480-488.

34. MELONI, G., D. C. FABRITIIS & A. M. CARELLA. 1990. Autologous bone marrow transplantation in patients with AML in first complete remission: Results of two different conditioning regimens after the same induction and consolidation therapy. Bone Marrow Transpl. **5:** 29-32.

35. CARELLA, A. M., E. GAOZZA, G. SANTINI *et al.* 1988. Autologous unpurged bone marrow transplantation for acute non-lymphoblastic leukemia in first complete remission. Bone Marrow Transplant. **3:** 537-541.

36. GORIN, N. C., P. AEGERTER & B. AUVERT *et al.* 1990. Autologous bone marrow transplantation for acute myelocytic leukemia in first remission: European survey of the role of marrow purging. Blood **75:** 1606-1614.

37. GORIN, N. C., M. LABOPIN, G. MELONI *et al.* 1991. Autologous bone marrow transplantation for acute myelocytic leukemia in Europe: Further evidence of the role of marrow purging by mafosfamide. Leukemia **5:** 896-904.

38. BRENNER, M. K., D. R. RILL, R. C. MOEN *et al.* 1993. Gene-marking to trace origin of relapse after ABMT. The Lancet **341:** 85-86.

39. GOLDMAN, J. M., R. P. GALE, M. M. HOROWITZ *et al.* 1988. Bone marrow transplantation for chronic myelogenous leukemia in chronic phase: Increased risk of relapse associated with T cell depletion. Ann. Intern. Med. **108:** 806-814.

40. JUTTNER, C. A., L. B. TO, D. N. HAYLOCK *et al.* 1985. Circulating autologous stem cells collected in very early remission from acute non-lymphoblastic leukemia produce prompt but incomplete haematopoietic reconstitution after high dose melphalan or supralethal chemoradiotherapy. Br. J. Haematol. **61:** 739-745.

41. KESSINGER, A., J. O. ARMITAGE, J. D. LANDMARK *et al.* 1988. Autologous peripheral hematopoïesis stem cell transplantation restores hematopoietic function following marrow ablative therapy. Blood **71:** 723-727.

42. KÖRBLING, M., T. M. FLIEDNER, R. HOLLE *et al.* 1991. Autologous blood stem cell (ABSCT) versus purged bone marrow transplantation (p ABMT) in standard risk AML: Influence of source and cell composition of the autograft on hemopoietic reconstitution and disease free survival. Bone Marrow Transplant. **7:** 343-349.

43. REIFFERS, J., M. LABOPIN, M. SANZ *et al.* 1994. Autologous blood stem cell transplantation (ABSCT) versus marrow transplantation (ABMT) for patients with acute myeloid leukemia (AML) in first complete remission: A retrospective analysis of the Bone Marrow Transpl EBMT registry. 20th annual meeting of the European group for BMT, Harrogate, UK, March 13-17, 1994. p 373a.

44. SANZ, M. A., J. DE LA RUBIA & G. F. SANZ. 1993. Busulfan plus cyclophosphamide followed by autologous blood stem-cell transplantation for patients with acute myeloblastic leukemia in first complete remission: A report from a single institution. J. Clin. Oncol. **11:** 1661-1667.

45. TAKAHUE, Y. 1994. Engraftment kinetics and interim therapeutic results after autologous peripheral blood stem cell transplantation (PBSCT) in children with cancer. Exp. Hematol. **22:** 782a.

46. ESTEY, E. H. 1994. Use of colony-stimulating factors in the treatment of acute myeloid leukemia. Blood **83:** 2015-2019.

47. FOA, R. 1993. Does Interleukin-2 have a role in the management of acute leukemia? J. Clin. Oncol. **11:** 1817-1825.

48. SLAVIN, S., E. NAPARSTEK, E. OR & L. WEISS. 1988. Prevention of GVHD and induction of graft versus leukemia effects: Will it ever be possible? Bone Marrow Transplant. Suppl 1: 208.

49. YEAGER, A. M., G. B. VOGELSANG, R. J. JONES *et al.* 1993. Cyclosporine-induced graft versus host disease after ABMT for acute myeloid leukemia. Leukemia-Lymphoma **11:** 215–220.

50. DOUAY, L., N. C. GORIN, J. P. LAPORTE, M. LOPEZ, A. NAJMAN & G. DUHAMEL. 1984. Asta Z 7557 (INN Mafosfamide) for the in vitro treatment of human leukemic bone marrow. Invest. New Drugs **2:** 187–190.

51. LOPEZ, M., M. C. DUPUY-MONTBRUN, L. DOUAY, J. P. LAPORTE & N. C. GORIN. 1985. Standardization and characterization of the procedure for in vitro treatment of human bone marrow with cyclophosphamide derivatives. Clin. Lab. Haematol. **7:** 327–334.

52. GORIN, N. C., G. HERZIG, M. I. BULL & R. C. GRAW. 1978. Long-term preservation of bone marrow and stem cell pool in dogs. Blood **51:** 257–265.

53. GORIN, N. C. & G. DUHAMEL. 1978. Conservation de cellules souches hématopoïétiques par congélation lente et élimination de la chaleur de fusion. C. R. Acad. Sci. Paris **286:** 547–550.

54. GORIN, N. C., R. ELGJO, F. STOUT & T. KNUTSEN. 1978. Long-term preservation of canine bone marrow: in vitro studies. Blood Cells **4:** 419–429.

55. GORIN, N. C. 1986. Collection, manipulation and freezing of haemopoïetic stem cells. Clin. Haematol. **15:** 19–48.

56. DOUAY, L., M. LOPEZ & N. C. GORIN. 1986. A technical bias: Differences in cooling rates prevent ampoules from being a reliable index of stem cell cryopreservation in large volumes. Cryobiology **23:** 296–301.

57. MELONI, G., M. VIGNETTI, C. ANDRIZZI *et al.* 1994. Autologous BMT in AML: The nine year experience at hematology university "La Sapienza" of Roma. 20th annual meeting of the European group for bone marrow transplantation. Harrogate, U.K., March 13–17, 529a.

58. GIRALT, S., S. ESCUDIER, H. KANTARJIAN *et al.* 1993. Preliminary results of treatment with filgrastim for relapse of leukemia and myelodysplasia after allogeneic bone marrow transplantation. N. Engl. J. Med. **329:** 757.

59. DOUAY, L., C. HU, M. C. GIARRATANA *et al.* 1995. Amifostine improves the antileukemic therapeutic index of mafosfamide: Implications for bone marrow purging. Blood. In press.

60. WILEY, J. M. & A. M. YEAGER. 1991. Predictive value of colony forming unit assays for engraftment and leukemia free survival after transplantation of chemopurged syngeneic bone marrow in rats. Exp. Hematol. **19:** 179–184.

61. ROWLEY, S. D., R. J. JONES, S. PIANTADOSI *et al.* 1989. Efficacy of ex-vivo purging for ABMT in the treatment of acute non-lymphoblastic leukemia. Blood **74:** 501–506.

62. MILLER, C. B., B. A. ZEHNBAUER, S. PIANTADOSI *et al.* 1991. Correlation of occult clonogenic leukemia drug sensitivity with relapse after ABMT. Blood **78:** 1–5.

63. GRANDE, M., V. BARBU, J. VAN DEN AKKER *et al.* 1994. Autologous bone marrow transplantation in ALL: Relapse linked to infusion of tumor cells with the back-up marrow. Bone Marrow Transplant. **14:** 477–480.

64. JUTTNER, C. A., L. B. TO, D. N. HAYLOCK *et al.* 1985. Circulating autologous stem cells collected in very early remission from acute non lymphoblastic leukemia produce prompt but incomplete haematopoïetic reconstitution after high dose melphalan or supralethal chemoradiotherapy. Br. J. Haematol. **61:** 739–745.

65. KESSINGER, A., J. O. ARMITAGE, J. D. LANDWARK *et al.* 1988. Autologous peripheral hematopoïesis stem cell transplantation restores hematopoïetic function following marrow ablative therapy. Blood **71:** 723–727.

66. KÖRBLING, M., T. M. FLIEDNER, R. HOLLE *et al.* 1991. Autologous blood stem cell (ABSCT) versus purged bone marrow transplantation (p ABMT) in standard risk AML:

Influence of source and cell composition of the autograft on hemopoietic reconstitution and disease free survival. Bone Marrow Transplant. **7:** 343–349.

67. REIFFERS, J., M. LABOPIN, M. SANZ *et al.* 1994. Autologous blood stem cell transplantation (ABSCT) versus BMT (ABMT) for patients with acute myeloid leukemia (AML) in first complete remission: A retrospective analysis of the EBMT registry. Bone Marrow Transplantation. 20th annual meeting of the European group for BMT. Harrogate, U. K. March 13–17, 373a.

68. BELL, A. J., T. J. HAMBLIN & D. G. OSCIER. 1986. Circulating stem cell autograft. Bone Marrow Transplant. **1:** 103–110.

69. CASTAIGNE, S., F. CALVO, L. DOUAY *et al.* 1986. Successful haematopoietic reconstitution using autologous peripheral blood mononucleated cells in a patient with acute prolymphocytic leukaemia. Br. J. Haematol. **63:** 209–211.

70. KÖRBLING, M., B. DORKEN, A. B. HO *et al.* 1986. Autologous transplantation of blood derived hemopoietic stem cells after myeloablative therapy in a patient with Burkitt's lymphoma. Blood **67:** 529–532.

71. REIFFERS, J., P. BERNARD, B. DAVID *et al.* 1986. Successful autologous transplantation with peripheral blood haematopoietic cells in a patient with acute leukaemia. Exp. Hematol. **14:** 321–315.

72. TO, L. B. & C. A. JUTTNER. 1987. Peripheral blood stem cell autografting: A new therapeutic option for AML? Br. J. Haematol. **66:** 285–288.

73. LAPORTE, J. P., N. C. GORIN, J. FEUCHTENBAUM *et al.* 1987. Relapse after autografting with peripheral blood stem cells (letter). Lancet **2:** 1393.

74. ANTHONY, T. R. S., J. L. CRAIG, K. LANGLANDS *et al.* 1993. Detection of tumor contamination by polymerase chain reaction analysis in peripheral blood stem cells collected from patients with leukaemia and lymphoma. 3rd international symposium on peripheral blood stem cell autografts, Bordeaux, France. 39a.

75. GORIN, N. C., M. LABOPIN, L. FOUILLARD *et al.* 1995. Retrospective evaluation of autologous bone marrow transplantation versus allogeneic bone marrow transplantation from an HlA identical related donor in acute myelocytic leukemia. A study of the European cooperative group for blood and marrow transplantation (EBMT). Submitted for publication.

76. GLUCKMAN, E., M. LABOPIN, M. ESPEROU-BOURDEAU *et al.* 1994. Comparison of allogeneic and autologous transplantation for acute lymphoblastic leukemia (ALL) in children and adults. Exp. Hematol. **22:** 765a.

77. FRASSONI, F., M. LABOPIN, E. GLUCKMAN, H. G. PRENTICE, G. GAHRTON, F. MANDELLI, A. M. CARELLA, P. HERVE, A. GRATWHOL, J. GOLDMAN, & N. C. GORIN on behalf of the Acute Leukemia Working Party of the European Group for Bone Marrow Transplantation (EBMT). 1994. Are patients with acute leukaemia, alive and well 2 years post-bone marrow transplantation cured? A European survey. Leukemia **8:** 924–928.

78. LABOPIN, M., O. RINGDEN, N. C. GORIN *et al.* 1995. A comparison of outcome after bone marrow transplantation using unrelated or autologous bone marrow in patients with acute leukemia. 21st Annual Meeting of the European Group for Blood and Marrow Transplantation (EBMT). Davos, Switzerland. March 18–23.

79. ZITTOUN, R. A., F. MANDELLI, R. WILLEMZE, T. DE WITTE *et al.* for the European Organization for research and treatment of cancer (EORTC) and the Gruppo Italiano Malattie Ematologiche Maligne dell'Adulto (GIMEMA). 1995. Autologous of allogeneic bone marrow transplantation compared with intensive chemotherapy in acute myelogenous leukemia. N. Engl. J. Med. **332:** 217–223.

80. ATTAL, M., D. BLAISE, G. MARRIT, M. MICHALLET, J. P. VERNANT *et al.* 1995. Consolidation treatment of adult acute lymphoblastic leukemia (ALL): A prospective study comparing allo BMT versus auto BMT and testing the impact of IL2 after auto BMT. Nouv. Rev. Fr. Hematol. **37:** 161a.

High Dose versus Standard Dose Chemotherapy for the Treatment of Breast Cancer

A Review of Current Concepts

KAREN K. FIELDS,[a,b] GERALD J. ELFENBEIN,[a]
JANELLE B. PERKINS,[a] AND LYNN C. MOSCINSKI[c]

[a]Division of Bone Marrow Transplantation
Department of Internal Medicine
and
[c]Department of Pathology
University of South Florida College of Medicine at the H. Lee
Moffitt Cancer Center and Research Institute
Tampa, Florida 33612

Standard therapy in the treatment of metastatic breast cancer remains disappointing, because virtually all patients eventually die of disease despite therapy.[1] Additionally, most patients with high risk stage II, stage III, and inflammatory breast cancer do not benefit from adjuvant chemotherapy administered in standard doses; high relapse rates and frequent cancer-related deaths are seen in these patients following therapy as well.[2] Higher doses of chemotherapy have been associated with increased response rates in both the *in vitro*[3] and the *in vivo* setting.[4,5] Autologous stem cells derived from bone marrow or peripheral blood permit the administration of high dose chemotherapy at maximum tolerated doses given with curative intent. Dose-limiting toxicities in this setting are nonhematopoietic.

High dose therapy in the treatment of breast cancer has been associated with increased response rates and improved disease-free survival compared to historical controls.[6] Breast cancer has become the most common indication for high dose therapy.[7] Given the myriad of high dose regimens used in the treatment of this disease, it is clear that the optimal regimen remains to be defined. Additionally, the optimal source of stem cells, bone marrow or peripheral blood, remains an area of active investigation, and improvements in our ability to detect minimal disease further compound the issues surrounding the stem cell product.

This communication describes several novel high dose chemotherapy regimens developed at a single institution to treat breast cancer. We summarize current literature-based data on treatment outcomes following standard therapy for the treatment of metastatic and high risk early stage breast cancer and compare these data to our

[b]Address for correspondence: Karen K. Fields, MD, Moffitt Cancer Center, University of South Florida, 12902 Magnolia Drive, Tampa, Florida 33612.

large, single institutional group of patients treated with high dose chemotherapy and autologous stem cell rescue. Additionally, the effects of dose intensity in the high dose setting are presented. Finally, the influence of the stem cell source on event-free survival and the clinical implications of contamination of the stem cell product with minimal metastatic disease detected using polymerase chain reaction techniques are discussed.

MATERIAL AND METHODS

The studies presented were conducted at the H. Lee Moffitt Cancer Center at the University of South Florida. All patients gave written informed consent for treatment according to protocols that were approved and are reviewed annually by the Institutional Review Board of the University of South Florida. Patients included in these analyses were treated from October 1989 through December 1994.

Patients

Patients, up to 65 years of age, with pathologically documented breast cancer were eligible to receive high dose therapy and autologous stem cell rescue and were treated with various protocols based on the stage of disease and responsiveness to previous therapy. Prior to high dose therapy, all patients underwent thorough evaluation to assess disease extent and physiologic function. Disease staging included CT scans of the head, chest, abdomen, and pelvis, nuclear medicine bone scans, serum chemistries and complete blood counts, disease-related tumor markers including CEA and CA15-3, and bilateral bone marrow aspirates and biopsies. Adequate physiologic function was required with a pulmonary diffusion capacity $\geq 60\%$ of predicted, a left ventricular ejection fraction $\geq 50\%$ (by MUGA), a measured creatinine clearance ≥ 60 ml/min, total serum bilirubin ≤ 2 mg/dl, serum transaminases ≤ 2.5 times normal, and a Karnofsky performance status of $\geq 80\%$. Patients with uncontrolled brain metastases or evidence of leptomeningeal involvement, HIV-positive patients, patients with an uncontrolled psychiatric disorder, and patients with a previous history of malignancy were excluded.

Response to therapy was defined as a complete or partial response (50% or greater decrease in the product of the sum of the two largest perpendicular diameters of the measurable lesions). In the case of bone only disease, response was defined as a decrease in the size or number of bone scan abnormalities or, in the absence of objective improvements in bone scan findings, the presence of two or more indicators including marked subjective improvement in bone pain, a 50% decrease in a measurable laboratory abnormality such as alkaline phosphatase or other tumor markers, and evidence of bone healing on plain radiographs of the area. Patients with brain metastases demonstrating a complete response to radiation therapy and stable for a minimum of 3 months were also eligible for high dose therapy on selected protocols.

Patients with metastatic breast cancer responsive to induction chemotherapy consisting of an anthracycline-based regimen were considered ''anthracycline-responsive'' patients. Patients with metastatic breast cancer unresponsive to anthracycline-based regimens were considered ''anthracycline refractory'' but were eligible for

TABLE 1. Treatment Protocols Based on Stage of Disease

Protocol	Maximum Tolerated Dose		Stages Treated
ICE	Ifosfamide	20,100 mg/m^2	Stage II, 8 or more + nodes
	Carboplatin	1,800 mg/m^2	Stage III, A and B
	Etoposide	3,000 mg/m^2	Stage IV, anthracycline responsive
			Stage IV, anthracycline responsive miniICE refractory
MITT	Mitoxantrone	90 mg/m^2	Stage IV, anthracycline refractory
	ThioTEPA	1,200 mg/m^2	Stage IV, anthracycline responsive
			Stage III, A and B
TNT	Taxol (paclitaxel)	360 mg/m^2	Stage IV, anthracycline refractory
	Mitoxantrone	75 mg/m^2	
	ThioTEPA	900 mg/m^2	
BUCY	Busulfan	16 mg/kg	Stage III, A and B
	Cyclophosphamide	120 mg/kg	

high dose therapy. Patients with a solitary metastatic lesion that was completely resected or patients rendered disease-free following radiation therapy were also eligible and considered anthracycline refractory if they had received prior therapy with anthracyclines. Patients with stage II breast cancer with eight or more axillary nodes positive for metastases and patients with stage III breast cancer, stages IIIA and IIIB, noninflammatory or inflammatory breast cancer, were eligible following standard adjuvant therapy which generally consisted of surgery (lumpectomy or mastectomy and axillary node dissection), 4 to 6 cycles of an anthracycline-based chemotherapy regimen given in standard doses, and radiation therapy as indicated to the remaining breast tissue or chest wall and axilla either prior to or following high dose therapy.

Treatment Protocols

Treatment protocols and disease-specific eligibilities are outlined in TABLE 1. Ifosfamide, carboplatin, and etoposide (ICE) were initially used for the treatment of patients with breast cancer in October 1989, and began as a phase I dose escalation trial to determine the maximum tolerated doses of these drugs given in combination.[8] Total doses of each drug were divided over 6 days and were escalated in successive groups of patients with doses ranging from ifosfamide 6,000–24,000 mg/m^2, carboplatin 1,200–2,100 mg/m^2, and etoposide 1,800–3,000 mg/m^2. The maximum tolerated doses of each drug were determined to be ifosfamide 20,100 mg/m^2, carboplatin 1,800 mg/m^2, and etoposide 3,000 mg/m^2. Dose-limiting toxicities were defined as central nervous system toxicity and acute renal failure. Patients treated at the maximum tolerated doses were considered evaluable for phase II studies assessing the activity of this regimen. Patients eligible for this study included patients with stage II breast cancer, eight or more positive nodes, stage III and inflammatory breast cancer, and metastatic breast cancer, responsive to an anthracycline-based regimen or, if anthracycline refractory, responsive to an abbreviated course of ICE (miniICE) given over 2-3 days.[9]

In patients with anthracycline- and miniICE-refractory metastatic breast cancer, another high dose regimen consisting of mitoxantrone and thiotepa (MITT) was explored to determine tolerance and efficacy. Patient accrual began in September 1990 and continues to the present time. These drugs were given over 3 days with doses of mitoxantrone ranging from 45-105 mg/m^2 and doses of thiotepa ranging from 900-1,350 mg/m^2 and with the maximum tolerated doses of mitoxantrone and thiotepa determined to be 90 mg/m^2 and 1,200 mg/m^2, respectively. Dose-limiting toxicities were defined as protracted mucositis and delayed hematologic recovery. Following a phase I evaluation for safety, marked activity was noted in patients with highly refractory metastatic breast cancer, including some patients with brain metastases.[10] Ongoing phase II studies of MITT include patients with anthracycline-responsive metastatic breast cancer and some patients with stage III and inflammatory breast cancer in complete remission following surgery, adjuvant chemotherapy with an anthracycline-based regimen, radiation therapy to the chest wall and axilla prior to beginning high dose therapy.

Since MITT appeared to be an active regimen in highly refractory and heavily pretreated patients with metastatic breast cancer, a third drug, paclitaxel (Taxol), was added in an attempt to increase the anticancer activity of this regimen. This regimen began accruing patients in March 1993 and consists of escalating doses of continuous infusion paclitaxel ranging from 120-360 mg/m^2 in combination with fixed doses of mitoxantrone (Novantrone, 75 mg/m^2) and thiotepa (900 mg/m^2) given in equally divided doses over 3 days (TNT). The maximum tolerated dose of paclitaxel administered in this manner appears to be 360 mg/m^2, and in a group of patients with anthracycline- and miniICE-refractory metastatic breast cancer, high response rates were seen with acceptable hematologic and nonhematologic toxicity.[11]

Finally, busulfan (16 mg/kg) and cyclophosphamide (120 mg/kg) (BUCY) were evaluated in a variety of malignancies including breast cancer.[12] Given the predictable hematopoietic recovery seen with this regimen and the tolerable nonhematopoietic toxicity, patients with stage III breast cancer, including inflammatory breast cancer, were treated with this combination in the adjuvant setting following surgery, standard anthracycline-based therapy, and radiation therapy. All patients received peripheral blood stem cell rescue with stem cells obtained following hematologic recovery after cyclophosphamide and etoposide followed by G-CSF.[13]

Stem Cell Source

Patients received autologous bone marrow stem cells, peripheral blood stem cells, or a combination of both based on clinical circumstances. Initially, all patients with no evidence of bone marrow metastases on routine histologic evaluation and adequate cellularity underwent autologous bone marrow harvesting, and patients with evidence of bone marrow metastases or inadequate cellularity underwent peripheral blood stem cell harvesting following a variety of "priming" regimens.[13] Recently, patients with no evidence of bone marrow involvement underwent both bone marrow harvesting and peripheral blood stem cell harvesting following priming with hematopoietic growth factors alone in a randomized trial evaluating the source of stem cells on hematopoietic reconstitution.[14]

Detection of Minimal Metastatic Breast Cancer Using Polymerase Chain Reaction Techniques

We used reverse transcriptase polymerase chain reaction techniques (RT-PCR) to detect message for the protein cytokeratin 19 (K19) in the bone marrows of patients undergoing autologous stem cell harvesting before high dose therapy.[15,16] Using this assay we were able to detect one breast cancer cell in 10^7 normal marrow cells with a high degree of sensitivity and specificity. We retrospectively studied patients at the time of routine histologic evaluation of bone marrow following standard therapy with 4-6 cycles of an anthracycline-based regimen before high dose therapy and autologous bone marrow harvesting. All bone marrows were histologically normal immediately prior to or at the time of harvesting.

RESULTS

We have treated over 250 patients with various stages of breast cancer including 183 patients on phase II protocols with the ICE, MITT, TNT, and BUCY regimens. The median age of all treated patients was 44 with an age range of 25-64 years. All patients were female. Treatment-related mortality for all patients was 14% with the highest treatment-related mortality in the anthracycline-refractory patients treated with MITT and TNT (26% and 15%, respectively). Anthracycline-responsive patients treated with MITT also had a high mortality rate (33%) in the face of an event-free survival in excess of 60%. Of 183 patients 78 remain event-free with a median follow-up of 17 months (range 5-58 months). FIGURE 1 illustrates the event-free survival time for all patients treated on phase II protocols based on the stage of disease, where an event represents relapse or death due to therapy.

For patients with metastatic breast cancer, anthracycline responsiveness was associated with an improved event-free survival when compared to that of patients with anthracycline-refractory disease. TABLE 2 illustrates the differences in median survival and actuarial and event-free survival at 2 years in 126 patients with metastatic breast cancer treated on various phase II protocols based on responsiveness to induction therapy following the development of metastatic disease. FIGURE 2A demonstrates the event-free survival of anthracycline-responsive patients compared to that of anthracycline-refractory patients (two-tailed $p = 0.0256$); FIGURE 2B divides anthracycline-refractory patients into patients who are responsive to salvage therapy with miniICE versus patients who are refractory to miniICE (two-tailed $p = 0.008$). Of note, patients who are refractory to primary anthracycline therapy but responsive to salvage therapy with miniICE and are treated with high dose ICE have an event-free survival of 20.5% at 2 years, suggesting that this subgroup of patients with anthracycline resistance can achieve clinically significant event-free survival.

Recently, anthracycline- and miniICE-resistant patients were treated on the TNT protocol. FIGURE 3 illustrates differences in outcome for these heavily pretreated patients following the addition of paclitaxel to the regimen, with MITT patients

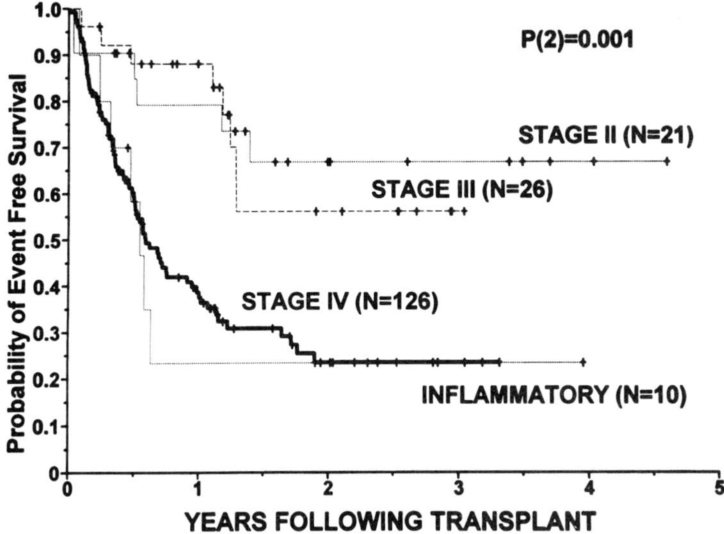

FIGURE 1. Event-free survival in 183 patients with all stages of breast cancer treated on all protocols (ICE, MITT, and TNT).

TABLE 2. High Dose Chemotherapy and Autologous Stem Cell Transplantation for Metastatic Breast Cancer: Experience at the H. Lee Moffitt Cancer Center from 1991–1994 in 126 Patients

Risk Category for Stage IV Pts/Regimen	Patients (n)	Median Survival (mo.)[a]	Actuarial Survival at Two Years[a]	Event-Free Survival at Two Years[a]
(1) Anthracycline responsive	27	36	59.6%	49.2%
(2) Anthracycline refractory but miniICE responsive	27	19	38.6%	20.5%
(3) Anthracycline refractory and miniICE refractory[b]	72	13.7	11.7%	5.2%

[a] From Kaplan-Meier plots, from the day of transplantation.

[b] Failed at least 2 regimens, up to 5 regimens, and a median of 3 regimens.

divided into two groups, patients treated at the lower dose levels (1–4) and patients treated at the upper dose levels (5–7; phase II patients). As can be seen, although the follow-up of the TNT-treated patients is shorter, event-free survival appears comparable to that of patients treated with MITT.

Effect of Stem Cell Source

Patients with evidence of bone marrow involvement or inadequate celluarity underwent peripheral blood stem cell harvesting as just noted. Event-free survival

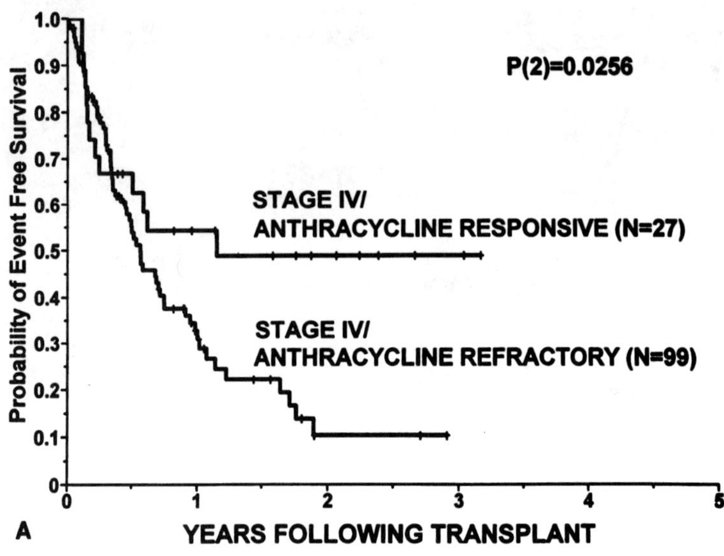

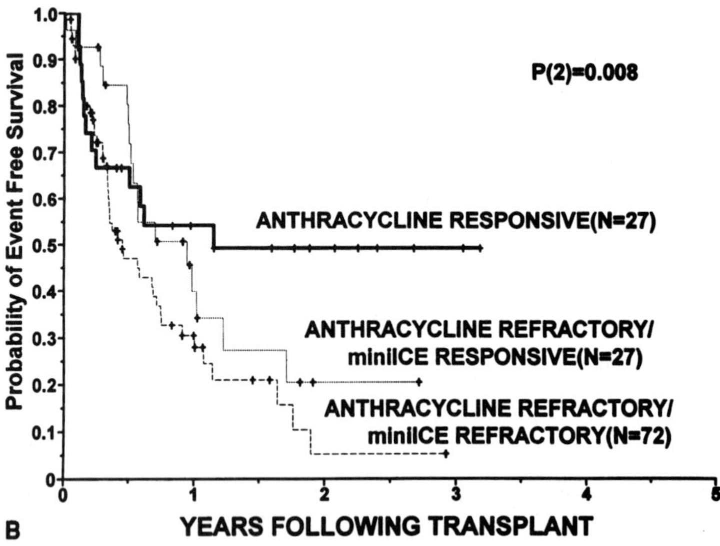

FIGURE 2. Event-free survival in 126 patients with stage IV breast cancer based on responsiveness to anthracyclines. (**A**) Anthracycline-responsive patients versus anthracycline-refractory patients. (**B**) Anthracycline-responsive patients versus anthracycline-refractory patients responding to salvage therapy with miniICE-versus anthracycline-refractory, miniICE-refractory patients.

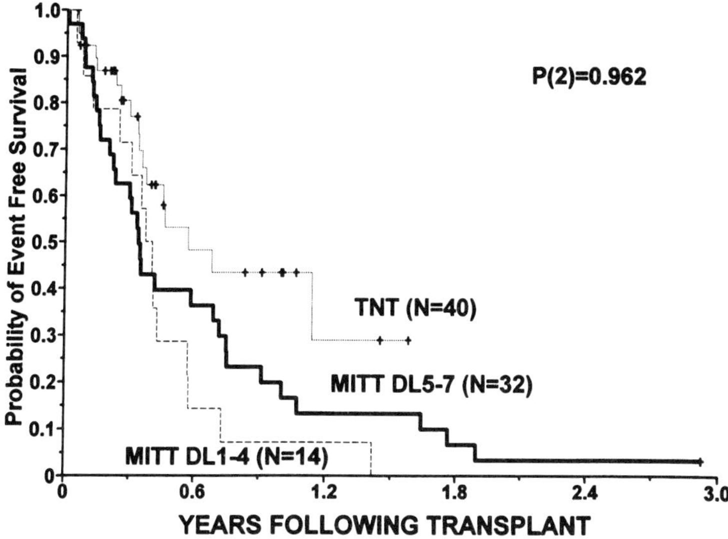

FIGURE 3. Event-free survival in 86 patients with stage IV breast cancer refractory to anthracyclines and miniICE following therapy with lower doses of MITT (DL 1-4), upper dose levels of MITT (DL 5-7), and TNT.

based on the source of stem cells, autologous bone marrow versus peripheral blood stem cells, was assessed for patients treated with ICE (FIG. 4A) and MITT (FIG. 4B). As can be seen, there is no significant difference in outcome based on the stem cell product.

Effect of Contamination of the Stem Cell Product

RT-PCR to detect K19 was used to evaluate the bone marrow of patients with stage II and stage III breast cancer.[17] The bone marrow of 13 patients with stage II breast cancer and 10 patients with stage III, noninflammatory breast cancer obtained at the time of bone marrow harvesting following standard adjuvant chemotherapy but prior to high dose therapy were retrospectively evaluated and found to be positive for K19 in 6 of 13 stage II patients and 5 of 10 stage III patients. All samples studied were considered to be histogically free of disease at the time of marrow harvesting. Event-free survival based on K19 positivity for stage II and III patients is illustrated in FIGURES 5A and B. The time to relapse based on K19 positivity for all patients is seen in FIGURE 6. It is important to note that no relapses have been seen among patients who have K19-negative bone marrow prior to high dose therapy, and the probability of relapse for patients with K19-positive bone marrow prior to high dose therapy is 30% at 3-4 years after stem cell transplant.

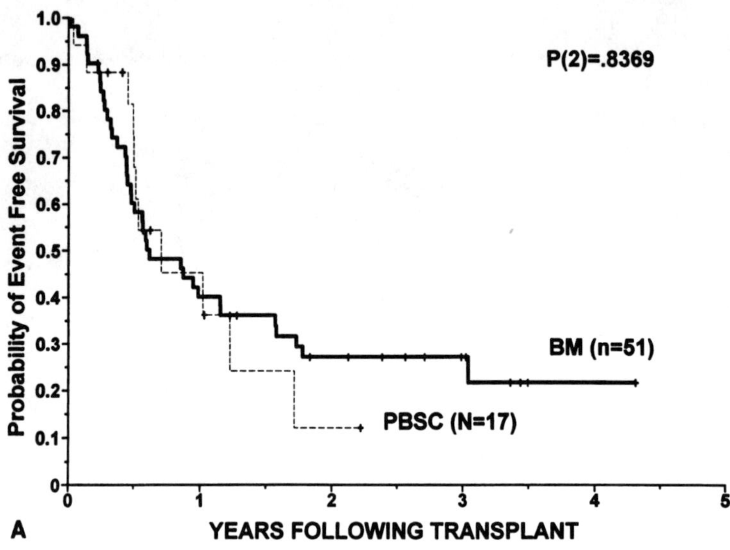

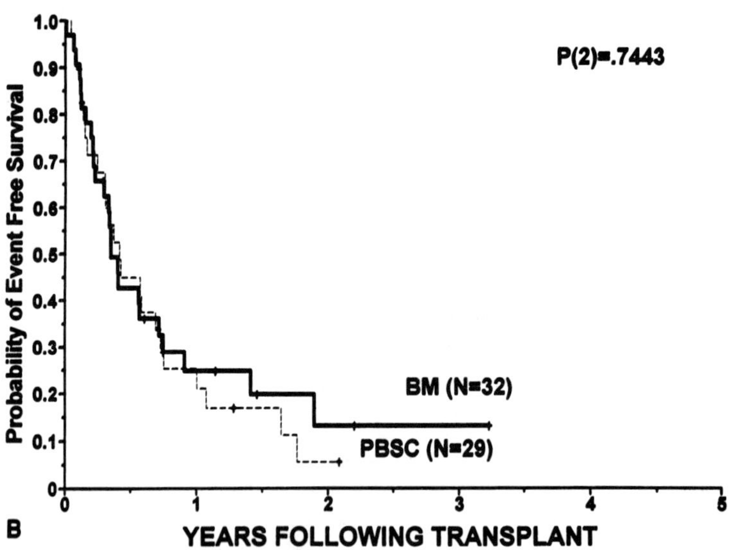

FIGURE 4. Event-free survival in patients with metastatic breast cancer based on the source of stem cells. (**A**) ICE patients. (**B**) MITT patients. BM = bone marrow; PBSC = peripheral blood stem cells; P(2) = two-tailed *p* value.

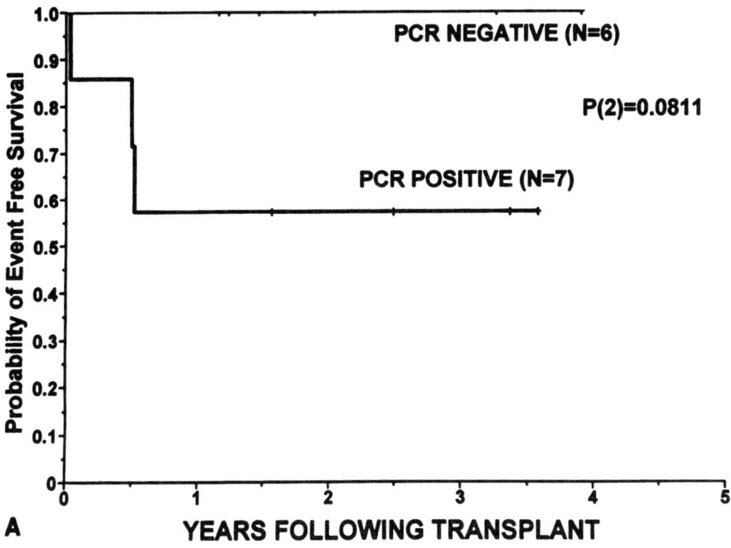

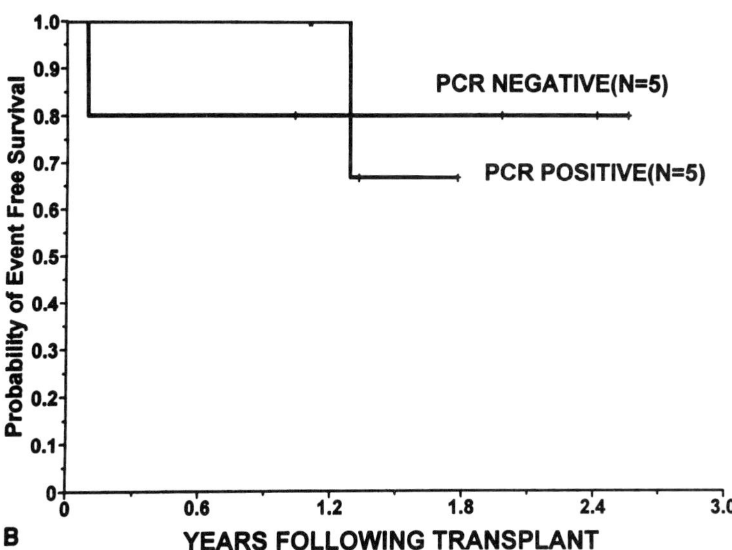

FIGURE 5. Event-free survival in patients based on the presence of K19 in the bone marrow. (A) Stage II breast cancer. (B) Stage III breast cancer. PCR negative = K19 negative; PCR positive = K19 positive.

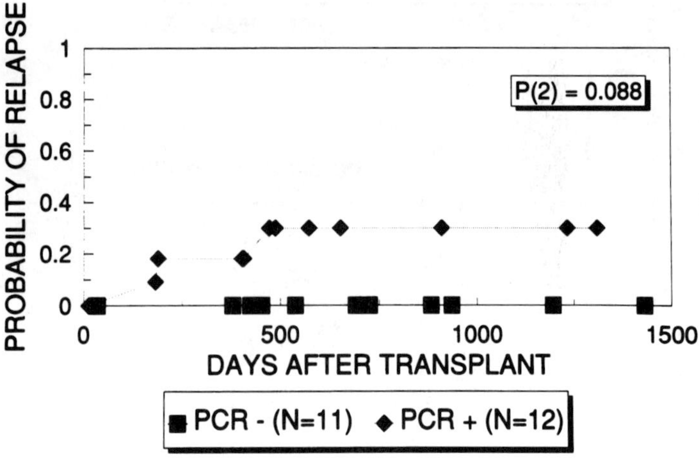

FIGURE 6. Time to relapse in stage II and stage III breast cancer patients based on PCR positivity for K19 (PCR +) versus PCR negativity for K19 (PCR −).

DISCUSSION

Although high dose therapy followed by autologous stem cell rescue has been used with increasing frequency for the treatment of breast cancer, several important questions concerning the optimal use of this therapy remain unanswered. Opponents of high dose therapy cite the lack of randomized prospective data to evaluate the benefits of high dose chemotherapy compared to standard chemotherapy and suggest that patients receiving high dose therapy are highly selected and not comparable to patients in large studies who are treated with standard therapy. They also suggest that the reports of outcomes following standard therapy used as historical controls do not reflect current outcomes following standard therapy.

Two examples of modern chemotherapy studies for the treatment of metastatic breast cancer are available from the literature for comparison. Muss *et al.*[18] published the results of a large randomized trial from the Piedmont Group to illustrate the differences in outcome following continuous or intermittent chemotherapy for the treatment of patients with newly diagnosed, metastatic breast cancer previously untreated with chemotherapy.[18] In this trial, 250 women with metastatic breast cancer received induction chemotherapy with 6 cycles of cyclophosphamide, doxorubicin, and fluorouracil (CAF) followed by randomization to either continuous therapy with cyclophosphamide, methotrexate, and 5-fluorouracil (CMF) or observation and reinduction (further treatment) with CMF at the time of symptom progression. The study demonstrated an improved disease-free survival for patients receiving continuous chemotherapy but no overall survival advantage in this group. The median time to progression was 9.4 months for the continuously treated patients and 3.2 months for the intermittently treated group with less than 5% disease-free survivors in either group at 30 months.

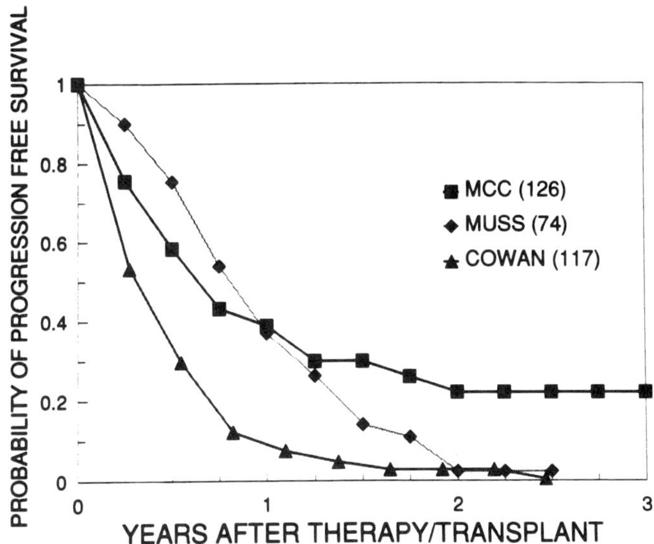

FIGURE 7. Progression-free survival in patients with metastatic breast cancer following high dose therapy or standard therapy. MCC = Moffitt Cancer Center; Muss and Cowan = standard therapy.

Another large study, reported by Cowan *et al.*[19] for the Southwest Oncology Group (SWOG), treated 411 women with metastatic breast cancer previously failing 1 cycle of nonanthracycline-based chemotherapy with single-agent chemotherapy consisting of either doxorubicin, mitoxantrone, or bisantrene.[19] No survival advantage was seen in any treatment arm, although doxorubicin was the most active single agent of the three drugs studied. The disease-free interval was less than 1 year for 97% of the patients in this study.

FIGURE 7 demonstrates disease-free survival for all patients with metastatic breast cancer treated on phase II high dose studies from our own institution and compares this group to the best treatment arms from both the Piedmont study and the SWOG study. Patients in the high dose group included anthracycline-responsive, anthracycline-refractory but miniICE-responsive patients, and patients refractory to all induction therapy and represents a more heavily pretreated group of patients than either group reported in the Piedmont or the SWOG study. As can be seen, however, high dose therapy appears to offer a disease-free survival advantage when compared to historical controls of patients receiving standard dose chemotherapy. Patients in all studies had similar pretreatment requirements concerning performance status and other physiologic criteria, making the patients in all groups comparable.

Peters *et al.*[20] conducted a similar analysis of patients with stage II and III breast cancer with 10 or more positive lymph nodes. They compared actuarial event-free survival of 85 women treated with induction chemotherapy consisting of CAF followed by high dose carmustine, cyclophosphamide, and cisplatin and autologous bone marrow support treated at their own institution to that of three historical or

TABLE 3. Doses of Chemotherapy in Patients with Metastatic Breast Cancer Treated with High Dose ICE

Drug	Dose Range (mg/m^2)	
	Dose Levels 1–10	Dose Levels 11–16
Ifosfamide	6,000–14,000	17,000–24,000
Carboplatin	1,200–2,100	1,800
Etoposide	1,800–2,100	2,100–3,000

concurrent Cancer and Leukemia Group B adjuvant chemotherapy trials of similar patients. The actuarial event-free survival for transplanted patients was 72% at 2.5 years of follow-up compared to between 38% and 52% at 2.5 years following completion of therapy for the nontransplanted patients. There was an event-free survival advantage for the transplanted group primarily related to a decrease in relapse rates for patients receiving high dose therapy.

As just illustrated, when similar groups of patients with stage II, stage III, and metastatic breast cancer were evaluated, high dose therapy appears to offer a progression-free survival advantage over standard therapy. Perhaps a more convincing demonstration of the importance of dose intensity is the event-free survival advantage of patients with metastatic breast cancer receiving higher doses of ICE. Because of the dose escalation nature of the ICE study, groups of patients were treated at multiple dose levels over a wide range of doses. Inasmuch as patients with metastatic breast cancer were comparable at all dose levels and included patients with disease responsive to either anthracyclines or miniICE, a comparison of event-free survival based on the dose of ICE received could be performed. Patients were divided into two groups based on doses received as described in TABLE 3. These groups were based on the published maximum tolerated doses of chemotherapy reported by other investigators compared to the maximum tolerated doses of ICE that we reported.[8] The upper dose levels represent dose levels of ICE given at greater than previously reported maximum tolerated doses. FIGURE 8 compares the event-free survival of patients treated at upper dose levels (dose levels 11–16) with that of patients treated at lower dose levels (dose levels 1–10). Patients receiving higher doses of ICE had improved event-free survival compared to patients treated at lower dose levels (two-tailed $p = 0.0264$), confirming the importance of administering escalated doses of chemotherapy to maximum levels. Regimen-related questions in terms of optimization of drug combinations and drug doses apparently remain. Definition of the optimal stem cell source remains a question as well. As illustrated in FIGURES 4A and B, the source of stem cells administered, bone marrow or peripheral blood, does not influence event-free survival. The absence of an advantage in patients with metastatic breast cancer receiving peripheral blood stem cell transplants contrasts with the findings in a recent publication concerning high dose therapy and autologous stem cell rescue in the treatment of non-Hodgkin's lymphoma.[21] This study demonstrated that peripheral blood stem cell transplantation was associated with superior freedom from progression in patients with good prognosis non-Hodgkin's lymphoma compared to autologous

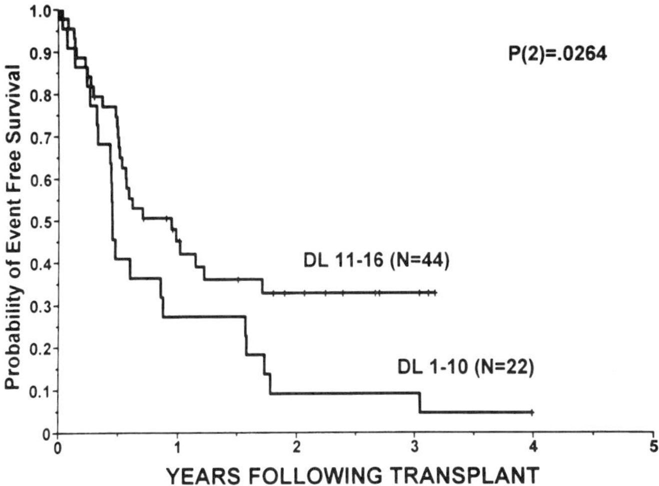

FIGURE 8. Event-free survival in patients with metastatic breast cancer treated with ICE based on the dose of chemotherapy received. DL = dose level.

bone marrow transplantation. Patients received peripheral blood stem cell transplants based on the same indications employed at our institution (i.e., evidence of bone marrow involvement or inadequate marrow cellularity for harvesting). Certainly, prospective trials to evaluate event-free survival in patients with various diseases receiving bone marrow or peripheral blood stem cell transplants are needed to determine the optimal stem cell source.

Another area of concern is that of contamination of the stem cell product with metastatic breast cancer cells. As we illustrated, PCR can be very sensitive in detecting minimal residual breast cancer in the bone marrow of patients thought to be free of metastases as determined by standard methods of detection. In this study, relapses were only seen in K19-positive patients; the absence of K19 as detected by RT-PCR methods was associated with no relapses following bone marrow transplantation, suggesting that evidence of cytokeratin 19 in the bone marrow of patients following adjuvant chemotherapy for early stage breast cancer predicts a poor outcome after high dose therapy. On the other hand, so far only a minority of K19-positive patients have had relapses.

Although it is generally assumed that peripheral blood contains fewer contaminating breast cancer cells than does bone marrow, several recent studies have demonstrated breast cancer cells in both bone marrow and peripheral blood, and at least one group of investigators has shown that these cells are viable and capable of clonogenic growth *in vitro*.[22] Other investigators have used RT-PCR methods to detect cytokeratin 19 using a different probe for K19 messenger RNA and have confirmed the presence of micrometastatic breast cancer in harvested bone marrow and peripheral blood stem cell collections of patients undergoing high dose therapy in the treatment of breast cancer.[23] Recently, messenger RNA for cytokeratin 18 has also been detected using RT-PCR methods in the blood of patients undergoing surgery in the primary treatment of breast cancer.[24]

The clinical importance of contamination of the stem cell product by breast cancer cells is currently unknown. One investigator, however, used genetic transduction studies to mark tumor cells contaminating the stem cell products of patients with neuroblastoma undergoing bone marrow transplantation and demonstrated that reinfused tumor cells can be associated with relapse.[25] In our own studies, relapses have not occurred in K19-positive breast cancer patients, suggesting that other factors also influence relapse, such as the inability to achieve complete cell kill in the remaining tumor. Further studies are needed to determine the significance of minimal metastatic disease in the bone marrow and peripheral blood stem cell products of patients undergoing high dose therapy and to define the role of manipulations to ''purge'' these contaminating cells.

In conclusion, high dose therapy is associated with improved progression-free survival compared to standard therapy in the treatment both of metastatic breast cancer and of early stage, high risk disease. We have identified several factors that influence event-free survival after treatment for metastatic breast cancer. Responsiveness to induction chemotherapy before high dose therapy, including responsiveness to anthracyclines and to ''salvage'' therapy with a regimen such as miniICE, apparently is one of the most important predictors of outcome; however, in our experience even highly refractory patients have had prolonged relapse-free survival. Dose intensity has proved to be important even within a regimen. The source of stem cells used does not influence outcome in our experience, but identification of breast cancer cells contaminating the stem cell product may predict a poorer event-free survival in some patients.

ACKNOWLEDGMENTS

The authors would like to acknowledge Walter L. Trudeau, Med Tech, for technical assistance in preparing this manuscript and Elizabeth Hubbell, Executive Secretary, for help in compiling this manuscript.

REFERENCES

1. CLARK, G., G. SLEDGE, C. K. OSBORNE & W. L. McGUIRE. 1987. Survival from first recurrence: Relative importance of prognostic factors in 1,015 breast cancer patients. J. Clin. Oncol. **5:** 55–56.
2. PETERS, W. P. 1991. High-dose chemotherapy and autologous bone marrow support for breast cancer. *In* Important Advances in Oncology. V. T. DeVita, S. Hellman & S. A. Rosenberg, Eds. : 135–150. Lippincott. Philadelphia.
3. FREI, E., B. A. TEICHER, S. A. HOLDEN *et al.* 1988. Preclinical studies and clinical correlation of the effect of alkylating dose. Cancer Res. **48:** 6417–6423.
4. BONADONNA, G. & P. VALGUSSA. 1981. Dose-response effect of adjuvant chemotherapy in breast cancer. N. Engl. J. Med. **302:** 1–15.
5. WOOD, W. C., D. R. BUDMAN, A. H. KORZUN *et al.* 1994. Dose and dose intensity of adjuvant chemotherapy for stage II, node-positive breast carcinoma. N. Engl. J. Med. **330:** 1253–1259.

6. ANTMAN, K., R. CORRINGHAM, E. DE VRIES *et al.* 1992. Dose intensive therapy in breast cancer. Bone Marrow Transplant. **10** (suppl): 67-73.

7. ARMITAGE, J. O. 1994. Research potential of the ABMTR database. Autologous Blood and Marrow Transplant Registry-North America Newsletter **1**: 2.

8. FIELDS, K. K., G. J. ELFENBEIN, H. M. LAZARUS *et al.* 1995. Maximum tolerated doses of ifosfamide, carboplatin, and etoposide given over six days followed by autologous stem cell rescue: Toxicity profile. J. Clin. Oncol. **13**: 323-332.

9. FIELDS, K. K., P. E. ZORSKY, J. W. HIEMENZ *et al.* 1994. Ifosfamide, carboplatin, and etoposide: A new regimen with a broad spectrum of activity. J. Clin. Oncol. **12**: 544-552.

10. FIELDS, K. K., G. J. ELFENBEIN, J. B. PERKINS *et al.* 1993. Two novel high-dose treatment regimens for metastatic breast cancer—Ifosfamide, carboplatin, plus etoposide and mitoxantrone plus thiotepa: Outcomes and toxicities. Semin. Oncol. **20** (suppl 6): 59-66.

11. FIELDS, K. K., J. B. PERKINS, G. J. ELFENBEIN *et al.* 1995. A phase I dose escalation trial of high dose Taxol, Novantrone, and thiotepa (TNT) followed by autologous stem cell rescue (ASCR). Toxicity. In press.

12. KLUMPP, T. R., K. F. MANGAN, L. D. GLENN & J. S. MACDONALD. 1993. Preliminary report. Phase II pilot study of high-dose busulfan and CY followed by autologous BM or peripheral blood stem cell transplantation in patients with advanced chemosensitive breast cancer. Bone Marrow Transplant. **11**: 337-339.

13. JANSSEN, W. E., R. SMILEE, R. CARTER *et al.* 1994. Mobilization of peripheral blood stem cells (PBSC): Comparing cyclophosphamide and growth factor based regimens. Prog. Clin. Biol. Res. **389**: 429-439.

14. JANSSEN, W. E., J. W. HIEMENZ, K. K. FIELDS *et al.* 1994. Peripheral blood "stem cells" do not always produce faster engraftment than bone marrow in autotransplantation. Exp. Hematol. **22**: 765.

15. FIELDS, K. K., L. C. MOSCINSKI, D. C. HEBEL, J. B. PERKINS & G. J. ELFENBEIN. 1993. Polymerase chain reaction (PCR) evaluation of bone marrow micrometastases in metastatic breast cancer. Breast Cancer Res. Treatment **27**: 144.

16. FIELDS, K., L. MOSCINSKI, W. TRUDEAU & G. ELFENBEIN. 1994. The use of polymerase chain reaction (PCR) for amplification of cytokeratin 19 (K19) to detect bone marrow (BM) micrometastases in breast cancer (CA). Proc. Am. Soc. Clin. Oncol. **13**: 115.

17. FIELDS, K. K., L. C. MOSCINSKI, W. L. TRUDEAU *et al.* 1994. High incidence of bone marrow micrometastases using the polymerase chain reaction technique in patients with high risk stage II and stage III breast cancer following adjuvant therapy: Clinical correlates. Breast Cancer Res. Treatment **32** (suppl): 63.

18. MUSS, H. B., L. D. CASE, F. RICHARDS *et al.* 1991. Interrupted versus continuous chemotherapy in patients with metastatic breast cancer. N. Engl. J. Med. **325**: 1342-1348.

19. COWAN, J. D., J. NEIDHART, S. MCCLURE *et al.* 1991. Randomized trial of doxorubicin, bisantrene, and mitoxantrone in advanced breast cancer. A Southwest Oncology Group study. J. Natl. Cancer Inst. **83**: 1077-1084.

20. PETERS, W. P., M. ROSS, J. J. VREDENBURGH *et al.* 1993. High-dose chemotherapy and autologous bone marrow support as consolidation after standard-dose adjuvant therapy for high-risk primary breast cancer. J. Clin. Oncol. **11**: 1132-1143.

21. VOSE, J., J. R. ANDERSON, A. KESSINGER *et al.* 1993. High-dose chemotherapy and autologous hematopoietic stem-cell transplantation for aggressive non-Hodgkin's lymphoma. J. Clin. Oncol. **11**: 1846-1851.

22. ROSS, A. A., B. W. COOPER, H. M. LAZARUS *et al.* 1993. Detection and viability of tumor cells in peripheral blood stem cell collection from breast cancer patients using immunocytochemical and clonogenic assay techniques. Blood **82**: 2605-2610.

23. DATTA, Y. H., P. T. ADAMS, W. R. DROBYSKI *et al.* 1994. Sensitive detection of occult breast cancer in the reverse-transcriptase polymerase chain reaction. J. Clin. Oncol. **12**: 475-482.

24. BROWN, D. C., A. D. PURUSHOTHAM, G. D. BIRNIE & W. D. GEORGE. 1995. Detection of intraoperative tumor cell dissemination in patients with breast cancer by use of reverse transcription and polymerase chain reaction. Surgery **117:** 96–101.
25. SHPALL, E. J., R. B. JONES, S. I. BEARMAN *et al.* 1994. Transplantation of enriched CD34-positive autologous marrow into breast cancer patients following high-dose chemotherapy: Influence of CD34-positive peripheral-blood progenitors and growth factors on engraftment. J. Clin. Oncol. **12:** 28–36.
26. BRUGGER, W., K. J. BROSS, M. GLATT *et al.* 1994. Mobilization of tumor cells and hematopoietic progenitor cells into peripheral blood of patients with solid tumors. Blood **83:** 636–640.
27. BRENNER, M. K., D. R. RILL, R. C. MOEN *et al.* 1993. Gene-marking to trace origin of relapse after autologous bone-marrow transplantation. Lancet **341:** 85.

Factors Influencing Prognosis after Dose-Intensive Therapy for Recurrent or Refractory Hodgkin's Disease

Results of Sequential Trials: A Case for Treating Patients with Resistant Disease

TAUSEEF AHMED,[a] DIANA LAKE, ERIC FELDMAN,
KAREN SEITER, LAWRENCE HELSON,
ABRAHAM MITTELMAN, CARMELO PUCCIO,
HOO CHUN, KATHLEEN GRIMA,
TANVEER AKHTAR, JEFFREY PERCHICK,
ZUBAIR NIAZI, ROBERT PRETI, STEVEN PAPISH,
STANLEY WAINTRAUB, MARTIN KATZ,
GREGORY BERK, MORTON COLEMAN, AND
MARIO BEER

Division of Oncology and Hematology
New York Medical College
Valhalla, New York 10595

Dose-intensive chemotherapy is now firmly established as appropriate therapy in patients with relapsed or recurrent Hodgkin's disease.[1-14] A number of factors appear to influence survival and disease-free survival after therapy for recurrent disease.[15,16] Patients with disease resistant to either initial or subsequent chemotherapy are often not treated with such therapies perhaps because of the poor results noted by several observers. Because of the occasional success with dose-intensive therapy and autologous marrow transplantation, in some patients with disease resistant to standard intensity therapy, we evaluated various factors that may be predictive of response to dose-intensive therapy. We also evaluated the impact of dose-intensive therapy on the overall prognosis of patients with recurrent resistant/refractory Hodgkin's disease who responded to one cycle of dose-intensive therapy. When possible, these patients were treated with a second cycle of dose-intensive therapy using chemotherapeutically dissimilar regimens to take advantage of non-cross-resistance between the regimens employed and also to reduce nonhematologic toxicity.

[a] To whom correspondence should be addressed.

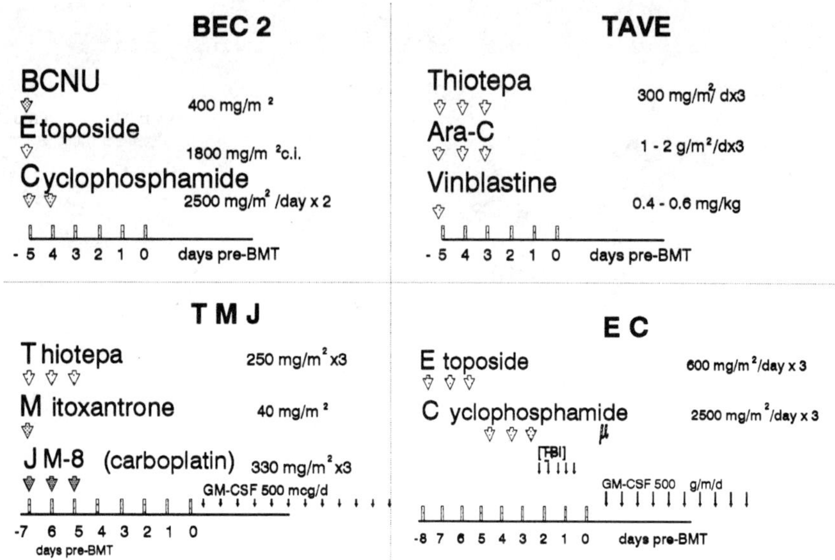

FIGURE 1. Chemotherapeutic regimens.

This report analyzes the effect of dose-intensive therapy in patients with Hodgkin's disease and evaluates the impact of various prognostic factors on outcome. Also, the impact of sequential cycles of dose-intensive therapy on the survival and disease-free survival of patients with refractory Hodgkin's disease is presented.

MATERIALS AND METHODS

Patients with histologically documented Hodgkin's disease who had not responded to or who relapsed after initial chemotherapy were eligible for dose-intensive therapy. Patients who had progression or persistence of Hodgkin's disease after initial therapy or who did not respond to salvage therapy were eligible to receive a second cycle of dose-intensive therapy if they had not exhibited progression after the first cycle of dose-intensive therapy and had adequate physiologic functions.

The chemotherapeutic regimens used are outlined in FIGURE 1. Patients were treated with these regimens along the schema outlined in TABLE 1. The first cohort of patients was treated with a combination of carmustine (BCNU) 400 mg/m², etoposide 1,800 mg/m², and cyclophosphamide 5 g/m² (BEC 2).[17] Patients with Hodgkin's disease responsive to salvage therapy (sensitive relapse) received one cycle of this therapy and autologous bone marrow/stem cell transplantation. Patients with disease refractory to initial or salvage therapy were treated with BEC 2. They were then eligible for a second cycle of dose-intensive therapy using thiotepa 900 mg/m², cytarabine 3-6 g/m², and vinblastine 0.4-0.6 mg/kg (TAVE). Because central and peripheral neurotoxicity was frequent with this regimen, patients in the latter portion

TABLE 1. Treatment Sequence

		First	Second		
Prior Response	None	BEC	None	TAVE	TMJ
Sensitive relapse		20	20	—	—
Refractory relapse		31	14	7	10
Primary refractory	2	16	5	5	6
		TMJ		EC	
Sensitive relapse		19	19	—	—
Refractory relapse	1	9	5	4	
Primary refractory	1	23	10	13	

Abbreviations: BEC = carmustine, etoposide, and oxylophosphamide; TC = etoposide and cyclophosphamide; TAVE = thiotepa, cytarabin, and vinblastine; TMJ = thiotepa, mitoxanthrone, and carboplatin.

of the BEC-2-based study were treated with a combination of thiotepa 750 mg/m^2, mitoxantrone 40 mg/m^2, and carboplatin 1,000 mg/m^2 (TMJ) and given a second infusion of autologous marrow. Cytokines were not available during this portion.

The second cohort of patients was treated with thiotepa, mitoxantrone, and carboplatin according to the schema just outlined and then an autologous marrow transplant. Patients with sensitive relapse were followed without additional therapy until evidence of progression. Patients with resistant disease were given a second course of therapy including either cyclophosphamide 5-7.5 g/m^2, etoposide 1,800-2,400 mg/m^2, and total body irradiation to 1000 cG (EC/TBI) and a second autologous marrow/stem cell transplant.

Cytokines were administered once they were available on a commercial or investigational basis.[18] Patients were treated in private or semiprivate rooms with HEPA-filtered air-handling systems. All patients received irradiated blood products. Patients seronegative for antibodies to cytomegalovirus received blood products screened for cytomegalovirus. All patients received prophylactic therapy for fungal, viral, and pneumocystis carinii infections. Broad spectrum antibiotics were given for therapy of episodes of nadir sepsis; prophylactic systemic antibiotics were not given. Total parenteral nutrition was administered in patients experiencing catabolic states secondary to oral mucositis. Intravenous morphine was given to control mucosal pain. Steroids were given for interstitial pneumonitis observed after BCNU administration.

All data were maintained in patient hospital/outpatient charts and in files in the secretariat office of the Division of Oncology and Hematology. Survival was measured from the first day of chemotherapy conditioning to the last day of followup or death. All patients were treated consecutively as part of these treatment programs. Data were entered, validated, and formated on commercially available programs, and statistical calculations were performed using the BMDP statistical package.[19] Differences between various subgroups were evaluated by chi-square and Fisher's exact tests, where appropriate, for categorical variables and by either Student's *t* test or

TABLE 2. Patient Characteristics

	Series			
	BEC		TMJ	
Total entered	69	refusal	53	122
Early progression	2		2	4
Age				
Range	16–61		19–61	4
Median	29		34	30
Sex				
Male	35		33	68
Female	34		20	54
Stage at first diagnosis				
I	1		1	2
II	20		18	38
III	27		20	47
IV	17		13	30
Undetermined	4		1	5
Prior chemotherapy regimens (*n*)				
1	7		6	13
2	33		25	58
3	22		16	39
>4	7		6	13
Prior radiation				
Yes	43		24	67
No	26		29	55
Prior response status				
Sensitive relapse	20		19	39
Refractory relapse	31		10	41
Primary refractory	18		24	42

nonparametric tests, as appropriate, after proper correction and testing for distribution.[20] The log rank test was used to evaluate differences between survival curves.[21] If not mentioned, test power is 80% or higher for negative comparisons.[22] All comparisons are for a two-sided alpha error of 5%. A stepwise multivariate analysis based on Cox's model was performed including, after appropriate coding, all singly significant or possibly significant pretreatment characteristics with regard to survival.[19]

RESULTS

Patient Characteristics

One hundred twenty-two patients were treated with the program just outlined. Their characteristics are listed in TABLE 2. Sixty-nine patients were entered on the

TABLE 3. Potentially Lethal Nonhematologic Toxicity

	Regimen	
	BEC 2 ($n = 67$)	TMJ ($n = 51$)
Lung	8	4
Liver	6	0
Cardiac	1	3
Sepsis	3	0
Fungal/Tbc	2	0
Ileus	1	0
CNS	1	0

BEC-based regimens and 53 patients signed consents for TMJ-based therapies. Two patients in each group did not receive transplants despite initial consent, two because they died before transplantation and two because they refused. They were, however, included in all outcome analyses. One hundred eighteen patients were treated with these regimens. The median age was 30 years (range 16-61), and 68 were male and 54 female. Two patients had stage I Hodgkin's disease at the time of initial diagnosis, while 38 had stage II Hodgkin's disease, 47 had stage III, and 30 had stage IV. The exact stage was unclear in five patients, four in the BEC group and 1 in the TMJ group. Twelve patients had no evidence of disease after salvage therapy, whereas an additional 27 had responsive disease, albeit with residual radiographic abnormalities. These two subgroups were broadly characterized as having sensitive relapse of Hodgkin's disease. Seventy-nine patients had refractory disease; of these, 40 had not responded to salvage therapy after having experienced a response to initial chemotherapy, and 39 had persistent disease or evidence of progression of the disease after initial induction therapy.

Toxicity

The major toxicities in patients receiving these therapies are outlined in TABLE 3. Patients receiving BEC-based therapy were more likely to develop interstitial pneumonitis than were patients treated with TMJ. In addition to the eight patients developing pulmonary dysfunction after initial BCNU-based therapy, four on BEC-based therapy who developed pulmonary dysfunction died as a result of supervening opportunistic infections during steroid therapy which was necessary to treat pneumonitis while clinically free of disease. Interstitial pneumonia was a frequent cause of mortality in patients with sensitive relapse of Hodgkin's disease receiving BEC therapy. This was not the case in patients with sensitive relapse who were treated with TMJ. In fact, it was unusual to encounter pulmonary dysfunction in TMJ-treated patients. Serious hepatic toxicity was more common with BEC therapies than with TMJ. This generally manifested itself with an increase in hepatic enzymes and bilirubin and was clinically associated with encephalopathy. Although no specific therapy was employed for hepatic abnormalities, with supportive therapy enzymes often returned to normal values. Hematologic toxicity was similar in both groups. The median time to blood count recovery was faster in patients receiving peripheral blood progenitor cells. Mucositis, however, was less common in BEC-treated patients after the advent of propantheline therapy for the group.[23] The median number of days in hospital was similar for both groups.

In the subset of patients receiving a second cycle of dose-intensive therapy, TAVE was used initially; however, prohibitive neurologic toxicity, severe myalgias requiring morphine, and ileus requiring surgery led to the adoption of TMJ as the conditioning regimen for the second transplant. Neurologic toxicity was markedly uncommon with TMJ as the second or initial therapy. Therapy-related mortality was more frequent with BCNU-containing regimens than with TMJ-based therapy, especially in patients with sensitive relapse of Hodgkin's disease receiving BEC compared to patients with sensitive relapse receiving TMJ.

Survival and Factors Associated with Improved Outcome

Absence of significant differences could not be established sufficiently in the overall survival of patients treated with BEC than in those receiving TMJ-based therapy, with, respectively, 49% and 70% actuarial survival probability at 2 years, even though there was an apparent advantage to being treated with TMJ than with BEC. This apparent difference could be related to factors other than the exact conditioning regimen, that is, use of cytokines, peripheral stem cells, and other differences in supportive techniques. Patients with sensitive relapse who were transplanted when there was no evidence of disease or evidence of residual disease by clinical criteria were equally likely to survive. Overall, patients with sensitive relapse receiving one transplant had superior survival to those with refractory relapse given two transplants who, in turn, did clearly better than did those with refractory disease given one transplant, that is, resistance to standard dose chemotherapy was associated with a worse outcome after dose intensive therapy. However, the number of prior regimens was not a significant factor in outcome after dose-intensive therapy. Thus, this analysis indicated that patients with disease that remained sensitive to standard intensity therapy are likely to respond favorably to dose-intensive therapy regardless of the number of prior regimens.

Besides resistance to standard dose therapy, factors associated with a poor outcome included prior radiation therapy. There was likewise a trend towards a worse outcome with initial stage II disease, which could represent an association with radiotherapy in stage II disease. Other factors identified as being significant in univariate analysis, such as age or sex (males worse than females), were not identified as independently significant variables in the multivariate analysis.

DISCUSSION

A number of regimens have been used to reinduce remission in patients with relapsing Hodgkin's disease in an attempt to cytoreduce and test chemosensitivity before more aggressive therapies.[18,24-29] A tremendous amount of interest has been generated in the use of dose intensity as curative therapy in the management of patients with malignant and nonmalignant disorders. Dose-intensive therapy has been effective in curing selected patients with Hodgkin's disease. Many factors affect survival after dose-intensive therapy. Analyses of prognostic variables are intrinsically affected by the regimens involved. Also, significant prognostic features in the untreated state[30,31] differ from those when radiation or standard intensity therapy has been used. Dose-intensive therapies should be used with a clear understanding of the principles involved and the rationale behind such therapies. Therapeutic strategies could thus lead to the identification of prognostic variables that are dissimilar to variables that are important with other therapies.[15,16] In this series sensitivity to standard intensity therapy apparently had an impact on the overall probability of survival after dose-intensive therapy. Also, dose-intensive therapy could be delivered in a sequential manner to patients with refractory disease, a subgroup often construed to be inappropriate for this type of therapy. It should be borne in mind that response to prior therapy did in fact influence progression-free survival, but a subset of these patients could be rendered free of disease. Patients with refractory disease could be successfully salvaged when dose-intensive therapy was administered sequentially.

The use of regimens not containing BCNU reduced the frequency of pulmonary dysfunction and its complications. High dose steroids are often essential in managing patients with the pulmonary complications of therapy.[17] Patients on long-term steroid therapy can develop life-threatening opportunistic infections.

The availability of better methods of supportive care, especially peripheral blood progenitor cells and cytokines, has allowed these types of therapy to be administered with relative facility.[6,18,32–35] Peripheral progenitor cell support helped increase blood counts rapidly and shortened the period of cytopenia, thus potentially having a favorable impact on the risk of morbidity and the probability of survival after dose-intensive therapy.[6,36]

The economic consequences of this therapy are not trivial. Patients and payers are under significant pressure as a result of these treatments. Hospitals have seized upon dose intensity as a means of enhancing reputation and income. As improved methods of supportive care have emerged and continue to develop, it is obvious that the next generation of therapies for this group of patients will address the question of the price, in human terms, of this type of therapy. The question of allocating scarce resources in an era of competing priorities, the cost of such therapies, the impact of these therapies in improving survival, disease-free survival, and quality of life issues must come to the forefront.

As improved supportive therapies and better conditioning regimens emerge, the therapeutic strategies employed in deciding therapy for individuals and patient groups will obviously change. Given our data, dose-intensive therapies applied appropriately are effective in enhancing disease-free and overall survival of patients with refractory, recurrent, and relapsed Hodgkin's disease. Patients with refractory disease can be effectively salvaged and can enjoy long-term disease-free survival if dose-intensive therapies are given repetitively.

REFERENCES

1. AHMED, T., D. CIAVARELLA, E. FELDMAN, J. ASCENSAO, F. HUSSAIN, C. ENGELKING, S. GINGRICH, A. MITTELMAN, M. COLEMAN & Z. A. ARLIN. 1989. High-dose, potentially

myeloablative chemotherapy and autologous bone marrow transplantation for patients with advanced Hodgkin's disease. Leukemia **3:** 19-22.

2. APPELBAUM, F. R., K. M. SULLIVAN, C. D. BUCKNER, R. A. CLIFT, H. J. DEEG, A. FEFER, R. HILL, J. MORTIMER, P. E. NEIMAN, J. E. SANDERS *et al.* 1987. Treatment of malignant lymphoma in 100 patients with chemotherapy, total body irradiation, and marrow transplantation. J. Clin. Oncol. **5:** 1340-1347.

3. ANDERSON, J. E., M. R. LITZOW, F. R. APPELBAUM *et al.* 1993. Allogeneic, syngeneic and autologous marrow transplantation for Hodgkin's disease: The 21 year Seattle experience. J. Clin. Oncol. **11:** 2342-2350.

4. CARELLA, A. M., A. CONGIU, P. CARLIER, G. MELONI, G. CIMINO, A. ANSELMI, P. MAZZA, L. MANGONI, A. PORCELLINI, N. LOCATELLI *et al.* 1989. Italian experience with autologous bone marrow transplantation in 104 advanced Hodgkin's lymphoma patients. Bone Marrow Transplant. **4** (Suppl. 4): 113-116.

5. CARELLA, A. M. & A. M. MARMONT. 1989. Treatment of resistant Hodgkin's lymphoma with bone marrow transplantation in Italy. Recent results. Cancer Res. **117:** 239-241.

6. KESSINGER, A., P. J. BIERMAN, J. M. VOSE & J. O. ARMITAGE. 1991. High-dose cyclophosphamide, carmustine and etoposide followed by autologous peripheral stem cell transplantation for patients with relapsed Hodgkin's disease. Blood **77:** 2322-2325.

7. RUSSELL, J. A., P. J. SELBY, B. A. RUETHER, E. K. MBIDDE, S. ASHLEY, G. ZULIAN, J. BERRY, B. HOUWEN, A. R. JONES, M. C. POON *et al.* 1989. Treatment of advanced Hodgkin's disease with high dose melphalan and autologous bone marrow transplantation. Bone Marrow Transplant. **4:** 425-429.

8. SPINOLO, J. A., S. JAGANNATH, K. A. DICKE, K. E. SMITH, F. CABANILLAS, F. B. HAGEMEISTER, L. J. HORWITZ, P. MCLAUGHLIN, F. SWAN & G. SPITZER. 1989. High-dose combination chemotherapy with cyclophosphamide, carmustine, etoposide, and autologous bone marrow transplantation in 60 patients with relapsed Hodgkin's disease: The M. D. Anderson experience. Recent Results Cancer Res. **117:** 233-238.

9. PHILLIPS, G. L., S. N. WOLFF, R. H. HERZIG, H. M. LAZARUS, J. W. FAY, H. S. LIN, D. C. SHINA, G. P. GLASGOW, R. C. GRIFFITH, C. W. LAMB *et al.* 1989. Treatment of progressive Hodgkin's disease with intensive chemoradiotherapy and autologous bone marrow transplantation. Blood **73:** 2086-2092.

10. WEAVER, C. H., F. R. APPELBAUM, F. B. PETERSON *et al.* 1993. High-dose cyclophosphamide, carmustine and etoposide followed by autologous bone marrow transplantation in patients with lymphoid malignancies who have received dose limiting radiation therapy. J. Clin. Oncol. **11:** 1329-1335.

11. YAHALOM, J., S. GULATI, B. SHANK, B. CLARKSON & Z. FUKS. 1989. Total lymphoid irradiation, high-dose chemotherapy and autologous bone marrow transplantation for chemotherapy-resistant Hodgkin's disease. Int. J. Radiat. Oncol. Biol. Phys. **17:** 915-922.

12. ZULIAN, G. B., P. SELBY, S. MILAN, A. NANDI, M. GORE, G. FORGESON, T. J. PERREN & T. J. MCELWAIN. 1989. High dose melphalan, BCNU and etoposide with autologous bone marrow transplantation for Hodgkin's disease. Br. J. Cancer **59:** 631-635.

13. REECE, D. E., M. J. BARNETT, J. M. CONNORS *et al.* 1991. Intensive chemotherapy with cyclophosphamide, carmustine, and etoposide followed by autologous bone marrow transplantation for relapsed Hodgkin's disease. J. Clin. Oncol. **9:** 1871-1879.

14. REECE, D. E., J. M. CONNORS, J. J. SPINELLI *et al.* 1994. Intensive therapy with cyclophosphamide, carmustine, etoposide +/- cisplatin and autologous bone marrow transplantation for Hodgkin's disease in first relapse after combination chemotherapy. Blood **5:** 1193-1199.

15. JAGANNATH, S., J. O. ARMITAGE, K. A. DICKE, S. L. TUCKER, W. S. VELASQUEZ, K. SMITH, W. P. VAUGHAN, A. KESSINGER, L. J. HORWITZ, F. B. HAGEMEISTER *et al.* 1989. Prognostic factors for response and survival after high-dose cyclophosphamide, carmus-

tine, and etoposide with autologous bone marrow transplantation for relapsed Hodgkin's disease. J. Clin. Oncol. **7:** 179-185.

16. LOHRI, A., M. BARNETT, R. N. FAIREY et al. 1991. Outcome of treatment of first relapse of Hodgkin's disease after primary chemotherapy: Identification of risk factors from the British Columbia experience 1970-1988. Blood **77:** 2292-2298.

17. BISHOP, M. R., R. ANDERSON, J. D. JACKSON et al. 1994. High dose therapy and peripheral progenitor transplantation. Effects of recombinant human granulocyte macrophage colony stimulating factor on the autograft. Blood **83:** 610-616.

18. DIXON, W. J., M. B. BROWN, L. ENGELMAN & R. I. JENNRICH (Eds.) 1990. BMDP Statistical Software Manual. University of California Press. Los Angeles. :135-144, 145-163, 231-310, 739-768.

19. DIXON, W. J. & F. J. MASSEY, Jr. 1983. Introduction to Statistical Analysis. 4th Ed. McGraw-Hill. New York.

20. MANTEL, N. 1966. Evaluation of survival data and two new rank order statistics arising in its consideration. Cancer Chemother. Rep. **50:** 163-170.

21. MACHIN, D. & M. J. CAMPBELL (Eds.). 1987. Statistical Tables for the Design of Clinical Trials. : 10-34, 54-59, 79-88, 132-168. Blackwell Scientific Publication. Oxford.

22. AHMED, T., C. ENGELKING, J. SZALYGA, L. HELSON, N. COOMBE, P. COOK, D. CORBI, C. PUCCIO, H. CHUN & A. MITTELMAN. 1993. Propantheline prevention of mucositis from etoposide. BMT **12:** 131-132.

23. AHMED, T., P. COOK, E. FELDMAN, N. COOMBE, C. PUCCIO, A. MITTELMAN, H. CHUN, M. COLEMAN & L. HELSON. 1994. Phase I-II trial of high dose Ara-C, carboplatinum, etoposide and steroids in patients with refractory or relapsed lymphomas. Leukemia **8:** 531-534.

24. BUZAID, A. C., S. M. LIPPMAN & T. P. MILLER. 1987. Salvage therapy of advanced Hodgkin's disease. Critical appraisal of curative potential. Am. J. Med. **83:** 523-532.

25. CABANILLAS, F., W. S. VELASQUEZ, P. McLAUGHLIN, S. JAGANNATH, F. B. HAGEMEISTER, J. R. REDMAN, F. SWAN & M. A. RODRIGUEZ. 1988. Results of recent salvage chemotherapy regimens for lymphoma and Hodgkin's disease. Semin. Hematol. **25** (Suppl. 2): 47-50.

26. LONGO, D. L., P. L. DUFFEY & R. C. YOUNG. 1992. Conventional dose salvage combination chemotherapy in patients relapsing with Hodgkin's disease after combination chemotherapy: The low probability of cure. J. Clin. Oncol. **10:** 210-218.

27. PFREUNDSCHUH, M. G., U. RUEFFER, B. LATHAN et al. 1994. Dexa-BEAM in patients with Hodgkin's disease refractory to multidrug chemotherapy regimens. A trial of the German Hodgkin's disease study group. J. Clin. Oncol. **12:** 580-586.

28. VELASQUEZ, W. S., F. CABANILLAS, P. SALVADOR, P. McLAUGHLIN, M. FRIDIK, S. TUCKER, S. JAGANNATH, F. B. HAGEMEISTER, J. R. REDMAN, F. SWAN & B. BARLOGIE. 1988. Effective salvage therapy for lymphoma with cisplatin in combination with high dose Ara-C and dexamethasone (DHAP). Blood **71:** 117-122.

29. STRAUSS, D. J., J. J. GAYNOR, J. MYERS et al. 1990. Prognostic factors among 185 patients with newly diagnosed advanced Hodgkin's disease treated with alternating potentially non-cross resistant chemotherapy and intermediate dose radiation therapy. J. Clin. Oncol. **8:** 1173-1186.

30. PROCTOR, S. J., P. TAYLOR, P. DONNAN et al. 1991. A numerical prognostic index for clinical use in identification of poor risk patients with Hodgkin's disease at diagnosis. Eur. J. Cancer **116:** 177-182.

31. DEVEREAUX, S., D. C. LINCH, J. G. GRIBBEN, A. McMILLAN, K. PATTERSON & A. H. GOLDSTONE. 1989. GM-CSF accelerates neutrophil recovery after autologous bone marrow transplantation for Hodgkin's disease. Bone Marrow Transplant. **4:** 49-54.

32. GIANNI, A., S. SIENA, M. BREGNI et al. 1989. Granulocyte macrophage colony stimulating factor to harvest circulating hematopoietic stem cells for auto transplantation. Lancet **1:** 580-595.

33. JONES, H. M., S. A. JONES, M. J. WATTS *et al.* 1994. Development of a simplified single apheresis approach for peripheral blood progenitor cell transplantation in previously treated patients with lymphoma. J. Clin. Oncol. **12:** 1693–1702.
34. AHMED, T., D. CIAVARELLA, P. COOK & D. WUEST. 1994. Blood progenitor cells: Collection techniques and applications. Cancer Invest. **12:** 421–424.
35. KORBLING, M., R. HOLLE, R. HASS *et al.* 1990. Autologous blood stem-cell transplantation in patients with advanced Hodgkin's disease and prior radiation to the pelvic site. J. Clin. Oncol. **8:** 978–985.

Relative Contributions of Marrow Microenvironment, Growth Factors, and Stem Cells to Hematopoiesis *in Vivo* in Man

Review of Results from Autologous Stem Cell Transplant Trials and Laboratory Studies at the Moffitt Cancer Center

GERALD J. ELFENBEIN,[a] WILLIAM E. JANSSEN,
AND JANELLE B. PERKINS

Division of Bone Marrow Transplantation
Department of Internal Medicine
University of South Florida College of Medicine at the H. Lee
Moffitt Cancer Center and Research Institute
Tampa, Florida 33612

Laboratory research over the last 30 years has defined the process of hematopoiesis rather clearly. We now know from animal studies and *in vitro* model systems that three critical components are responsible for hematopoiesis in all vertebrates studied: (1) stem cells, (2) growth factors, and (3) marrow microenvironment. In any system studied, these three components participate in an interactive manner, and the resulting hematopoietic outcome is a product of these three factors and not just the consequence of any single one acting independently. Autologous stem cell transplantation after myeloablative chemotherapy or chemoradiotherapy is an ideal model system for the study of hematopoiesis *in vivo* in man. By studying the recovery of granulopoiesis from the null state, we can determine the relative roles and interactive characteristics of each of the three components contributing to hematopoiesis.

High dose chemotherapy or chemoradiotherapy has become an extremely valuable tool in the therapeutic arsenal for patients with malignant diseases that are responsive to therapy but not curable at conventional doses or not curable as frequently at conventional doses. High dose therapy uses cytotoxic agents at doses well beyond the tolerance of the bone marrow, that is, high dose therapy is myeloablative. High dose therapy can only be given because a salvage procedure from myeloablation, that is, hematopoietic stem cell transplantation, is available. High dose therapy was first widely used for malignancies of the bone marrow, such as leukemias, and then for malignancies of the immune system, such as lymphomas. It is now being employed

---

[a] Address for correspondence: Gerald J. Elfenbein, MD, Moffitt Cancer Center, University of South Florida, 12902 Magnolia Drive, Tampa, FL 33612.

more often for solid tumors, as in breast cancer, where no known aberration in hematopoiesis or immune function is caused by the malignant disease.

High dose chemotherapy for solid tumors followed by autologous stem cell transplantation in man provides the opportunity to confirm *in vivo* the interactive roles of the three components contributing to hematopoiesis. This communication reviews the results of clinical trials and the supporting laboratory studies at a single institution that demonstrates that the process of granulopoiesis, especially after high dose chemotherapy and autologous stem cell transplantation, involves all three components in an interactive manner. These observations have clearcut clinical relevance. As we strive to achieve faster and faster granulopoiesis (to reduce treatment toxicity) by modulating stem cells and altering growth factors, we must also be aware that optimizing the antineoplastic activity of high dose chemotherapy (by altering doses or changing cytotoxic agents) may have profound consequences on the process of granulopoiesis as well. After all, it is cure of cancer that is our primary objective with less toxicity as the secondary goal.

MATERIALS AND METHODS

Patients. The data that are presented herein come from clinical trials that were approved by the Scientific Review Committee of the H. Lee Moffitt Cancer Center and Research Institute and approved and reviewed annually by the Institutional Review Board of the University of South Florida in Tampa, Florida. All patients involved in these trials gave written informed consent to participate. The principal goal of these trials was to develop high dose chemotherapy that was more effective for specific neoplastic diseases, such as breast cancer, to achieve improved long-term freedom from disease, with the secondary goal of these trials being reduction in the toxicity of high dose chemotherapy, such as shortening the period of aplasia after autologous stem cell transplantation, to reduce death from infection while neutropenia was still present. TABLE 1 shows the cumulative stem cell transplant experience of the Bone Marrow Transplant Program at the Moffitt Cancer Center since its inception in October 1989 through the end of February 1995.

Regimens. Four high dose chemotherapy regimens were employed, three of which are novel. The first one developed was the ICE regimen which employs high doses of ifosfamide, carboplatin, and etoposide.[1-3] The second one developed was the MITT regimen which employs high doses of mitoxantrone and thio-TEPA.[4] The third one developed was the TNT regimen which added Taxol to Novantrone (mitoxantrone) and thio-TEPA.[5] The fourth one, which was adopted, was the BUCY2 regimen which employs high doses of busulfan and cyclophosphamide. The ICE, MITT, and TNT regimens were all phase I dose escalation trials that were converted to phase II trials once the maximum tolerated doses (MTD) of the drugs in combination were determined. Summaries of these three regimens are shown in TABLE 2. The BUCY2 regimen was the first Ohio State modification of the original Johns Hopkins protocol[6] and is also shown in TABLE 2.

Growth Factors. Hematopoietic growth factors were employed in two circumstances. The first use was to stimulate more rapid recovery of granulopoiesis after autologous stem cell transplantation. Recombinant human granulocyte-macrophage

TABLE 1. Annual and Cumulative Hematopoietic Stem Cell Transplants Through February 28, 1995

Calendar Year (Time Frame)	Autologous				Allogeneic		HSCT Totals	Breast Cancer
	BMT	PBSCT	Both	Random Trial	HLA-Identical (and Syngeneic)	MRD and MUD		
1989 (2 mo)	5	0	0	0	0	0	5	3
1990	30	3	1	0	13	5	52	20
1991	44	16	0	0	10	4	74	44
1992	57	27	0	1	14 (1)	5	104	55
1993	21	29	18	25	23	2	118	60
1994	5	67	26	24	16 (1)	7	145	63
1995 (2 mo)	0	11	6	2	0	0	18	12
Totals	160	153	51	52	76 (2)	23	515	257

Abbreviations: BMT = bone marrow transplant; PBSCT = peripheral blood stem cell transplant; Both = both bone marrow transplant and peripheral blood stem cell transplant; Random Trial = randomized to either PBSCT or BMT, both collected after growth factor stimulation; MRD = mismatched related donor allogeneic BMT; MUD = matched unrelated donor allogeneic BMT; HSCT = hematopoietic stem cell transplant.

TABLE 2. Autologous Stem Cell Transplant Regimens

Regimen (Ref.)	Drugs (Cumulative Doses)			Dose Levels	Drug Delivery
ICE (1–3)	Ifosfamide (I)	Carboplatin (C)	Etoposide (E)	16	E: Continuous infusion over 6 days
Starting	6.0 g/m^2	1.2 g/m^2	1.8 g/m^2		
Highest	24.0 g/m^2	2.1 g/m^2	3.0 g/m^2		I & C: 6 daily boluses
MTD	20.1 g/m^2	1.8 g/m^2	3.0 g/m^2		
MITT (4)	Mitoxantrone (Mi)	ThioTEPA (TT)		7	Mi & TT: 3 daily boluses
Starting	45 mg/m^2	0.9 g/m^2			
Highest	105 mg/m^2	1.35 g/m^2			
MTD	90 mg/m^2	1.2 g/m^2			
TNT (5)	Taxol[a] (Tax)	Novantrone[b] (Nov)	ThioTepa	5	Nov & TT: 3 daily boluses
Starting	120 mg/m^2	90 mg/m^2	1.2 g/m^2		Tax: Continuous infusion over same 3 days
Highest	360 mg/m^2	90 mg/m^2	1.2 g/m^2		
BUCY2 (6)	Busulfan (Bu)	Cyclophosphamide (Cy)		—	Bu: Oral over 4 days
	16 mg/kg	120 mg/kg			Cy: Boluses over subsequent 2 days

Abbreviation: MTD = maximal tolerated dose.

[a] Taxol = paciltaxel.

[b] Novantrone = mitoxantrone.

colony stimulating factor (GM-CSF; sargramostim) was given intravenously at a dose of 250 μg/m^2 per day starting 1 day after stem cell infusion and continuing until the granulocyte count was greater than 1,000/μL for 3 consecutive days. Recombinant human granulocyte colony stimulating factor (G-CSF; filgrastim) was given intravenously at a dose of 10 μg/kg per day starting 1 day after stem cell infusion and continuing until the granulocyte count was greater than 1,000/μl for 3 consecutive days.

The second use was to assist in the enrichment of the stem cell content of peripheral blood mononuclear cell collections to reduce the number of leukaphereses necessary to collect a sufficient number of stem cells to serve as an adequate stem cell source for restoring hematopoiesis after myeloablative chemotherapy. This process has been termed "mobilization." Chemotherapy alone can mobilize stem cells and, in so doing, can also provide an additional antineoplastic effect. Growth factors alone can rapidly mobilize stem cells when given for a brief period before leukaphereses. We used GM-CSF alone for 5 days at a dose of 250 μg/m^2 per day before initiating leukapheresis and continued GM-CSF through the penultimate day, that is, the day before the last leukapheresis. We used G-CSF alone at a dose of 16 μg/kg per day before initiating leukaphereses and continued G-CSF through the penultimate day. We also used G-CSF at a dose of 10 μg/kg per day starting 1 day after completing chemotherapy with either cyclophosphamide (CY) alone (50 mg/kg per day for 2 days) or CY (same dose and schedule) in combination with etoposide (VP16; 300 mg/m^2 per day for 2 days by continuous infusion on the same days as CY administration). Leukaphereses were begun as early as the day the leukocyte count first reached 1,000/μL. G-CSF was continued until the penultimate day. Under all three circumstances, the median number of aphereses was five with a range of four to eight with the number of aphereses determined by the desire to collect the minimally acceptable number of CD34 positive (+) cells (more than 0.5 $\times$ 10^6 cells/kg) to assure engraftment, as measured by direct immunofluorescence microscopy (to be described).

Stem Cells. Two sources of hematopoietic stem cells were used, unpurged bone marrow stem cells (BMSC) and unmanipulated peripheral blood stem cells (PBSC).[7] The techniques for collecting BMSC and PBSC are well known and were previously reported.[3,8] Two different sets of criteria for choice of stem cell product were employed at two different times. The first set of criteria are the same as those used at the University of Nebraska in Omaha. Specifically, if bilateral bone marrow biopsies obtained on two separate occasions were all morphologically free of tumor cells, that is, "never positive," sufficiently cellular, and free of significant fibrosis, then BMSC were collected from the patient in the "resting" state, that is, at least 4 weeks after the last chemotherapy or growth factor administration. If any of the four biopsies showed evidence of tumor cells, that is, "ever positive," or if the most recent bone marrow biopsies after chemotherapy were insufficiently cellular or showed significant fibrosis, then PBSC were collected after mobilization either with chemotherapy alone, with chemotherapy followed by G-CSF, or after growth factors alone.

The second (and current) set of criteria are as follows: If bone marrow biopsies were ever positive or marrow was otherwise unharvestable (because of poor cellularity or significant fibrosis), than PBSC were collected after chemotherapy with CYVP16 followed by G-CSF (CYVPG) during recovery from neutropenia. If bone marrow biopsies were never positive, marrow was harvestable and the patient was to be treated with ICE or MITT, then the patient was eligible to participate in a prospective, controlled trial in which both products would be collected, and at the scheduled time of stem cell infusion, the patient would receive one or the other stem cell product on a randomized basis. In the first phase of this randomized trial, patients were pretreated with GM-CSF before harvesting BMSC on day 5 of growth factor, and PBSC were harvested daily on days 6 through 10 of growth factor. In the second phase of this trial, G-CSF replaced GM-CSF. The objective of this trial was to determine if BMSC collected under ''stimulating'' conditions, that is, those used to mobilize stem cells for PBSC collection with growth factors, were as effective as mobilized PBSC in accelerating granulopoiesis after stem cell infusion. In this trial the control arm was the PBSC arm. It was theoretically possible for stimulated BMSC to be as effective as mobilized PBSC or inferior to mobilized PBSC. Furthermore, it was also possible for stimulated BMSC to be, in fact, inferior to resting BMSC. This, however, could only be demonstrated by comparison with historical data. If the patient chose not to participate in the randomized stem cell trial, then we collected resting BMSC, which was our standard practice.

Statistics. The endpoints of the clinical studies insofar as hematopoiesis is concerned were the first days after stem cell infusion at which the granulocyte count exceeds $500/\mu L$, the platelet count exceeds $20,000/\mu L$, and the platelet count exceeds $50,000/\mu L$. To test for significance between groups, when two groups were being compared, a log-rank test was applied. When three or more groups were being compared, Mantel's generalization of Gehan's Wilcoxan log-rank test was used. All statistical manipulations were performed using the Statistica software package (StaSoft, Tulsa, Oklahoma).

Hematopoietic Assessment.[9–12] To measure the fraction of cells that bore on their surface the CD34 antigen, 5×10^5 cells to be assayed suspended in 0.1 ml of Dulbecco's phosphate-buffered saline solution (DPBS) (GIBCO, Grand Island, New York) were admixed with 20 μl of phycoerythrin-tagged anti-CD34 (HPCA-2, Becton-Dickinson, San Jose, California). After 30 minutes of incubation on ice, cells were thrice washed with cold DPBS and resuspended in 0.1 ml. The cell suspension was placed on a microscope slide, and CD34[+] cells were scored by eye using fluorescence microscopy. In more recent studies, flow cytometric evaluation has supplanted visual enumeration. To measure the presence of granulocyte/macrophage colony-forming cells (CFU-GM), 2×10^5 cells were plated in 35 mm petri dishes containing 1 ml of Iscove's medium containing 0.8% or, in later studies, 1.15% methylcellulose (Stem Cell Technologies, Vancouver, British Columbia) and supplemented with 20% fetal bovine serum and 1 ng GM-CSF (Genzyme, Boston, Massachusetts). After 14 days of incubation, colonies of greater than 25 cells were scored.

RESULTS

Marrow Microenvironment. Five bodies of data illustrate that patient-specific circumstances, that is, those that are not growth factor related or stem cell dependent, determine the pace of hematopoiesis after autologous stem cell infusion following high dose chemotherapy. These circumstances we deem marrow microenvironmental, whether they are soluble or cellular in nature.

The first set of data come from the phase I portion of the high dose ICE trial in which resting BMSC were used as the source of reconstituting hematopoietic stem cells. We made a curious observation. At lower dose levels of ICE (1-9), recovery of the platelet count to 20,000/μl (untransfused and self-sustained) actually preceded the recovery of granulocytes to 500/μl (FIG. 1A).[8] In fact, recovery of the platelet count to 50,000/μl occurred simultaneously with the recovery of granulocytes to 500/μl (data not shown).

Subsequently, we observed at the higher dose levels of ICE (9-16) that the time to recover a platelet count of 20,000/μl was longer than that at the lower dose levels of ICE (1-9) and that platelet counts recovered after granulocyte counts (FIG. 1B-D).[8] Patients who received dose levels 1-9 received no growth factor; patients who received dose levels 9-16 received GM-CSF; and subsequent patients who received dose level 16 (the MTD) received G-CSF. The earlier recovery of granulocytes despite higher dose levels of ICE is undoubtedly due to the use of growth factors, details of which are to be described. The later recovery of platelets at higher dose levels of ICE may be a negative effect because of the use of granulopoietic growth factors; however, this is felt to be unlikely, especially with the growth factor G-CSF. Thus, we have the first bit of evidence suggesting that a patient-specific factor, in this case the dose intensity of chemotherapy, may have an impact on the pace of recovering hematopoiesis, in this case thrombopoiesis, from the null state.

The second body of data comes from the phase I portion of the high dose MITT trial when viewed in the context of the parallel ICE trial.[12] In both studies, there were patients for whom resting BMSC were used to reconstitute hematopoiesis. In both studies, there were sequential patients for whom G-CSF was used after autologous stem cell infusion to accelerate granulopoiesis. As can readily be seen from FIGURE 2A, the slope of the curve (which we will term "kinetics") of granulocyte recovery is different for the two different regimens, and the median day or midpoint of the curve (which we will term "pace") of granulocyte recovery is vastly different for the two different regimens. No measurable differences were evident in either the CD34[+] cell count or the CFU-GM growth potential of the BMSC collected from these two groups of patients to account for either the differences of slope or midpoint of the sigmoid-shaped curves of granulocyte recovery after BMSC infusion following high dose chemotherapy.

Patients were prospectively assigned to the ICE regimen[4] if their disease was sensitive to an anthracycline-based induction regimen or, failing that, if their disease was sensitive to an abbreviated version of high dose ICE, the "mini-ICE" regimen.[1,13] Patients who were refractory to both an anthracycline-based regimen and mini-ICE were assigned to receive the MITT regimen (and later in time the TNT regimen, see below). The differences in pace of granulopoiesis may be due to either the extent of prior chemotherapy,[14] which was clearly different between the two groups,[4] the different high dose regimens themselves, or both circumstances. In any event we have the second bit of evidence suggesting that a patient-specific factor, in this case chemotherapy (remote and/or recent), may have an impact on the pace of hematopoiesis, in this case granulopoiesis, from the null state.

The third body of data also comes from the phase I portions of the ICE and MITT trials and from the phase II portion of the BUCY2 trial.[12] In all three studies, there were patients for whom mobilized PBSC were used to reconstitute hematopoie-

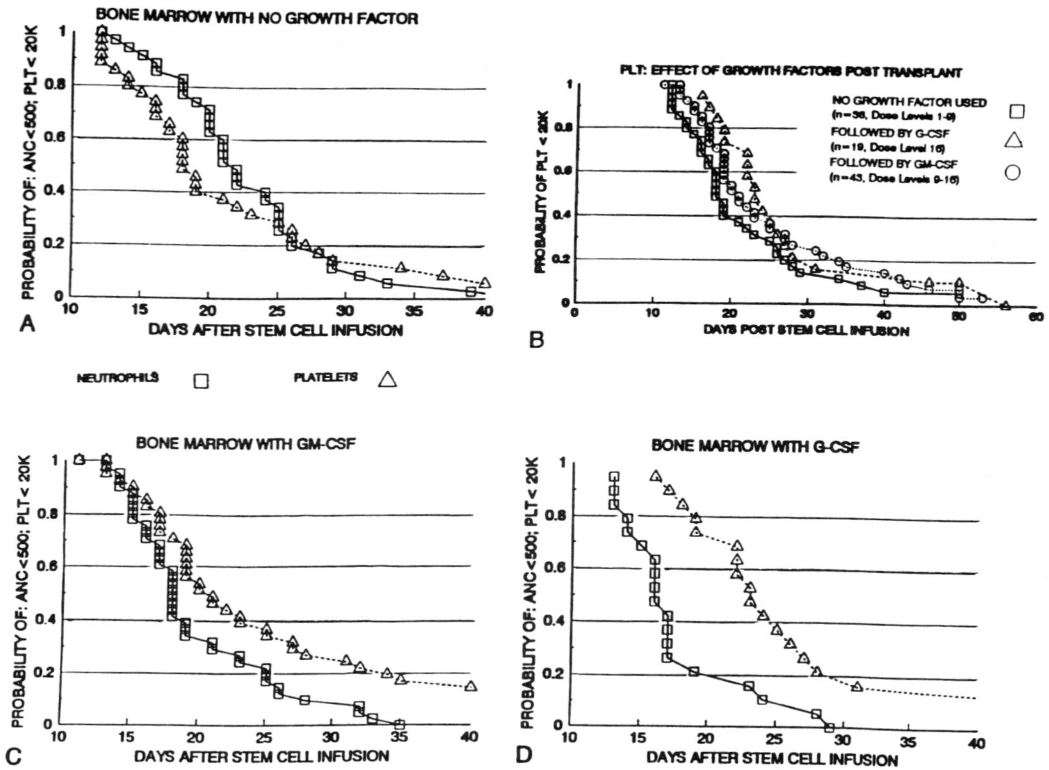

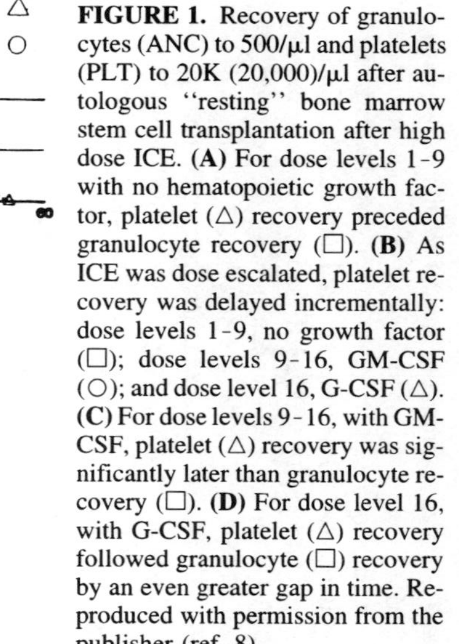

FIGURE 1. Recovery of granulocytes (ANC) to 500/µl and platelets (PLT) to 20K (20,000)/µl after autologous ''resting'' bone marrow stem cell transplantation after high dose ICE. (**A**) For dose levels 1–9 with no hematopoietic growth factor, platelet (△) recovery preceded granulocyte recovery (□). (**B**) As ICE was dose escalated, platelet recovery was delayed incrementally: dose levels 1–9, no growth factor (□); dose levels 9–16, GM-CSF (○); and dose level 16, G-CSF (△). (**C**) For dose levels 9–16, with GM-CSF, platelet (△) recovery was significantly later than granulocyte recovery (□). (**D**) For dose level 16, with G-CSF, platelet (△) recovery followed granulocyte (□) recovery by an even greater gap in time. Reproduced with permission from the publisher (ref. 8).

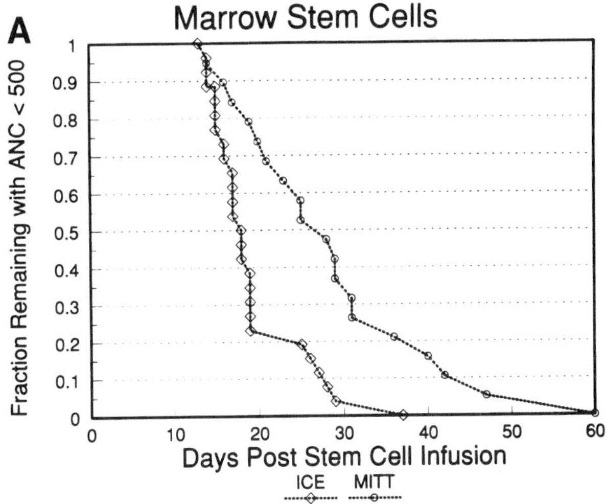

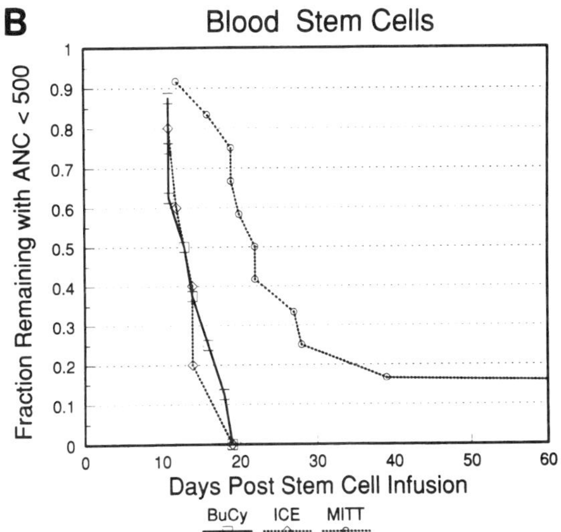

FIGURE 2. Recovery of granulocytes (ANC) after autologous stem cell transplantation after high dose chemotherapy. (**A**) ''Resting'' bone marrow stem cells after ICE ($\Diamond$) or MITT ($\bigcirc$). The slope and median for recovery after MITT are both significantly different than for recovery after ICE. (**B**) Peripheral blood stem cells ''mobilized'' with a cyclophosphamide-based mobilization regimen after BUCY ($\square$, BUCY2), ICE ($\Diamond$), and MITT ($\bigcirc$). Recovery after BUCY2 and ICE is identical and significantly faster than that after MITT. The shallower slope and delayed recovery for PBSC after MITT (**B**) resembles that for BMSC after MITT (**A**). Reprinted (with modifications) from ref. 12, p 413 by courtesy of Marcel Dekker, Inc.

sis. These PBSC were mobilized with CY $\pm$ VP16 $\pm$ G-CSF. All patients received G-CSF after stem cell infusion to accelerate granulopoiesis. As also can be seen from FIGURE 2B, the kinetics of granulocyte recovery are the same for BUCY2 and ICE which are, however, different from the kinetics for MITT. Furthermore, the relative slopes and midpoint positions of the granulocyte recovery curves for ICE and MITT are the same whether the stem cell source is resting BMSC or mobilized PBSC (compare FIG. 2B with FIG. 2A). As with the studies with BMSC just discussed, no differences were noted in the numbers of CD34$^+$ cells or the CFU-GM content of PBSC infusions to explain differences between granulocyte recovery after MITT and granulocyte recovery after ICE or BUCY2. Finally, differences were noted between the median granulocyte recovery times for PBSC as compared to BMSC, which will be discussed in detail. This is the third bit of evidence suggesting that a patient-specific factor, such as chemotherapy again, may be important in determining the pace of granulopoiesis from the null state. These data also serve to confirm the second bit of evidence just described.

The fourth body of data comes from our more recent experiences with the MITT regimen.[15] The marked efficacy of the MITT regimen (in phase I studies), especially in highly chemorefractory breast cancer, has induced us to use the MITT regimen at the MTD in metastatic, that is, stage IV, and locally advanced, that is, stage III and inflammatory, breast cancer that is responsive to anthracycline-based regimens (in phase II studies). Because of the delayed recovery of hematopoiesis observed at the MTD of MITT and the possibility that mitoxantrone blood levels may persist longer than expected (in the phase I study), we delayed the infusion of stem cells from 4 days after the end of high dose chemotherapy to 7 days after chemotherapy (in the phase II study). All patients in this comparison received MITT at the MTD and all patients received G-CSF after stem cell infusion to accelerate granulopoiesis. As shown in FIGURE 3, median granulocyte recovery time is faster in patients in the phase II portion of the MITT study than in patients in the phase I portion of the MITT study. Interestingly, the kinetics of granulocyte recovery are the same for the two patient groups. Although we cannot ascribe this significant improvement in granulocyte recovery to just one parameter, that is, less prior chemotherapy or longer delay after high dose MITT before stem cell infusion, it is still clear that modifying a patient-specific factor and not a growth factor related or stem cell dependent factor has changed the pace of granulocyte recovery from the null state. This, then, is the fourth bit of evidence that patient-specific factors make an impact on granulopoiesis after high dose chemotherapy followed by autologous stem cell transplantation.

The fifth body of evidence has most recently come to light.[16] When the MITT regimen was advanced to front-line therapy in patients with breast cancer responsive to anthracyclines, we initiated the TNT regimen for refractory malignancies. In this phase I protocol, we escalated the dose of the new drug Taxol in the setting of dose level 3 of the older MITT regimen (TABLE 2). In patients who received resting BMSC after TNT we found a significantly delayed recovery of granulopoiesis as compared to that in equivalent patients who received resting BMSC after dose level 3 of MITT, as shown in FIGURE 4. Patients who received TNT received, on average, 200 $\mu g/m^2$ of Taxol and had a 7-day delay between their last chemotherapy drug administration and stem cell infusion. Patients who received dose level 3 of MITT obviously received no Taxol and had only a 4-day delay between last drug and stem cell infusion.

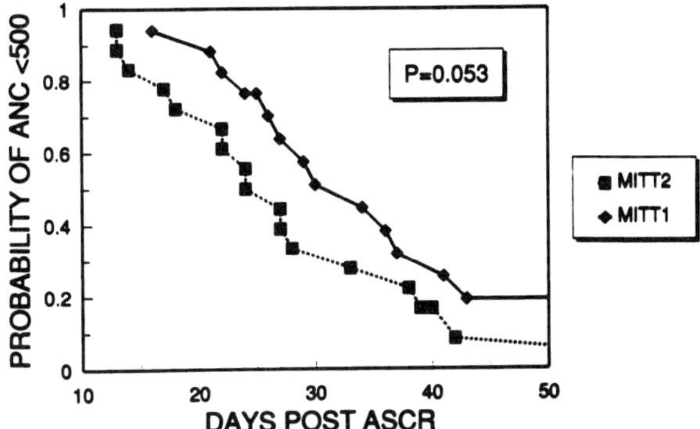

FIGURE 3. Neutrophil (ANC, granulocyte) recovery after autologous bone marrow transplantation after high dose MITT. MITT1 vs MITT2. Patients eligible for MITT1 had highly refractory malignancies and received autologous stem cell rescue (ASCR) 4 days after completion of the MITT regimen. Subsequent patients eligible for MITT2 had anthracycline-responsive malignancies and received ASCR 7 days after completion of MITT. All patients received BMSC; all patients received the same dose level of MITT. Recovery for MITT2 patients was significantly quicker than for MITT1 patients (see ref. 15).

These results are remarkable in that they indicate that despite further delay between chemotherapy and stem cell infusion, the addition of another drug to an established regimen altered (delayed) the pace of granulopoiesis for resting BMSC followed by G-CSF after stem cell infusion. This, then, is the fifth bit of evidence that patient-specific factors make an impact on granulopoiesis.

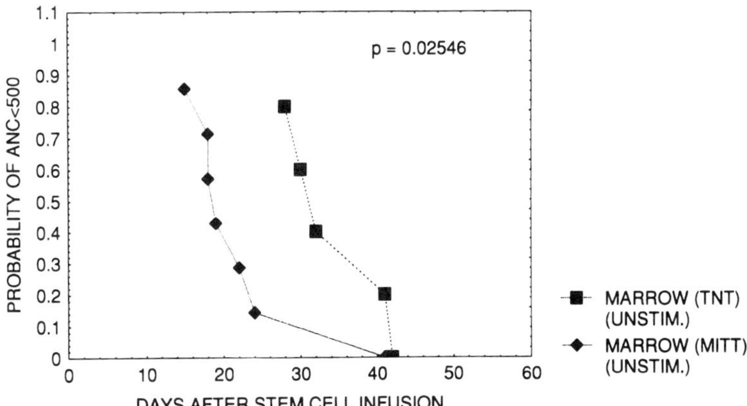

FIGURE 4. Neutrophil (ANC, granulocyte) recovery following autologous stem cell infusion after high dose MITT or TNT. Effect of graft type and priming and conditioning. "Resting" (unstim.) BMSC were given to all patients after either MITT (dose level 3) or TNT (■, Taxol, added to dose level 3 of MITT). An average of 200 mg/m^2 Taxol was given. Taxol significantly delayed granulopoiesis (see ref. 16).

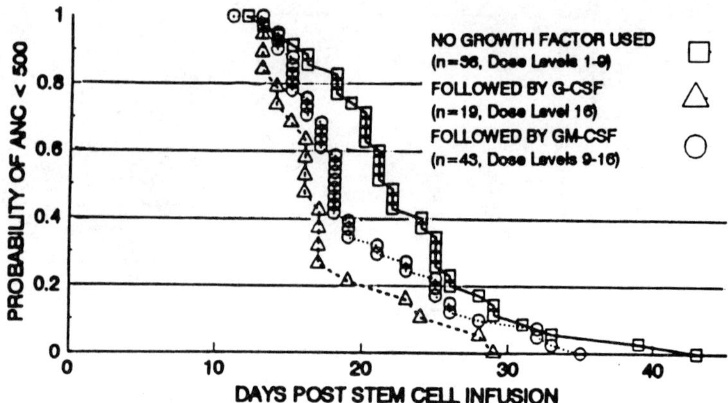

FIGURE 5. Neutrophil (ANC, granulocyte) recovery following autologous stem cell infusion after high dose ICE. "Resting" BMSC were given to all patients after ICE. Depicted are patients who received dose levels 1-9 with no hematopoietic growth factor (□), dose levels 9-16 with GM-CSF (○), and dose level 16 with G-CSF (△) after stem cell infusion. Growth factors significantly shortened the period of neutropenia; G-CSF yielded significantly faster granulopoiesis than did GM-CSF (see ref. 8).

Growth Factors. Recovery of granulopoiesis from the null state after stem cell infusion following high dose chemotherapy is influenced by the use of hematopoietic growth factors. We have two bodies of data that speak to this observation and also demonstrates the relative values of the two currently commercially available growth factors with respect to their ability to accelerate granulopoiesis.

The first body of data comes from the phase I portion of the ICE study.[8] When hematopoietic growth factors first became available, we employed GM-CSF in patients receiving dose levels 9-16, as just described. Subsequently, we employed G-CSF in a series of consecutive patients on dose level 16 of ICE. Patients on dose levels 1-9 received no growth factor. All patients in the three groups presented received resting BMSC as the source of stem cells for hematopoietic reconstitution. FIGURE 5 shows the recovery of granulopoiesis in the three groups of patients described. It is evident that GM-CSF shortened the duration of aplasia, as compared to that of historical controls (dose level 1-9) who received no growth factor despite the increased dose intensity of ICE that might have the propensity of lengthening the period of aplasia as it did the period of thrombocytopenia (FIG. 1B). Furthermore, it is evident that G-CSF shortened the period of aplasia as compared to that in historical controls. Remarkably, G-CSF also shortened the period of aplasia as compared to that with GM-CSF, despite the fact that G-CSF was given only to patients at the MTD of the ICE regimen. The three curves shown in FIGURE 5 are significantly different from one another. The relative difference between GM-CSF and G-CSF cannot be explained by schedule or route but may be explained by dose as about 40% more micrograms of G-CSF per square meter were given to patients than was GM-CSF. Of course, other potential interpretations for these results may be operative including the possibility that G-CSF is a superior growth factor for accelerating the

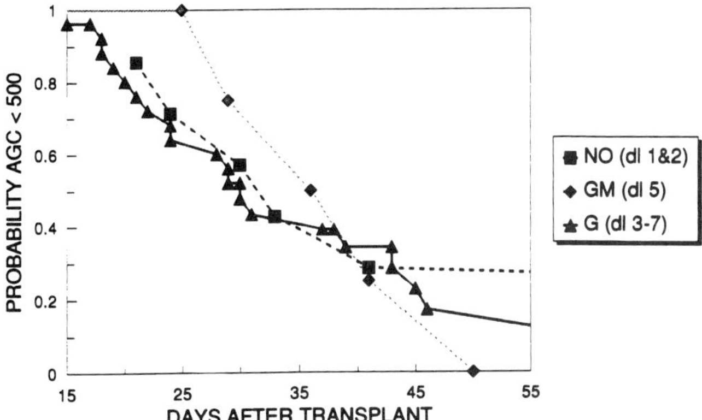

FIGURE 6. Granulocyte (AGC) recovery following autologous bone marrow transplantation after high dose MITT. All patients received "resting" BMSC. For dose levels 1 and 2 (■) of MITT no hematopoietic growth factor or colony-stimulating factor (CSF) was given; for dose levels 3-7 (▲), G-CSF was given; and at the maximal tolerated dose of MITT (dose level 5 [◆]), GM-CSF was given. G-CSF appeared to overcome the delaying effect of increased dose intensity of MITT (unpublished observations).

recovery of granulopoiesis from the null state after stem cell infusion following high dose chemotherapy.

The second body of data comes from the phase I portion of the MITT study.[4] Consecutive patients who received dose levels 1-2 did not receive any growth factor. When hematopoietic growth factors first became available, we employed G-CSF in patients on dose levels 3-7. For subsequent, consecutive patients treated at the MTD (dose level 5) we employed GM-CSF. All patients received resting BMSC as the source of hematopoietic stem cells to reconstitute hematopoiesis. Several interesting observations are presented in FIGURE 6. First, the delaying effect of increased dose intensity of MITT can be seen by comparing the granulocyte recovery curves for no growth factor (dose level 1 and 2) with that of GM-CSF (dose level 5). This confirms the observation from our dose escalation studies of ICE in which recovery of thrombopoiesis was delayed by higher doses of ICE (FIG. 1B). Second, G-CSF can reverse the delaying effect of dose escalation but cannot accelerate the recovery of granulopoiesis any further. This latter limitation may be overcome with a higher dose of G-CSF. Finally, G-CSF is superior to GM-CSF in accelerating the pace of granulopoiesis after MITT. This latter observation is not due to the different dose intensities of MITT delivered. When we examined the granulocyte recovery curves for both G-CSF and GM-CSF, restricting our attention to only dose levels 5, we still observed more rapid recovery after G-CSF (data not shown). Alternative explanations are that in patients treated with high dose MITT, GM-CSF is not particularly active at accelerating granulopoieses or that at the dose of GM-CSF employed, GM-CSF cannot overcome the granulocyte recovery delaying effect that very dose-intense MITT produces. This would, of course, be in contrast to our observations for G-CSF which, after both high dose ICE and MITT, clearly overcame the granulocyte recovery delaying effect of very dose intense therapy.

Stem Cells. It is now widely touted that PBSC are superior to BMSC in the rapidly of recovery of granulopoiesis from the null state after autologous stem cell infusion following high dose chemotherapy. This is based predominantly on phase II trials with comparisons to historical controls. We have five bodies of data that can speak to this issue. Two of these bodies of data come from retrospective analyses of clinical trials and one from a prospective, randomized, controlled, phase III clinical trial. Additionally, two of these bodies of data come from the laboratory where *in vitro* hematopoietic assessment studies were performed on stem cell collections to correlate with *in vivo* hematopoietic reconstitution results.

The first body of data comes from the phase I and phase II portions of the ICE and MITT studies.[4] In these studies we employed the first set of criteria (discussed in Materials and Methods) to determine which stem cell product to use as a source of stem cells to reconstitute hematopoiesis after high dose chemotherapy. Furthermore, there were sequential patients in both studies for whom PBSC were collected after mobilization with either CY $\pm$ VP16 $\pm$ G-CSF, that is, "chemo-mobilized", or GM-CSF alone. All BMSC employed were collected in the resting state. The data shown in FIGURE 7A and B are granulocyte recovery profiles from patients who received resting BMSC followed by G-CSF, patients who received chemo-mobilized PBSC followed by G-CSF, and patients who received GM-CSF mobilized PBSC followed by GM-CSF. After stem cell infusion, growth factors were given to accelerate recovery of granulopoiesis from the null state produced by high dose chemotherapy. As can be seen in FIGURE 7A and B, chemo-mobilized PBSC produced much more rapid recovery of granulopoiesis than did resting BMSC even though both groups of patients received the same growth factor after stem cell infusion, that is, G-CSF.[12] By contrast, patients who received GM-CSF mobilized PBSC showed slower recovery of granulopoiesis than did patients who received chemo-mobilized PBSC.[12] More remarkably, GM-CSF mobilized PBSC were even slower at restoring granulopoiesis than were resting BMSC. These observations were identical for both ICE and MITT high dose chemotherapy regimens. Although patients who received GM-CSF mobilized PBSC also received GM-CSF after stem cell infusion, it is little likely that the growth factor given after stem cell infusion is responsible for the tardy granulocyte recovery observed for GM-CSF mobilized PBSC. The major drawback of these studies is that they are retrospective.

On the other hand, these studies are supported by a second, substantial body of hematopoietic progenitor content data that illustrate differences in the content of the three types of stem cell products.[12] FIGURE 8A displays the total nucleated stem cell content of the PBSC collected after mobilization with chemotherapy alone, after chemotherapy followed by G-CSF, and after GM-CSF alone. FIGURE 8B and C also displays the total CD34$^+$ cell count and the total CFU-GM content of the various PBSC products. The major findings from these data may be summarized as follows: CYVPG mobilized PBSC contain more cells, more CD34$^+$ cells, and more CFU-GM than do PBSC mobilized with CY alone, CYVP16, CYG-CSF, or GM-CSF. In that sense, CYVPG produces the superior PBSC product. More intriguingly, however, is the observation that although GM-CSF mobilizes adequate numbers of nucleated and CD34$^+$ cells, it is notably deficient in mobilizing CFU-GM than the other mobilizing regimens studied. The reduced number of CFU-GM collected after GM-CSF may be the *in vitro* correlate of our *in vivo* observation that GM-CSF mobilized stem

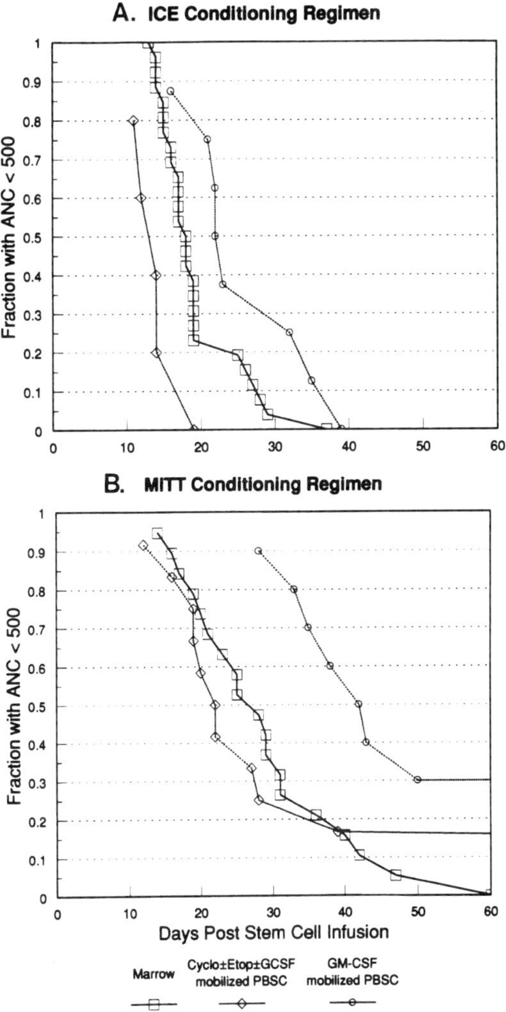

FIGURE 7. Recovery of granulocytes (ANC) following autologous stem cell infusion after high dose ICE or MITT. Patients receiving "resting" bone marrow stem cells (□) were treated with G-CSF after stem cell infusion. Patients whose PBSC were "mobilized," with chemotherapy (cyclophosphamide [cyclo] with or without etoposide [etop]) with or without G-CSF (◇), also received G-CSF after stem cell infusion. Finally, patients whose PBSC were "mobilized" with GM-CSF (○) received GM-CSF after stem cell infusion. **(A)** ICE conditioning regimen. **(B)** MITT conditioning regimen. Within treatment regimens all three stem cell products have the same slope. The relative order of positions of midpoints is the same for all three stem cell products for both treatment regimens. Chemotherapy ± G-CSF-mobilized PBSC reproducibly and significantly produced earlier granulopoiesis than did resting BMSC. GM-CSF-mobilized PBSC yielded reproducibly and significantly slower granulopoiesis than did both chemotherapy ± G-CSF-mobilized PBSC and resting BMSC. Reprinted (with modifications) from ref. 12, p 413, by courtesy of Marcel Dekker, Inc.

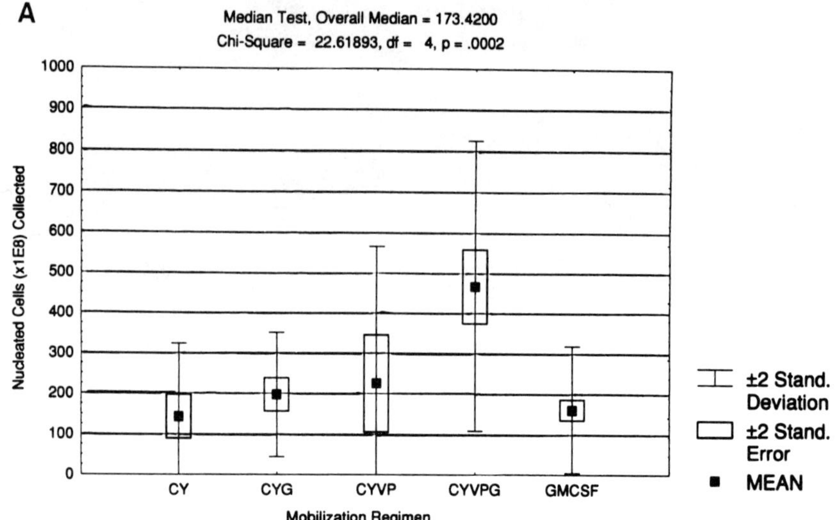

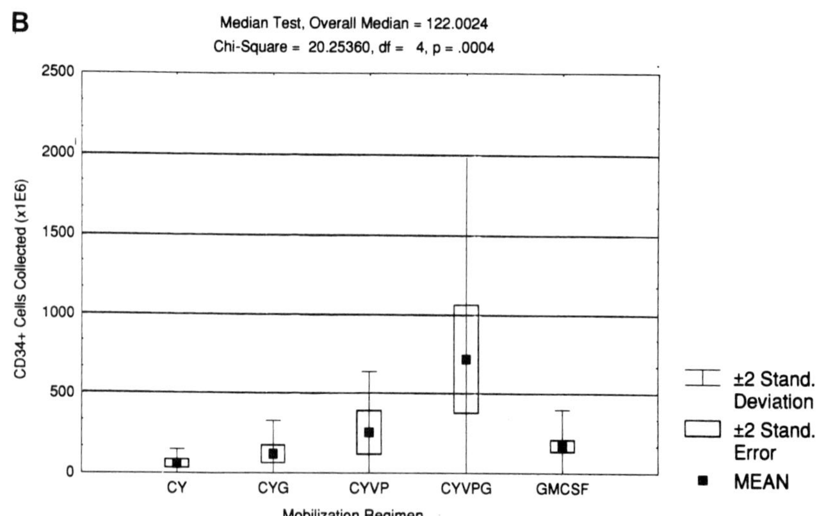

FIGURE 8A and B.

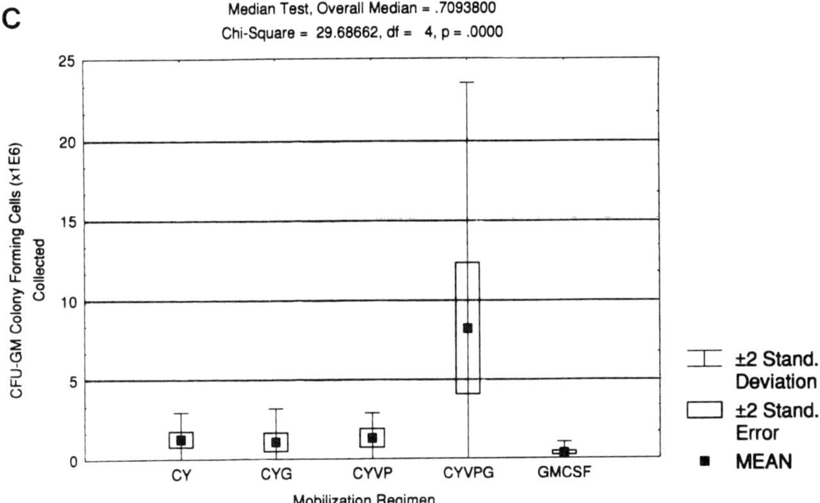

FIGURE 8. Different methods of mobilizing PBSC. (**A**) Nucleated cells collected. (**B**) CD34[+] cells collected. (**C**) CFU-GM colony-forming cells collected. Mobilizing regimens were CY = cyclophosphamide; CYG = cyclophosphamide and G-CSF; CYVP = cyclophosphamide and etoposide; CYVPG = cyclophosphamide, etoposide and G-CSF, and GM-CSF. CYVPG yielded the richest PBSC collections. GM-CSF-mobilized PBSC contained significantly fewer CFU-GM. Reprinted (with modifications) from ref. 12, p. 411, by courtesy of Marcel Dekker, Inc.

cells are slow to produce granulocyte recovery. These data lend more credence to the retrospective data from the clinical trials just discussed.

More convincingly, however, may be the third body of data that we just recently collected.[17,18] In the phase II portions of the ICE and MITT studies, when patient bone marrow biopsies were never positive and when patients had harvestable marrow and gave informed consent, we collected both BMSC and PBSC after treatment with either GM-CSF, in the first set of consecutive patients, or G-CSF, in the second set of consecutive patients. At the time that stem cell infusion was scheduled, patients received one stem cell product or the other on a randomized basis after stratification for the high dose regimen employed and whether the patients had breast cancer or other malignant disease. Those patients who received GM-CSF mobilized PBSC received GM-CSF after stem cell infusion to accelerate granulopoiesis. Those patients who received G-CSF mobilized PBSC received G-CSF after stem cell infusion. As can be seen in FIGURE 9A-C, from prospective, randomized, controlled, phase III studies, no difference in granulocyte recovery profiles, neither midpoint nor slope, was noted for mobilized PBSC and stimulated BMSC. Differences between ICE and MITT in the granulocyte recovery profiles seen in the retrospective studies persist in the prospective studies. Finally, G-CSF apparently is superior to GM-CSF as a growth factor alone mobilizer of PBSC.

The fourth body of data comes from our experience with laboratory evaluations of GM-CSF and G-CSF mobilized PBSC.[19] FIGURE 10A, B, and C compares total

A
All Patients in Trial
120
100
80
60
40
20
0
Cumulative Percent with ANC < 500
0 10 20 30 40 50
Days After Stem Cell Infusion
PBSC
BMSC

B
Comparison of MITT vs. ICE Regimens
120
100
80
60
40
20
0
Cumulative Percent with ANC < 500
0 10 20 30 40 50
Days After Stem Cell Infusion
MITT
ICE

C
Comparison of GM-CSF & G-CSF Mobilization
120
100
80
60
40
20
0
Cumulative Percent with ANC < 500
0 10 20 30 40 50
Days After Stem Cell Infusion
GCSF
GMCSF

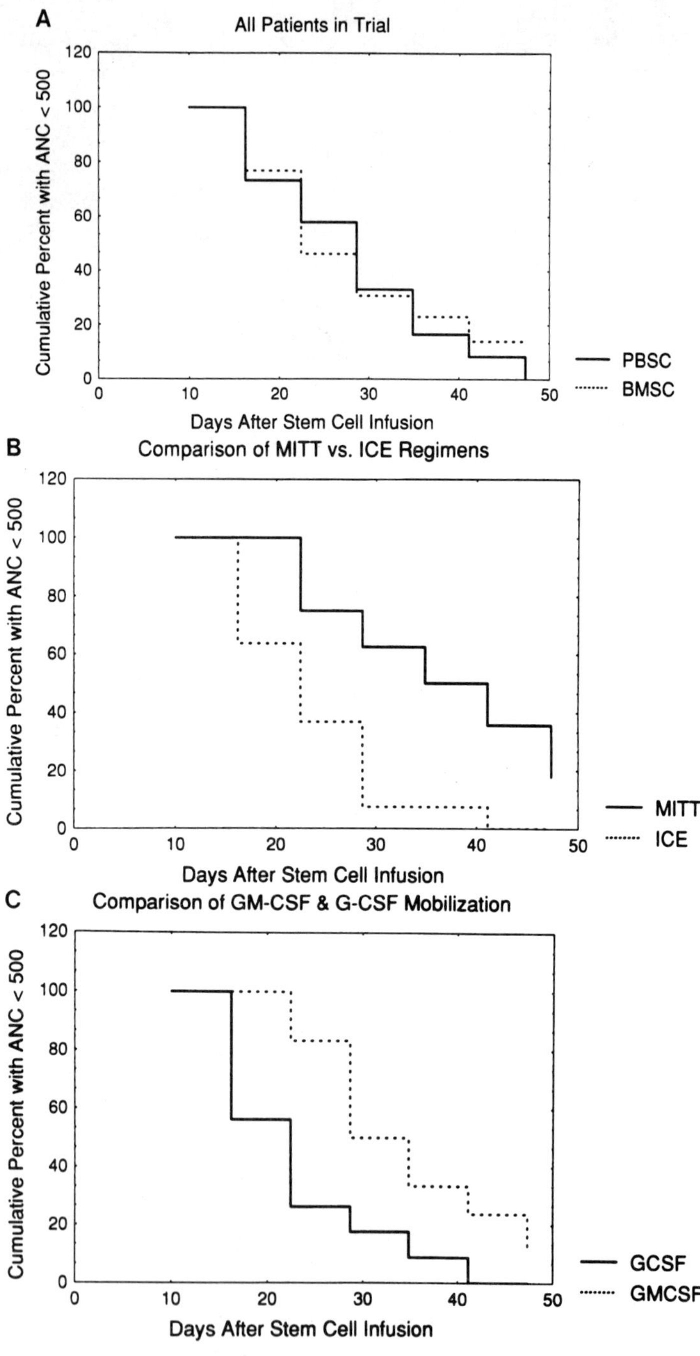

FIGURE 9.

nucleated cell, CD34[+] cell, and CFU-GM content for PBSC mobilized by either GM-CSF or G-CSF. G-CSF mobilized more nucleated cells (the increase was predominantly juvenile and polymorphonuclear leukocytes), the same number of CD34[+] cells, and more CFU-GM than did GM-CSF. It is altogether possible that the latter observation is responsible for the faster pace of granulopoiesis produced by PBSC mobilized by G-CSF (FIG. 10D). Under the circumstances we employed (dose and schedule of growth factor), G-CSF is superior to GM-CSF as a mobilizer for PBSC. These data suggest that how stem cells are activated may be critical in determining how they perform as reconstitutors of hematopoiesis.

The fifth body of data comes from the phase I study of the TNT regimen[16] where we made a second, intriguing observation. For patients who were "ever positive" we collected PBSC after CYVPG treatment. For patients who were "never positive" we collected both BMSC and PBSC after treatment with G-CSF exactly as we did on the randomized trial just presented. We hypothesized that a double transplant (PBSC and BMSC) would be superior to a single transplant (PBSC) especially as all stem cells would be collected under stimulating/mobilizing conditions with G-CSF. Furthermore, there were already reports from other investigators that double transplants (mobilized PBSC and resting BMSC) were superior (in terms of recovery of hematopoiesis) to single transplants (resting BMSC) from sequential phase II trials and randomized phase III trials. As shown in FIGURE 11, we found that CYVPG-mobilized PBSC produces earlier recovery of granulopoiesis than did G-CSF-stimulated BMSC plus G-CSF-mobilized PBSC. These results were not from a randomized but from an allocated trial. The patients who received chemo-mobilized PBSC had malignant cells in their bone marrow before stem cell collection, whereas those who received growth factor-stimulated stem cells did not. However, in all other regards, these two patient populations are the same, even to the extent of receiving the same average dose of Taxol (data not shown). We believe that these data lend further credence to the hypothesis that it is how the patient is treated before collecting stem cells rather than from what anatomic source(s) stem cells are derived that determines the pace of granulopoiesis after autologous stem cell infusion following myeloablative chemotherapy.

DISCUSSION

This summary of data from studies at a single institution was intended to illustrate that several factors could be characterized and attributed to one of three components

FIGURE 9. Recovery of granulocytes (ANC) following stratified, randomized, prospective controlled trial of BMSC vs PBSC. All patients had both BMSC and PBSC collected under the same pretreatment (activation/mobilization) conditions. (**A**) BMSC vs PBSC, all patients in trial. (**B**) Comparison of MITT and ICE regimens. (**C**) Comparison of GM-CSF and G-CSF mobilization. Multifactorial analysis confirms that only high dose chemotherapy treatment regimen and stem cell mobilization/activating growth factor influence the pace of granulopoiesis, not the anatomic compartment of origin of stem cells. Reproduced with permission of the publisher (ref. 17).

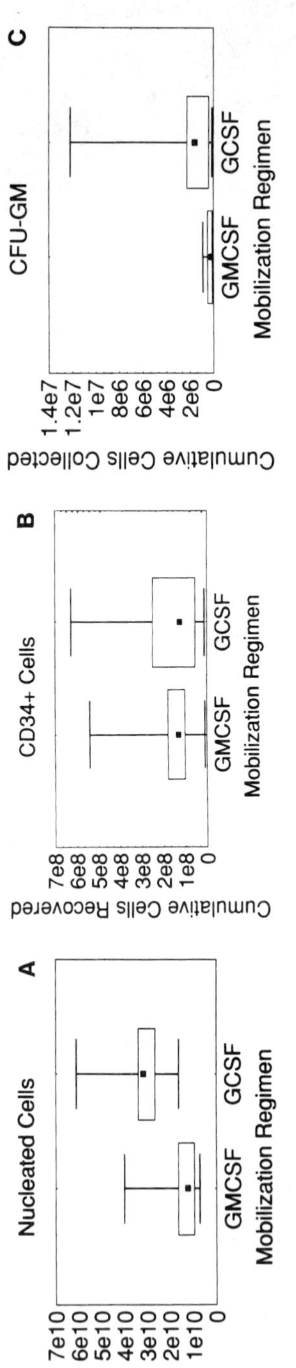

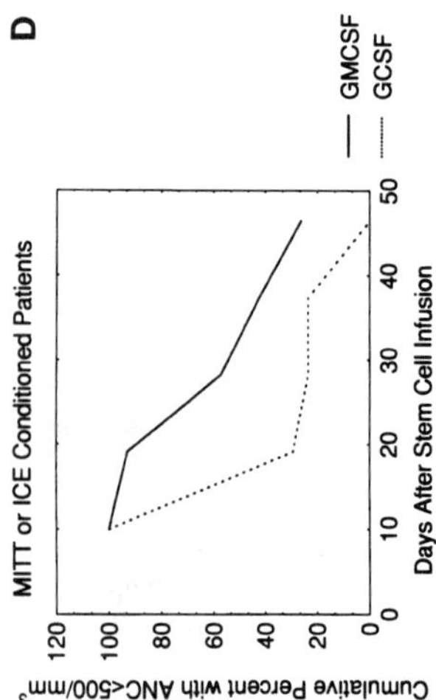

FIGURE 10. Comparison of mobilized PBSC produced by different growth factors. (A) Cumulative nucleated cells recovered. (B) Cumulative CD34$^+$ cells recovered. (C) Cumulative CFU-GM colony-forming cells recovered. G-CSF mobilized significantly more nucleated cells and more CFU-GM than did GM-CSF, but mobilized no more CD34$^+$ cells than did GM-CSF. (D) Comparison of recovery of granulocytes (ANC) in all patients receiving MITT or ICE and GM-CSF or G-CSF–mobilized PBSC. G-CSF PBSC yielded significantly faster granulopoiesis than did GM-CSF PBSC. Reproduced with permission of the publisher (ref. 19).

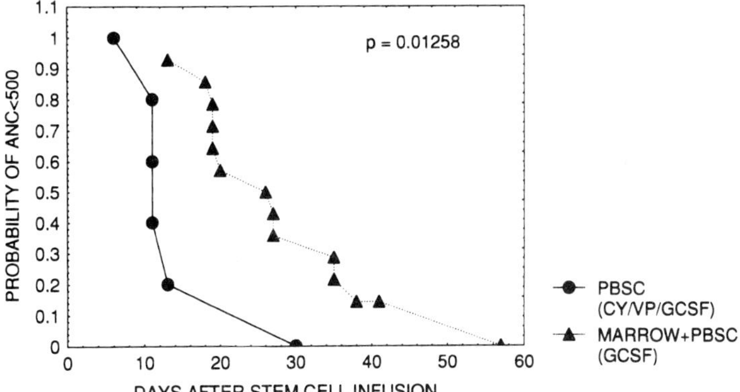

FIGURE 11. Neutrophil (ANC, granulocyte) recovery following autologous stem cell infusion(s) after high dose TNT. Effect of graft type and priming and conditioning. Patients with harvestable (see Materials and Methods) bone marrow received G-CSF and then had BMSC and PBSC collected sequentially. Double (simultaneous) transplants with marrow and PBSC were performed (▲). Patients with nonharvestable bone marrow received cyclophosphamide, etoposide, and G-CSF (CY/VP/GCSF) and had PBSC collected during recovery from leukopenia. Single PBSC transplants were performed (●). Both groups received, on average, 300 mg/m² of Taxol. Chemo-growth factor-mobilized PBSC yielded significantly faster granulopoiesis than did growth factor-mobilized PBSC plus growth factor ''activated'' BMSC (see ref. 16).

of the hematopoietic system that influence events after stem cell infusion following high dose chemotherapy when granulopoiesis was recovering from the null state. These components are marrow microenvironment, growth factors, and stem cells. These are precisely the same three components that have been known from years of work with animals and laboratory model systems. That these are seen in the autologous stem cell transplant model system in man is, therefore, no great surprise and is reassuring to us as basic and clinical scientists.

We were able to demonstrate that high dose chemotherapy given before stem cell infusion can influence the pace of recovery of granulopoiesis from the null state. The precise drugs used in high dose may determine the kinetics of recovery (slope of the curve), and the dose intensity of the chemotherapy may determine the pace of recovery (midpoint of the curve). Prior conventional dose chemotherapy may also influence the pace of recovery as may the interval between the end of high dose chemotherapy and the start of stem cell infusion. Adding a new drug to an established regimen may alter the pace of granulopoiesis. We take these observations to be indicative of the effects of various states of the patient's marrow microenvironment on the process of hematopoiesis after high dose chemotherapy and autologous stem cell infusion.

We have shown that hematopoietic growth factors can influence the pace of recovery (midpoint) without altering the kinetics of recovery (slope). We have also shown that different growth factors may have different effects on granulopoiesis. It is possible but little likely that the difference we observed between the two growth factors was due to dose alone as the dose difference was only approximately a factor of 1.4 (i.e., the square root of 2). The effect of growth factors is smaller than that of marrow microenvironment on recovering granulopoiesis. What other hematopoietic growth factors can do in this setting remains to be determined in future phase II and III trials.

Finally, we have shown that different mobilizing regimens for collection of PBSC produce stem cell products that are different with respect to their *in vitro* hematopoietic progenitor content and, more importantly, their ability to reconstitute hematopoiesis from the null state *in vivo*, that is, the pace of granulopoiesis. We have also shown that when PBSC and BMSC are collected under identical mobilization or stimulation conditions, no obvious difference exists in the pace or kinetics of granulocyte recovery. Differences in the two sources of stem cells that have previously been ascribed to anatomic source are more likely due to the mobilization regimen used to collect PBSC, because BMSC were traditionally collected in the resting state. Finally, the observation that chemotherapy-growth factor mobilized PBSC produced earlier granulopoiesis than did G-CSF-mobilized PBSC plus G-CSF-stimulated BMSC strongly supports the hypothesis that the state of activation of stem cells is more important than the anatomic source of stem cells.

From these observations, we infer that for every modification we make in the treatment plan for the malignancy we are attempting to cure, that is, the high dose chemotherapy regimen, for every change in the growth factor given after stem cell infusion, for every PBSC-mobilizing regimen that we employ, and for every decision we make about which stem cell source to use, we must carefully evaluate our reason(s) for making the alteration(s) and even more carefully observe the consequence(s) of the alteration(s) in terms of recovery of hematopoieses. Ultimately, the most important outcome is progression-free survival. The question of whether one source of stem cells will be responsible for better disease-free survival remains open (see ref. 20). It is now clear that we may not simply adapt what has been observed from other treatment circumstances to our own treatment circumstances without thorough evaluation. We must test each regimen and stem cell choice critically (see ref. 21).

ACKNOWLEDGMENTS

The authors would like to acknowledge the many substantive contributions to the planning, execution, and analysis of the clinical trials and laboratory studies summarized herein. These individuals include Drs. Oscar Ballester, Karen Fields, Steven Goldstein, John Hiemenz, and Paul Zorsky, nurses Mary Foody, Lori Kronish, Bonnie Beach, and Linda Meulemans, laboratory technicians Carlos Lee, Renee Smilee, Darlene Rahn, Enid Ferguson, Deana Thompson, Randy Carter, Mary Jane Farmelo, and Gail Mueller, and office staff LaVerne Machesney, Elizabeth Hubbell, and Diane Gougelet.

DEDICATION

This communication is dedicated to the memory of the first author's father, Robert Lawrence Elfenbein (1904–1994), who lay mortally ill as the first author wrote this review at the foot of his deathbed. He is now with his beloved wife; may they both rest in peace.

REFERENCES

1. FIELDS, K., G. ELFENBEIN, R. SALEH, P. ZORSKY, W. JANSSEN, J. PERKINS, T. SALEH, J. PIAZZA, L. KRONISH, M. MACHAK & G. LYMAN. 1992. Ifosfamide, carboplatin, and etoposide in combination for induction and high-dose chemotherapy: Focus on breast cancer and lymphoma. Hematol. Oncol. **10:** 61-74.

2. FIELDS, K. K., J. P. PERKINS, J. W. HIEMENZ, P. E. ZORSKY, W. E. JANSSEN, L. E. KRONISH, M. C. MACHAK & G. J. ELFENBEIN. 1993. Intensive dose ifosfamide, carboplatin, and etoposide followed by autologous stem cell rescue: Results of a phase I/II study in breast cancer patients. Surg. Oncol **2:** 87-95.

3. FIELDS, K. K., G. J. ELFENBEIN, H. M. LAZARUS, B. C. COOPER, J. B. PERKINS, R. J. CREGER, O. F. BALLESTER, J. W. HIEMENZ, W. E. JANSSEN & P. E. ZORSKY. 1995. Maximum tolerated doses of ifosfamide, carboplatin, and etoposide given over six days followed by autologous stem cell rescue: Toxicity profile. J. Clin. Oncol. **13:** 322-332.

4. FIELDS, K. K., G. J. ELFENBEIN, P. B. PERKINS, J. W. HIEMENZ, W. E. JANSSEN, P. E. ZORSKY, O. F. BALLESTER, L. E. KRONISH & M. C. FOODY. 1993. Two novel high dose treatment regimens for metastatic breast cancer: Ifosfamide, carboplatin plus etoposide (ICE) and mitoxantrone plus thiotepa (MITT): Outcomes and toxicities. Semin. Oncol. **20** (suppl. 6): 59-66.

5. FIELDS, K., J. PERKINS, G. ELFENBEIN, O. BALLESTER, J. HIEMENZ, S. GOLDSTEIN, P. ZORSKY & L. KRONISH. 1995. A phase I dose escalation trial of high dose TAXOL®, NOVANTRONE®, and thioTEPA (TNT) followed by autologous stem cell rescue (ASCR): Toxicity. Prog. ASCO **14:** 322.

6. TUTSCHKA, P. J., G. W. SANTOS & G. J. ELFENBEIN. 1980. Marrow transplantation in acute leukemia following busulfan and cyclophosphamide. *In* Immunobiology of Bone Marrow Transplantation. S. Thierfelder, H. Rodt & H. J. Kolb, Eds. (Suppl. 25 to BLUT). : 375-380. Springer. New York.

7. KORBLING, M., P. BURKE, H. G. BRAINE, G. J. ELFENBEIN, G. W. SANTOS & H. KAIZER. 1981. Successful engraftment of blood derived normal hemopoietic stem cells in chronic myelogenous leukemia. Exp. Hematol. **9:** 684-690.

8. FIELDS, K. K., G. J. ELFENBEIN, J. B. PERKINS, W. E. JANSSEN, O. F. BALLESTER, J. W. HIEMENZ, P. E. ZORSKY, L. E. KRONISH & M. C. FOODY. 1994. High-dose ifosfamide/carboplatin/etoposide: Maximum tolerable doses, toxicities, and hematopoietic recovery after autologous stem cell reinfusion. Semin. Oncol. **21** (suppl. 12): 86-92.

9. JANSSEN, W. E., M. J. FARMELO, C. LEE, R. SMILEE, L. KRONISH & G. J. ELFENBEIN. 1992. The CD34+ cell fraction in bone marrow and blood is not universally predictive of CFU-GM. Exp. Hematol. **20:** 528-530.

10. JANSSEN, W. E., C. LEE, R. SMILEE, M. J. FARMELO, K. BARTH, K. K. FIELDS, P. E. ZORSKY & G. J. ELFENBEIN. 1992. Use of CD34+ cell fraction as measure of hematopoietic stem cells in bone marrow and peripheral blood: Comparison with the CFU-GM assay. Prog. Clin. Biol. Res. **377:** 513-521.

11. JANSSEN, W. E., R. SMILEE, R. CARTER, D. RAHN, M. CAIRO, J. W. HIEMENZ, P. E. ZORSKY, K. K. FIELDS, O. BALLESTER, J. PERKINS, L. KRONISH & G. J. ELFENBEIN. 1994. Mobilization of peripheral blood stem cells (PBSC): Comparing cyclophosphamide and growth factor based regimens. Prog. Clin. Biol. Res. **389:** 429-439.

12. JANSSEN, W. E. & G. J. ELFENBEIN. 1995. Mobilization of peripheral blood stem cells: Are all regimens created equal? *In* Hematopoietic Stem Cells: Biology and Therapeutic Applications. D. Levitt & R. Mertelsmann, Eds.: 403-419. Marcel Dekker, New York.

13. FIELDS, K. K., P. E. ZORSKY, J. W. HIEMENZ, L. E. KRONISH & G. J. ELFENBEIN. 1994. Ifosfamide, carboplatin, and etoposide: A new regimen with a broad spectrum of activity. J. Clin. Oncol. **12:** 544-552.

14. GRAHAM-POLE, J., A. GEE, S. EMERSON, J. GALLO, C. LEE, J. LUZINS, W. E. JANSSEN, T. PICK, D. WORTHINGTON-WHITE, G. ELFENBEIN, S. GROSS & R. WEINER. 1991. Myeloablative chemoradiotherapy and autologous bone marrow transplant for treatment of neuroblastoma: Factors influencing engraftment. Blood **78:** 1607-1614.

15. PERKINS, J. B., K. A. CREMERS, K. K. FIELDS, W. E. JANSSEN, O. F. BALLESTER, S. C. GOLDSTEIN, J. W. HIEMENZ, P. E. ZORSKY & G. J. ELFENBEIN. 1994. Differences in engraftment rate between two groups of breast cancer patients treated with the same high dose chemotherapy regimen: Potential contributing factors for hematopoietic recovery. Exp. Hematol. **22:** 782.

16. ELFENBEIN, G. J., J. B. PERKINS, K. K. FIELDS, O. F. BALLESTER, S. C. GOLDSTEIN, J. W. HIEMENZ, W. E. JANSSEN & P. E. ZORSKY. 1994. Hematologic recovery after high dose Taxol, Novantrone, Thiotepa (TNT) and autologous stem cell transplant: Evaluation of the effects of stem cell source and Taxol. Blood **84** (suppl. 1): 707a.

17. JANSSEN, W. E., J. W. HIEMENZ, K. K. FIELDS, P. E. ZORSKY, O. F. BALLESTER, S. C. GOLDSTEIN & G. J. ELFENBEIN. 1994. Stem cells from bone marrow and blood for transplant: A comparative review. Cancer Control **1:** 225-230.

18. JANSSEN, W. E., J. W. HIEMENZ, K. K. FIELDS, P. E. ZORSKY, O. F. BALLESTER, S. C. GOLDSTEIN, R. SMILEE, L. KRONISH & G. J. ELFENBEIN. 1994. Peripheral blood "stem cells" do not always produce faster engraftment than bone marrow in autotransplantation. Exp. Hematol. **22:** 765.

19. JANSSEN, W. E., G. J. ELFENBEIN, K. K. FIELDS, J. W. HIEMENZ, P. E. ZORSKY, O. F. BALLESTER, S. C. GOLDSTEIN, R. SMILEE, L. KRONISH, B. BEACH & G. LEPARC. 1995. Comparison of cell collections and rates of post-transplant granulocyte recovery when G-CSF and GM-CSF are used as mobilizers of peripheral blood stem cells for autotransplantation. *In* Autologous Bone Marrow Transplantation, Proceedings of the 7th International Symposium. K. A. Dicke & A. Keating, Eds. 527-539. Arlington, Texas.

20. FIELDS, K. K., D. P. AGALIOTIS, W. E. JANSSEN, J. B. PERKINS, O. F. BALLESTER, J. W. HIEMENZ, P. E. ZORSKY & G. J. ELFENBEIN. 1994. High dose chemotherapy and the treatment of metastatic breast cancer: Selecting the regimen and the source of stem cells. Cancer Control **1:** 213-218.

21. ELFENBEIN, G. J. 1994. Hematopoietic stem cells for transplantation: Marrow or peripheral blood? Cancer Control **1:** 188-189.

Abrogation of Graft-versus-Host Disease Following Allotransplantation of Cytotoxically Deficient Bone Marrow across Major Histocompatibility Barriers

GENNARO SELVAGGI,[a] LUCA INVERARDI,[a]
ROBERT B. LEVY,[b] MATHIAS D. BRENDEL,[a]
JULIE SPIELMAN,[b] DANIEL H. MINTZ,[a]
ECKHARD R. PODACK,[b] AND CAMILLO RICORDI[a,c]

[a]Diabetes Research Institute
Cell Transplant Center
and
[b]Department of Microbiology and Immunology
University of Miami School of Medicine
Miami, Florida 33136

Graft-versus-host disease (GVHD) represents one of the major complications of bone marrow transplantation protocols, especially across Class I and II MHC barriers.[1] Although many mechanisms underlying the development of this disease still remain unknown, it is now commonly accepted that GVHD pathogenesis is linked to the presence of a mature, donor-derived T-cell population contained in bone marrow inoculum.[2]

T-cell activation in an allogeneic environment, according to some authors, leads to a massive release of cytokines and other soluble factors, creating a so-called "cytokine storm," responsible for the clinical symptoms of GVHD[3]; other investigators, on the other hand, consider cell-mediated cytotoxicity as the leading mechanism in GVHD development.[4]

Several techniques have been successful in preventing the onset of GVHD, such as T-cell depletion,[5,6] and the administration of interleukin-2 (IL-2) or of immunosuppressive drugs (cyclosporine A, FK 506, and others).[7–9] Unfortunately, all of these strategies have some disadvantages such as a low rate of bone marrow engraftment, recurrence of malignancies, and toxic side effects of the immunosuppressive regimens.[10,11]

In the present study, we explored the role of the perforin pathway of cytotoxicity in the development of GVHD. Perforin is contained in granules of activated cytotoxic T cells and is released in the intercellular space as a monomer upon contact with

---

[c]To whom correspondence should be addressed.

TABLE 1. Animal Survival and Incidence of Lethal GVHD after Transplantation of 4×10^7 Bone Marrow Cells (BMC)

Description	n	Survival Days	MST $\pm$ SD	Incidence of Lethal GVHD	
Irradiation controls	5	4, 4, 5, 6, 11	6 $\pm$ 2.9	0/5	(0%)
Syngeneic controls	5	>160	>160	0/3	(0%)
B6 P+/+ → BALB/c	6	22, 27, 61, 62, 63, 64	49.8 $\pm$ 19.7	6/6	(100%)
B6 PKO → BALB/c	8	>160	>160	0/8	(0%)

ABBREVIATIONS: MST = mean survival time (in days); SD = standard deviation.

the target cell.[12] The monomers then polymerize to form a transmembrane channel that allows massive influx of water, ions, and other cytotoxic molecules, such as granzymes, leading to cell death. Other perforin-independent pathways of cytotoxicity exist, such as apoptosis induced on target cells by the interaction of the Fas-ligand molecule on effector cells and Fas molecule on targets,[13] but the perforin pathway is thought to be prevalent, at least under physiological conditions.[14]

To investigate the role of perforin in the establishment of GVHD we used perforin knock-out mice derived from the C57BL/6 strain (B6 PKO). B6 PKO mice, obtained by gene disruption via DNA homologous recombinant techniques, have severely impaired cytotoxicity *in vitro*.[15] CD8$^+$ T cells and natural killer (NK) cells fail to lyse sensitive targets; in particular, cytotoxic T cells appear incapable of killing allogeneic fibroblastoid targets, and NK cells do not mediate any significant lysis of the NK-sensitive target YAC-1. Furthermore, *in vivo* clearance of the lymphocytic choriomeningitis virus is severely impaired. Lymphocytes from these animals still possess cytolytic activity, and this is most probably due to the presence of an intact Fas pathway, as shown by significant lysis of Fas-positive target cells. The existence of other pathways of cytotoxicity, the importance of which is yet to be established, cannot at this time be excluded.

We used a model to induce GVHD across complete Class I and II MHC barriers by means of bone marrow transplantation from wild-type, perforin-producing C57BL/6 mice (B6 P+/+) or perforin-negative B6 PKO mice (H-2^b) into lethally irradiated BALB/c mice (H-2^d). We monitored the incidence, timing, severity, and histopathological features of GVHD in the two experimental groups.[16]

RESULTS

In the first set of experiments, BALB/c mice were reconstituted 24 hours postirradiation (9.25 Gy) with 4×10^7 bone marrow cells (BMC). Recipients of B6 P+/+ BMC developed lethal GVHD with an onset of clinical signs (weight loss, diarrhea, dermatitis, hunchback position, and fur loss) starting 2-3 weeks after bone marrow transplantation (BMT); the disease progressed, leading to the death of all animals within 64 days posttransplant (TABLE 1). Histopathological assessment of the specimens derived from the affected animals showed marked mononuclear infiltration in

TABLE 2. Animal Survival following Bone Marrow Cells (BMC) + Splenocyte (SC) Transplantation

Description	n	Transplanted Cells	Survival Days	MST $\pm$ SD
BALB/c $\rightarrow$ BALB/c	5	4×10^7 BMC + 4×10^7 SC	>160	>160
B6 P+/+ $\rightarrow$ BALB/c	4	4×10^7 BMC + 2×10^7 SC	18, 19, 19, 20	19 ± 0.8
B6 P+/+ $\rightarrow$ BALB/c	5	4×10^7 BMC + 4×10^7 SC	7, 11, 12, 15, 16	12.2 ± 3.5
B6 PKO $\rightarrow$ BALB/c	4	4×10^7 BMC + 2×10^7 SC	25, 27, 41, 45	34.5 ± 9.9
B6 PKO $\rightarrow$ BALB/c	9	4×10^7 BMC + 4×10^7 SC	19, 21, 23, 33, 34, 38, 38, 38, 38	31.3 ± 8

the periportal spaces of the liver, in the alveolar tissue of the lungs, as well as in the tongue. The clinical observation of dermatitis was confirmed by histological examination of skin specimens which showed heavy mononuclear infiltrates in the dermoepidermal junction. The weight of these animals gradually declined, in parallel with the clinical signs of progressing GVHD.

Conversely, when the same amount of BMC (4×10^7) was harvested from B6 PKO donors, recipient animals did not develop any clinical signs of GVHD as late as 160 days after BMT (TABLE 1). Histologic evaluation was also performed in selected animals from this group at various time points, but no signs of GVHD were detectable. Moreover, recipients of B6 PKO BMT, after the first phase of weight loss due to the irradiation regimen, rapidly returned to weight values comparable to those of syngeneically reconstituted BALB/c animals, and such values were maintained as long as 70 days posttransplantation (further measurements were not performed).

A direct correlation is reported to exist between the number of mature T cells infused on bone marrow transplantation and the time of onset of GVHD and its severity.[2] Because GVHD had been observed only in B6 P+/+ BMC recipients and not in the recipients of B6 PKO BMC, we decided to explore the influence of high inocula of mature T lymphocytes in our experimental system. As a source of mature T cells, freshly harvested splenocytes were infused at different doses concomitant to the infusion of BMC.

When BALB/c recipients received 4×10^7 BMC + 2×10^7 splenocytes from B6 P+/+ donors, an accelerated onset of severe GVHD was observed in the recipients, leading to the death of all animals within 20 days (TABLE 2). This effect was even more evident when 4×10^7 splenocytes were administered together with 4×10^7 BMC, and no animal survived longer than 16 days. The administration of large numbers of splenocytes together with BMC from B6 PKO donors also induced lethal GVHD, but the onset of the disease was significantly delayed, and at least in the first period, clinical signs were somewhat milder than those observed in the previous groups (TABLE 2). BALB/c receiving 2×10^7 splenocytes in addition to the BMC inoculum survived up to 45 days (p <0.002 when compared to the recipients of P+/+ BMC + splenocytes), and animals receiving 4×10^7 splenocytes survived 38 days posttransplant (p <0.04).

To exclude the possibility that the lack of clinical and histopathological GVHD in the allogeneic recipients of B6 PKO BMC could be accounted for by defective engraftment of transplanted marrow, we analyzed the newly developed cell subpopulations in the reconstituted animals. First, we assessed the presence and percentage of donor-derived cells. BALB/c recipients of B6 PKO BMC were investigated for chimerism 30 days after BMT. Peripheral blood lymphocytes or, alternatively, splenocytes were incubated with saturating concentrations of mouse monoclonal antibodies specific for MHC Class I determinants of BALB/c (H-2K^d, FITC conjugated) and B6 (H-2K^b, PE conjugated) strains, then analyzed by flow cytometry on FACS fluorimeter. All animals showed complete reconstitution with H-2K^b-positive cells, with percentages that varied between 95 and 98%, defining them as full allogeneic chimeras (B6 PKO → BALB/c chimeras). Further analysis of T-cell subsets (CD3$^+$, CD4$^+$, and CD8$^+$ cells) and B cells (sIg$^+$ cells) showed no gross alteration of percentages and absolute numbers compared to those of untransplanted B6 PKO animals, proving that complete engraftment, at least for these cell subpopulations, had indeed been achieved.

It has been shown that achievement of a state of full allogeneic chimerism is paralleled by acceptance of donor-derived grafted tissues and organs, whereas reactivity towards third party tissues is largely preserved.[17] To determine if B6 PKO → BALB/c chimeras that had not developed GVHD would behave similarly, we analyzed the immune competence of these chimeric animals by means of full-thickness skin graft (FTSG).[18] B6 PKO → BALB/c chimeras were therefore grafted with both donor-derived B6 skin grafts and third party, B10.BR (H-2^k) skin grafts. Chimeric animals were able to maintain their B6 grafts indefinitely, proving that donor-specific unresponsiveness had been obtained. Conversely, third party skin grafts were rejected with an MST of 24.8 ± 10.1 days ($n = 9$). It must be noted, however, that rejection occurred with delayed kinetics, which could be explained by the generalized immune incompetence previously reported as a characteristic of fully allogeneic chimeras.[19]

DISCUSSION

Perforin seems to play a key role in the development of GVHD. Its absence in the bone marrow inoculum prevents the development of clinical and histopathological signs of GVHD when BMC only are administered; on the other hand, the addition of spleen cells to the inocula indeed leads to fatal GVHD. One possible explanation of these contradictory results is that a quantitative effect is responsible for what was observed: when only BMC are infused, not enough mature T-cells are present in the inoculum to trigger clinical GVHD, whereas this threshold is reached and surpassed when splenocytes (as a source of T cells) are added. To formally prove that a quantitative effect is responsible for the development of GVHD when splenocytes are added to the BMC inoculum, we are performing experiments in which BMC are supplemented with discrete numbers of highly purified T cells or T-cell subpopulations.

Alternatively, it is possible that a qualitative difference could account for the observed effect. This is to say, a yet undefined population(s) could be administered with splenocytes and not with BMC inoculum and be responsible for the development of GVHD.

Although ongoing studies will attempt to clarify the relative role of BMC and/or splenocytes in the pathogenesis of GVHD, the encouraging results so far obtained set the basis for the extension of this model towards functional inactivation of the perforin pathway in large animal models for eventual transfer to the clinical setting.

REFERENCES

1. STORB, R. & E. D. THOMAS. 1983. Allogeneic bone marrow transplantation. Immunol. Rev. **71:** 77-102.
2. KORNGOLD, R. & J. SPRENT. 1982. Features of T cells causing H-2 restricted lethal graft versus host disease across minor histocompatibility barriers. J. Exp. Med. **155:** 872-883.
3. FERRARA, J. L. M. 1993. Cytokine disregulation as a mechanism of graft versus host disease. Curr. Opin. Immunol. **5:** 794-799.
4. THIELE, D. R., M. R. CHARLEY, J. A. CALOMENI & P. E. LIPSKEY. 1987. Lethal graft-versus-host disease across major histocompatibility barriers: Requirement for leucyl-leucine methyl ester sensitive cytotoxic T cells. J. Immunol. **138:** 51-57.
5. KORNGOLD, R. & J. SPRENT. 1978. Lethal graft versus host disease following bone marrow transplantation across minor histocompatibility barriers in mice: Prevention from removing mature T cells from marrow. J. Exp. Med. **148:** 1687-1698.
6. VALLERA, D. A. & B. R. BLAZER. 1989. T cell depletion for graft versus host disease prophylaxis. Transplantation **47:** 751-760.
7. RINGDEN, O., M. M. HOROWITZ, P. SONDEL, R. P. GALE, J. C. BIGGS, R. E. CHAMPLIN, H. J. DEEG, K. DICKE, T. MASAOKA & R. L. POWLES. 1993. Methotrexate, cyclosporine, or both to prevent graft-versus-host disease after HLA-identical sibling bone marrow transplants for early leukemia? Blood **81:** 1094-1101.
8. MARKUS, P. M., X. CAI, W. MING, A. J. DEMETRIS, J. J. FUNG & T. E. STARZL. 1991. Prevention of graft-versus-host disease following allogeneic bone marrow transplantation in rats using FK506. Transplantation **52:** 590-594.
9. FABIAN, M. A., S. M. DENNING & R. R. BOLLINGER. 1992. Rapamycin suppression of host-versus-graft and graft-versus-host disease in MHC-mismatched rats. Transplant. Proc. **24:** 1174-1176.
10. GOLDMAN, J. M., R. P. GALE, M. M. HOROWITZ, J. C. BIGGS, R. E. CHAMPLIN, E. GLUCKMAN, R. G. HOFFMAN, S. J. JACOBSEN, A. M. MARMONT & P. B. McGLACE. 1988. Bone marrow transplantation for chronic myelogenous leukemia in chronic phase: Increased risk of relapse associated with T-cell depletion. Ann. Intern. Med. **108:** 806-810.
11. MARTIN, P. J., J. A. HANSEN, B. TOROK-STORB, D. DURNAM, D. PRZEPIORKA, J. O'QUIGLEY, J. SANDERS, K. M. SULLIVAN, R. P. WITHERSPOON & H. J. DEEG. 1988. Graft failure in patients receiving T cell-depleted HLA identical allogeneic marrow transplants. Bone Marrow Transplant. **3:** 445-456.
12. PODACK, E. R., J. D. YOUNG & Z. A. COHN. 1985. Isolation and biochemical and functional characterization of perforin 1 from cytolytic T-cell granules. Proc. Natl. Acad. Sci. USA **82:** 8629-8633.
13. ROUVIER, E., M. F. LUCIANI & P. GOLSTEIN. 1988. Fas involvement in Ca^{++}-independent T-cell mediated cytotoxicity. J. Exp. Med. **177:** 195-200.
14. YOUNG, J. D., C. LIU, P. M. PERSECHINI & Z. A. COHN. 1988. Perforin dependent and independent pathways of cytotoxicity mediated by lymphocytes. Immunol. Rev. **103:** 160-202.
15. KAGI, D., B. LEDERMANN, K. BURKI, P. SEILER, B. ODERMATT, K. J. OLSEN, E. R. PODACK, R. M. ZINKERNAGEL & H. HENGARTNER. 1994. Cytotoxicity mediated by T cells and natural killer cells is greatly impaired in perforin-deficient mice. Nature **369:** 31-37.
16. RAPPAPORT, H., A. KHALIL, O. HALLE-PANNENKO, L. PRITCHARD, D. DANTCHEV & G. MATHE. 1979. Histopathological sequence of events in adult mice undergoing lethal

graft-versus-host reaction developed across H-2 and/or non-H-2 histocompatibility barriers. Am. J. Pathol. **96:** 121-142.

17. ILDSTADT, S. T. & D. H. SACHS. 1984. Reconstitution with syngeneic plus allogeneic or xenogeneic bone marrow leads to specific acceptance of allografts. Nature **307:** 168-170.

18. BILLINGHAM, R. E. 1961. Free skin grafting in mammals. *In* Transplantation of Tissues and Cells. R. E. Billingham & W. R. Silvers, Eds. : 1. Wistar Institute Press. Philadelphia.

19. ZINKERNAGEL, R. M., A. ALTHAGE, G. CALLAHAN & R. M. WELSH. 1980. On the immunocompetence of H-2 incompatible irradiation bone marrow chimeras. J. Immunol. **124:** 2356-2365.

Multiple Bone Marrow Infusions to Enhance Acceptance of Allografts from the Same Donor

CAMILLO RICORDI,[a] THEODORE KARATZAS,
GENNARO SELVAGGI, JOSE NERY, MARC WEBB,
HUGO FERNANDEZ, PHILLIP RUIZ,
SHEN-SHEN KONG, VIOLET ESQUENAZI,
JOSHUA MILLER, EUGENE SCHIFF, AND
ANDREAS G. TZAKIS

*Diabetes Research Institute and
Departments of Surgery, Medicine, and Pathology
University of Miami School of Medicine
Miami, Florida 33136*

Two major drawbacks of organ transplantation are the continuous requirement for immunosuppressive drugs and the incidence of rejection episodes that acutely, or over time, contribute to the loss and/or decrease in the function of the allograft. In fact, even kidney allograft recipients who, in some centers (ours included), have ~90% probability of maintaining a functioning graft 1 year after transplantation, experience a progressive decrease in organ survival of 30-40% at 10 years posttransplant. The development of strategies to allow organ allograft survival without rejection episodes and/or the potential of progressively decreasing and even discontinuing immunosuppressive therapy would represent an incredible benefit to the patient and would substantially decrease the cost of posttransplant patient care. Donor-specific transplantation tolerance has been achieved in animal models using several approaches that include infusion of donor-specific bone marrow derived cells. However, the induction of permanent graft acceptance without continuous recipient immunosuppression remains elusive in large animals, including humans. Even before human organ transplantation was introduced, it was shown that the induction of specific immunological tolerance could be induced in inbred rodent strains by infusing allogeneic bone marrow derived cell suspensions with resultant permanent acceptance of donor-specific skin grafts.[1,2] Infusion of donor-type immune cells was performed during the first 24 hours of neonatal life.

Until recently, attempts to use human bone marrow to induce tolerance have met with critical skepticism in clinical investigation. Monaco *et al.*[3] performed donor-specific bone marrow transplants simultaneously with kidney transplantation using

[a] Address for correspondence: Camillo Ricordi, MD, Cell Transplant Center, Diabetes Research Institute, University of Miami School of Medicine, 1450 N.W. 10th Avenue, Miami, FL 33136.

antilymphocyte globulin "induction" therapy[3] in a protocol similar to one they had described in inbred mice.[4] In a discussion of his results,[3] Monaco acknowledged the learning experience from pretransplant blood transfusion studies, which highlight the importance of the number of transfusions and the time interval between them as critical variables in allograft outcome. Barber *et al.*,[5,6] in a series of cases from the University of Alabama, reported encouraging results with kidney plus bone marrow from human cadaver organ donors. Recently, Thomas *et al.*[7,8] reported donor-specific graft acceptance in a primate model in which recipients were treated with donor bone marrow cells.

It has been widely accepted that cytoablative treatment of recipients is generally required to "make space" for newly transplanted bone marrow components. This dogma has been challenged recently, indicating that it is possible to infuse a high dose of donor marrow to successfully and permanently repopulate a recipient without the need for radiation treatment.[9,10] These observations offer extraordinary clinical investigative opportunities to explore many variables such as cell number, route of administration, inductive immunosuppression, and timing that could affect the outcome of bone marrow transplantation in patients in whom cytoablation is not required because of the nature of the underlying disease (i.e., hematologic malignancy). The enthusiasm for bone marrow cell transfusion without cytoablation arises from the enormous clinical possibilities if the risks of cytoablation can be circumvented. Recent results indicate that even in large animals such as the dog bone marrow engraftment can be obtained without any cytoablative treatment,[11] confirming previous observations in a murine model.[12]

Following the description of long-term persistence of donor bone marrow derived cells (DBMC) in recipients of organ allografts,[13-20] we reported the initial results in trials of donor bone marrow infusion for tolerance induction.[21] These trials demonstrated that one bone marrow infusion at day 0 with a dose of 3×10^8/kg DBMC did not prevent rejection episodes that occurred in most liver allograft recipients.

In consideration of our own preliminary experience[21] and of the recent results of Quesenberry's group,[9] we decided to proceed with a clinical trial to test the effect of a higher dose of DBMC with an additional infusion of DBMC at day 11 following liver allografting. Donor bone marrow cells were harvested at the end of multiorgan procurement from heart-beating cadaveric donors. After retrieval of solid organs, the surgical field was prepared for resection of the vertebral column. Nine to twelve vertebral bodies were harvested from each donor, and the retrieved vertebral column was divided at the intervertebral disk level into two or three segments for transport to the processing laboratory in cold preservation solution. The protocol employed to harvest vertebral bone marrow is a modification (Method in Cell Tx, in press) of the protocol previously described by Strong *et al.*[22] Briefly, with aseptic techniques, the vertebral column was separated into individual vertebra and divided along the sagittal craniocaudal axis. The cancellous bone was chipped-off by rongeurs and placed in modified RPMI medium for passive release of bone marrow cells. This cell suspension was then filtered through two consecutive stainless steel screens (450 and 180 μm, respectively), centrifuged at 300/*g* for 10 minutes, and the cell pellet was resuspended in 300 ml of RPMI solution. To release cells trapped within the trabecular framework of the marrow, cancellous chips retained on the filter were reprocessed by gentle shaking in the processing medium twice for 30 minutes each. The cell suspension

TABLE 1. Characteristics of Donor Blood Marrow Cell (DBMC) Source, Number, Infusion Timing, and Immunosuppression in Recipients of Liver Allografts

DBMC Source	Vertebral Bodies
DBMC number	$5\text{-}10 \times 10^8$/kg
Number and timing of DBMC infusions	1 or 2: at day 0 or days 0 and 11
Base immunosuppression	FK-506 + steroids
Induction immunosuppression	None or OKT3 (5 mg/day 0-10)

was then centrifuged and processed as just mentioned. Cell count and viability were assessed by trypan blue exclusion, and the cells were finally resuspended at 10^8 cells ml^{-1}. Samples for progenitor cell assay (colony-forming units), microbial surveillance, and flow cytometric analysis were retained from the final cell preparation.

The characteristics of DBMC dose, timing, and recipient immunosuppression are summarized in TABLE 1. Our initial results in liver allograft recipients with random HLA matching and with negative cross-matching are summarized in TABLE 2. The 17 patients who received two DBMC infusions did not experience any rejection episode following the second DBMC infusion, the only two episodes occurring at day 8. By contrast, patients receiving only one DBMC infusion, with or without OKT3 induction, had an incidence of rejection that was higher than that of the control group. Allograft survival in recipients of either one DBMC (89%) or two DBMC (100%) infusions was significantly better, than that in the controls (74%) at 4-month follow-up. Rejection episodes never occurred in the four patients receiving two DBMC infusions and OKT3.

Statistical analysis with chi-square, likelihood ratio chi-square, and Fisher's exact test revealed that the overall incidence of rejection in the controls and in recipients of one DBMC infusion was significantly different from that in recipients of two

TABLE 2. Recipient Age, Follow-up, and Incidence of Rejection Episodes following Liver Allograft Alone (No DBMC) or after combined Liver Allograft and One (1 DBMC) or Two (2 DBMC) Infusions of Donor Bone Marrow (DBMC)

				Rejection Episodes	
	n	Age (yr)	Follow-up (days)	Before Postoperative Day 11	After Postoperative Day 11
No DBMC	23	41 ± 17	104 ± 42	2/23	7/23
No DBMC + OKT3	1	36	73	0/1	0/1
1 DBMC	4	47 ± 6	108 ± 55	0/4	3/4
1 DBMC + OKT3	5	45 ± 7	143 ± 36	0/5	3/5
2 DBMC	13	33 ± 18	131 ± 57	2/13	0/13
2 DBMC + OKT3	4	46 ± 18	137 ± 63	0/4	0/4

DBMC infusions. Further analysis revealed that these differences were not related to early events (before the second bone marrow infusion). Even excluding all cases of rejection occurring before day 11, the difference between patients receiving two DBMC infusions and either the controls or patients receiving one DBMC infusion was still significant (Fisher's exact test). The higher incidence of rejection in patients receiving one DBMC infusion than in the controls barely missed the level of significance with Fisher's exact test. Most importantly, Kaplan-Meier survival analysis also revealed a significant difference in graft survival among the three groups. The best graft survival occurred in recipients of two DBMC infusions (0 graft loss, 0 death), followed by the groups receiving one DBMC (0 graft loss, 1 death) and the control group (3 graft losses, 2 deaths). Despite the very encouraging observations on the incidence of rejection and graft survival, our preliminary results did not reveal a significant difference between groups in either the dose of steroids or the dose and level of FK-506. Also, no significant difference in HLA matching (including DR matches) was noted between groups. In contrast to the results in patients with a negative cross-match, DBMC infusion in patients with a positive cross-match did not prevent rejection episodes that were more frequent than in the control group (liver allograft alone). The presence of a positive cross-match may therefore contraindicate intravascular infusion of donor-derived cells at the time of liver allograft. We are currently exploring whether delayed first infusion of DBMC in positive cross-match cases will be more effective.

In the Pittsburgh trial,[21] the incidence of rejection was comparable to that in our groups receiving one DBMC infusion (>50%). However, in the Pittsburgh experience, the incidence of rejection in DBMC recipients was lower than that in the control group without DBMC (>60%). In our experience in Miami, the incidence of rejection in the control group was approximately 30%. The difference in our observations could be due to our shorter follow-up or to the higher dose of DBMC used in patients treated with a single DBMC infusion in this study. Of interest is that we have not yet observed any significant graft versus host reaction despite the higher DBMC dose.

As in our preliminary experience in Pittsburgh,[21] we were unable to establish a direct correlation between the degree of chimerism and the presence or absence of rejection episodes. The results are still preliminary, and longer follow-up together with more sensitive methods to analyze lineages of donor cells will allow us to determine whether and what kind or degree of chimerism is associated with a lower incidence of chronic rejection.

Nevertheless, the results obtained with two DBMC infusions are encouraging. The reason that one DBMC infusion appeared to increase rejection while two infusions reduced the incidence of rejection episodes is not yet understood. One possibility is that the first DBMC infusion induced the immune activation that was important for subsequent inhibition of the immune response by the second DBMC infusion. Alternatively, the second infusion could have enhanced the number of donor stem cells that engrafted as per the hypothesis of Quesenberry's group on the positive effect of multiple infusions of donor bone marrow on stem cell engraftment. Finally, the first infusion could be completely irrelevant, and the second infusion at day 11 could be the one responsible for the favorable effect. In fact, the beneficial effect of a DBMC infusion at day 11 posttransplant has been already reported by Thomas *et al.*[23] It is of interest that graft survival was better in patients receiving a single infusion of DBMC than in the controls, even though these recipients experienced more rejection episodes than did recipients of a liver allograft alone. In contrast to protocols of bone marrow transplantation for treatment of hematologic malignancies, DBMC infusion to promote or enhance allograft acceptance does not require aggressive cytoablative conditioning of the recipients. In the absence of recipient cytoablation, variables such as dose, timing, route of administration, and inductive immunosuppressive treatment may constitute critical maneuverable components that could affect DBMC engraftment and induction of donor-specific graft acceptance. Our preliminary observations with two DBMC infusions on liver allograft recipients support the observations of Quesenberry's group in the murine model[9] and may be of assistance in defining strategies of multiple donor bone marrow infusions in clinical trials of allotransplantation.

REFERENCES

1. BILLINGHAM, R. E., L. BRENT & P. B. MEDAWAR. 1953. Actively acquired tolerance of foreign cells. Nature **172:** 603-606.
2. BILLINGHAM, R. E. & L. BRENT. 1954. Quantitative studies of tissue transplantation immunity. II. The origins, strengths and duration of actively and adoptively acquired immunity. Proc. R. Soc. B. **143:** 58-80.
3. MONACO, A. P., A. W. CLARK, M. L. WOOD, A. L. SAHYOUN, S. D. CODISH & R. W. BROWN. 1976. Possible active enhancement of a human cadaver renal allograft with antilymphocytic serum (ALS) and donor bone marrow: Case report of an initial attempt. Surgery **79:** 384-392.
4. MONACO, A. P., M. L. WOOD & P. S. RUSSEL. 1966. Studies on heterologous anti-lymphocyte serum in mice. III. Immunologic tolerance and chimerism produced across the H-2 locus with adult thymectomy and anti-lymphocyte serum. Ann. N. Y. Acad. Sci. **129:** 190-206.
5. BARBER, W. H., J. A. MANKIN, D. A. LASKOW, M. H. DEIERHOI, B. A. JULIAN, J. J. CURTIS & A. G. DIETHELM. 1991. Long-term results of a controlled prospective study with transfusion of donor-specific bone marrow in 57 cadaveric renal allograft recipients. Transplantation **51:** 70-75.
6. McDANIEL, D. O., J. NAFTILAN, K. HULVEY, S. SHANEYFELT, J. A. LEMONS, S. LAGOO-DEENADAYALAN, S. HUDSON, A. G. DIETHLEM & H. BARBER. 1994. Peripheral blood chimerism in renal allograft recipients transfused with donor bone marrow. Transplantation **57:** 852-856.
7. THOMAS, F. T., F. M. CARVER & M. B. FOIL. 1983. Long-term incompatible kidney survival in outbred higher primates without chronic immunosuppression. Ann. Surg. **198:** 370.
8. THOMAS, J. M., F. M. CARVER & M. B. FOIL. 1983. Renal allograft tolerance induced with ATG and donor bone marrow in outbred rhesus monkeys. Transplantation **36:** 104.
9. STEWART, F. M., R. B. CRITTENDEN, P. A. LOWRY, S. PEARSON-WHITE & P. J. QUESENBERRY. 1993. Long-term engraftment of normal and post-5-fluorouracil murine marrow into normal mice. Blood **81:** 2566.
10. HARRISON, D. E. 1993. Competitive repopulation in unirradiated normal recipients. Blood **81:** 2473-2474.
11. BIENZLE, D., A. C. G. ABRAMS-OGG, S. A. KRUTH, J. ACKLAND-SNOW, R. F. CARTER, J. E. DICK, R. M. JACOBS, S. KAMEL-REID & I. D. DUBE. 1994. Gene transfer into hematopoietic stem cells: Long-term maintenance of in vitro activated progenitors without marrow ablation. Proc. Natl. Acad. Sci. USA **91:** 350-354.

12. CARTER, R. F., A. C. G. ABRAMS-OGG, J. E. DICK, S. A. KRUTH, V. E. VALLI, S. KAMEL-REID & I. A. DUBE. 1992. Autologous transplantation of canine long term marrow culture cells genetically marked by retroviral vectors. Blood **79:** 356-364.

13. STARZL, T. E., A. J. DEMETRIS, M. NORIKO, S. T. ILDSTAD, C. RICORDI & M. TRUCCO. 1992. Cell migration, chimerism, and graft acceptance. Lancet **339:** 1579-1582.

14. STARZL, T. E., A. J. DEMETRIS, M. TRUCCO, I. I. RAMOS, A. ZEEVI, W. A. RUDERT, M. KOCOUA, C. RICORDI, S. ILDSTAD & N. MURASE. 1992. Systemic chimerism in human female recipients of male livers. Lancet **340:** 876-877.

15. STARZL, T. E., A. J. DEMETRIS, N. MURASE, A. W. THOMSON, M. TRUCCO & C. RICORDI. 1993. Donor cell chimerism permitted by immunosuppressive drugs: A probable basis of organ transplant acceptance and tolerance. Immunol. Today **14:** 326-332.

16. STARZL, T. E., A. J. DEMETRIS, M. TRUCCO, A. ZEEVI, H. RAMOS, P. TERASAKI, W. A. RUDERT, M. KOCOVA, C. RICORDI, S. T. ILDSTAD & N. MURASE. 1993. Chimerism and donor specific nonreactivity 27 to 29 years after kidney allotransplantation. Transplantation **55:** 1272-1277.

17. STARZL, T. E., A. J. DEMETRIS, M. TRUCCO, N. MURASE, C. RICORDI & S. ILDSTAD. 1993. Cell migration and chimerism after whole organ transplantation: The basis of graft acceptance. Hepatology **17:** 1127-1152.

18. STARZL, T. E., A. J. DEMETRIS, M. TRUCCO, C. RICORDI, N. MURASE & A. W. THOMSON. 1993. The role of cell migration and chimerism in organ transplant acceptance and tolerance induction. Transplant Sci. **3:** 47-50.

19. STARZL, T. E., A. J. DEMETRIS, M. TRUCCO, C. RICORDI, S. T. ILDSTAD, N. MURASE & R. S. KENDALL. 1993. Chimerism after liver transplantation in patients with Type IV glycogen storage disease. N. Engl. J. Med. **328:** 745-749.

20. STARZL, T. E., N. MURASE, A. J. DEMETRIS, S. ILDSTAD, C. RICORDI & M. TRUCCO. 1993. Allograft and xenograft acceptance under FK506 and other immunosuppressive treatment. Ann. N. Y. Acad. Sci. **685:** 46-51.

21. FONTES, P., A. RAO, A. J. DEMETRIS, A. ZEEVI, M. TRUCCO, P. CARROLL, W. RYBKA, C. RICORDI, F. DODSON, R. SHAPIRO, A. TZAKIS, S. TODO, K. ABU-ELMAGD, M. JORDAN, J. J. FUNG & T. E. STARZL. 1994. Augmentation with bone marrow of donor leukocyte migration for kidney, liver, heart, and pancreas islet transplantation. Lancet **344:** 151-155.

22. STRONG, M. 1992. Seattle Protocol: Vertebral body recovery for bone marrow. (PRO-550G) 1-5.

23. THOMAS, J. M., F. M. CARVER, J. KASTEN-JOLLY, C. E. HAISCH, L. M. REBELLATO, U. GROSS, S. J. VORE & F. T. THOMAS. 1994. Further studies of veto activity in rhesus monkey bone marrow in relation to allograft tolerance and chimerism. Transplantation **57:** 101-115.

Newborn Blood Used as a Source of Donor Cells in a Murine Model of Transplantation across Non-MHC Antigens[a]

VÉRONIQUE DE LA SELLE AND
MARTINE BRULEY-ROSSET

INSERM U267
Groupe hospitalier Paul Brousse
Villejuif, France

Bone marrow transplantation is widely used in the treatment of malignant and non-malignant disorders, but it is often complicated by graft-versus-host disease (GVHD).[1] The elimination of mature T cells from bone marrow graft reduces GVHD but increases graft failure and malignant relapse.[2] In addition, suitable marrow from HLA identical sibling donor is often unavailable, justifying the prospect of new sources of cells for transplantation.

The use of umbilical cord blood (CB) for therapeutic reconstitution was proposed from the experimental observations of Boyse[3] who obtained successful reconstitution of lethally irradiated mice with syngeneic neonatal blood.[3] Furthermore, *in vitro* studies have shown that CB contains large numbers of hematopoietic progenitors with a high proliferative potential.[3-5] Another theoretical advantage of CB is the reduced risk of GVHD from the relative immaturity of T cells.[6,7] Preliminary results of CB transplantation in pediatric patients[8,9] are encouraging, but many questions remained unanswered because *in vivo* experimental models are lacking.

In this work, we used newborn blood (NBB) as a murine model for human CB transplantation and studied the immuno-hematologic reconstitutive capacity of NBB cells derived from B10.D2 donors when grafted to lethally irradiated H-2 compatible (DBA/2 × B10.D2)F1 recipients. In this genetic combination, donor and recipient differ in multiple DBA/2 minor histocompatibility Ags (mHAgs), and lethal GVHD developed in nearly 100% of (DBA/2 × B10.D2)F1 recipients[10] engrafted with bone marrow and lymphoid cells from adult B10.D2 mice. We evaluated the number of NBB cells required to achieve engraftment and studied the resulting survival and degree of chimerism. We also investigated the risk of GVHD development across mHAgs.

MATERIAL AND METHODS

Mice. B10.D2 (H-2^d), DBA/2 (H-2^d) (DBA/2 × B10.D2)F1 (H-2$^{d/d}$), and (BALB/c × C57B1/6)F1 (H-2$^{d/b}$) mice were prepared in our own facilities.

[a] This work was supported by Agence Française du sang/INSERM grant 3FSO2.

Blood Collection. Blood from newborn B10.D2 mice was collected the day of birth on Calciparin. Cells were either left unseparated or separated on Ficoll/Hypaque gradient (1090, Pharmacia). White and red blood cell counts were performed on a Technicon H-2 system (Bayer Diagnostics).

Graft Procedure. Cells from NBB or bone marrow (10^7) and spleen (8×10^6) were obtained from B10.D2 donor mice and grafted intravenously into lethally irradiated (9,5 Gy) (DBA/2 × B10.D2)F1 recipients.

Phenotype Characterization. FITC or PE-conjugated anti-CD4, anti-CD8, and anti-TCR α/β monoclonal antibodies (mABs) were obtained from Pharmingen (Clinisciences) and anti-Thy-1 mAb from Coulter. Unconjugated mAbs against stem cell antigen (SCA-1) were provided by Pharmingen and revealed by FITC-conjugated goat anti-rat Ig (Coulter). To analyze the chimerism, 5×10^5 lymph node cells from B10.D2, DBA/2, and NBB engrafted F1 mice were incubated 30 minutes at 4°C with unconjugated anti-Lyt-1.1 mAb (specific for DBA/2 mice). Cells were washed and incubated for 30 minutes at 4°C with FITC-conjugated (Coulter) goat anti-mouse Ig (Coulter) and PE-conjugated anti-CD4 and anti-CD8. One- or two-color fluorescence analysis was performed on 5,000–10,000 cells using a cell analyzer (Profile-Coulter), and the percentage of single- or double-positive cells was calculated.

Mixed Lymphocyte Reaction (MLR). Spleen cells (4×10^5 per well) from normal B10.D2 mice or NBB engrafted F1 mice collected 2–3 months after transplantation were cultured in the presence of irradiated stimulator cells (4×10^5 per well) from different mouse strains. Proliferation was evaluated 3 days later by [³H]thymidine incorporation in the last 18 hours of culture.

Cytotoxic Assay (CTL). After a 5-day mixed lymphocyte reaction in the presence of irradiated DBA/2 (specific for mHAgs) or C57Bl/6 (H-2 unrelated) cells, spleen cells from normal B10.D2 or NBB engrafted F1 mice were incubated at different effector-to-target ratios with ⁵¹Cr-labeled P815 (DBA/2 specific) or ⁵¹Cr-EL4 (C57Bl/6, H-2 unrelated) target cells. Four hours later, the amount of ⁵¹Cr released was measured in the supernatants and used to calculate the percentage of cytotoxicity.

In Vivo Transfer Experiments. Both 10^7 bone marrow cells and 8×10^6 spleen cells collected from NBB engrafted F1 mice were injected in either lethally irradiated (BALB/c × C57Bl/6)F1 recipients incompatible for H-2^b or (DBA/2 × B10.D2) F1 recipients incompatible for DBA/2 mHAgs. The following rate and incidence of lethal GVHD were measured.

RESULTS

Characteristics of Newborn Blood Collection

Data on the collection of blood of newborns on the day of birth are summarized in TABLE 1 and represent the mean of 6–8 individual blood samples. The volume of collected blood ranged from 40–50 µl, and the number of nucleated cells was evaluated as approximatively $4–5 \times 10^5$ per sample. Cytologic examination revealed that unfractionated blood contained around 57% mature lymphocytes, 3% immature lymphocytes, 6% monocytes, and 34% polymorphonuclear cells (not shown).

TABLE 1. Characteristics of Newborn Blood Collection[a]

	Value
Median volume of newborn blood	40–50 µl
Mean number of white blood cells	$9.5 \pm 2.8 \ 10^3/\mu l$
Mean number of red blood cells	$1.7 \pm 0.3 \ 10^6/\mu l$

[a] Values are mean $\pm$ SD of 6–8 blood samples.

Phenotype Characterization of Newborn Blood Cells

Cytofluorometric analysis of NBB cells was performed after Ficoll/Hypaque gradient purification to obtain enrichment in mononuclear cells and was compared to that of adult lymph node cells (TABLE 2). The mean results of 5–7 samples indicated that T cells from NBB express a double-positive CD4+CD8+ immature phenotype (30%) with only a few T cells expressing a single-positive CD4+ (2.8%) or CD8+ (1.9%) phenotype, whereas T cells from adult lymph nodes exhibit a mature phenotype with single-positive CD4+ (33.1%) and CD8+ (23.7%) cells and no double-positive T cells. Lymph nodes contain a few SCA-1+ (stem cell antigen) cells, while cells from NBB contain a mean percentage of 15% SCA-1+ cells. In addition, a typical histogram (FIG. 1) indicated that double-positive CD4+CD8+ T cells are TcRα/β^{low} and Thy-1^{high} and that SCA-1+ cells were not stained by anti-Thy-1 mAb.

Survival and GVHD Incidence in NBB Engrafted F1 Recipients

Unfractionated blood from one newborn mouse or pooled blood from two or three newborn mice was injected to lethally irradiated (B10.D2 × DBA/2)F1 recipients. Survival of NBB engrafted mice was compared to that of the same recipients receiving 10^7 bone marrow together with 8×10^6 spleen cells derived from a B10.D2 donor (FIG. 2). As described previously, all F1 recipients engrafted with bone marrow and

TABLE 2. Comparison of the Phenotype of Cells from Different Origins

Cell Origin	Mean Percentage $\pm$ SD of Positive Cells						
	CD3+	CD4+CD8−	CD4−CD8+	CD4+CD8+	TCRαβ+	THY-1+	SCA-1+
Lymph nodes	58.7 ± 1.5^a	33.1 ± 0.6	23.7 ± 1.4	ND[b]	58.7 ± 2.8	49.8 ± 2.9	2.6 ± 0.6
Newborn blood	NT[c]	2.8 ± 0.5	1.9 ± 0.4	30.0 ± 7.1	3.7 ± 0.9	33.2 ± 11.4	14.7 ± 4.3

[a] Values are mean $\pm$ SD of 5–7 donor samples.
[b] Not detected.
[c] Not tested.

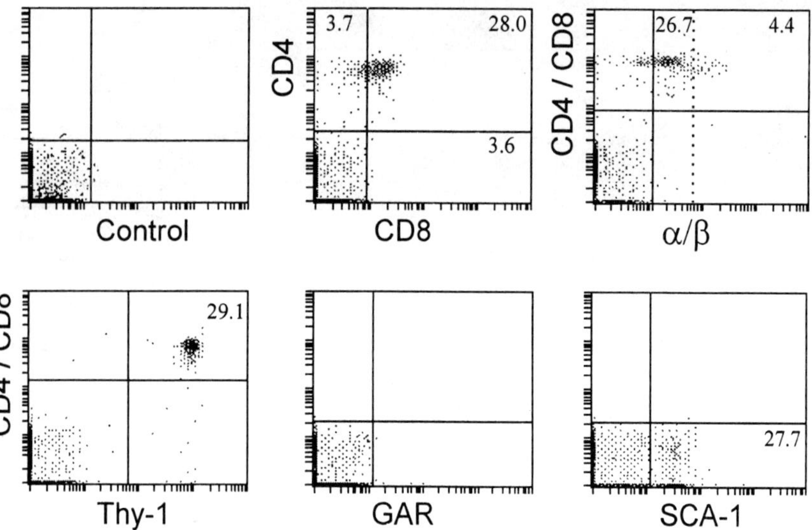

FIGURE 1. Typical cytofluorometric analysis of an individual newborn blood sample. Mononuclear cells were isolated and stained with different monoclonal antibodies. Percentage of single- or double-positive cells is shown for each indicated Ag. GAR = goat-anti-rat Igs; SCA = stem cell antigen.

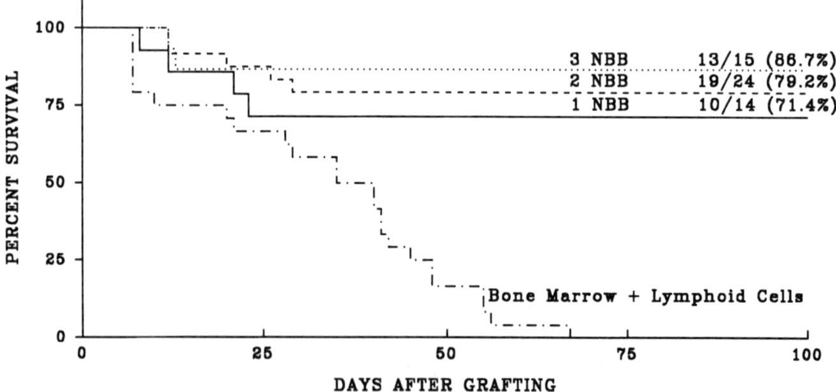

FIGURE 2. Survival and graft-versus-host disease *in vivo*. Lethally irradiated (DBA/2 × B10.D2)F1 mice were reconstituted with bone marrow and lymphoid cells (–··–) or with one (-), two (- - -), or three (···) pooled samples of newborn blood (NBB) and mortality was recorded daily.

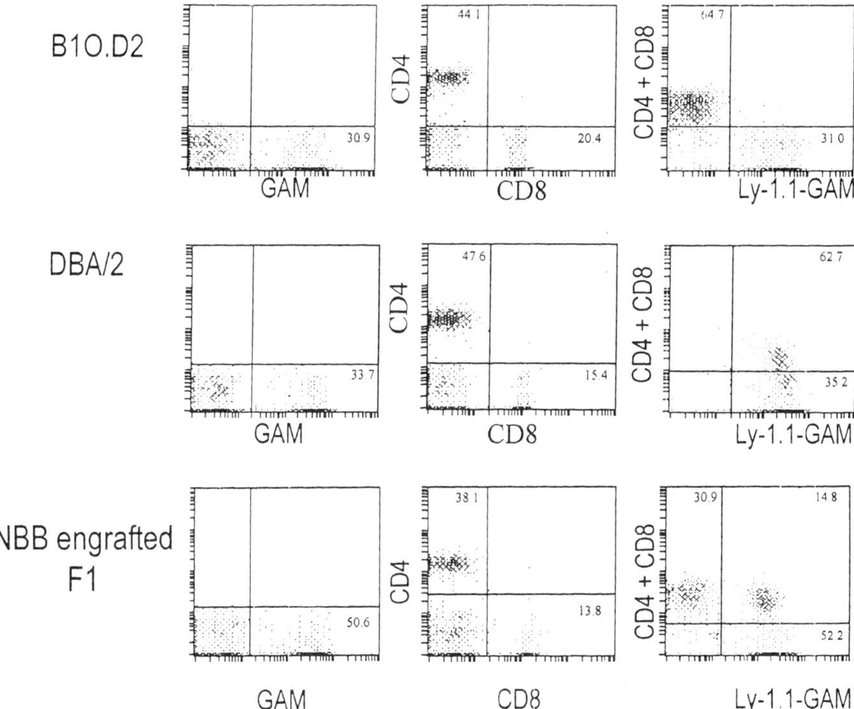

FIGURE 3. Chimerism evaluation. Lymph node cells from B10.D2 (donor), DBA/2 (recipient), and newborn blood (NBB) engrafted F1 mice were stained with anti-Lyt 1.1 monoclonal antibody (mAb) and revealed by FITC-conjugated goat–anti-mouse (GAM) mAb and further incubated with PE-conjugated anti-CD4 and anti-CD8 mAbs. The percentage of single- or double-positive cells was measured by flow cytometry.

spleen cells developed lethal GVHD across DBA/2 mHAgs. Interestingly, NBB perfectly engrafted F1 mice, and the percentage of survival seems to depend on the dose of cells infused: 71% survival for one NBB sample to 86% for three NBB samples injected to F1 recipients. These mice survived more than 100 days with no clinical signs of GVHD.

Evaluation of the Degree of Chimerism in NBB Engrafted F1 Mice

We next verified that reconstitution was achieved by cells of donor origin and not by radioresistant cells of host origin. F1 recipients infused with bone marrow and spleen cells were already shown to be fully chimeric. Engraftment of NBB was assessed in two-color fluorescence analysis in lymph node cells of F1 recipients using a mAb against lyt-1.1, an allele-specific T-cell marker. FIGURE 3 shows that lyt-1.1 was expressed only on recipient DBA/2 and not on donor B10.D2 CD4[+] and

TABLE 3. Establishment of Chimerism in Newborn Blood (NBB) Engrafted F1 Mice

Number of NBB Injected to (DBA/2xB10.D2)F1	Percentage of Donor Origin T Cells		
	Time after Grafting		
	13–15 Days	18–19 Days	60–120 Days
1 NBB	40.2 ± 25.3[a]	44.0 ± 10.2	66.8 ± 2.3
2 NBB	60.9 ± 12.0	62.4 ± 4.7	67.9 ± 4.6
3 NBB	71.7 ± 7.9	67.7 ± 1.3	68.1 ± 5.4

[a] Values are mean ± SD of three individual recipients for each time point.

$CD8^+$ T cells. With this method we found that 2 months after the graft, both lyt-1.1$^+$ and lyt-1.1$^-$ were detected within the T-cell subset, indicating that a mixed chimerism (approximately 69%) was achieved in long-term surviving F1 mice engrafted with NBB.

We further demonstrated that the rate of chimerism established but not the degree of chimerism depend on the initial dose of NBB cells injected: TABLE 3 shows that maximum chimerism (60-70%) was reached in the lymph node of F1 recipients as early as 13-15 days after the graft of three NBB pooled samples, while at the same time the injection of one NBB sample resulted in only 40% chimerism.

Establishment of Host-Specific Tolerance in Newborn Blood Engrafted Mice

Two to three months after the graft, the proliferative and cytotoxic capacity of spleen cells from NBB engrafted F1 mice was evaluated in response to DBA/2 host mHAgs and to H-2^b third party Ag and compared to that of normal B10.D2 mice. TABLE 4 indicates that cells from normal B10.D2 mice incorporated tritiated thymidine

TABLE 4. Proliferative Response of Newborn Blood Engrafted F1 Mice

Irradiated Stimulating Cells	Incompatibility for:	Thymidine Incorporation into Cells from: (mean cpm ± SD)		
		Normal B10.D2	NBB1 Engrafted F1	NBB2 Engrafted F1
B10.D2	—	6,281 ± 414	2,819 ± 433	3,471 ± 450
DBA/2	Minor + Mls[a]	**12,277 ± 231***	2,866 ± 476	3,486 ± 128
C57BL/6	H-2^b	**29,658 ± 7,059**	**12,288 ± 903**	**20,746 ± 531**

*This result represents a typical experiment in which each culture was performed in triplicate. Significant proliferation is indicated by *bold type*.

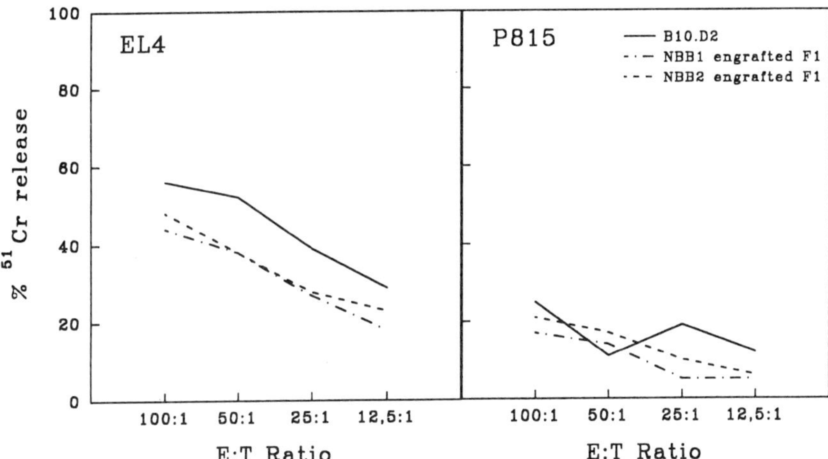

FIGURE 4. Cytotoxic activity. Spleen cells from normal B10.D2 or from newborn blood (NBB) engrafted F1 mice were incubated at a different effector-to-target (E:T) ratio with ^{51}Cr-labeled EL4 (H-2^b) or P815 (H-2^d) target cells. ^{51}Cr release was measured 4 hours later and the percentage of specific cytotoxicity calculated.

when stimulated *in vitro* with DBA/2 and C57B/6 irradiated cells. Conversely, cells from two NBB engrafted F1 mice were unresponsive to DBA/2 cells but still respond to C57B/6 cells.

Similarly, cytotoxic assay reactivity of NBB engrafted F1 mice against H-2^b third party Ags expressed on EL4 targets was similar to that of spleen cells of normal B10.D2 mice (FIG. 4). By contrast, low or no cytotoxicity was detected against DBA/2 mHAgs expressed on P815 targets, whatever the origin of effector cells. Indeed, cytotoxic assay activity against mHAgs could be raised not after primary *in vitro* cultures alone but only after immunization *in vivo* or in engrafted mice.

In addition, spleen cells from long-term surviving NBB engrafted F1 mice, when grafted together with bone marrow cells, retained their ability to induce lethal GVHD in irradiated (BALB/c × C57BL/6)F1 × recipients incompatible for H-2^b third party Ag (FIG. 5). By contrast, the same cells injected to irradiated (DBA/2 × B10.D2)F1 recipients incompatible for DBA/2 mHAgs were unable to initiate a lethal GVHD over a 3-month period of observation. Altogether, data demonstrated that NBB engrafted F1 recipients developed a host-specific tolerance which preserved immunocompetence against H-2 unrelated Ags.

DISCUSSION

Since the early work of Boyse,[3] no further studies on the blood of newborn mice have been performed, and this analysis confirms and extends previous observations that NBB cells can perfectly engraft H-2-compatible murine recipients. This source of cells was chosen, because we believe that it likely represents the best equivalent

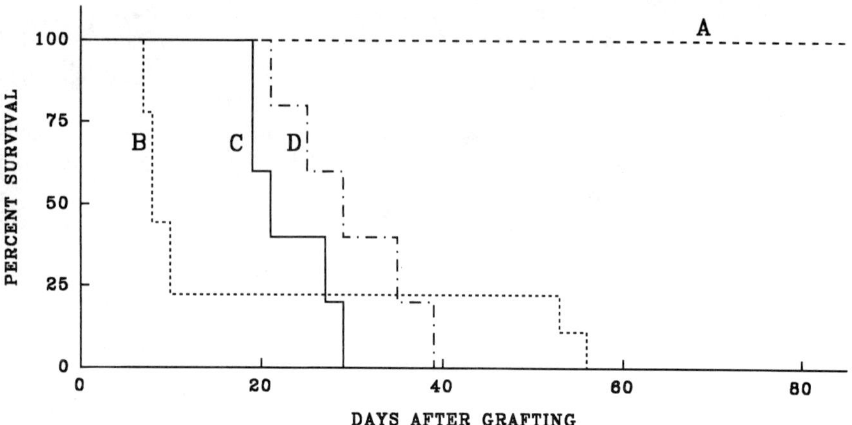

FIGURE 5. *In vivo* transfer experiments. Lethally irradiated (DBA/2 × B10.D2)F1 recipients (**A** and **D**) or (BALB/c × C57BL/6)F1 recipients (**B** and **C**) were engrafted with bone marrow and spleen cells from normal B10.D2 (**C** and **D**) or newborn blood engrafted F1 mice (**A** and **B**), and mortality was recorded daily.

of human CB cells. The results indicate that more than 70% of lethally irradiated F1 recipients survived after the injection of one NBB sample and that this percentage is improved by increasing the initial dose of cells infused. As FACS analysis determined that NBB contained approximately 15% of SCA-1$^+$ stem cells, as few as 6 to 7×10^4 progenitor cells apparently were sufficient to repopulate the host hematopoietic system. Survival data obtained in our *in vivo* murine model are consistent with human data suggesting that CB contains hematopoietic stem cells with long-term repopulating capacity.[4] A recent work reports that stable human long-term hematopoiesis was observed in CB transplanted SCID mice for at least 3 months, indicating engraftment of early hematopoietic progenitor cells.[5]

Donor engraftment evaluated by the proportion of lyt-1.1 T cells of recipient origin revealed that all NBB engrafted F1 mice became mixed chimera with approximately 69% of cells of donor origin 2–3 months after transplantation and that the rate of engraftment but not the degree of chimerism depended on the initial dose of NBB cells injected. To explain the mixed chimerism, we hypothesized that radioresistant stem cells from recipient bone marrow compete for restoration with stem cells from donor NBB which would be more primitive than those derived from bone marrow. This hypothesis is supported by *in vitro* data showing that CB stem cells have a higher proliferative potential[5–11] than do bone marrow stem cells and that they can be maintained in liquid cultures for many weeks.[12] Moreover, CB contains a higher percentage of primitive CD34$^+$ CD38$^-$ (4%) stem cells than does bone marrow (1%).[13]

Newborn blood engrafted F1 mice survived more than 100 days without clinical signs of GVHD, and the lack of GVHD induction is likely to be related to the immaturity of NBB T cells which in the majority express double-positive CD4$^+$ CD8$^+$ phenotype with low levels of T-cell receptor α/β. It is interesting that if these immature

T cells were unable to initiate GVHD, their presence may be sufficient to promote the engraftment of stem cells, and this characteristic represents an advantage of NBB over T-cell-depleted bone marrow. However, despite the fact that features of phenotypic immaturity were also described for T cells isolated from CB,[8,9] T cells from NBB appeared to be more immature. Finally, NBB T cells become tolerant to host mHAgs, but the mechanism is still unknown.

In conclusion, these preliminary experimental data emphasize the potential of NBB as a source of cells for transplantation by showing that a small number of progenitor stem cells is necessary to achieve full engraftment of recipients and thus support the assumption of several investigators[6,14,17] that a single CB collection might be sufficient to reconstitute adult patients. In addition, we believe that our experimental model should be helpful in answering questions on the degree of mismatching acceptable in regard to the risk of GVHD and the preservation of a graft-versus-leukemia effect. However, definitive conclusions on the putative advantage of NBB cells over bone marrow cells would require careful comparison of their respective capacity to reconstitute the immunohematological system of the recipients and to induce GVHD. Moreover, because of the phenotypic and functional differences between murine NBB cells and human CB cells, these experimental data should be extrapolated with caution to clinical CB transplantation.

SUMMARY

Cells derived from human cord blood instead of bone marrow were recently used for transplantation. However, several questions concerning the potential of this source of cells to reconstitute the hematopoietic and immunologic system of the recipient and to induce graft-versus-host disease (GVHD) remain unanswered. We used newborn blood (NBB) cells from B10.D2 mice to engraft lethally irradiated (DBA/2 × B10.D2)F1 recipients incompatible for multiple non-H-2 antigens. The median volume of NBB collected from one mouse ranged between 40 and 50 μl and the number of nucleated cells was approximately 4-5 × 10^5 per sample. We first established that NBB contains around 10-20% of stem cells (SCA-1$^+$) and 30% of CD4$^+$CD8$^+$ Thy-1$^+$ immature T cells. The injection of blood pooled from one to three newborn mice resulted in engraftment of 71%-86% of F1 recipients that survived more than 100 days. Long-term surviving mice exhibited mixed chimerism ($\approx$69% of cells of donor origin) 2-4 months after transplantation, and clinical signs of GVHD across minor histocompatibility Ags (mHAgs) were never observed. Additionally, mixed lymphocyte reaction and cytotoxic assay responses of those mice against host antigens were undetectable, while reactivity against unrelated H-2 Ag was normal. The establishment of host-specific tolerance in NBB engrafted mice was confirmed by *in vivo* transfer experiments.

In conclusion, NBB cells reconstituted the lymphohematopoietic system of lethally irradiated mice without inducing GVHD. However, the question of the presence of an active antileukemic effect remains to be answered.

ACKNOWLEDGMENTS

We wish to thank Pr. E. Gluckman for helpful discussion and J. Roué for typing the manuscript.

REFERENCES

1. THOMAS, E. D., R. STORB, R. A. CLIFT *et al.* 1975. Bone marrow transplantation. N. Engl. J. Med. **292:** 832–843.

2. MARTIN, P. J., J. A. HANSEN, C. D. BUCKNER, J. E. SANDERS, H. J. DEEG, P. STEWART, F. R. APPELBAUM, R. CLIFT, A. FEFER, R. P. WITHESRPOON, M. S. KENNEDY, K. M. SULLIVAN, N. FLOURNOY, R. STORB & E. D. THOMAS. 1985. Effects of in vitro depletion of T cells in HLA-identical allogeneic marrow grafts. Blood **66:** 664–672.

3. BROXMEYER, H. E., J. KURTZBERG, E. GLUCKMAN, A. D. AUERBACH, G. DOUGLAS, S. COOPER, J. H. F. FALKENBURG, J. BARD & E. A. BOYSE. 1991. Umbilical cord blood hematopoietic stem and repopulating cells in human clinical transplantation. Blood Cells **17:** 313–329.

4. BROXMEYER, H. E., G. HANGOC, S. COOPER, R. C. RIBEIRO, V. GRAVES, M. YODER, J. WAGNER, S. VADHAN-RAJ, L. BENNINGER, P. RUBISTEIN & E. R. BROUN. 1992. Growth characteristics and expansion of human umbilical cord blood and estimation of its potential for transplantation in adults. Proc. Natl. Acad. Sci. USA **89:** 4109–4113.

5. VORMOOR, J., T. LAPIDOT, F. PFLUMIO, G. RISDON, B. PATTERSON, H. E. BROXMEYER & J. E. DICK. 1994. Immature human cord blood progenitors engraft and proliferate to high levels in severe combined immunodeficient mice. Blood **83:** 2489–2497.

6. GERLI, R., A. BERTOTTO, S. CRUPI, C. ARCANGELI, I. MARINELLI, F. SPINOZZI, C. SPINOZZI, C. CERNETTI, P. ANGELELLA & P. RAMBOTTI. 1989. Activation of cord T lymphocytes. I. Evidence for a defective T cell mitogenesis induced through the CD2 molecule. J. Immunol. **142:** 2583–2589.

7. HARRIS, D. T., M. J. SCHUMACHER, J. LOCASCIO, F. J. BESENCON, G. B. OLSON, D. DELUCA, L. SHENKER, J. BARD & E. A. BOYSE. 1992. Phenotypic and functional immaturity of human umbilical cord blood T lymphocytes. Proc. Natl. Acad. Sci. USA **89:** 10006–10010.

8. GLUCKMAN, E., H. E. BROXMEYER, A. D. AUERBACH, H. FRIEDMAN, G. W. DOUGLAS, A. DEVERGIE, H. ESPEROU, D. THIERRY, G. SOCIE, P. LEHN, S. COOPER, D. ENGLISH, J. KURTZBERG, J. BARD & E. A. BOYSE. 1989. Hematopoietic reconstitution in patients with Fanconi anemia by means of umbilical cord blood from an HLA identical sibling. N. Engl. J. Med. **321:** 1174–1178.

9. APPERLEY, J. F. 1994. Umbilical cord blood progenitor cell transplantation. Bone Marrow Transplant. **14:** 187–196.

10. HALLE-PANNENKO, O., L. L. PRITCHARD, R. MOTTA & G. MATHE. 1978. Non-H-2 antigens can induce high GVH mortality in adult recipients of normal cells. Biomedicine **29:** 253–255.

11. LU, L., M. XIAO, R. N. SHEN, S. GRIGSBY & H. E. BROXMEYER. 1993. Enrichment, characterization and responsiveness of single primitive CD34$^+$ umbilical cord blood hematopoietic progenitors with high proliferative and replating potential. Blood **81:** 41–48.

12. SALAHUDDIN, S. Z., P. D. MARKHAM, F. W. RUSCETTI & R. C. GALLO. 1981. Long-term suspension culture of human cord blood myeloid cells. Blood **58:** 931–938.

13. CARDOSO, A. A., M. L. LI, P. BATARD, A. HATZFELD, E. L. BROWN, J. P. LEVESQUE, H. SOOKDEO, B. PANTERNE, S. C. CLARK & J. HATZFELD. 1993. Release from quiescence of CD34$^+$ CD38$^-$ human umbilical cord blood cells reveals their potentiality to engraft adults. Proc. Natl. Acad. Sci. USA **90:** 8707–8711.

Immunogenicity and Stem Cell Content of Class II Depleted Human Vertebral Body Bone Marrow

NORMA S. KENYON, XIU-MIN XU,
ALLIE GARCIA-SERRA, AND CAMILLO RICORDI

Diabetes Research Institute
University of Miami School of Medicine
1450 N.W. 10th Ave.
Miami, Florida 33136

The application of islet cell transplantation as a cure for Type I diabetes is limited by the requirement for immunosuppressive agents to prevent rejection, because these drugs are considered more harmful to the individual than is the administration of exogenous insulin. The only patients eligible for islet cell transplantation are therefore those who are already receiving immunosuppressive treatment for a previous or concurrent solid organ transplant, that is, patients who have advanced diabetes and its complications.

Recent observations of microchimerism in long-term, solid organ transplant recipients who have discontinued immunosuppression have led to the concept that chimerism is critical to the establishment of donor-specific tolerance, and precursor dendritic cells have been postulated to play a key role in this process.[1,2] Our goal is to transplant a minimally immunogenic, progenitor-rich bone marrow preparation at the time of or subsequent to solid organ and/or islet cell transplantation, to enhance the potential for the development of chimerism.

This study assesses the effect, on immunogenicity and stem cell content, of depleting directly immunogenic, Class II bright cells from vertebral body marrow (VBM). Therefore, before and after bead-based depletion of Class II bright cells, we analyzed the stem cell content (% CD34$^+$, colony-forming capacity), % Class II positive cells, and mixed lymphocyte culture stimulating capacity of whole VBM versus VBM cells obtained after density gradient centrifugation over ficoll-paque (to enrich for the mononuclear cells) and 14.5 g% metrizamide (to enrich for putative dendritic cells, DC). Beads coated with two monoclonal antibodies specific for human Class II antigens (I2 and I3, Coulter Corporation, Miami, Florida) were used to deplete Class II bright cells from VBM populations. Direct immunoflourescent staining with CD34-FITC and DR-PE (Becton Dickinson, Mountain View, California), plus the appropriate isotype controls, was followed by flow cytometric analysis on a Coulter EPICS XL flow cytometer. Mixed lymphocyte cultures were established with peripheral blood lymphocytes obtained from healthy volunteers, serving as responder cells; irradiated VBM populations served as stimulators. Cultures were pulsed with 1 μCi tritiated thymidine on day 5 and harvested and counted on day 6. Colony-forming capacity was determined by plating the various populations in methylcellulose media

TABLE 1. Colony-Forming Capacity after Elimination of Class II Bright Cells

	Whole Bone Marrow		Ficoll Interface		Matrizamide Interface	
	Pre	Post	Pre	Post	Pre	Post
CFU-E/BFU-E	114	142	140	236	116	176
CFU-GM	72	100	166	52	128	104
CFU-GEMM	6	6	4	4	4	4
CFU-DC	20	36	20	44	48	36

(StemCell Technologies, Inc., Vancouver, British Columbia) containing recombinant growth factors. Colonies were enumerated on day 14.

Flow cytometric analysis revealed that cells obtained after density gradient separation of VBM contained a higher percentage of CD45/CD34 dual positive cells (% ± SD, whole VBM = 1.9 ± 0.4 ficoll interface [FI] = 3.6 ± 0.6, metrizamide interface [MI] = 4.1 ± 1.4, $n = 6$). The increased percentage of CD34$^+$ cells obtained after fractionation was reflected by greater colony-forming capacity of ficoll and metrizamide interface cells compared to whole VBM. In addition, the percentage of DR-positive cells was significantly greater for FI and MI cells (% ± SD, whole VBM = 12.6 ± 1.8, *FI = 20.8 ± 2.7, *MI = 27.4 ± 3.6, *p <0.05 compared to whole VBM, $n = 7$), with corresponding significant increases in mixed lymphocyte culture stimulatory capacity for FI and MI cell populations.

Treatment of various fractions with anti-Class II coated beads consistently resulted in removal of the Class II bright cells including a small population of CD34/DR bright VBM. A corresponding decrease in the more mature CFU-GM colonies was sometimes observed, whereas other colonies, including dendritic cells, were still abundant, and erythroid colonies were actually increased (See TABLE 1 for representative example.) As might be expected, because of the decrease in the total percentage of HLA-DR positive cells, the mixed lymphocyte culture stimulatory capacity of gradient-enriched cells was significantly decreased after elimination of the Class II bright cells (numbers in parentheses = after Class II depletion, *p <0.05 compared to untreated fraction, expressed as counts per minute ± SD): whole VBM 5,510 ± 3,045 (4,022 ± 3,105, $n = 10$), *FI 11,072 ± 5,919 (3,820 ± 3,671, $n = 6$), and *MI 15,837 ± 6,109 (4,560 ± 647, $n = 4$).

If therefore appears that elimination of the bright Class II positive cells from donor bone marrow effectively decreases the directly immunogenic potential of VBM while maintaining the progenitors required for the establishment and maintenance of chimerism.

REFERENCES

1. STARZL, T. E., A. J. DEMETRIS, M. TRUCCO *et al.* 1993. Chimerism and donor specific nonreactivity 27 to 29 years after kidney allotransplantation. Transplantation **55:** 1272-1277.
2. STARZL, T. E., A. J. DEMETRIS, N. MURASE *et al.* 1993. Donor cell chimerism permitted by immunosuppressive drugs: A probable basis of organ transplant acceptance and tolerance. Immunol. Today **14:** 326-332.

Automation of Human Vertebral Body Bone Marrow Isolation

RITA BOTTINO, ELINA LINETSKY,
GENNARO SELVAGGI, SHEN-SHEN KONG,
TIE QIAN, AND CAMILLO RICORDI

Cell Transplant Center
Diabetes Research Institute
University of Miami School of Medicine
Miami, Florida 33136

To discontinue immunosuppression remains an elusive goal in the field of transplantation. On the basis of results from experimental studies in mice and analysis of long-term transplant recipients who discontinued their immunosuppressive medications, it was proposed that the establishment of chimerism may lead to the induction of donor-specific tolerance to subsequent solid organ or tissue grafts.[1-3] Although the concept remains to be proven in humans, interest in the use of donor bone marrow infusion to induce a state of chimerism, and hopefully tolerance, is increasing. Vertebral bodies from cadaver donors provide a rich source of bone marrow, with high cell yield and no contamination from peripheral blood. To facilitate the isolation of vertebral body marrow (VBM), we developed an automated method for preparation of VBM and compared the cells obtained to those isolated by a manual method.[4]

Vertebral bodies were retrieved from multiorgan cadaver donors. Fat, muscles, ligaments, and intervertebral disks were removed, and the vertebral bodies were divided into several segments. At this point, the chips were processed either manually, with rongeurs, or automatically, in a machine designed to crush the segments. The resulting fragments were placed into processing medium (RPMI 1640 with 10% human serum albumin, 1% gentamicin, 10,000 units of heparin, and 0.2% HEPES) and shaken gently by hand (circular motion) to release cells from the trabecular framework of the bone. The suspension was filtered through two consecutive stainless steel screens (450 μm followed by 180 μm) and briefly centrifuged to eliminate bone fragments; this was done by bringing the centrifuge up to a speed of $300 \times g$ and then stopping. Cell viability was subsequently assessed by trypan blue exclusion and was determined to be greater than 95% in all cases.

FIGURE 1 demonstrates the results obtained with isolation of VBM from four different donors; in each experiment, donor vertebral bodies were divided equally, with half processed automatically and the other half processed manually. Similar cell yields were obtained in all cases.

Because cell yield and viability were comparable when vertebral bodies from the same donor were concurrently processed by the manual or the automated method, we used the machine to isolate all of the VBM from eight consecutive donors and compared the results obtained with those from eight previous isolations performed with the manual method. Results are given in TABLE 1. No significant difference in

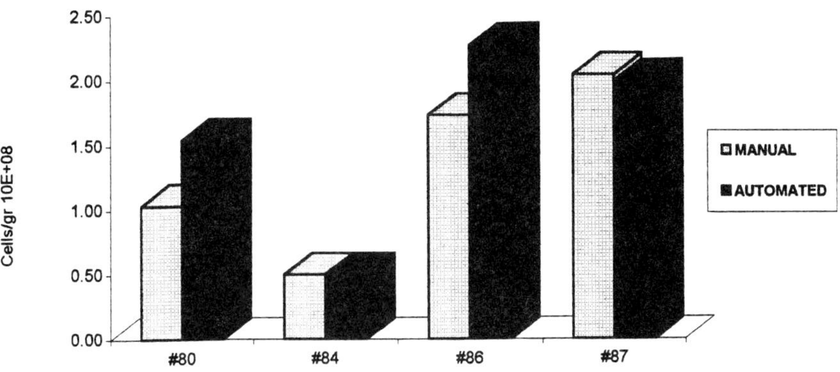

FIGURE 1. Bone marrow cells/gr of vertebrae: manual versus automated.

TABLE 1. Results of Isolation of Vertebral Body Marrow

	Manual ($n = 8$)	Automated ($0 = 8$)	Significance
Vertebral bodies (n)	10.8 ± 2.6	12 ± 1.0	NS
Weight of vertebral bodies	305.5 ± 126.1	344.9 ± 110.7	NS
Total no. of bone marrow cells			
(10^{10})	5.3 ± 3.3	5.2 ± 1.3	NS
Cells/gr (10^8)	1.6 ± 0.5	1.6 ± 0.4	NS
Processing time (h)	5.7 ± 0.8	3.2 ± 0.7	0.004

starting material or cell yield was observed. Processing time, however, was significantly decreased. The excellent cell yield and viability, decreased processing time, and decreased risk of contamination have led us to continue our clinical trials with VBM processed with the automated method.

REFERENCES

1. STARZL, T. E., A. J. DEMETRIS, N. MURASE, A. W. THOMSON, M. TRUCCO & C. RICORDI. 1993. Immunol. Today 14(6): 326–332.
2. STARZL, T. E., A. J. DEMETRIS, M. TRUCCO, A. ZEEVI, H. RAMOS, P. TERASAKI, W. A. RUDERT, M. KOCOVA, C. RICORDI, S. ILDSTAD & N. MURASE. 1993. Transplantation 55: 1272–1277.
3. FONTES, P., A. RAO, A. J. DEMETRIS, A. ZEEVI, M. TRUCCO, P. CARROLL, W. RYBKA, C. RICORDI, F. DODSON, R. SHAPIRO, A. TZAKIS, S. TODO, K. ABU-ELMAGD, M. JORDAN, J. J. FUNG & T. E. STARZL. 1994. Lancet 344: 151–155.
4. STRONG, M. 1992. Seattle Protocol: Vertebral body recovery for bone marrow (PRO-550G).

Perforin-Deficient T Cells Can Induce Acute Graft-versus-Host Disease after Transplantation of MHC-Matched or MHC Disparate Allogeneic Bone Marrow

R. B. LEVY, M. BAKER, AND E. R. PODACK

Department of Microbiology and Immunology
University of Miami School of Medicine
Miami, Florida 33101

The precise role of cytotoxicity in the development and expression of graft-versus-host disease (GVHD) remains difficult to define.[1] We approached this question by using T cells from genetically engineered or mutant mice that are deficient in the ability to mediate cytotoxic function. To definitively determine the role of perforin-mediated cytotoxicity in the development of GVHD, allogeneic bone marrow transplantation was performed in which lethally irradiated BALB/c ($H-2^d$) mice received donor inocula from perforin-deficient (perforin 0/0) or normal (perforin +/+) C57BL/6 ($H-2^b$) mice containing varying numbers of T cells.[2] Recipient mice were monitored for clinical signs of GVHD including weight loss, alopecia, hunched posture, and death. Recipients of 2.5×10^6 T cells from normal donors developed clinical signs of severe GVHD with 100% mortality and median survival time of 35.4 days. Interestingly, all recipients of 2.5×10^6 T cells from perforin 0/0 donors also developed clinical signs of severe acute GVHD which was ultimately lethal. However, the onset of these signs was delayed and the median survival time was significantly increased to 75.8 in the recipients of perforin 0/0 T cells. Histopathologic analysis of skin and liver tissues from recipients of normal or perforin 0/0 T cells exhibited severe acute dermatitis and cholangitis. These studies conclusively demonstrate that perforin-deficient donor T cells are indeed capable of inducing severe acute lethal GVHD across major histocompatibility disparities.

To examine the significance of perforin-mediated cytotoxicity in a model for HLA-matched allogeneic bone marrow transplantation (BMT), we transplanted 1×10^7 B6-perforin 0/0 or normal B6 T cells into MHC-matched lethally irradiated LP ($H-2^b$) recipients. Following BMT with perforin 0/0 T cells, the onset of clinical signs of severe acute GVHD including weight loss, hunched posture, alopecia, and diarrhea was delayed as in MHC-disparate BMT; however, mortality was reduced. Thus, perforin-deficient T cells can also induce severe, acute GVHD across non-MHC genetic differences.

366

TABLE 1. Incidence of Clinical Signs of Graft-versus-Host Disease and Median Survival Time (MST) in BALB/c Recipients after Allogeneic BMT with Wild-Type or Perforin-Deficient T Cells

Donor	T Cells ($\times 10^6$)	Alopecia	Diarrhea	Hunched Posture	MST
BALB/c	2.5	No	No	No	>130
C57BL/6	2.5	Yes	Yes	Yes	35.4 days
B6-Perforin 0/0	2.5	Yes	Yes	Yes	75.8 days

Together, perforin- and Fas-mediated killing appears to constitute most cell-mediated cytotoxicity.[3] Therefore, we also began to examine the capacity of Fas-ligand defective T cells from B6.C3H-*gld* mice to induce GVHD across minor transplantation barriers. LP/J strain recipients of B6.C3H-*gld* T cells exhibited a pattern of weight loss, hunched posture, and mortality similar to those of recipients of normal B6 T cells. Notably, no skin or coat involvement or any evidence of histopathologic damage in the liver was observed in these recipients. Therefore, if Fas- and perforin-dependent cytotoxicity is not required for GVHD, inflammatory cytokines, such as gamma interferon and tumor necrosis factor, will be strongly implicated as the critical effector molecules in this disease.[4]

REFERENCES

1. FERRARA, J. L. M. & H. J. DEEG. 1991. N. Engl. J. Med. **324:** 667–674.
2. KÄGI, D., B. LEDERMANN, K. BÜRKI *et al.* 1994. Nature **369:** 31–37.
3. KÄGI, D., F. VIGNAUX, B. LEDERMANN *et al.* 1994. Science **265:** 528–530.
4. JADUS, M. R. & H. T. WEPSIC. 1992. Bone Marrow Transplant. **10:** 1–14.

Fas and Perforin Cytotoxic Pathways Are Not the Major Effector Mechanisms in Allogeneic Resistance to Bone Marrow

M. BAKER, E. R. PODACK, AND R. B. LEVY

Department of Microbiology and Immunology
University of Miami School of Medicine
Miami, Florida 33101

Failure to engraft is a major complication in allogeneic bone marrow transplantation when T cell-depleted donor marrow is transplanted. Previous work implicated radioresistant host natural killer cells and CD3[+] T cells as primary effectors mediating resistance to allogeneic bone marrow.[1] To precisely characterize the role of perforin and Fas-mediated cytotoxic function in the rejection of bone marrow allografts, we used Fas ligand-defective (B6.C3H-*gld*), perforin-deficient (B6-perforin 0/0), and normal B6 (H-2[b]) mice as recipients of marrow allografts from DBA/2 (H-2[d]) mice.

Recipient mice received 900cGy total body irradiation and were infused 12-24 hours later with 2×10^6 T cell-depleted bone marrow cells from allogeneic or syngeneic donors. On day 5 posttransplant, spleen cell cultures were established at 1×10^5 cells/ml/well in the presence of 50 U/ml rm GM-CSF. Large colonies (>25 cells) were scored after 4 days in culture. This short-term assay provides an accurate prediction of long-term engraftment or rejection of marrow allografts.[2]

Cultures of spleen cells from syngeneic recipients produced many colonies (~100/well), whereas cultures from normal and Fas ligand-defective B6 recipients of allogeneic marrow failed to produce any colonies, indicating strong allogeneic resistance. Notably, a small number of colonies (0-12/well) grew in cultures from perforin-deficient recipients.

The C3H/HeJ → B6 donor-recipient combination exhibits relatively weak allogeneic resistance following primary bone marrow transplantation.[3] We reasoned that this strain combination should provide a more sensitive measure of the role of perforin-mediated cytotoxic function in allogeneic resistance. Although cultures from syngeneic recipients produced large numbers of colonies (69 ± 22), normal and perforin-deficient B6 recipients exhibited equivalent degrees of resistance to C3H/HeJ allogeneic marrow (TABLE 1) as indicated by essentially identical numbers of colonies (18 ± 3 and 16 ± 5, respectively).

The present findings demonstrate that allogeneic resistance remains largely intact in mice that lack perforin- or Fas-mediated cytotoxic function. Therefore, Fas and perforin pathways of cell-mediated cytotoxicity do not appear to be the principal effector mechanisms in marrow allograft rejection. Previous work has suggested that cytokines produced by host radioresistant natural killer, lymphokine-activated killer, and T cells such as gamma-interferon and tumor necrosis factor can strongly inhibit

TABLE 1. Resistance to Allogeneic Marrow by Normal and Perforin-Deficient Recipients

Donor	Recipient	*n*	CFU-GM
C3H/HeJ	C3H/HeJ	3	69 ± 22
C3H/HeJ	B6	3	18 ± 3
C3H/HeJ	B6-perforin 0/0	3	16 ± 5

the growth of hematopoietic stem cells.[4] Serum levels of these cytokines are elevated in the early period after clinical allogeneic bone marrow transplantation.[5,6] On the basis of our present findings and previous work, we hypothesize that gamma-interferon and tumor necrosis factor are critical effector molecules in allogeneic resistance.

REFERENCES

1. MURPHY, W. J., V. KUMAR & M. BENNETT. 1987. J. Exp. Med. **166:** 1499–1509.
2. MURPHY, W. J., M. BENNETT, V. KUMAR *et al.* 1992. J. Immunol. **148:** 2953–2960.
3. DENNERT, G., C. G. ANDERSON & J. WARNER. 1985. J. Immunol. **135:** 3729–3734.
4. CLERIGUE, M., P. PISA, L. TSAI *et al.* 1990. Clin. Exp. Immunol. **81:** 459–465.
5. NIEDERWIESER, C., M. HEROLD *et al.* 1990. Transplantation **50:** 620–625.
6. HOLLER, E., H. J. KOLB, A. MÖLLER *et al.* 1990. Blood **75:** 1011–1016.

Use of Control Cells to Standardize Enumeration of CD34⁺ Stem Cells

PATRICIA ROTH, JOHN MAPLES, JANET HALL, AND
TESS DAILEY

Immunology Research and Technology
Coulter Corporation
Miami, Florida 33116-9015

The CD34 antibodies define heavily glycosylated membrane antigens expressed selectively on immature hematopoietic and endothelial cells. Although function of the CD34 molecules has remained elusive, such antibodies have become important reagents in leukemia phenotyping and hematopoietic stem cell identification and selection, the latter being extremely important for bone marrow transplantation.[1-3]

The KG1a cell line, often used as a model for the binding of CD34 monoclonal antibodies, expresses the CD34 antigen at a density many times greater than that in immature hematopoietic cells. The high expression of CD34 antigen on KG1a cells has made them unsuitable as control cells in the analysis of normal immature hematopoietic cells. Frozen clinical specimens have been used in clinical studies, but these provide only limited standardization. There are currently no satisfactory cell controls for testing with anti-CD34 antibody.

When 18 anti-CD34 mAbs submitted to the Fifth Workshop were tested against KG1a cells treated with various enzymes, distinct clustering of reactivity was demonstrated. The CD34 epitopes could be clustered into at least three groups, depending on the reactivity of the mAb after treatment of the KG1a cells with neuraminidase, *Pasteurella haemolytica* glycoprotease, or chymopapain. Antibodies that detect epitopes removed by neuraminidase treatment are called Class I antibodies. Monoclonal antibodies that detect epitopes destroyed by the *P. haemolytica* glycoprotease or chymopapain and not by neuraminidase are designated as Class II. Antibodies that recognize epitopes not sensitive to either treatment are designated as Class III. Class III epitopes are likely to be protein rather than carbohydrate in nature.[1-3]

KG1a cells can be treated with a combination of various enzymes to decrease the expression of Class I and Class II epitopes. Protein-modifying agents are used to decrease the expression of Class III epitopes. The resulting KG1a cells would then express the CD34 epitopes at a density similar to that of clinically detected cells and thus could be used as suitable controls for CD34 antigen detection.

MATERIALS AND METHODS

KG1a cells were grown to approximately 1×10^6/ml, harvested, and centrifuged to a pellet. Paraformaldehyde (4.5% in phosphate-buffered saline solution) was added to the cells and incubated overnight, washed, and tested for Class I, II, and III antibody binding. These same cells were then washed and treated with a 1.0, 0.5, or

0.1 mg/ml solution of chymopapain (Sigma Cat. C9007) for 1 hour and, after washing, were tested for Class I, II, and III antibody binding. Finally, cells were lyophilized in 10% isotonic trehalose and reconstituted. These cells were mixed with lyophilized and reconstituted mouse myeloma cells (CD34 negative) at a final concentration of 5% (KG1a:mouse myeloma). The mixture was tested for Class I, II and III antibody binding. CD34 epitope expression was targeted based on expression in normal bone marrow, from which cells were stained with Class I, II, or III CD34 antibody (phycoerythrin [PE]-labeled) and was analyzed on an HLA-DR⁺-gated population. In addition, an aliquot of KG1a cells directly from culture was lyophilized in 10% isotonic trehalose.

The PE-labeled antibodies were utilized according to manufacturer's instructions: Class I = clone Immu-133 (ImmunoTech, Westbrook, Maine); Class II = clone QBEnd10 (ImmunoTech, Westbrook, Maine); and Class III = clone HPCA2 (Becton Dickinson, San Jose, California).

RESULTS

Lyophilization of KG1a cells with decreased CD34 antigen density produces a stabilized CD34 antigenic cell control suitable for use with anti-CD34 testing. These antigen control cells may be used to standardize methods used in the detection and enumeration of hematopoietic stem cells. HLA-DR-gated bone marrow cells stained with Class I, II, or III antibodies demonstrates the low percentage and low mean channel of CD34⁺ cells. Staining of KG1a cells with the same panel of antibodies demonstrates that for all antibodies used, the intensity of staining is much greater in these cells than in bone marrow cells (TABLE 1).

TABLE 1. Expression of CD34 Epitopes on Bone Marrow and KG1a Cells

	Class I		Class II		Class III	
	%+	MC	%+	MC	%+	MC
Bone marrow	3.0	0.851	2.8	0.759	4.6	0.904
Untreated KG1a[a]	99.4	93.4	99.6	27.4	100.0	103.3
Modified KG1a[b]	2.9	3.12	1.9	3.03	3.7	13.7

Abbreviation: MC = mean channel.
[a] Cells lyophilized directly from culture.
[b] 5% modified cells + 95% CD34 negative cells.

Treatment of KG1a cells with paraformaldehyde (4.5%) dramastically reduces staining with a Class III antibody. However, staining with antibodies to Class I and II epitopes showed little or no change (TABLE 2). Studies have shown that a reduction of these epitopes requires treatment with enzymes that effect carbohydrate moieties.[1-3] Treatment of KG1a cells with various concentrations of chymopapain is required to produce a reduction of Class I and II epitopes. This decrease is directly proportional to the concentration of enzyme used (TABLE 2). An unexpected effect of enzyme treatment is an increase in the (paraformaldehyde-reduced) expression of Class III epitopes. This increase is also directly proportional to the enzyme concentration and is likely due to exposure of the protein-dependent epitopes on cleavage of carbohydrate residues.

TABLE 2. Effect of Chemical and Enzymatic Modification of KG1a Cells

	Mean Channel		
	Class I	Class II	Class III
Untreated	93.4	27.4	102.3
Paraformaldehyde (only)	71.2	26.6	1.8
Chymopapain			
1 mg/ml	4.1	1.5	9.76
0.5 mg/ml	7.94	3.14	8.60
0.1 mg/ml	38.4	10.1	7.76

Lyophilization of paraformaldehyde/chymopapain-treated KG1a cells provides a stable reagent which exhibits consistent staining with CD34 antibodies. While the staining intensity of these antibodies can be controlled by appropriate chemical and enzyme treatments, the desired level of positive cells in the population (% positive) is achieved by mixing the modified KG1a cells with cells that are negative for CD34 antigen. Values for modified, diluted KG1a cells, for which a 5% mixture of treated KG1a cells and mouse myeloma cells was stained with Class I, II, or III antibodies, are shown in TABLE 1. The level of CD34 positivity in both percent positive and mean channel was thus reduced, demonstrating that it is possible to make a stable CD34 cell control with the desired staining intensity as well as percent positivity.

CONCLUSIONS

The goal of this study was to demonstrate that a stable control cell with a consistent CD34 staining pattern can be manufactured by modification of antigens on existing cell lines. The desired pattern was chosen to produce densities for Class I, II, and III antigens that resemble that seen in normal bone marrow. This was achieved by modifying the cell surface of high CD34-expressing KG1a cells at both the protein and the carbohydrate level to control expression of the different classes of CD34 epitopes. Lyophilization of modified cells provides a reagent with the long-term stability needed for successful inter- and intralaboratory control and the establishment of standardization in the detection and enumeration of CD34+ cells.

REFERENCES

1. SUTHERLAND, D. R., K. M. ABDULLAY, P. I. CYOPICK & A. MELLORS. 1992. Cleavage of the cell-surface O-sialoglycoproteins CD34, CD43, CD44 and CD45 by a novel glycoprotease from *Pasteurella haemolytica*. J. Immunol. **148:** 1458.
2. SUTHERLAND, D. R., J. C. W. MARSH, J. DAVIDSON, M. A. BAKER, A. KEATING & A. MELLORS. 1992. Differential sensitivity of CD34 epitopes to cleavage by *Pasteurella haemolytica* glycoprotease: Implications for purification of CD34-positive progenitor cells. Exp. Haematol **20:** 590.
3. WOUTER, M., G. MARJOLEIN DAAMS, M. DE HAAS, A. VON DEM BORNE & E. VAN DER SCHOOT. 1995. M10.2 Characterization of the CD34 Cluster. *In* Leukocyte Typing V. S. F. Schlossman, L. Boumsell, W. Gilks, J. M. Harlan, T. Kishimoto, C. Morimoto, J. Ritz, S. Shaw, R. L. Silverstein, T. A. Springer, T. F. Tedder & R. F. Todd, Eds. Oxford University Press. Cambridge.

LF 08-0299 Protects Murine Recipients of Minor Antigen Disparate Donor Marrow from Lethal Graft-versus-Host Disease

M. BRULEY-ROSSET,[a] E. CHURAQUI,[a] J. ANNAT,[b]
AND P. DUTARTRE

Laboratoires Fournier S.C.A.
Daix, France

[a]*Inserm U267*
Groupe Hospitalier Paul Brousse
Villejuif, France

Graft-versus-host disease (GVHD) results from T-cell activation in response to allogeneic MHC or non-MHC antigens in an immunocompromised host. Despite advances in preventing GVHD in humans by combining immunosuppressive prophylactic agents, GVHD still remains a major complication after bone marrow transplantation (BMT), and therefore new therapeutics are required.[1]

LF 08-0299 is a new stable immunosuppressive analog of 15-deoxyspergualin (DSG) obtained by organic chemical synthesis. It was selected for further evaluation after an *in vivo* screening program in mice and rats demonstrated its potent effects. It controlled alloreactivity in a fully MHC mismatched rat cardiac transplant model and also induced donor-specific long-lasting unresponsiveness.[2]

The present study investigates the ability of LF 08-0299 to prevent murine GVHD induced across non-H-2 Ag and to bring about a state of specific tolerance to host antigens. B10.D2 bone marrow and spleen cells were injected into lethally irradiated (DBA/2 × B10.D2)F1 recipients. In this combination, donors and recipients differ for multiple minor histocompatibility antigens and for Mls-1[a] and Mls-2[a] superantigens.[3] Grafted mice were treated with LF 08-0299, and clinical signs of GVHD and survival of the mice were analyzed according to dosage and schedule of LF 08-0299 administration. Long-term surviving mice were examined for their degree of chimerism and for their immune mixed lymphocyte reaction and cytotoxic T-cell response towards host antigens and unrelated H-2 Ag. Additionally, the establishment of specific tolerance to host antigens was assessed by *in vivo* transfer experiments.

RESULTS AND DISCUSSION

This study demonstrates that posttransplant LF 08-0299 therapy effectively protected mice from lethal GVHD in a dose-related manner. The dose schedule finding

[b] Address for correspondence: Jocelyne Annat, Laboratoires Fournier, Département Immunologie, 50 rue de Dijon, 21121 Daix, France.

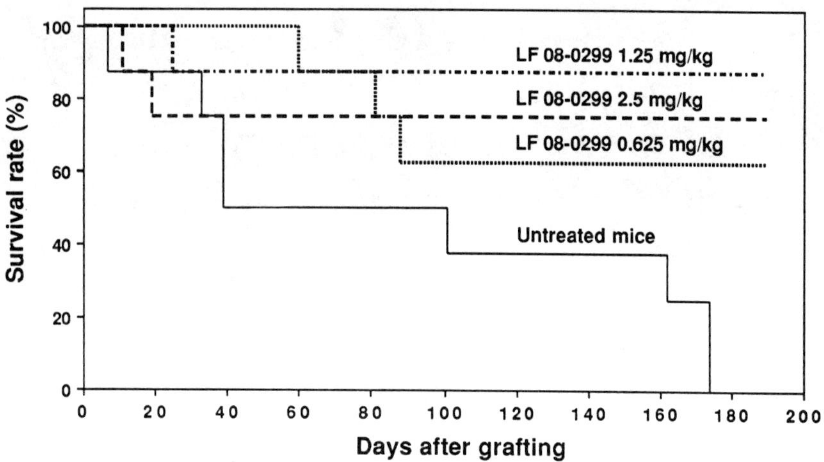

FIGURE 1. LF 08-0299 protects mice from lethal graft-versus-host disease.

study showed that an efficacious dosage ranged between 1.25 and 2.5 mg/kg, when the compound was administrated intraperitoneally for 20 days post-BMT, and it led to an 80-90% survival of mice for 5 months without clinical evidence of GVHD (FIG. 1). Moreover, 10 days of treatment seemed as effective as 3 weeks of therapy, indicating that even a very short treatment period protected against GVHD.

Peripheral lymphoid cell reconstitution was examined in long-term surviving LF 08-0299-treated mice. Flow cytometry analysis demonstrated that all mice were complete chimeras. Furthermore, no significant reduction in either CD4+ or CD8+ lymph node cell populations occurred. We further investigated both mixed lymphocyte reaction and cytotoxic T-cell reactivity and found that anti-host antigen responsiveness was reduced, whereas response against unrelated H-2 antigen was normal or slightly diminished (not significantly), depending on mice. In addition, *in vivo* transfer experiments showed that spleen cells from long-term survivors treated with LF 08-0299 retained the ability to induce lethal GVHD in an irradiated (BALB/c × C57B1/6)F1 recipient, incompatible for H-2b, demonstrating that host immune competence was preserved. In contrast, the same cells injected into an irradiated (DBA/2 × B10.D2)F1 recipient, incompatible for DBA/2 minor H antigens, were unable to induce lethal GVHD over the 3-month period of observation (FIG. 2), suggesting that long-term surviving LF 08-0299-treated F1 mice were specifically tolerant to host antigens. Hence, LF 08-0299 might exert a GVHD protective effect by preventing the activation and/or expansion of CD4+ and CD8+ T cells. Alternatively, it could induce counterregulatory cells or deletion of donor-specific T-cell clones.

Cyclosporine A, FK 506,[4] DSG,[5] and rapamycine have all been reported to ameliorate the GVHD-free interval and survival in murine models of lethal GVHD. However, following these treatments, mice often developed a chronic form of GVHD or an autoimmune-like syndrome.[6] Long-term surviving LF 08-0299-treated mice, on the other hand, did not display such syndromes over the study period. Nevertheless,

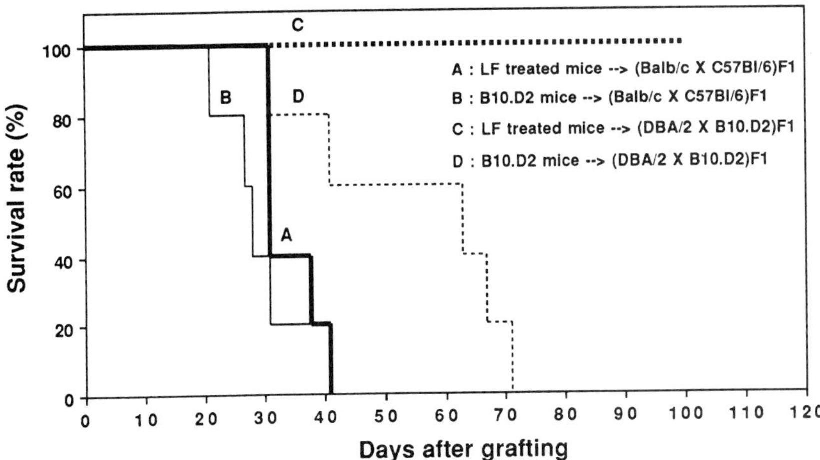

FIGURE 2. LF 08-0299 induces host-specific tolerance and preserves host immune competence.

the mechanism by which LF 08-0299 induces tolerance remains unknown and needs to be investigated further.

In conclusion, we demonstrated that transient LF 08-0299 therapy is efficient for GVHD prophylaxis in mice and that long-term donor-specific immune tolerance is induced. Hence, this compound deserves further investigation for preclinical development, as it may be effective in reducing the incidence of GVHD in human BMT.

REFERENCES

1. VOGELSANG, G. B. & A. D. HESS. 1994. Blood **84:** 2061–2067.
2. DUTARTRE, P., J. ANNAT & P. DERREPAS. 1995. Transplant. Proc. **27:**440–442.
3. MICONNET, I., R. HUCHET, D. BONARDELLE, R. MOTTA, C. CANON, E. GARAY-ROJAS, M. KRESS, M. REYNES, O. HALLA-PANNENKO & M. BRULEY-ROSSET. 1990. J. Immunol. **145:** 2123–2131.
4. BLAZER, B. R., P. A. TAYLOR, W. E. FITZSIMMONS & D. A. VALLERA. 1994. J. Immunol. **153:** 1836–1846.
5. NEMOTO, K., M. HAYASHI, J. ITO, Y. SUGAWARA, T. MAE, H. FUJII, F. ABE, A. FUJII & T. TAKEUCHI. 1991. Transplantation **51:** 712–715.
6. BLAZER, B. R., P. A. TAYLOR, D. C. SNOVER, S. N. SEHGAL & D. A. VALLERA. 1993. J. Immunol. **151:** 5726–5741.

Recipient T-Cell Immune Reconstitution in X-linked SCID after Haploidentical Maternal Bone Marrow Transplant

M. T. DE LA MORENA, A. S. WAYNE, N. K. DAY,
M. M. HAAG, K. R. HINDS-FREY, R. P. NELSON,
M. J. SUTCLIFFE, AND R. A. GOOD

All Children's Hospital
University of South Florida College of Medicine
St. Petersburg, Florida 33701

Bone marrow transplantation (BMT) continues to be the only cure for most forms of human severe combined immunodeficiency (SCID).[1-3] The case report of a patient with SCID is described.

A male infant with a half-brother who had died of SCID at 10 months was diagnosed with X-linked SCID at 8 weeks of age. The patient had severely depressed T cells with the presence of B cells, absence of lymphocyte proliferative responses to mitogens, and hypogammaglobulinemia (IgA and IgM were undetectable; IgG was 400 mg/dl which probably reflects maternal antibodies). At 2 months of age the patient received a maternal haploidentical T-cell–depleted bone marrow transplant (cell dose 1.24×10^8/kg after soybean agglutination and sheep RBC rosetting). The immediate post-BMT course was complicated by transient alloimmune neutropenia. Post-BMT immune parameters demonstrated recipient T cells 6 months after BMT, which continue to be present 22 months later. Lymphocyte proliferative responses to mitogens (phytohemagglutinin, concanavalin A, and pokeweed) and antigens (Candida, Tetanus, and Staphylococcus) were also present. Delayed type hypersensitivity to Candida, Tetanus, and Trichophyton is absent. Humoral immunity continues to be depressed.

Transient donor chimerism as documented by karyotype analysis was only noted 9 months post-BMT, while restriction fragment length polymorphism of blood and bone marrow failed to detect donor DNA. Twenty-two months after BMT no evidence of donor chimerism is present, and partial immune reconstitution persists despite loss of donor chimerism. The absence of donor chimerism leaves unexplained the mechanism of the long-term T-cell reconstitution attributable to recipient cells. Possible mechanisms include the patient's SCID as a transient condition secondary to maternal alloimmunity, but this seems unlikely, especially considering the family history. Transient donor chimerism may have been sufficient to promote autologous T-cell development by an unknown mechanism. Transfer of soluble or cellular maternal elements could have promoted either T-lymphocyte migration and maturation through a functioning thymus and/or essential T- and B-cell cooperation. Further analysis to define the mechanism of recipient T-cell immune reconstitution in this patient is essential.

REFERENCES

1. BUCKLEY, R. H., S. E. SCHIFF, R. I. SCHIFF *et al.* 1993. Haploidentical bone marrow stem cell transplantation in human severe combined immunodeficiency. Semin. Hematol. **30:** 92-104.
2. VAN LEEVWEN, J. E. M., M. J. D. VAN TOL, A. M. JOOSTEN *et al.* 1994. Relationships between patterns of engraftment in peripheral blood and immune reconstitution after allogeneic bone marrow transplantation for (severe) combined immunodeficiency. Blood **84:** 3936-3947.
3. ROSEN, F., M. EIBL, C. GRISCELLI, F. AIUTI, T. KISHIMOTO, I. B. REZNIK, L. A. HANSON, R. A. THOMPSON, M. D. COOPER, R. A. GEHA, R. A. GOOD & T. A. WALDMANN. 1995. Primary immunodeficiency diseases. Report of a WHO Scientific Group. Clin. Exp. Immunol. **99** (Suppl. 1-24).

Hematopoietic Stem Cell-Chemotactic Factor Production by Bone Marrow and Thymic Stromal Cells

CHERRY,[a,b] S. IKEHARA,[a] AND R. A. GOOD[b]

[a]1st Department of Pathology
Kansai Medical University
Moriguchi-City, Osaka, Japan

[b]University of South Florida
All Children's Hospital
St. Petersburg, Florida 33701

When hematopoietic stem cells are injected into irradiated mice, they migrate into the spleen, thymus, and bone marrow, where they form colonies. However, it is still unknown why hematopoietic stem cells are home to these organs.

We analyzed chemotactic factor production by stromal cells in the bone marrow and thymus. These factors demonstrated the ability to attract bone marrow cells with stem cell characteristics. The biochemical nature of these factors differed from that of previously described chemotactic factors. Other hematopoietic factors and growth hormones do not have such capabilities. These findings strongly suggest that stromal cells produce chemotactic factors that attract hematopoietic stem cells.

Mature CD4[+] Cells Help Lineage-Negative but Not More Purified, MHC Class I Bright Marrow Cells to Cross the MHC Transplantation Barrier

BING-YAN WANG, KAZUNORI ONOÉ,[a] AND
ROBERT A. GOOD

All Children's Hospital
University of South Florida
St. Petersburg, Florida 33701

[a]*Institute of Immunological Science*
Hokkaido University
Sapporo, Hokkaido, Japan

Highly purified bone marrow stem cells alone cannot produce long-lived allogeneic bone marrow chimeras across the major histocompatibility complex (MHC) barrier. Purified marrow stem cells plus mature CD4[+] donor cells were transplanted into allogeneic recipients to determine if CD4[+] cells can assist purified stem cells to cross the MHC barrier. Low density, lineage-negative cells (CD4[-], CD8[-], CD71[-], B220[-], Mac-1[-], and Gr-1[-] cells) and low density, lineage-negative, class I highly positive, Elite sorted cells from 5-fluoracil-treated donors were mixed with normal CD4[+] lymph node T cells from B6 donor mice and transplanted into lethally irradiated AKR recipients. (AKR → AKR) → AKR bone marrow cells were used as compromised cells to permit long-term experiments.

All chimeric mice survived more than 10 weeks without showing signs of graft-versus-host disease. The lineage-negative plus mature CD4[+] cell transplantation group showed chimerism similar to that of Thy-1 depleted whole bone marrow transplants. Control (lineage-negative stem cells without CD4[+] helper cells) produced poor chimerism. However, even when transplanted with CD4[+] lymphocytes, low density, lineage-negative, MHC class I high stem cells did not repopulate recipient mice. Lymphoid cells in this group were of recipient origin. Mature CD4[+] cells help low density, lineage-negative cells, but not more purified class I highly positive cells, to cross the MHC barrier.

Application of Stem Cell-Enriched Bone Marrow Transplants to Prevent the Development of Coronary Vascular Disease in WB/F1 Autoimmune-Prone Mice

R. P. KIRZNER, R. W. ENGELMAN, AND
R. A. GOOD

University of South Florida
All Children's Hospital
St. Petersburg, Florida 33701

In an effort to employ bone marrow transplantation (BMT) to prevent the development of coronary vascular disease in an aggressive autoimmune model, ongoing studies have focused on male WB/F1 mice. WB/F1 mice transplanted with haploidentical whole bone marrow or purified stem cell populations from normal B6C3 donors demonstrated a reduction in the onset and severity of the disease. Autoantibodies to cardiolipin and dsDNA were markedly decreased near normal levels by the haploidentical bone marrow transplants. Immunohistochemistry of heart and kidneys revealed significant amelioration of degenerative coronary vascular disease and glomerulonephritis in WB/F1 recipients.

Likewise, normal B6C3 mice transplanted with bone marrow from WB/F1 mice demonstrated the development of autoimmunity. B6C3 recipients had elevated levels of both anti-cardiolipin and anti-dsDNA antibodies. In addition to significant hepatosplenomegaly, histologic studies of heart and kidneys showed progression of degenerative coronary vascular disease and glomerulonephritis. Flow cytometric analysis of splenocytes demonstrated donor phenotypes in both WB/F1 and B6C3 mice that had received bone marrow from haploidentical donors.

Subject Index